Small Animal Practice
Client Handouts

Rhea V. Morgan, DVM
Diplomate, American College of Veterinary Internal Medicine
Diplomate, American College of Veterinary Ophthalmology
Smoky Mountain Veterinary Services
Walland, Tennessee;
Ophthalmology Services at Village Veterinary Medical Center
Farragut, Tennessee

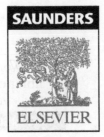

SAUNDERS

ELSEVIER

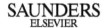

SAUNDERS
ELSEVIER

3251 Riverport Lane
Maryland Heights, Missouri 63043

SMALL ANIMAL PRACTICE CLIENT HANDOUTS   ISBN: 978-1-4377-0850-9

Notice

Knowledge and best practice in this field are constantly changing. As new research and experience broaden our understanding, changes in research methods, professional practices, or medical treatment may become necessary.

Practitioners and researchers must always rely on their own experience and knowledge in evaluating and using any information, methods, compounds, or experiments described herein. In using such information or methods they should be mindful of their own safety and the safety of others, including parties for whom they have a professional responsibility.

With respect to any drug or pharmaceutical products identified, readers are advised to check the most current information provided (i) on procedures featured or (ii) by the manufacturer of each product to be administered, to verify the recommended dose or formula, the method and duration of administration, and contraindications. It is the responsibility of practitioners, relying on their own experience and knowledge of their patients, to make diagnoses, to determine dosages and the best treatment for each individual patient, and to take all appropriate safety precautions.

To the fullest extent of the law, neither the Publisher nor the authors, contributors, or editors, assume any liability for any injury and/or damage to persons or property as a matter of products liability, negligence or otherwise, or from any use or operation of any methods, products, instruction, or ideas contained in the material herein.

The Publisher

Library of Congress Cataloging-in-Publication Data
Small animal practice client handouts / [edited by] Rhea V. Morgan.
    p. ; cm.
  Includes index.
  ISBN 978-1-4377-0850-9 (pbk. : alk. paper)
  1. Pet medicine.   I. Morgan, Rhea Volk.
  [DNLM: 1. Dog Diseases—Handbooks. 2. Cat Diseases—Handbooks. 3.
Veterinary Medicine—Handbooks. SF 981 S635 2011]
  SF981.S63 2011
  636.089—dc22   2009049755

Vice President and Publisher: Linda Duncan
Publisher: Penny Rudolph
Senior Developmental Editor: Shelly Stringer
Editorial Assistant: Leah Guerrero
Publishing Services Manager: Patricia Tannian
Project Manager: Kristine Feeherty
Design Direction: Maggie Reid

Working together to grow
libraries in developing countries

www.elsevier.com | www.bookaid.org | www.sabre.org

ELSEVIER   BOOK AID International   Sabre Foundation

Printed in the United States of America

Last digit is the print number: 9 8 7 6

The *Small Animal Practice Client Handouts* text is dedicated:

In honor of two people who greatly influenced my choice of careers:

Sister Nancy Folkl, Academy of Our Lady
my high school biology teacher and mentor

Warren D. Nichols, DVM, Washington Veterinary Clinic
who gave me my first job in veterinary medicine when I was sixteen

and

In memory of my dear friend and neighbor:

Kay McWilliam (1904–2008)
who lived to be 104 years young

SECTION EDITORS

Joseph W. Bartges, DVM, PhD, DACVIM (Small Animal), DACVN
Professor of Medicine and Nutrition
The Acree Endowed Chair of Small Animal Research
Department of Small Animal Clinical Sciences
College of Veterinary Medicine
The University of Tennessee
Knoxville, Tennessee
Nutritional Disorders

Ronald M. Bright, DVM, MS, DACVS
Staff Surgeon
VCA—Veterinary Specialists of Northern Colorado
Loveland, Colorado
Respiratory System
Reproductive System

Lynette K. Cole, DVM, MS, DACVD
Associate Professor of Dermatology
Veterinary Clinical Sciences
College of Veterinary Medicine
The Ohio State University
Columbus, Ohio
Diseases of the Ear

Rebecca E. Gompf, DVM, MS, DACVIM (Cardiology)
Associate Professor of Cardiology
Department of Small Animal Clinical Sciences
College of Veterinary Medicine
The University of Tennessee
Knoxville, Tennessee
Cardiovascular System

Lynn F. Guptill, DVM, PhD, DACVIM (Small Animal)
Associate Professor
Department of Veterinary Clinical Sciences
School of Veterinary Medicine
Purdue University
West Lafayette, Indiana
Infectious Diseases

Marc Kent, DVM, DACVIM (Small Animal and Neurology)
Associate Professor
Department of Small Animal Medicine & Surgery
College of Veterinary Medicine
The University of Georgia
Athens, Georgia
Neurologic System

Cathy E. Langston, DVM, DACVIM (Small Animal)
Staff Veterinarian
Nephrology and Urology
Animal Medical Center
New York, New York
Urinary System

Kristi S. Lively, DVM, DABVP
Owner
Village Veterinary Medical Center
Farragut, Tennessee
Hemolymphatic System

Rhea V. Morgan, DVM, DACVIM (Small Animal), DACVO
Smoky Mountain Veterinary Services
Walland, Tennessee;
Ophthalmology Services at Village Veterinary Medical Center
Farragut, Tennessee
Procedures and Techniques
Endocrine System
Immune System
Diseases of the Eye
Behavioral Disorders
Environmental Disorders

Mark C. Rochat, DVM, MS, DACVS
Professor and Chief, Small Animal Surgery
Department of Veterinary Clinical Sciences
Center for Veterinary Health Sciences
Oklahoma State University
Stillwater, Oklahoma
Musculoskeletal System

Emily Rothstein, DVM, DACVD
Owner
Animal Allergy and Dermatology Service of Connecticut, LLC
Plantsville, Connecticut
Dermatologic System

Craig G. Ruaux, BVSc, PhD, DACVIM (Small Animal)
Assistant Professor, Small Animal Medicine
Department of Clinical Sciences
College of Veterinary Medicine
Oregon State University
Corvallis, Oregon
Digestive System

Petra A. Volmer, DVM, MS, DABVT, DABT
Manager of Veterinary Services, Pharmacovigilance
Summit VetParm
Champaign, Illinois
Toxicology

CONTRIBUTORS

Anisa D. Dunham, AS, RVT
Registered Veterinary Technologist
Department of Veterinary Clinical Sciences
School of Veterinary Medicine
Purdue University
West Lafayette, Indiana
Infectious Diseases

A. Courtenay Freeman, DVM
Neurology Intern
Department of Small Animal Medicine & Surgery
College of Veterinary Medicine
The University of Georgia
Athens, Georgia
Neurologic System

Russell W. Fugazzi, DVM
Resident, Small Animal Surgery
Washington State University
Pullman, Washington
Respiratory System
Reproductive System

Simon R. Platt, BVM&S, MRCVS, DACVIM (Neurology), DECVN
Associate Professor
Department of Small Animal Medicine & Surgery
College of Veterinary Medicine
The University of Georgia
Athens, Georgia
Neurologic System

Donna M. Raditic, DVM, CVA
Department of Small Animal Clinical Sciences
Veterinary Teaching Hospital
College of Veterinary Medicine
The University of Tennessee
Knoxville, Tennessee
Nutritional Disorders

Scott J. Schatzberg, DVM, PhD, DACVIM (Neurology)
Assistant Professor
Department of Small Animal Medicine & Surgery
College of Veterinary Medicine
The University of Georgia
Athens, Georgia
Neurologic System

Elizabeth A. Shull, DVM, DACVB, DACVIM (Neurology)
Practice Owner
Appalachian Veterinary Specialists
Knoxville, Tennessee
Behavioral Disorders

PREFACE

Welcome to the *Small Animal Practice Client Handouts* book. This text is composed of client education handouts on 450 diseases, tests, and procedures. Each disease handout is divided into two major sections, covering Basic Information and Treatment Options. Easy-to-understand information is given on the description of the disease/condition, clinical signs, diagnostic tests, treatment options, patient follow-up, and prognosis. Numerical data in the handouts are derived from the *Handbook of Small Animal Practice,* Fifth Edition, published by Elsevier Saunders. Feel free to examine the references in this book for further details.

These handouts are provided in both print and digital (CD-ROM) formats. The print version of the handouts is in English. The CD-ROM contains the handouts in both English and Spanish. Files on the CD-ROM can be downloaded to your practice's computers. Space has been provided at the top of each page, to the left of the subject title, for clinic contact information. Space has also been allotted at the bottom of each page for Special Instructions that pertain to the individual patient. In addition to the handouts, the CD-ROM contains approximately 100 images that we believe will be helpful in explaining diseases, conditions, and procedures to your clients. We hope these educational tools will make it easier for clients to understand their pet's medical problem, the rationale behind your recommendations, and the potential outcomes.

I would like to recognize the section editors for their help in organizing the 19 sections of this text and for choosing the subjects to be covered. I would also like to thank all the authors of these handouts for their hard work, dedication, and expertise. It has been a pleasure working with Penny Rudolph and Shelly Stringer at Elsevier again. It is worth noting that both the authors and editorial team encountered numerous personal challenges during the preparation of this text, and it was very gratifying that we still managed to conclude the project on time. Thank you to the entire team!

Sincerely,
Rhea Morgan

CONTENTS

SECTION 1: Procedures and Techniques

Section Editor: Rhea V. Morgan, DVM, DACVIM (Small Animal), DACVO

Amputation, Limb, 2
Arthrodesis, 3
Blood Pressure Measurement, Indirect, 4
Bone Marrow Aspiration and Evaluation, 5
Bronchoscopy, 6
Castration of Male Cats, 7
Castration of Male Dogs, 8
Chemotherapy and Your Pet, 9
Dialysis, 10
Echocardiography, 11
Electrocardiography: Intermittent and Continuous, 12
Femoral Head and Neck Ostectomy, 13
Fluid Therapy, 14
Fracture Repair: Casts and Splints, 15
Fracture Repair: External Skeletal Fixation, 16
Fracture Repair: Internal Fixation, 17
Kidney Transplantation in Cats, 18
Laboratory Tests of Kidney Function, 19
Nutritional Management of Chronic Kidney Disease, 20
Oxygen Therapy, 21
Physical Rehabilitation, 22
Preoperative Evaluation, 23
Rhinoscopy, 24
Sterilization of Female Cats, 25
Sterilization of Female Dogs, 26
Subcutaneous Fluid Administration, 27
Total Hip Arthroplasty, 28
Transfusion Therapy in Cats, 29
Transfusion Therapy in Dogs, 30
Triple Pelvic Osteotomy for Hip Dysplasia, 31
Urine Protein Assays in Dogs, 32

SECTION 2: Cardiovascular System

Section Editor: Rebecca E. Gompf, DVM, MS, DACVIM (Cardiology)

Arrhythmogenic Right Ventricular/Cardiomyopathy in Boxers, 34
Arterial Thromboembolism, Peripheral, 35
Atrial Fibrillation, 36
Atrial Premature Contractions and Tachycardia, 37
Atrioventricular Valve Degeneration in Dogs, 38
Cardiac Tumors, 39
Cardiopulmonary Resuscitation, 40
Congestive Heart Failure in Dogs, Left-Sided, 41
Congestive Heart Failure in Dogs, Right-Sided, 42
Dilated Cardiomyopathy in Cats, 43
Dilated Cardiomyopathy in Dogs, 44
Endocarditis, 45
Heartworm Disease in Cats, 46
Heartworm Disease in Dogs, 47
Hypertrophic Cardiomyopathy in Cats, 49

Occult Cardiomyopathy in Doberman Pinschers, 50
Patent Ductus Arteriosus, 51
Pericardial Effusion, 52
Peritoneopericardial Diaphragmatic Hernia, 53
Persistent Right Aortic Arch, 54
Pulmonary Hypertension, 55
Pulmonic Stenosis, 56
Second- and Third-Degree Heart Block, 57
Sick Sinus Syndrome and Atrial Standstill, 58
Sinus Arrhythmia, 59
Sinus Bradycardia, 60
Subaortic Stenosis, 61
Systemic Hypertension, 62
Tetralogy of Fallot, 63
Tricuspid and Mitral Valve Dysplasia, 64
Ventricular and Atrial Septal Defects, 65
Ventricular Fibrillation and Cardiac Arrest, 66
Ventricular Premature Contractions and Tachycardia, 67

SECTION 3: Respiratory System

Section Editor: Ronald M. Bright, DVM, MS, DACVS

Acute Respiratory Distress Syndrome, 69
Allergic Bronchitis in Cats, 70
Allergic Bronchitis in Dogs, 71
Brachycephalic Syndrome, 72
Bronchitis, Acute, 73
Bronchitis, Chronic, 74
Bullous Lung Disease, 75
Diaphragmatic Hernia, 76
Flail Chest, 77
Laryngeal Collapse in Dogs, 78
Laryngeal Paralysis, 79
Laryngeal and Tracheal Neoplasia, 80
Laryngitis and Tracheitis, 81
Lung Lobe Torsion, 82
Lung Tumors, 83
Mediastinal Masses, 84
Nasal and Nasopharyngeal Polyps in Cats, 85
Nasal Tumors, Malignant, 86
Pleural Effusion, 87
Pneumonia, Aspiration, 88
Pneumonia, Bacterial, 89
Pneumonia, Fungal, 90
Pneumothorax, 91
Pulmonary Contusions, 92
Pulmonary Edema, 93
Rhinitis and Sinusitis in Cats, 94
Rhinitis and Sinusitis in Dogs, 95
Tracheal Collapse in Dogs, 96
Tracheal Obstruction, 97
Tracheal Trauma, 98

SECTION 4: Neurologic System

Section Editor: Marc Kent, DVM, DACVIM (Small Animal and Neurology)

Atlantoaxial Subluxation in Dogs, 100
Botulism, 101
Brachial Plexus Avulsion, 102
Brain Tumors, 103
Canine Distemper Neurologic Disease, 104
Caudal Cervical Spondylopathy (Wobbler Syndrome), 105
Caudal Occipital (Chiari-like) Malformation and Syringohydromyelia, 106
Degenerative Myelopathy, 107
Discospondylitis, 108
Fibrocartilaginous Embolic Myelopathy, 109
Granulomatous Meningoencephalitis and Necrotizing Encephalitis, 110
Head Trauma, 111
Hydrocephalus, 112
Idiopathic Facial Nerve Paralysis, 113
Idiopathic Peripheral Vestibular Disease, 114
Idiopathic Trigeminal Neuropathy, 115
Intervertebral Disc Disease, 116
Ischemic Brain Injury (Stroke), 118
Lumbosacral Disease, Degenerative, 119
Myasthenia Gravis, 120
Peripheral Nerve Sheath Tumors, 121
Polyradiculoneuritis in Dogs, Acute, 122
Seizures: Causes and Diagnosis, 123
Seizures: Idiopathic Epilepsy, 124
Seizures: Treatment, 125
Seizures: Treatment of Resistant Cases, 126
Spinal Cord Trauma, 127
Spinal Tumors, 128
Spondylosis Deformans, 129
Steroid-Responsive Meningeal Arteritis, 130
Tick Paralysis, 131
Tremor Syndrome, 132

SECTION 5: Digestive System

Section Editor: Craig G. Ruaux, BVSc, PhD, DACVIM (Small Animal)

Anal Sac Diseases, 134
Cholangiohepatitis in Cats, 135
Cleft Palate, 136
Colitis, Acute, 137
Colitis, Chronic, 138
Copper Storage Hepatopathy in Dogs, 139
Epulis in Dogs, 140
Esophageal Foreign Body, 141
Esophagitis and Esophageal Stricture, 142
Exocrine Pancreatic Insufficiency, 143
Fecal Incontinence, 144
Gall Bladder Disease in Dogs, 145
Gastric Dilatation-Volvulus, 146
Gastric Foreign Body, 147
Gastric Neoplasia, 148
Gastritis, Acute, 149
Gastritis, Chronic, 150
Gastrointestinal Ulceration, 151
Gingivitis, 152
Hemorrhagic Gastroenteritis in Dogs, 153

Hepatic Encephalopathy, 154
Hepatic Lipidosis in Cats, 155
Hepatitis in Dogs, Chronic, 156
Inflammatory Bowel Disease in Cats, 157
Inflammatory Bowel Disease in Dogs, 158
Intestinal Neoplasia, 159
Intestinal Obstruction, 160
Intestinal Parasites, 161
Lymphoplasmacytic Stomatitis in Cats, 162
Megacolon in Cats, 163
Megaesophagus, 164
Oral Melanoma in Dogs, 165
Oral Squamous Cell Carcinoma in Cats, 166
Pancreatitis in Cats, 167
Pancreatitis in Dogs, 168
Perianal Fistula in Dogs, 169
Perianal Tumors, 170
Perineal Hernia in Dogs, 171
Portosystemic Vascular Anomalies, 172
Protein-Losing Enteropathy, 173
Salivary Mucocele in Dogs, 174

SECTION 6: Endocrine System

Section Editor: Rhea V. Morgan, DVM, DACVIM (Small Animal), DACVO

Diabetes Insipidus, 176
Diabetes Mellitus in Cats, 177
Diabetes Mellitus in Dogs, 178
Hyperadrenocorticism (Cushing's Disease) in Dogs, 179
Hypercalcemia, 180
Hyperlipidemia, 181
Hyperthyroidism in Cats, 182
Hypoadrenocorticism (Addison's Disease), 183
Hypoglycemia, 184
Hypothyroidism in Dogs, 185

SECTION 7: Urinary System

Section Editor: Cathy E. Langston, DVM, DACVIM (Small Animal)

Acute Kidney Failure, 187
Anemia of Chronic Kidney Disease, 188
Benign Prostatic Hypertrophy in Dogs, 189
Bladder Cancer, 190
Bladder Stones in Cats, 191
Bladder Stones in Dogs, 192
Bladder Trauma, 193
Chronic Kidney Disease in Cats, 194
Chronic Kidney Disease in Dogs, 195
Cystitis in Cats, 196
Cystitis in Dogs, 197
Ectopic Ureter in Dogs, 198
Fanconi Syndrome in Dogs, 199
Kidney Dysplasia in Dogs, 200
Kidney Stones in Cats, 201
Kidney Toxins (Nephrotoxicosis), 202
Perinephric Pseudocysts in Cats, 203
Polycystic Kidney Disease in Cats, 204
Prostate Cancer in Dogs, 205
Prostatic and Paraprostatic Cysts in Dogs, 206
Prostatitis and Prostatic Abscessation in Dogs, 207
Protein-Losing Nephropathy in Dogs, 208

Pyelonephritis (Kidney Infection), 209
Renal Neoplasia, 210
Ureteral Obstruction in Cats, 211
Urethral Obstruction in Cats, 212
Urethral Prolapse in Dogs, 213
Urethritis, 214
Urinary Incontinence in Dogs, 215

SECTION 8: Reproductive System

Section Editor: Ronald M. Bright, DVM, MS, DACVS

Agalactia, 217
Cryptorchidism in Dogs and Cats, 218
Dystocia in Dogs and Cats, 219
Eclampsia in Dogs, 220
Infertility in Bitches, 221
Infertility in Male Dogs, 222
Infertility in Queens, 223
Infertility in Toms, 224
Mammary Fibroadenomatous Hyperplasia, 225
Mammary Tumors in Cats, 226
Mammary Tumors in Dogs, 227
Mastitis, 228
Ovarian Remnant Syndrome, 229
Paraphimosis in Dogs, 230
Penile Tumors in Dogs, 231
Phimosis, 232
Pregnancy Loss in Bitches, 233
Pseudocyesis, 234
Pyometra Complex, 235
Subinvolution of Placental Sites in Dogs, 236
Testicular Tumors in Dogs, 237
Uterine Prolapse, 238
Vaginal Edema in Dogs, 239
Vaginitis in Dogs, 240

SECTION 9: Hemolymphatic System

Section Editor: Kristi S. Lively, DVM, DABVP

Acute Lymphocytic Leukemia, 242
Anemia in Dogs and Cats, 243
Anticoagulant Rodenticide Toxicity, 244
Aplastic Anemia, 245
Babesia Infection in Dogs, 246
Chronic Lymphocytic Leukemia, 247
Coagulopathy Associated with Liver Disease, 248
Disseminated Intravascular Coagulation, 249
Fever of Unknown Origin, 250
Hemobartonellosis in Cats, 251
Hemophilia A, 252
Hemophilia B, 253
Hypercalcemia Associated with Cancer, 254
Immune-Mediated Hemolytic Anemia, 255
Immune-Mediated Thrombocytopenia, 256
Lymphedema, 257
Lymphoma in Cats, 258
Lymphoma in Dogs, 259
Mastocytosis, 260
Primary and Secondary Polycythemia, 261
Splenic Hemangiosarcoma, 262
Splenic Torsion, 263
Splenomegaly, 264
Thrombocytopenia: Other Causes, 265
Thrombosis, 266
Von Willebrand Disease, 267

SECTION 10: Immune System

Section Editor: Rhea V. Morgan, DVM, DACVIM (Small Animal), DACVO

Allergic Reactions, 269
Extramedullary Plasmacytoma, 270
Malignant Histiocytosis and Histiocytic Sarcoma, 271
Multiple Myeloma, 272
Systemic Lupus Erythematosus in Dogs: Systemic Aspects, 273

SECTION 11: Musculoskeletal System

Section Editor: Mark C. Rochat, DVM, MS, DACVS

Angular Limb Deformities in Dogs, 275
Bicipital Tendinopathy, 276
Bone Tumors, 277
Calcaneal Tendon Injury, 278
Carpal and Tarsal Shearing Injuries, 279
Cranial Cruciate Ligament Disease, 280
Elbow Incongruency, 281
Elbow Luxation, Traumatic, 282
Fibrotic Myopathies, 283
Fragmented Medial Coronoid Process Disease, 284
Hip Dysplasia in Dogs, 285
Hip Luxation, 286
Hypertrophic Osteodystrophy in Dogs, 287
Hypertrophic Osteopathy in Dogs, 288
Immune-Mediated Arthritis, 289
Juvenile Carpal Hyperextension/Hyperflexion Disorder, 290
Legg-Calvé-Perthes Disease, 291
Mandibular Fractures, 292
Masticatory Myositis, 293
Nutritional Bone Diseases, 294
Osteoarthritis: Medical Management, 295
Osteochondrosis (Osteochondritis Dissecans), 296
Osteomyelitis, 297
Panosteitis, 298
Patella Luxation, 299
Sacroiliac Luxation, 300
Scapular Luxation, 301
Septic Arthritis, 302
Shoulder Luxation, 303
Stifle Luxation, 304
Ununited Anconeal Process Disease, 305

SECTION 12: Dermatologic System

Section Editor: Emily Rothstein, DVM, DACVD

Acne in Cats, 307
Acute Moist Dermatitis in Dogs, 308
Alopecia X, 309
Atopic Dermatitis in Dogs, 310
Atypical Mycobacteriosis, 311
Benign Skin Tumors in Dogs, 312
Cheyletiellosis, 313
Claw (Toenail) Disease, Asymmetrical, 314
Claw (Toenail) Disease, Symmetrical, 315

Cutaneous or Discoid Lupus Erythematosus, 316
Cutaneous (Epitheliotropic) T-Cell Lymphoma, 317
Cyclical Flank Alopecia, 318
Deep Bacterial Pyoderma and Furunculosis, 319
Demodicosis in Dogs, 320
Dermatophytosis, 321
Eosinophilic Granuloma Complex in Cats, 322
Exfoliative Cutaneous Lupus Erythematosus, 323
Flea Allergic Dermatitis, 324
Food Reactions, Adverse, 325
Juvenile Cellulitis, 326
Lipomas in Dogs, 327
Malassezia Dermatitis, 328
Mast Cell Tumors in Cats, 329
Mast Cell Tumors in Dogs, 330
Nasal Depigmentation, 331
Notoedric Mange, 332
Pemphigus Complex, 333
Pinnal Seborrhea, 334
Plasma Cell Pododermatitis in Cats, 335
Primary Seborrhea, 336
Sarcoptic Mange, 337
Sebaceous Adenitis in Dogs, 338
Skin Fold Pyoderma (Intertrigo), 339
Sporotrichosis, 340
Subcutaneous Abscesses and Cellulitis, 341
Superficial Bacterial Folliculitis in Dogs, 342
Systemic Lupus Erythematosus: Dermatologic Aspects, 343
Vaccine-Associated Vasculitis in Dogs, 344
Vitamin A–Responsive Dermatosis, 345
Zinc-Responsive Dermatosis, 346

SECTION 13: Diseases of the Eye
Section Editor: Rhea V. Morgan, DVM, DACVIM (Small Animal), DACVO

Anterior Uveitis, 348
Cataracts, 349
Chorioretinitis and Optic Neuritis, 350
Collie Eye Anomaly, 351
Conjunctivitis, 352
Corneal Ulceration, 353
Distichiasis and Ectopic Cilia, 354
Ectropion, 355
Entropion, 356
Eyelid Tumors, 357
Feline Corneal Sequestration, 358
Feline Eosinophilic Keratitis, 359
Feline Herpesvirus Keratoconjunctivitis, 360
Glaucoma in Cats, 361
Glaucoma in Dogs, 362
Horner's Syndrome, 363
Hypertensive Retinopathy, 364
Hyphema, 365
Intraocular Tumors, 366
Iridociliary Cysts, 367
Iris Melanosis of Cats, 368
Keratoconjunctivitis Sicca (Dry Eye), 369
Lens Luxation and Subluxation, 370
Lipid Keratopathy, 371
Orbital Cellulitis and Abscessation, 372

Orbital Tumors, 373
Pannus, 374
Persistent Corneal Erosions, 375
Pigmentary Keratitis, 376
Progressive Retinal Atrophy, 377
Prolapse of the Gland of the Third Eyelid, 378
Proptosis of the Eye, 379
Retinal Detachment, 380
Retinal Dysplasia, 381
Sudden Acquired Retinal Degeneration, 382
Taurine Retinopathy, 383

SECTION 14: Diseases of the Ear
Section Editor: Lynette K. Cole, DVM, MS, DACVD

Aural Hematoma, 385
Deafness, 386
Otitis Externa, 387
Otitis Interna, 388
Otitis Media, 389

SECTION 15: Infectious Diseases
Section Editor: Lynn F. Guptill, DVM, PhD, DACVIM (Small Animal)

Bartonellosis, 391
Blastomycosis, 392
Borreliosis (Lyme Disease), 393
Brucellosis in Dogs, 394
Campylobacteriosis, 395
Canine Distemper Virus, 396
Canine Infectious Tracheobronchitis (Kennel Cough), 397
Canine Influenza, 398
Coccidioidomycosis, 399
Coccidiosis, Enteric, 400
Cryptococcosis, 401
Cryptosporidiosis, 402
Cytauxzoonosis, 403
Ehrlichiosis and Anaplasmosis in Dogs, 404
Feline Coronavirus, 405
Feline Immunodeficiency Virus, 406
Feline Leukemia Virus, 407
Feline Upper Respiratory Infection, 408
Giardiasis, 409
Helicobacteriosis, 410
Hepatozoonosis in Dogs, 411
Histoplasmosis, 412
Leishmaniasis, 413
Leptospirosis, 414
Methicillin-Resistant *Staphylococcus* Infections, 415
Neosporosis in Dogs, 416
Parvovirus in Cats, 417
Parvovirus in Dogs, 418
Protothecosis in Dogs, 419
Pythiosis, 420
Rabies, 421
Rocky Mountain Spotted Fever, 422
Tetanus, 423
Toxoplasmosis, 424
Tritrichomoniasis in Cats, 425

SECTION 16: Behavioral Disorders

Section Editor: Rhea V. Morgan, DVM, DACVIM (Small Animal), DACVO

Aggression Among Household Cats, 427
Dominance Aggression in Dogs, 428
Elimination Problems in Cats, 429
Elimination Problems in Dogs, 431
Fear and Anxiety Disorders in Dogs, 432
Petting Intolerance and Status Aggression in Cats, 433
Play Aggression in Cats, 434
Possessive and Territorial Aggression in Dogs, 435

SECTION 17: Nutritional Disorders

Section Editor: Joseph W. Bartges, DVM, PhD, DACVIM (Small Animal), DACVN

Feeding Trials for Possible Food Allergy, 437
Homemade Diets, 438
Obesity in Cats, 439
Obesity in Dogs, 440
Overnutrition of Large-Breed Dogs, 441
Taurine Deficiency, 442

SECTION 18: Toxicology

Section Editor: Petra A. Volmer, DVM, MS, DABVT, DABT

Acetaminophen Toxicosis, 444
Amitraz Toxicosis, 445
Antifreeze Poisoning, 446
Avermectin Toxicosis, 447

Bread Dough Poisoning, 448
Chocolate and Methylxanthine Toxicosis, 449
Cholecalciferol Rodenticide Poisoning, 450
Grape and Raisin Toxicosis in Dogs, 451
Herbal Poisonings, 452
Lead Poisoning, 454
Macadamia Nut Toxicosis in Dogs, 455
Metaldehyde Poisoning, 456
Nonsteroidal Anti-Inflammatory Drug Toxicosis, 457
Organophosphorus and Carbamate Insecticide
    Poisoning, 458
Paintball Toxicosis, 459
Poisoning from Illicit Human Drugs: Depressants, 460
Poisoning from Illicit Human Drugs: Opioids and
    Stimulants, 462
Pyrethrin and Pyrethroid Toxicosis, 464
Strychnine Poisoning, 465
Xylitol Toxicosis in Dogs, 466
Zinc Toxicosis, 467

SECTION 19: Environmental Disorders

Section Editor: Rhea V. Morgan, DVM, DACVIM (Small Animal), DACVO

Burns, 469
Electrical Cord Injury, 470
Heat Prostration, 471
Shock, 472
Venomous Snake Bites, 473

SECTION 1

Procedures and Techniques

Section Editor: Rhea V. Morgan, DVM, DACVIM (Small Animal), DACVO

Amputation, Limb
Arthrodesis
Blood Pressure Measurement, Indirect
Bone Marrow Aspiration and Evaluation
Bronchoscopy
Castration of Male Cats
Castration of Male Dogs
Chemotherapy and Your Pet
Dialysis
Echocardiography
Electrocardiography: Intermittent and Continuous
Femoral Head and Neck Ostectomy
Fluid Therapy
Fracture Repair: Casts and Splints
Fracture Repair: External Skeletal Fixation
Fracture Repair: Internal Fixation

Kidney Transplantation in Cats
Laboratory Tests of Kidney Function
Nutritional Management of Chronic
    Kidney Disease
Oxygen Therapy
Physical Rehabilitation
Preoperative Evaluation
Rhinoscopy
Sterilization of Female Cats
Sterilization of Female Dogs
Subcutaneous Fluid Administration
Total Hip Arthroplasty
Transfusion Therapy in Cats
Transfusion Therapy in Dogs
Triple Pelvic Osteotomy for Hip Dysplasia
Urine Protein Assays in Dogs

Amputation, Limb

Mark C. Rochat, DVM, MS, DACVS

Purpose of Procedure

Limb (leg) amputation is the removal of a portion of a limb. Dogs and cats, in general, function extremely well following amputation. Poor candidates for amputation include very large dogs, obese dogs, and dogs with orthopedic or neurologic disorders that affect the other legs.

Amputations may be performed for numerous reasons, including trauma, infection, and cancer. Certain neurologic diseases (paralysis of one or more nerves to the leg) and severe, painful osteoarthritis (degenerative joint disease) may also be treated by limb amputation. In some instances, such as trauma or bacterial infection (osteomyelitis), amputation is curative. In cases of bone tumors, amputation is done to relieve pain but rarely cures the underlying cancer.

Description of Technique

Amputation of the front leg is generally performed by removing the entire limb and scapula (shoulder blade). This approach results in a good cosmetic result. Amputation through the shoulder joint or at the level of the upper arm is generally of no benefit and less cosmetic. Amputation of the rear limb is usually done at the level of the mid-thigh. This approach results in a more cosmetic appearance and affords some degree of protection to the groin. When neoplasia (cancer) or infection involves the femur (the long bone of the thigh), amputation through the hip joint is done. Amputation at a point lower on the leg (front or rear) is rarely done, because prosthetic devices are not usually available, are very expensive, and are generally unnecessary.

Preparation of Animal

Radiographs (x-rays) of the limb and routine laboratory tests are usually recommended initially to further define the nature and extent of the limb problem and identify anesthetic risks, such as liver or kidney dysfunction. Other diagnostic tests are based on the suspected underlying condition or cause of the lameness. If trauma or cancer is suspected, chest x-rays are taken.

Potential Complications

Although rare, the most serious complication that can occur during amputation is severe bleeding. Other complications include failure of the incision to heal properly or premature opening (dehiscence) of the incision, infection at the surgical site, and recurrence of cancer at the incision site. Painful neuromas where the limb nerves were severed during the procedure and phantom pain after the amputation are extremely rare.

Postoperative/Follow-up Care

Upon discharge from the hospital, restricted exercise (leash walking) is usually prescribed until the surgery site has healed. Notify your veterinarian if any swelling or excessive redness occurs at the surgery site or if there is any drainage from the incision. Pain-relieving medications are commonly dispensed when the animal is discharged. Depending on the reason for the amputation, antibiotics may also be prescribed. Chemotherapy for treating cancer is often delayed until the incision has healed.

Follow-up consists of removal of the sutures or staples when the skin is fully healed, generally 10-14 days after surgery. Other postoperative instructions are tailored to address the underlying reason for the amputation.

SPECIAL INSTRUCTIONS:

Arthrodesis

Mark C. Rochat, DVM, MS, DACVS

Purpose of Procedure

Arthrodesis is the surgical fusion of a joint. With the exception of the hip, all major joints of the dog and cat can be fused. Commonly fused joints include the carpus (wrist), hock (ankle), and elbow. Less commonly fused joints include the stifle (knee) and shoulder. Other joints that are occasionally fused are the joints of the paw and the spine.

Arthrodesis results in loss of the function of the joint, but its primary goal is elimination of joint pain that is often severe and untreatable by other methods. Fusion of the carpus or hock usually has a minimal impact on overall limb function. Fusion of the elbow, shoulder, or knee results in significant changes in limb function.

Arthrodesis is indicated for treatment of joint injuries or disorders that cannot be controlled by other methods and are expected to lead to irreversible joint injury or osteoarthritis (degenerative joint disease).

Description of Technique

When arthrodesis of a joint is performed, any remaining cartilage in the joint is surgically removed, a bone graft is placed in the joint space, and the joint is secured with orthopedic devices (typically plates and screws or external fixators) at a functional angle until the bones have fused.

Preparation of Animal

Radiographs (x-rays) of the limb and routine laboratory tests are usually recommended initially to further define the nature and extent of the joint problem and identify anesthetic risks, such as liver or kidney dysfunction. Other diagnostic tests are based on the suspected underlying condition or cause of the lameness. If trauma is suspected, chest x-rays are taken to identify risk factors for anesthesia, such as pulmonary contusions (lung bruising) or diaphragmatic hernia. An electrocardiogram may also be performed to identify abnormal heart rhythms if trauma is suspected.

Potential Complications

In addition to anesthetic risks, complications of arthrodesis include failure of the joint to fuse, breakage of the surgical implants used to hold the bones in place, failure of the incision to heal or dehiscence (premature opening) of the incision, infection, nerve damage, and improper alignment of the leg. Rare complications include chronic infections that develop in association with the surgical implants, cancer at the surgical site, and lameness in cold weather from the effects of cold on the surgical implants.

Postoperative/Follow-up Care

Bandage changes are performed as needed, depending on the type of orthopedic device that was used and the nature of the injury or disease. X-rays are taken to assess healing at the arthrodesis site and are repeated every 4-6 weeks until healing is complete. Surgical implants usually are removed only if problems associated with the implants occur.

SPECIAL INSTRUCTIONS:

Blood Pressure Measurement, Indirect

Rhea V. Morgan, DVM, DACVIM (Small Animal), DACVO

Purpose of Procedure

Arterial or systemic blood pressure (BP) is the pressure exerted within the arteries of the body. Two time points are used when measuring BP: the time immediately after the heart contracts and pumps blood into the arteries (systolic pressure) and the time between beats when the heart is relaxed and pressure is at its lowest (diastolic pressure). BP results are given as systolic/diastolic. The average of the two values is mean arterial pressure (MAP).

BP measurements are used to diagnose and monitor systemic hypertension (high pressure). BP monitoring is also useful in conditions in which hypotension (low pressure) may occur, such as during shock, surgery, loss of blood or body fluids, or cardiac arrest and resuscitation. BP measurements are also helpful in making decisions about fluid therapy and what drugs and dosages to use for circulatory problems.

Description of Technique

BP may be measured with either direct or indirect methods in animals. Direct methods require that an intravenous catheter be inserted into an artery, with the catheter attached to a machine that measures pressure. This method is reserved for hospitalized patients that need continuous BP monitoring.

Indirect BP measurement is performed with the use of an inflatable cuff and either oscillometric (electronic pressure sensor) or Doppler (ultrasound-based) instruments to detect arterial blood flow. The arteries of companion animals are too small for a standard human BP cuff, sphygmomanometer, and stethoscope to be used. The equipment used for small animals is similar to that used for neonatal human infants.

Common sites used for indirect BP measurement in small animals include the peripheral arteries of the front and hind legs and the coccygeal artery at the base of the tail. Depending on the blood vessel used, the animal may be positioned on its side, in a sitting position, or standing. The same site and position are often used for repeated measurements for the sake of comparison.

Oscillometric instruments usually provide systolic, diastolic, and MAP pressures. Doppler instruments may provide only systolic BPs. Oscillometric instruments may have difficulty measuring pressures in very small animals (less than 10 lb or 4.5 kg), so they are sometime frustrating to use in cats. Doppler instruments work consistently in most small animals.

With the Doppler technique, electrode or ultrasound gel is applied over the artery. The pressure transducer (detector) is positioned over the point where arterial flow is best heard. An inflatable cuff is wound around the limb or tail above the transducer (closer to the heart). The cuff is manually inflated until the sound made by the blood flow stops. The cuff is then slowly deflated until arterial flow begins again, which is the point at which systolic BP is recorded.

With the oscillometric technique, an inflatable cuff is placed around the limb or tail over the artery. The oscillometric machine automatically inflates and deflates the cuff at specified time intervals. With both techniques, several measurements are taken to improve accuracy.

Preparation of Animal

Sedation is avoided when BPs are measured for the purpose of diagnosing or treating hypertension or hypotension, because sedation usually alters BP. Unless the measurement is being performed during surgery, animals are usually awake and a minimal amount of restraint is used. Every effort is made to keep the animal as relaxed as possible.

Fur may be shaved over the site of the arterial pulse, especially in long-haired animals.

Potential Complications

Complications are rare. There are no documented side effects associated with BP measurement by intermittent, indirect methods.

Some animals may be frightened by the sounds made by the machines and may resist or struggle, which can make the measurements inaccurate. Obtaining accurate BP measurements can be a challenge, because many animals are nervous and stressed while at the clinic or hospital.

Interpretation of Measurements

When measured by the indirect method in an awake animal, systolic BP values normally range from 110 to 140 mm Hg (millimeters of mercury), and diastolic values from 55 to 100 mm Hg. Hypertension is defined as pressures greater than 170-180 systolic or 95-110 diastolic in most dogs and cats. Hypotension is defined as BPs lower than 90/50 mm Hg in the awake animal. BPs tend to be lower in animals undergoing anesthesia and surgery. Trends in repeated measurements are more significant than single BP values, especially in awake animals.

SPECIAL INSTRUCTIONS:

Bone Marrow Aspiration and Evaluation

Kristi S. Lively, DVM, DABVP

 Purpose of Procedure

Bone marrow aspiration and biopsy are important diagnostic procedures for investigating the cause of an abnormal complete blood count (CBC), which can occur with many different diseases. Bone marrow may be adversely affected by many cancers, infections, and certain abnormalities of cell growth.

These procedures may be recommended when an abnormality in blood cells is suspected, because evaluation of the bone marrow yields important information about the production and maturation of different blood cell lines. Bone marrow aspiration may be performed in animals with unexplained anemias, platelet disorders, unexplained low or high white blood cell counts, or abnormal blood cells (such as leukemia cells) in the circulation, and for the detection of certain infectious organisms. It may also be done for staging of certain malignant cancers, such as lymphoma. *Staging* is the term used when a search is undertaken to determine which tissues of the body may contain cancer cells.

Preparation of Animal

Most bone marrow aspirates can be obtained with use of a local anesthetic and mild sedation. The position of the patient during the procedure depends on the site being aspirated or biopsied. The most commonly used sites are the pelvic bone in front of the hip (ilium), the rear leg bone below the hip joint (femur), and the front leg bone near the shoulder joint (humerus). Less commonly, a rib or the sternum (breast bone) may be aspirated.

Hair is shaved from the site, and the skin is scrubbed as for a sterile procedure. A local anesthetic, such as lidocaine, is injected into the area to be aspirated so that the site becomes numb, which minimizes the patient's discomfort.

 Description of Technique

Once the site has been clipped and prepared, a small incision is made in the skin. The biopsy needle is advanced through this incision, through the outer layer of the bone, and into the hollow marrow cavity in the center of the bone. A sample of marrow is aspirated into the syringe attached to the bone marrow needle and submitted for analysis. If a thicker sample is desired, a core biopsy needle may be used. Core needles retrieve small clumps of material rather than only fluid. Once a good sample has been obtained, the needle is removed, and the small incision in the skin is sutured, glued together, or left to heal by itself.

A CBC is often submitted along with the marrow sample to provide the pathologist with a more complete picture of the clinical condition.

Potential Complications

Complications from bone marrow aspiration and biopsy are rare but include reactions to the sedative used and damage to surrounding tissues from passage of the needle. The sciatic nerve in the hind leg runs close to the site of entry into the bone; temporary paralysis of this nerve can result from the lidocaine injection or damage from the needle. Bleeding may occur from laceration of adjacent blood vessels. Rarely, with aspiration from a rib or the sternum, air may be introduced into the chest, causing a pneumothorax.

Follow-up Care

Recovery from the sedative usually takes only a few hours. If sutures were placed, they are typically removed in 10-14 days. Results of the bone marrow analysis are often available in several days.

SPECIAL INSTRUCTIONS:

Bronchoscopy

Ronald M. Bright, DVM, MS, DACVS

 Purpose of Procedure

Bronchoscopy allows direct visualization of the lining of the respiratory tract through a fiberoptic viewing scope. It is used to obtain tissue or fluid (via bronchoalveolar lavage) for further diagnostic tests, including analysis of cells for inflammation, cancer, or presence of bacteria. If bacteria are found, the sample may also be submitted for culture and testing to identify an appropriate choice of antibiotics.

Bronchoscopy can be very helpful in rendering an accurate prognosis, because it helps identify irreversible changes to the anatomy of the airway. It is also used to retrieve foreign bodies and can be repeated as a follow-up procedure to monitor the response to therapy.

 Description of Technique

Although bronchoscopes can be either rigid or flexible, the latter type is most commonly used by veterinarians because of its versatility and maneuverability. It also allows examination of the nose and of tissues above the soft palate during the same procedure. With the animal under anesthesia, the bronchoscope is slowly passed into the airway, as far as it can reach. It is withdrawn after samples are obtained.

Bronchoscopy is usually accomplished within 30-45 minutes. Oxygen is delivered to the patient during the procedure and oxygen levels in the blood are constantly monitored. An electrocardiogram is used to monitor heart rate and rhythm during the procedure. Other vital signs may also be measured or monitored during the procedure.

Preparation of Animal

Bronchoscopy stimulates a number of protective reflexes, including sneezing, coughing, head shaking, and collapse of the airway; therefore, it can be done only with the animal under general anesthesia.

An endotracheal tube cannot be used during the procedure, so a soft tube is gently placed into the nose to allow delivery of 100% oxygen, and anesthesia is maintained with short-acting injectable drugs. An intravenous catheter is usually inserted in a vein of the leg for administration of anesthetic agents and intravenous fluids. The animal undergoing bronchoscopy is usually placed on its sternum for the procedure.

Potential Complications

Although the advantages of bronchoscopy far outweigh potential disadvantages, there are some instances in which it is not indicated, such as in patients with a known bleeding problem, severe oxygen depletion in the blood, or severe heart disease with an unstable heart rhythm (serious arrhythmia). Also at some risk are patients with severe respiratory disease, because they may have trouble waking up from anesthesia, and those with pulmonary hypertension or severe kidney disease.

For animals considered to be at low risk for bronchoscopy, some potential complications exist, although they have a low rate of occurrence. Potential complications include excessive stimulation and spasm of the larynx and bronchus resulting in coughing, bleeding into the airway, collapse of a portion of the lung, and delivery of low oxygen levels to the blood during the procedure.

 Follow-up Care

Most follow-up care pertains to the underlying respiratory disease rather than the bronchoscopy. If recovery is smooth, the animal may be discharged from the hospital on the same day.

SPECIAL INSTRUCTIONS:

Castration of Male Cats

Ronald M. Bright, DVM, MS, DACVS

 ## Purpose of Procedure

Castration is performed in cats to
- Reduce overpopulation and unwanted cats
- Decrease male aggressiveness, fighting with other tom cats, and roaming behavior
- Lessen the likelihood of cat bite abscesses from fighting with other cats
- Decrease the incidence of undesirable urination behaviors
- Prevent, eliminate, or remove tumors involving the testes or scrotum
- Repair traumatic wounds when surgery may not be able to preserve the scrotum or testes
- Control certain type of hormonal (endocrine) abnormalities

 ## Description of Technique

Castration, or *orchiectomy*, is surgical removal of the testicles. Incisions are made directly over the scrotum. If one or both testicles are located in the abdomen (retained testicle or cryptorchidism), an abdominal exploratory surgery is necessary. Another site where one or both testicles may be retained is under the skin near the last nipple or groin area of the abdomen. In these cases, incisions are made in the skin overlying the testicles.

No skin sutures are used for most routine scrotal castrations in the cat. External skin sutures may or may not be used when the testicles are removed from other locations. Scrotal ablation (removal of the scrotum and the testes) is necessary in some instances of cancer, trauma, or infection.

Preparation of Animal

Your veterinarian will instruct you to withhold food and sometimes water for a certain period of time, depending on the anesthesia to be used for the surgery.

Potential Complications

Complications following castration are uncommon.
- Excessive licking may occur, and some type of restraint device, such as an Elizabethan collar, is required to prevent trauma to the incision.
- A small amount of blood may be noted at the edges of the scrotal incision.
- Some cats that are castrated because of roaming or behavioral problems have no significant improvement after castration.
- Similarly, the incidence of cat bite abscesses may not decrease noticeably.

 ## Postoperative/Follow-up Care

It is advisable to avoid granular, clay, or clumping kitty litter for several days, until the scrotal incisions have healed. If an abdominal surgery was done, the cat should be kept quiet for 10-14 days or until the sutures have been removed. If possible, the cat should be kept inside in a clean and dry environment until the incisions have healed. No recheck visits may be needed if external sutures were not used.

SPECIAL INSTRUCTIONS:

Castration of Male Dogs

Ronald M. Bright, DVM, MS, DACVS

 Purpose of Procedure

Castration is performed in dogs to
- Reduce overpopulation and unwanted dogs
- Decrease male aggressiveness and roaming behavior
- Decrease the incidence of undesirable urination behaviors
- Reduce diseases of the prostate and possible tumors of the perianal area
- Help prevent the occurrence of perineal hernias in the older male (or recurrence of a hernia following surgical hernia repair)
- Prevent, eliminate, or remove tumors involving the testes or scrotum
- Repair traumatic wounds when surgery may not be able to preserve the scrotum or testes
- Repair hernias involving the scrotum
- Alleviate or prevent obstruction of the urethra from bladder stones (as a component of prescrotal urethrostomy surgery)
- Control certain hormonal (endocrine) abnormalities
- Prevent propagation of puppies that might inherit certain defects or diseases

Description of Technique

Castration, or *orchiectomy*, is surgical removal of the testicles. For dogs with both testicles in the scrotum, a single incision is made in the skin just in front of the scrotum. If one or both testicles are located in the abdomen (retained testicle or cryptorchidism), abdominal exploratory surgery is necessary. If the testicle is located near the sheath (prepuce) or in the groin (inguinal testicle), a skin incision is made directly over the testicle.

Most castration incisions are closed with buried sutures to decrease the tendency for licking. These sutures do not have to be removed. Scrotal ablation or removal of the entire scrotum (at the same time as the testes) is necessary in cases of cancer, trauma, or infection or if the scrotum is extremely pendulous (large and baggy).

Preparation of Animal

Your veterinarian will instruct you to withhold food and sometimes water for a certain period of time, depending on the anesthesia to be used for the surgery. Most dogs undergoing an elective castration are healthy and require minimal laboratory testing. If castration is done as part of therapy for another disease, more involved diagnostic tests may be done prior to castration.

Potential Complications

Most dogs do well after surgery, with no or minimal complications.
- Excessive licking requires some type of restraint device, such as an Elizabethan collar, to prevent trauma to the incision.
- A small amount of bloody fluid may collect within the remaining scrotal sac and usually disappears within 2 weeks. Rarely, a more significant amount of fluid accumulates and a second surgery is needed to remove the scrotum.
- Not all dogs castrated for roaming or behavioral problems show significant improvement after castration.

Postoperative Follow-up Care

The dog should be kept quiet for 10-14 days or until the sutures are removed, especially if an abdominal surgery was done. Restrict play and exercise to leash walking. If possible, except for going outside for elimination purposes, the dog should be kept inside in a clean and dry environment until the incisions have healed. No recheck visits may be needed if external sutures were not used.

SPECIAL INSTRUCTIONS:

Chemotherapy and Your Pet

Kristi S. Lively, DVM, DABVP

 ## Purpose of Procedure

The use of chemotherapy depends on several factors, including the type and location of the tumor, the condition of the patient, and the presence of metastases (spread of the cancer), as well as personal decisions, such as financial constraints. Chemotherapy may be used alone or with surgery or radiation therapy, depending on the tumor type and location. Positive responses to chemotherapy range from partial remission and slowing progression of the disease to complete remission (elimination of all cancer cells and clinical signs). Most cancers are not completely cured by chemotherapy and many recur at some time in the future.

Chemotherapy works by damaging rapidly growing cells. Rapidly dividing cancer cells are typically more sensitive to chemotherapy than normally dividing healthy cells. The effective use of chemotherapy is a balance between killing cancer cells and minimizing side effects that arise from killing healthy cells in the patient.

 ## Description of Technique

Chemotherapeutic agents are commonly administered together in specific protocols that maximize destruction of tumor cells, minimize resistance of tumor cells to medications, and minimize side effects to the patient. The protocols may be altered to fit the needs of the individual patient or changed based on the tumor type, the patient's health status, the veterinarian's experience, and the owner's constraints. Discuss your pet's protocol with your veterinarian to be sure you understand possible side effects, the treatment schedule, and costs, as well as the monitoring and follow-up care required. Some of the most commonly used chemotherapeutic drugs are
- Vincristine—injection given directly into a vein
- L-Asparaginase—injection given in the muscle
- Cyclophosphamide—injectable or pill form (wear latex gloves when administering)
- Doxorubicin—injection given slowly into a vein
- Cisplatin/carboplatin—injection given slowly into a vein
- Prednisone—a pill, to be given at home

Preparation of Animal

The protocol established for your pet often includes a calendar of treatment dates. Some treatments are administered at home, whereas others are administered at the veterinary hospital. Medications that minimize the side effects of chemotherapy, such as antinausea drugs, may be started a few days prior to the treatment date.

Many chemotherapy treatments can be given at the hospital over a few hours. Laboratory tests are often rechecked before chemotherapy is given. An intravenous catheter may be placed to allow safe delivery of the medication into the vein. Fluid therapy, sedatives, or antinausea medications may also be given during the hospital stay to maximize your pet's comfort and minimize side effects.

Potential Complications

Chemotherapeutic drugs affect the fastest dividing cells in the body, which include not only cancer cells but also some healthy cells, especially those of the bone marrow and gastrointestinal tract. Common side effects include suppression of healthy bone marrow cells, which results in a low white blood cell count, low red blood cell count (anemia), and/or low platelet count. Gastrointestinal effects include nausea, vomiting, decreased appetite, and diarrhea.

Pets rarely lose their hair as human patients undergoing chemotherapy do; however, hair may not regrow after it has been shaved. Some breeds, such as terriers and sheepdogs, are more susceptible to hair loss. Since lower doses of chemotherapeutic drugs are used in animals than in people, pets tend to tolerate their chemotherapy much better than people do. The side effects that develop in most pets are not typically as severe as those seen in people.

It is important for you to be aware of the potential side effects of the specific medications your pet is receiving. For example, some medications may cause a severe irritation at the injection site. If side effects occur, contact your veterinarian immediately so that these effects may be treated promptly and managed proactively in the future.

Issues that affect your pet's quality of life, such as pain management, meeting nutritional needs, and expected response to treatment, should also be discussed. Questions that arise once you are home can be written down and addressed with your veterinarian.

 ## Follow-up Care

Careful monitoring is required to check for side effects of chemotherapy, to monitor effects of the medications on other organ systems, to monitor response of the cancer to the chemotherapy, and to watch for spread of the cancer. Depending on the cancer type and the chemotherapeutic drugs used, monitoring may involve repeated physical examinations, laboratory tests, radiographs (x-rays), and abdominal ultrasound examinations.

SPECIAL INSTRUCTIONS:

Dialysis

Cathy E. Langston, DVM, DACVIM (Small Animal)

 ## Purpose of Procedure

Dialysis is a method of treating kidney disease. It is most commonly used to treat reversible causes of acute kidney failure. Causes of acute kidney failure include infections (such as pyelonephritis in cats or leptospirosis in dogs), poisonings (such as accidental ingestion of antifreeze or certain drugs), and situations that cause poor blood flow to the kidneys (such as anesthesia or low blood pressure). Kidney stones causing blockage of urine flow are becoming a common cause of kidney failure in cats, and some sort of dialysis may be needed to stabilize the cat in preparation for surgery to remove the blockage.

 ## Description of Technique

Peritoneal dialysis involves placing a catheter directly into the abdominal (belly) cavity. Fluid is delivered into the abdomen through the catheter. Toxins from the blood diffuse (flow) into the fluid, and then the fluid is drained and discarded. More fresh fluid is administered, and the process is repeated. In the early stages of treatment, the fluid may be drained and fresh fluid added every hour. As the patient improves, the fluid exchanges may be performed every 2-8 hours.

Hemodialysis involves placing a double-sided catheter in the large vein of the neck (jugular vein). This catheter allows blood to be withdrawn from one side and sent through a machine that clears out the toxins. The blood is returned to the body through the other side of the catheter. Hemodialysis can be intermittent (several hours a day) or continuous (24 hours a day). Continuous dialysis is usually called *continuous renal replacement therapy* (CRRT). Typically, different machine are used for intermittent versus continuous therapy. Hemodialysis is available at a limited number of veterinary hospitals.

Preparation of Animal

Peritoneal dialysis and both forms of hemodialysis are intensive treatments. It is important to have realistic expectations so that appropriate decisions can be made by the patient's family and the healthcare team about which animals are good candidates for treatment. Whenever possible, the cause of kidney failure is determined before deciding whether to start dialysis, because the possibility of recovery is usually best with acute renal failure. Chronic kidney failure is not a reversible condition. Blood tests, urine tests, abdominal radiographs (x-rays), and an ultrasound examination are frequently performed to help determine the cause. In most cases, acute disease can be differentiated from chronic disease.

Potential Complications

Complications of peritoneal dialysis include the following:
- Leakage of fluid under the skin in the area of the catheter
- Infection of the catheter or abdomen
- Clogging of the catheter
- Low blood protein levels

Complications of hemodialysis (intermittent or continuous) include the following:
- Bleeding associated with the blood thinner used during treatment
- Clotting of blood in tubes outside the body
- Blood clots in the catheter
- Seizures, coma, brain swelling
- Low blood pressure

 ## Follow-up Care

In people, peritoneal dialysis can be performed at home (without assistance) to provide continuous treatment for chronic, irreversible kidney disease. Because of the numerous technical complications associated with peritoneal dialysis in animals, it is usually performed in the veterinary hospital. When kidney values in the blood return to normal, the fluid exchanges are stopped. If the kidney values remain normal, then kidney function has recovered, and the catheter can be removed. Timing of recheck evaluations varies for each individual case.

With intermittent hemodialysis, some patients are stable after the first week or two and can go home between dialysis treatments. If kidney function has not completely recovered, the patient is usually returned to the hospital 3 days a week for dialysis treatments. Treatments typically take 4-6 hours. Most patients that are going to recover kidney function do so within 1 month.

With continuous dialysis treatment, the patient is hooked to the dialysis machine 24 hours a day, so the animal must remain hospitalized in an intensive care unit. After a few days of continuous therapy, the animal may be stable enough to be transferred to a facility with intermittent hemodialysis.

Both peritoneal dialysis and hemodialysis are reserved for patients with severe kidney failure that has not responded to other forms of medical therapy. Therefore, only the sickest animals receive dialysis. Success (survival) rates are approximately 50%. Of those animals that live, about half recover full kidney function, and about half have some degree of permanent kidney damage that can be managed with special diets and medications.

SPECIAL INSTRUCTIONS:

Echocardiography

Rebecca E. Gompf, DVM, MS, DACVIM (Cardiology)

 ## Purpose of Procedure

Echocardiography is performed when heart disease is suspected or chest radiographs (x-rays) show that the heart is enlarged. The echocardiogram (echo) shows the size of the heart chambers and how well the left side of the heart is functioning. It shows whether the heart valves are normal or thickened. An echo can detect the presence of extra fluid in the pericardial sac around the heart and sometimes the presence of tumors in the heart that are causing the extra fluid.

 ## Description of Technique

Echocardiography is a type of ultrasound examination. All types of ultrasounds bounce sound waves off an object and record the returning sound waves. Special probes are placed on the animal's chest. These probes send and receive the sound waves or echoes. The echo machine converts these sounds waves into images of the heart.

It takes special training and months of experience to become proficient in performing echocardiograms. Echo machines are expensive, so they are not available in all veterinary practices. Your pet may be referred to a specialist, such as a veterinary cardiologist, radiologist, or internist, for this procedure.

Several types of echocardiography exist and may be performed in sequence. Two-dimensional (2D) echocardiography shows the heart as it is moving, as well as the inner chambers and outer walls of the heart. Echo in 2D allows gross (major) abnormalities to be detected and identifies areas of the heart to be examined more closely. Tumors, extra fluid in the pericardial sac, and clots in the heart can be found with this technique. Abnormal heart rhythms (arrhythmia) can be identified, and most echo machines have built-in electrocardiographic capability, so the arrhythmia can be examined or recorded during the echo procedure.

Once the heart has been examined with 2D echo, an area is selected for examination with M-mode echo. This form of echocardiography is used to measure the chambers of the heart and to determine how well the left heart is functioning. Because M mode freezes the motion of the heart, it makes measuring the different areas easier. M-mode measurements must be done properly, because inaccurate measurements can underestimate or overestimate problems.

Doppler echocardiography uses color to map the blood flow in the heart. Doppler echo is used to determine whether the blood flow is too fast in certain areas, such as with subaortic stenosis or pulmonic stenosis (congenital heart defects that cause narrowing of the openings that blood flows through). Doppler echo can determine the severity of the defect by measuring the velocity of blood flowing through these narrowed areas. Doppler echo also can detect holes in the wall of the heart, such as occur with ventricular and atrial septal defects. Doppler echo can also detect leakage of the heart valves.

Three-dimensional (3D) echocardiography is available on some echo machines. It gives an accurate image of the heart but currently is used mainly for teaching purposes.

Preparation of Animal

Little preparation is needed for an echo examination. A few animals need to be tranquilized, but most do not. Aggressive cats that cannot be handled easily when awake may require general anesthesia or sedation to perform this procedure. It is best not to feed your animal on the morning of the procedure, just in case sedatives are needed.

In order to get the best possible contact between the echo transducer and the skin, the hair is usually shaved on both sides of the chest. Animals with thin hair coats may not be clipped, but if the hair is not clipped, the quality of the echo image may not be sufficient to make a diagnosis.

Most animals are required to lie on their sides for this procedure. More experienced ultrasonographers may perform the examination with the animal standing or sitting up. The procedure is done in a quiet room, with a minimal amount of stress to the animal.

Potential Complications

Echocardiography is a very safe procedure with no long-term or short-term side effects. The only potential complications are those that may arise from administration of tranquilizers, sedatives, or general anesthesia. Side effects of these drugs are uncommon.

 ## Follow-up Care

Repeated echo studies may be required to monitor the progression of your animal's heart disease. The frequency of these examinations and other follow-up visits is based on the underlying heart disease.

SPECIAL INSTRUCTIONS:

Electrocardiography: Intermittent and Continuous

Rebecca E. Gompf, DVM, MS, DACVIM (Cardiology)

 ## Purpose of Procedure

Electrocardiography is performed if an abnormal heart rhythm (arrhythmia) is suspected or unexplained collapsing or fainting episodes occur. Intermittent electrocardiograms (ECGs) can identify continuous or constant arrhythmias. If the arrhythmia is not present at all times, it may be recommended that your animal wear a Holter monitor or an event monitor at home. Continuous monitoring may also be done in the hospital, especially if the arrhythmia is frequent or is being treated.

 ## Description of Technique

An ECG is a recording of the electrical activity of the heart; it does not give information on how well the heart is contracting. An ECG machine is attached to the animal by special alligator clips that have been filed down and bent outward so that they do not pinch the skin too forcefully. Several clips and leads may be applied to the legs and the chest. A *routine ECG* is run for a few minutes and is printed out so that your veterinarian can read it or send it to a specialist for interpretation. Several telephone transmission services are available for sending an ECG to a specialist for interpretation. Some veterinarians are very experienced in reading ECGs and are comfortable interpreting them.

In *telemetry monitoring*, a transmitter is attached to the animal's chest and sends the ECG signal to a monitor located nearby. The ends of the ECG electrodes are snapped onto a sticky patch that is attached to the animal's skin (after hair is shaved from the site so that the patch will stick), making the device comfortable enough for continuous use. Telemetry is used for hospitalized animals, and it allows 24-hour continuous ECG monitoring without having the animal physically attached to an ECG machine. Telemetry units have limited range, usually several meters. They come with audible alarms that are triggered if an abnormal heart rhythm occurs.

A *Holter monitor* is a device used for recording the ECG on an outpatient basis. It contains either a tape or a digital recorder and is attached to the animal for 24 hours. The ECG leads are attached to the animal by a method similar to telemetry monitoring. The Holter monitor is taped and bandaged to the animal's chest (small animals) or worn in a specially designed jacket (larger dogs). Some of the devices are too big for very small animals to carry around.

The Holter monitor continuously records the ECG for 24 hours; it is then removed, and the entire tracing is printed out. While your animal is wearing a Holter monitor, it is very important to keep a diary of your pet's activities. The person interpreting the 24-hour tracing needs to know when your animal was sleeping, when it was active and running around, and when it had a fainting episode. The diary is returned with the monitor. Without a record of the exact times of these events, the Holter tracings cannot be accurately interpreted.

An *event monitor* is a smaller device that is attached to the animal in a fashion similar to a Holter monitor. Because of its smaller size, it can be used in cats and small dogs. It is used when an animal is not having a daily problem but might be having fainting episodes every few days to once weekly. An event monitor does not record the ECG unless a button is pushed. If the animal is observed having a problem, the button is pushed, and the monitor then records the ECG for 2 minutes. Up to four events can be recorded over 2 weeks. The event monitor is then removed and attached to a machine that prints out the ECG tracings for examination by your veterinarian or a specialist.

Preparation of Animal

Little preparation is needed for any of these ECG methods. If sticky patches are used, a small area of fur will be shaved where the patch attaches to the skin.

Potential Complications

Electrocardiography is a very safe procedure. The most common complications are removal of the electrodes by the animal or loosening of the bandage holding the monitor or transmitter to the chest.

 ## Follow-up Care

Frequent ECGs or repeat monitoring may be done to evaluate how well anti-arrhythmia medications are working, especially until the arrhythmia is controlled. The frequency of other follow-up visits and testing is based on the cause of the arrhythmia.

SPECIAL INSTRUCTIONS:

Femoral Head and Neck Ostectomy

Mark C. Rochat, DVM, MS, DACVS

 Purpose of Procedure

Femoral head and neck ostectomy (FHO) is considered a salvage procedure. FHO is performed to restore some normal function to a hip joint that has a problem that cannot be surgically corrected.

FHO is done in dogs and cats that have severe fractures of the hip; hip dysplasia that is not responsive to medical management; degenerative conditions of the hip that are not correctable by other surgical procedures, such as hip dysplasia and Legg-Calves-Perthes disease; or chronic dislocations of the joint. Financial limitations may also influence the decision of whether to perform an FHO.

Because the limb function that results from FHO is less predictable in large and giant breeds, this technique is often reserved for small dogs and cats. However, FHO can result in noticeably improved limb function in approximately 50% of large dogs.

 Description of Technique

FHO is a surgical procedure that involves cutting off the femoral head (ball of the thigh bone) that fits into the hip socket. A fibrous (scar) tissue junction then develops between the femur (thigh bone) and the pelvis. This procedure allows improved range of movement of the hip and eliminates the bone-on-bone pain that is often associated with the conditions mentioned. Alternative muscle sling techniques are generally discouraged.

Preparation of Animal

Any underlying problems associated with the original injury or disease must be identified and addressed prior to surgery. Routine laboratory tests are used to identify any risks that may affect general anesthesia. Your veterinarian will provide detailed instructions on withholding food and water prior to surgery.

Potential Complications

Complications include a continued, unacceptable degree of lameness, infection, severe bleeding, and nerve damage. With careful operating technique and proper choice of candidates for the surgery, these complications are uncommon.

 Postoperative/Follow-up Care

The incision is inspected daily for evidence of infection (excessive redness, pain, discharge), and the sutures or staples are removed after 10-14 days. The dog or cat is encouraged to use the leg as much as possible and as soon as possible, to enhance the quality of scar tissue that develops at the joint and to preserve as much movement as possible. Dogs that are allowed to carry the leg for the first few weeks often have significant loss of hip motion. Physical rehabilitation therapy often greatly improves the functional outcome.

SPECIAL INSTRUCTIONS:

Fluid Therapy

Rhea V. Morgan, DVM, DACVIM (Small Animal), DACVO

 Purpose of Procedure

Animals maintain a normal fluid balance in the body by drinking and taking in fluids in their foods to offset the fluids lost in urine and feces and from the respiratory tract (panting). When fluid balance is severely disrupted, dehydration and shock may occur.

Supplemental fluids may be needed if fluid intake decreases, losses increase, or both occur. Loss of appetite and less drinking lower the intake of fluids. Increased losses occur with vomiting, diarrhea, panting, kidney diseases, bleeding, or surface burns. Fluids may also be given for excessively high protein levels (hyperproteinemia, hyperviscosity) or for high numbers of red blood cells in the circulation (polycythemia). Fluid therapy involves administering fluids or supplementing body electrolytes, such as sodium and potassium, by injection.

 Description of Technique

Fluids are most commonly given by the subcutaneous (under the skin, SQ or SC) or the intravenous (into a vein, IV) route. SC fluids are often given between or near the shoulder blades. (See the handout on **Subcutaneous Fluid Administration**.) Only limited amounts of fluids can be given SC, because it takes 6-24 hours for fluids to be absorbed into the body from this space. Fluids given SC must be compatible with the surrounding tissues; they cannot be too concentrated or contain extra electrolytes or glucose (sugar). SC fluids are given when small amounts of fluids are needed infrequently (every 1-7 days) and the need is not immediate (acute).

IV fluids are given through a needle (one-time administration) or through a catheter (repeated administrations) inserted into the vein. IV catheters are most commonly inserted in the veins of the front or rear legs, but the jugular vein in the neck may also be used. Large amounts of IV fluids can be administered quickly, making this an ideal route when the need for fluids is urgent. A variety of fluids and electrolyte mixtures, as well as many medications, can be given IV.

Some puppies and kittens are so small that IV catheters cannot be inserted in their veins. In these instances, fluids are sometimes given intraperitoneally (into the abdominal cavity, IP) or intraosseously (into the bone marrow cavity of the long bone in the rear leg, IO). Special catheters and needles are available for administering fluids IO.

Numerous types of fluid solutions are available for use in animals. Crystalloid solutions have about the same consistency as the watery part of blood and can contain varying amounts of electrolytes. Glucose and other medications may be added to crystalloid fluids. Crystalloids can be administered via any of the routes described. Colloid solutions contain substances that attract water similar to normal blood proteins. Colloids are used primarily when blood proteins are low, to keep water from leaving the bloodstream. Colloid solutions can be irritating, so they are usually administered IV in a large vein.

Fluids may be administered continuously or intermittently, through open drip lines or through a syringe or IV pump that strictly controls the rate and amount to be given.

Preparation of Animal

For SC and IP fluid therapy, sterile needles are used, and the skin should be clean at the site of penetration. For IV and IO fluid therapy, fur is clipped from the skin at the site of catheter insertion, and the skin is cleaned with an antiseptic solution and alcohol until all dirt and debris are removed. After the catheter is inserted and a cap or plug is applied, it is bandaged to the skin. The leg or the neck is then wrapped in gauze, and a surface bandage is applied. An Elizabethan collar might be used if the animal licks or bothers the catheter or IV drip line.

Potential Complications

Complications are uncommon but can include infection (especially with SC or IP fluids) and temporary bleeding where the needle is inserted (SC fluids). Most infections arise from bacterial contamination of the fluid or entry site. Complications of IV administration include premature removal of the catheter, bleeding from the catheter port or insertion site, irritation to the vein (phlebitis), and loss of the catheter into the bloodstream (extremely rare). Overdosage of fluids can aggravate existing heart disease and lead to accumulation of fluid in the lungs and abdomen.

 Follow-up Care

Notify your veterinarian if any redness or swelling develops at the site where a needle or catheter has been removed.

SPECIAL INSTRUCTIONS:

Fracture Repair: Casts and Splints

Mark C. Rochat, DVM, MS, DACVS

Purpose of Procedure

Casts are external devices used to treat bone fractures or temporarily immobilize a joint. Casts are used for only certain types of fractures, typically those that are simple, closed (no exposure of the bone through the skin surface), and located below the elbow or stifle (knee). Casts are commonly made of fiberglass resin.

Splints are most often used as temporary devices to immobilize a broken bone or joint before surgery. If support for the leg after a surgical procedure is required, a padded splint may be applied. Splints are usually a combination of soft bandage materials and a strip of rigid metal or fiberglass.

Support bandages can also help reduce the pain and swelling associated with bone fractures or surgery. The Robert Jones bandage does not have a rigid splint in it but relies on a large amount of cotton padding to stabilize the leg. The Robert Jones bandage is commonly used if the injured area is below the elbow or stifle. If the area is above those joints, a spica splint is usually applied.

Description of Technique

Casts are applied while the animal is anesthetized. Casts encircle the limb and extend from the toes to just above the elbow or stifle, regardless of where the break is located. Splints are often applied following surgery, while the animal is anesthetized. After trauma, they may be applied while the animal is awake.

Preparation of Animal

Because other injuries might have occurred during the trauma that created the broken bone, extensive evaluation of the animal is often done prior to anesthesia. As a part of the pre-anesthetic evaluation, laboratory tests, radiographs (x-rays) of the chest, an electrocardiogram (to identify abnormal heart rhythms), and an ultrasound examination of the abdomen may be recommended. X-rays of the affected limb are also taken. No special, local preparation for a cast or splint is required except for the occasional need to shave very long hair from the leg before applying a cast.

Potential Complications

Complications are common and include toe swelling and slipping of the cast or splint, which often leads to pressure sores. Sometimes in a young animal, even with proper care, rapid growth requires application of a new cast periodically.

Postoperative/Follow-up Care

Casts require diligent, daily observation to avoid problems. The toes must be inspected at least daily to quickly identify toe swelling (toes spread apart when they become swollen), odor, discharge, or slipping of the cast. If any of these signs occur, if apparent irritation (animal chewing or licking at the cast) is seen, or if the cast gets wet, the cast should be immediately examined by a veterinarian. Severe skin ulceration or other problems can occur if veterinary care is delayed.

The end of the cast or splint must be covered with a plastic bag when the animal goes outside to keep the cast or splint from getting wet. Casts and splints cannot be fully dried and must be changed if they get wet. Splints are cared for in a similar manner as casts.

SPECIAL INSTRUCTIONS:

Fracture Repair: External Skeletal Fixation

Mark C. Rochat, DVM, MS, DACVS

 Purpose of Procedure

External skeletal fixation (ESF) is a method of stabilizing a broken bone to allow healing. ESF can be applied to a variety of fractures and can be used for fusing joints (See the handout on **Arthrodesis**.) ESF can also be used for temporary immobilization of joints and correction of bone growth deformities. ESF is often used for treating open fractures (when the bone is exposed).

 Description of Technique

ESF is a fracture repair method that connects a number of pins, which are inserted through the skin and into the bone, to an external rod using clamps.

Preparation of Animal

Because other injuries might have occurred during the trauma that created the broken bone, extensive evaluation of the animal is often done prior to surgery. As a part of the presurgical evaluation, laboratory tests, radiographs (x-rays) of the chest, an electrocardiogram (to identify abnormal heart rhythms), and an ultrasound examination of the abdomen may be recommended. X-rays of the affected limb are also taken.

Potential Complications

When ESF is properly done, complications are infrequent and mild. Potential complications include bleeding, nerve damage, loss of muscle mass (muscle atrophy), pin loosening, pin breakage, delays in healing, improper alignment of the bone, and infection.

 Postoperative/Follow-up Care

Once the animal is at home, the places where the pins enter the skin are cleaned with cotton swabs and an antiseptic once daily. Oral analgesic (pain-relief) medications are also usually given. If signs of inflammation (excessive redness, pain, swelling, or discharge) are observed, notify your veterinarian.

Until the fracture has healed, the animal is restricted to short leash walks only. Physical rehabilitation helps maintain muscle tone and joint mobility during healing. X-rays are taken every 4-6 weeks to evaluate the healing process. After healing of the bone is complete, the animal is sedated, and the external fixator device is removed.

SPECIAL INSTRUCTIONS:

Fracture Repair: Internal Fixation

Mark C. Rochat, DVM, MS, DACVS

 ## Purpose of Procedure

Internal fixation refers to a number of different methods of repairing broken bones with devices that are placed beneath the skin. These devices include intramedullary pins and cerclage wires, other pinning techniques, bone plates and screws, and interlocking nails. These devices are also used for arthrodesis (fusing a joint), corrective osteotomies (cutting the bone to correct abnormally angled or shortened bones), and treatment of certain joint disorders.

Description of Technique

Because these devices are unique and very different from one another, a detailed description of each would be too long for this handout. Please ask your veterinarian if you would like more details about a specific type of device.

Preparation of Animal

Because other injuries might have occurred during the trauma that created the broken bone, extensive evaluation of the animal is often done prior to surgery. As a part of the presurgical evaluation, laboratory tests, radiographs (x-rays) of the chest, an electrocardiogram (to identify abnormal heart rhythms), and an ultrasound examination of the abdomen may be recommended. X-rays are also taken of the affected bone or joint.

Potential Complications

Potential complications are uncommon but include infection, excessive bleeding, and damage to nerves and soft tissues (such as tendons or muscles). Failure of the implants (breakage or loosening), dehiscence (opening of the incision before it has healed), seroma formation (fluid buildup beneath the skin at the surgical site), lameness in cold weather related to the metal in the device, and delays or failure to heal can also occur.

 ## Postoperative/Follow-up Care

Oral analgesic (pain-relief) medications are commonly given before and after surgery. If signs of inflammation (excessive redness, pain, swelling, or discharge) are observed at the incision, notify your veterinarian.

Until the fracture has healed, the animal is restricted to short leash walks only. Running, jumping, and playing are prohibited until healing is complete. Healing may take 4-12 weeks or longer, depending on age of the animal, location of the fracture, and type of surgery performed, and presence of other factors that affect healing.

Physical rehabilitation helps maintain muscle tone and joint mobility during healing. X-rays are taken every 4-6 weeks to evaluate the healing process. Intramedullary pins are often removed after healing of the bone is complete. Other devices are usually left in place unless there is a specific problem related to the implant.

SPECIAL INSTRUCTIONS:

Kidney Transplantation in Cats

Cathy E. Langston, DVM, DACVIM (Small Animal)

🐾 Purpose of Procedure

Kidney transplantation is a method of treating chronic kidney failure in cats when standard medical management has failed. One half of one kidney can provide enough kidney function to maintain normal blood values. Cats who donate one kidney still have ample kidney function to live a normal life. The family of the transplanted cat adopts the donor cat.

➕ Description of Technique

Kidney transplantation is available only at a few veterinary hospitals. The kidney donor cat is anesthetized first, and the kidney to be donated is removed. While one team operates on the donor cat, another surgery team prepares the recipient cat. The kidney is attached to the large blood vessels in the abdomen (belly) of the recipient cat. The two poorly functional kidneys are left in place unless there is a medical reason to remove them.

Preparation of Animal

Several tests are performed to determine whether a cat is a good candidate for kidney transplantation. If diseases other than kidney disease are present, the risk of complications increases. Most feline transplant programs require the following tests on both the recipient and the donor:

- Biochemistry panel, complete blood count, urinalysis, urine culture
- Chest and abdominal radiographs (x-rays), abdominal ultrasound examination, echocardiogram (heart ultrasound)
- Blood typing
- Blood tests for toxoplasmosis, feline leukemia virus, and feline immunodeficiency virus

In the week or so before the scheduled surgery, a blood cross-match test is performed with several potential donor cats. One to three days before surgery, oral cyclosporine (an immune suppressant) is started so that blood levels of the drug will be high enough at the time the new kidney is transplanted to prevent rejection of the donated kidney.

If kidney infection is suspected as the cause of kidney failure, cyclosporine along with prednisone (a steroid drug) may be started 2 weeks before surgery to determine whether the recipient cat develops a urinary infection while on these drugs. If infection develops, transplant surgery is cancelled, because the risk is too high. If an active or latent (inactive) viral upper respiratory infection may be present, cyclosporine and prednisone are also started 1 week before surgery. If severe symptoms (sneezing, discharge from the nose) develop, transplant surgery is cancelled.

Potential Complications

Of cats that undergo a kidney transplantation, 80% live through the surgery and hospitalization period. Severe hypertension (high blood pressure), seizures, urine leakage, obstruction of the ureter (the tube that carries urine from the kidney to the bladder), and delayed function of the transplanted kidney are some of the most common postoperative complications.

Within the first 6 months of surgery, the most common complications include rejection of the kidney (if the levels of drugs used to suppress the immune system are too low) and infection (if the drug levels are too high). Other complications include obstruction of the kidney with scar tissue, hemolytic uremic syndrome (anemia from destruction of red blood cells), and diabetes mellitus. More than 60% of cats that receive a kidney transplant are still doing well 6 months after surgery.

After the first 6 months, the rate of complications decreases. Long-term complications include diabetes mellitus, cancer, and rare infections. About 40% of cats that receive a kidney transplant are healthy 3 years after surgery.

🐾 Postoperative/Follow-up Care

After discharge from the hospital, many rechecks are necessary to adjust the medications. The rechecks may be performed by the local veterinarian, who then relays the information to the transplant team. Each recheck includes (at a minimum) a physical examination, body weight, laboratory tests of kidney function and to monitor for anemia, blood cyclosporine measurement (usually sent to the transplant center or specialty laboratory), and a urine specific gravity test (measurement of urine concentration) on a urine sample collected at home by the owner (ideally). To decrease the risk of urinary infections, veterinarians caring for transplanted cats usually avoid collecting urine with a needle or catheter.

Recheck visits are scheduled for a few days after discharge, then weekly for 1 month, then every other week for 1 month, and then monthly until all parameters (assessments) are stable. Thereafter, rechecks usually occur at least every 3 months.

Cats with a transplanted kidney require medications every day for the rest of their life to prevent rejection of the kidney. Because they are at risk for infections, they should not be exposed to other cats in boarding facilities and should remain indoors.

SPECIAL INSTRUCTIONS:

Laboratory Tests of Kidney Function

Cathy E. Langston, DVM, DACVIM (Small Animal)

Blood Urea Nitrogen (BUN)

BUN is a waste product produced from the breakdown of protein. Blood urea is removed from the body via the urine, so BUN levels increase as kidney function decreases. Any increase in protein introduced into the intestines to be digested (such as a very high protein diet of meat or blood proteins from a bleeding ulcer) can increase BUN in the blood. Dehydration also increases the BUN value. BUN is measured as a simple blood test.

Creatinine

Creatinine is a waste product of muscle turnover. Creatinine also increases as kidney function decreases. Few influences outside the kidney affect creatinine concentration, so it is a better marker of kidney function than BUN. One thing that does affect creatinine is muscle mass. Dogs and cats that are very thin because of muscle wasting may have artificially low creatinine levels compared to the actual functioning capacity of their kidneys. Creatinine is measured as a simple blood test.

Urine Specific Gravity

Urine specific gravity is a measure of the ability of the kidneys to concentrate urine (decrease its water content) or to dilute urine (increase water content). There is no normal value, because normal kidneys should be able to make a large volume of dilute urine if the dog or cat drinks a large volume of water and to concentrate the urine if water intake is restricted. Despite the range of concentrating and diluting ability of the kidneys, under typical circumstances the urine specific gravity is usually greater than 1.025.

If the kidneys are damaged, the urine will have a specific gravity in a fixed range (usually between 1.008 and 1.012). Kidney damage affects the ability to concentrate urine before blood markers of kidney function become elevated. In early kidney disease, the only abnormal finding may be poorly concentrated urine, but many other diseases can also cause poorly concentrated urine. Specialized tests to determine the cause of the urine concentrating problem are recommended based on the specific details of the individual case.

Glomerular Filtration Rate (GFR)

Although BUN and creatinine are routine tests of kidney function, kidney function must be impaired by more than 75% before their values become abnormal. With damage of 66% or greater, the kidneys are unable to adequately concentrate urine, and the urine specific gravity remains midrange. If kidney disease is suspected but standard blood tests are normal, a more specific test of kidney function, the GFR test, can be performed. There are several ways to measure GFR, including iohexol clearance, creatine clearance, and renal scintigraphy (nuclear scan).

The *iohexol clearance test* is performed by giving an intravenous injection of a contrast agent—the same agent that is used for many x-ray and computed tomography (CT scan) studies. Blood samples are drawn hourly for 4 hours and sent to a specialized laboratory for analysis. The risk of an allergic reaction to the iodine in the contrast agent is very small.

In the *creatinine clearance test*, creatinine is injected intravenously, and blood samples are drawn over the next 10 hours. The creatinine concentration can be measured by a local laboratory, and the GFR rate is calculated from a software program. Although this test is used to assess the severity of kidney failure, creatinine is not toxic to the body, and the injection does not cause the animal to feel bad. The patient's creatinine level returns to the baseline by the end of the test in most cases, or within 24 hours if kidney function is severely impaired. Although results of this test are reported rapidly, creatinine that is pure enough for injection is not readily available.

Renal scintigraphy is the only method that allows the function of each individual kidney to be determined. A specially tagged radioactive substance (radioisotope) is injected intravenously, and the amount of this substance taken up by each kidney is measured with a gamma camera, which detects the low level of radiation given off by the radioisotope. After this test, the patient usually stays in the hospital overnight while the substance is eliminated from the body. Few veterinary hospitals have the equipment necessary to perform this test.

SPECIAL INSTRUCTIONS:

Nutritional Management of Chronic Kidney Disease

Cathy E. Langston, DVM, DACVIM (Small Animal)

Purpose of the Diets

Dietary management is one of the most effective methods of slowing the progression of chronic kidney disease (CKD). Kidney diets double the survival time of many animals with CKD and dramatically decrease the need for hospitalization.

Description of Dietary Components

- *Protein:* Kidney diets have less protein than standard adult maintenance diets. The protein that is present must be easily used by the body. The best protein is from animal sources such as egg, milk, beef, or chicken, and not from vegetable sources such as tofu. The minimum protein contents shown on labels of pet food containers cannot be directly compared, because those values are affected by the amount of moisture in the diet and by the caloric content, which vary widely. Labels also do not indicate the biologic value of the protein, which is a measure of how fully the protein can be used by the body. Animal proteins have higher biologic value than vegetable proteins, and egg whites have the highest biologic value.
- *Phosphate:* Phosphate restriction is an important part of formulating a kidney diet. Protein contains phosphate, so protein restriction also reduces phosphate.
- *Fatty acids:* Most commercial kidney diets are supplemented with omega-3 fatty acids, which may have a beneficial effect on kidney function.
- *Sodium:* Although sodium restriction is commonly recommended for people with CKD, the role of salt (sodium chloride) in CKD of dogs and cats is not completely understood. Excessive salt supplementation or restriction may be detrimental; moderate salt restriction is common in most kidney diets.
- *Potassium:* Because the kidneys are unable to conserve potassium, low blood levels of potassium may develop in dogs and cats with CKD. Kidney diets, especially for cats, are frequently supplemented with potassium to account for the extra urinary losses. In some patients, particularly those on chronic dialysis and those receiving medications that may increase blood potassium, high blood levels of potassium (hyperkalemia) may develop while the animal is on a kidney diet.
- *Vitamins:* The B vitamins are water soluble, so they can be lost in urine. Kidney diets typically contain increased levels of B vitamins compared to maintenance diets.

Indications for Dietary Therapy

Kidney diets are generally recommended if the blood creatinine concentration is greater than 2.0 mg/dL (milligrams per deciliter) in dogs or 2.8 mg/dL in cats. Dogs and cats with acute kidney failure may need more protein than most kidney diets provide.

Follow-up Care

Changing Diets

Animals with CKD frequently have decreased appetite, and rapid diet changes are rarely well accepted. It may take weeks for your pet to accept the new diet, so patience is necessary. A simple way to change the diet is to offer the new food in the cat's usual container (bowl) next to the usual offering, while using a different container for the old product. If you can put both products in similar containers, the diet change may be easier. If the cat does not eat a new canned food within 1 hour, take it up until the next feeding time.

Once the cat has been exposed to the food for a day or two, offer the new food first, when the cat is the hungriest. After the cat has eaten some of the new food or has initially refused it, offer the old diet. Repeat this process until the cat is eating the new diet. Once the cat is eagerly eating the new diet, you can start decreasing the old diet until you are no longer feeding the old food. You may decrease the old food in increments of ¼ cup until the change is complete. This same process can be used for dogs.

Appetite stimulants may be helpful for cats while changing the diet, on a continual basis, or as needed. If a cat with CKD will not eat the kidney diet or does not eat enough to sustain normal body weight, a feeding tube may be inserted so that an adequate amount of the right kind of food can be fed easily. In addition, medications and fluids can be given through the feeding tube, decreasing the stress on both patient and caretaker.

SPECIAL INSTRUCTIONS:

Oxygen Therapy

Rhea V. Morgan, DVM, DACVIM (Small Animal), DACVO

Purpose of Procedure

Oxygen therapy is delivery of high concentrations of oxygen into the respiratory tract to increase oxygen levels in the blood so that more oxygen reaches the tissues. Oxygen therapy may be indicated any time blood oxygen levels fall to a dangerous level, such as with heart and respiratory diseases, anemia, metabolic diseases, and shock. Red blood cells normally carry oxygen to the tissues, but if their numbers are low, delivery of high levels of oxygen into the lungs can increase the amount of oxygen that is absorbed directly into the bloodstream.

Description of Technique

If an animal is unconscious, a tube may be placed in its mouth and trachea (windpipe) and attached to a direct source of oxygen. If the animal is awake, oxygen may be administered through a mask, a hood, an oxygen cage, or a catheter inserted into the nose or trachea.

Masks are used when oxygen therapy is needed for only a short period, such as immediately before or after surgery. Most animals resist wearing a mask, so an assistant is usually needed to hold the mask in place.

Oxygen cages are ideal for small patients that require continuous oxygen over a long period. Hoods can be made by placing plastic over the opening of an Elizabethan collar. A lot of oxygen escapes into the environment with this method, so it is not as effective as insertion of an oxygen catheter. Hoods can be used if catheters are not available or not tolerated by the animal.

Nasal catheters are passed part way into the nose and then sutured to the skin of the head. Soft, rubber catheters are commonly used and may be left in place for several days. Usually a single catheter is inserted, but two can be placed simultaneously, one through each nostril.

Tracheal catheters, such as tracheostomy tubes, are primarily used in animals with an obstruction of the upper airway (nose, larynx, trachea). An incision is initially made in the skin and muscles of the neck. A small incision is then made between two rings in the windpipe, and the tracheostomy tube is inserted and sutured to the skin.

Continuous or long-term oxygen therapy requires that the oxygen be humidified so that the respiratory passages do not dry out. Oxygen cages have built-in humidifiers. Specially manufactured or homemade humidifiers may be attached to oxygen lines when other methods are used.

Preparation of Animal

When a mask, hood, or oxygen case is used, no preparation is needed. Nasal catheters and tubes can usually be inserted in awake animals, using a topical anesthetic solution or gel dripped into the nose. For some animals, light sedation may be needed. Insertion of an endotracheal tube through the mouth or a tracheostomy tube into the neck requires general anesthesia. If time allows, fur is clipped from the insertion site in the neck, and the skin is cleaned with an antiseptic solution and alcohol.

Potential Complications

Hoods, nasal catheters, and oxygen cages are generally well tolerated. A potential disadvantage of a hood is inadequate delivery of oxygen. If flow rates are too high through nasal catheters, small ulcers can develop in the nose where the tube ends, and air may be swallowed, which can cause the stomach to bloat.

The temperature and humidity levels in some oxygen cages can be difficult to control, especially if the animal is large for the size of the enclosed space. Careful monitoring is needed to ensure that the animal does not become overheated. In some oxygen cages, it is difficult to maintain consistently high levels of oxygen if the demand is great or if the door to the cage must be opened frequently for treatments to be performed.

The openings of tracheostomy tubes must be suctioned every few hours and cleaned, or they may become plugged with mucus. Both nasal catheters and tracheostomy tubes may become dislodged. An Elizabethan collar helps prevent dislodgment in animals with nasal catheters. Lack of proper humidification of the oxygen causes dryness of the respiratory passages.

Follow-up Care

Once the underlying problem resolves and the animal is weaned from the supplemental oxygen, little after care is needed. Blood oxygen levels may be monitored for several days to ensure that they are adequate while the animal is breathing only room air.

SPECIAL INSTRUCTIONS:

Physical Rehabilitation

Mark C. Rochat, DVM, MS, DACVS

 Purpose of Procedure

Physical rehabilitation (called *physical therapy* in people) is the manipulation of the muscles and joints of one or more legs to improve healing and mobility of joints and muscles, to decrease loss of muscle mass (reduce muscle atrophy), to improve balance and coordination, and to reduce pain. Physical rehabilitation is an effective tool for improving the function of dogs affected by various orthopedic and neurologic conditions. It may be done in conjunction with surgery or as a sole method of improving the function of one or more legs and joints, depending on the circumstances.

Description of Technique

Numerous therapies are available, such as the following:
- Passive range-of-motion exercises, which are done by gently moving a joint or limb through its normal arc of motion
- Stretching exercises, which are done by gently stretching portions of a leg or body part
- Therapeutic, active exercises, such as standing and balancing exercises, sit-to-stand and stand-to sit exercises, gait training, exercises around and over obstacles, and water treadmill exercises
- Electrical stimulation, which involves stimulating muscles by applying different types of currents through electrodes attached to the skin
- Ultrasound therapy, which is often done to warm deeper tissues
- Massage of muscles
- Heat and cold therapy for muscles
- Braces and orthotics

Preparation of Animal

Little preparation is needed for most of these activities, and most are performed with the animal awake.

Potential Complications

In the hands of a trained rehabilitator, complications are mild and infrequent. Care must be taken when applying heat and cold to avoid burns and frostbite. Passive range-of-motion exercises are not performed in limbs with unstable fractures or joints, or after certain skin-grafting procedures. Therapeutic exercises must be done cautiously in animals with heart or respiratory disease or unstable fractures. Treadmill exercises may be avoided in animals that are fractious or may bite. Aquatic exercises are not performed in the presence of open wounds, casts or splints, or external skeletal fixation devices and are often avoided for animals that fear water.

 Follow-up Care

Follow-up care is directed at the specific disease or condition being treated. Various exercises may be performed at home in conjunction with rehabilitation delivered at the veterinary hospital to obtain further improvement or to maintain the level of function achieved by a rehabilitation program.

SPECIAL INSTRUCTIONS:

Preoperative Evaluation

Rhea V. Morgan, DVM, DACVIM (Small Animal), DACVO

✚ Description

Patients are evaluated prior to general anesthesia to maximize the safety of the procedure and to ensure that anesthesia-related drugs and their dosages are modified based on the animal's needs. Although age (old or young) is no longer a contraindication to anesthesia, it is one factor that affects the protocol chosen. Other factors that may be taken into consideration include breed, reproductive status, body size, presence of concurrent illnesses, and medications being given. Be sure to provide your veterinarian with a detailed medical history on your pet.

Preoperative Testing

A physical examination is performed on the animal, and the body weight and vital signs are recorded. The animal's overall body condition is noted, as well as the presence of any pain or anxiety.

The overall health of the animal and the surgical procedure to be performed will determine whether laboratory or other preanesthetic testing should be considered. Laboratory tests may be recommended to assess the red and white blood cell counts, blood protein levels, kidney function, liver function, blood sugar level, and other parameters. A routine complete blood count, biochemistry profile, and urinalysis are sometimes referred to as the *baseline* or *minimum database*. If surgery is scheduled for a later date, these tests may be run on an outpatient basis prior to surgery. Sometimes laboratory tests are performed on the day of surgery.

Chest radiographs (x-rays) may also be recommended, especially if the animal is older or has a history of lung or heart disease or recent trauma, if cancer is suspected, or if the lung sounds are abnormal when listened to with a stethoscope.

Other tests may be needed to evaluate the status of concurrent illnesses, to assess the effects of recent trauma or prior surgeries, or for the sake of planning the best approach to the present surgery. Such tests may include, but are not confined to, the following:

- Abdominal x-rays or ultrasound examination
- Blood clotting tests or blood gas analysis
- Blood pressure measurement
- Evaluation of the heart by electrocardiography or echocardiography (heart ultrasound)
- X-rays of affected bones, the spine, or the skull

Classification of Anesthetic Risk

Several classification schemes are available to categorize the risk of anesthesia, of which the following is an example:

- Class 1—Animals have minimal risk for anesthesia-associated problems. They have a normal health status, with no underlying diseases. Examples include animals scheduled for routine spay, castration, or declaw surgery and those to be sedated for x-rays or other procedures.
- Class 2—Animals have a mild risk. They may be fragile, have mild health problems or laboratory abnormalities, or have diseases that are under control. Examples include very young and older animals, animals with mild obesity, and those with well-controlled diabetics. The surgery to be performed is often an uncomplicated procedure, such as skin mass removal, cystotomy, or wound repair.
- Class 3—Animals have a moderate risk. They often have active signs of disease or illness or moderate abnormalities on their physical examination and preoperative test results. Examples include animals with anemia, dehydration, fever, mild heart or lung disease, or controlled kidney disease.
- Class 4—Animals have a high risk of anesthesia-related problems. They are often significantly ill, and some have serious compromise of certain organ functions. Examples include animals that are in shock, have kidney failure or moderate heart or lung disease, or have experienced recent serious trauma.
- Class 5—Animals have a grave risk of succumbing while under anesthesia. Examples include animals that are comatose and those that have multiple organ failure, severe anemia, or blood clotting abnormalities.

℞ Treatment Options

Many different drugs are available for use as tranquilizers, preoperative sedatives, induction agents, and anesthetic maintenance agents. Most healthy animals undergoing general anesthesia are given preanesthetic drugs to sedate them; unconsciousness is then induced with an intravenous medication, and they are maintained on gaseous anesthesia during surgery.

Many alternative protocols are available, however, including elimination of preanesthetic drugs, use of only injectable medications throughout surgery, and induction with gas anesthetics through a mask or induction tank.

Your veterinarian will give you instructions on how long to withhold water and food before anesthesia and what modifications should be made in the medications the animal is currently receiving.

Prognosis

Great progress has been made in the development of anesthetic protocols that are safe for use in a wide variety of animals and circumstances.

SPECIAL INSTRUCTIONS:

Rhinoscopy

Ronald M. Bright, DVM, MS, DACVS

 Purpose of Procedure

Rhinoscopy is examination of the nasal cavity with a fiberoptic viewing scope. It is a minimally invasive technique that assists with the diagnosis and treatment of nasal diseases in the dog and cat. Rhinoscopy confirms immediately whether the nasal cavity is the area of concern. It is used to determine the exact location of the disease, the degree of involvement, and the changes present within the nasal cavity. Because many different types of nasal disease have the same signs, rhinoscopy also helps narrow the list of possible causes. Before rhinoscopy became available, the only adequate method to examine the nasal cavity was through invasive surgery.

In addition to visualizing the inside of the nasal cavities, the veterinarian can collect samples of tissue and liquid discharge and submit them for microscopic analysis and culture. Rhinoscopy can sometimes be used to find and potentially remove foreign bodies that are lodged in the nasal cavity. Since an endotracheal tube is in place in the windpipe, the nasal cavity can be flushed to help dislodge debris.

In some instances, rhinoscopy has been used to remove masses associated with fungal disease or to decrease the size of a tumor (debulking). Repeated rhinoscopy can be done to monitor response to therapy.

Description of Technique

Rhinoscopy involves insertion of a rigid or flexible fiberoptic viewing scope through the nostril into the nasal cavity. A flexible scope can also be inserted into the back of the mouth and retroflexed to examine the posterior part of the nasal cavity above the soft palate. The presence of fluid, masses, and any distortion of the tissues lining the nasal cavities are documented. If any abnormality is located, a biopsy of the tissue can be taken with special biopsy forceps.

Most of the nasal cavity in medium to large dogs can be visualized. Some limitations exist in cats and smaller dogs because their nasal cavities are so small. On occasion, the frontal sinuses can be accessed and evaluated; however, this is not routinely possible. Use of a flushing solution to enhance visualization and a rigid endoscope instead of a flexible one may increase the chances of achieving adequate examination of the front part of the nasal cavities, but a flexible scope is better at examining the posterior nasal cavity.

Preparation of Animal

Many patients scheduled for rhinoscopy are geriatric and require careful evaluation of their risk for anesthesia. Routine laboratory tests and chest radiographs (x-rays) may be done before anesthesia. X-rays of the nasal cavity and surrounding tissues (brain, throat) are also taken prior to the procedure, because rhinoscopy can cause some bleeding into the nasal cavity that distorts the findings on the x-rays. Computed tomography (CT scan) and magnetic resonance imaging (MRI) may also be performed prior to rhinoscopy or several days after the procedure.

Because of the sensitivity of the lining of the nose and the presence of a strong sneeze reflex, the patient must be under general anesthesia during the examination. A cuffed tube is placed in the trachea (endotracheal tube) for delivery of gas anesthetics and to prevent aspiration of liquid that may be flushed into the nasal cavity during rhinoscopy.

An intravenous catheter is often inserted prior to anesthesia for administration of intravenous medications and fluids. The animal is usually positioned on its sternum, with the head elevated on a towel or sand-bag.

Potential Complications

Bleeding from the nose (epistaxis) and sneezing are the most common complications following rhinoscopy. Epistaxis is not usually serious but can require hospitalization for rest and observation for a day or two.

Although rhinoscopy alone is helpful when assessing the nasal cavity, it does not always provide a diagnosis. Excessive bleeding during the procedure can obscure abnormalities and make biopsy difficult. Some tumors are difficult to identify because deep biopsy specimens cannot be taken with this technique. However, rhinoscopy is successful in diagnosing nasal conditions in about 90% of cases, without the need for surgery.

 Follow-up Care

It is important to keep the animal quiet after it is discharged, or epistaxis may worsen temporarily. Dogs should be discouraged from pulling hard against their collar and leash; consider using a harness instead. Sporadic sneezing of bloody liquid is to be expected for 1-3 days after rhinoscopy. Notify your veterinarian if bleeding increases, if coughing occurs, or if your pet has any trouble breathing.

SPECIAL INSTRUCTIONS:

Sterilization of Female Cats

Ronald M. Bright, DVM, MS, DACVS

 Purpose of Procedure

Elective sterilization is done primarily to prevent estrus (heat) cycles and unwanted pregnancies and offspring. This goal is accomplished by removing the ovaries, alone or in combination with removal of the uterus.

Ovariohysterectomy is the treatment of choice for uterine diseases, including pyometra (uterine infection), metritis, cystic changes of the uterus, rupture of the uterus, and tumors of the uterus. Vaginal prolapse, uterine prolapse, and some hormonal (endocrine) problems, such as diabetes mellitus, may benefit from a sterilization procedure.

Pregnancy termination is another indication for removal of the ovaries and uterus. Owners of some cats elect to have their queen sterilized at the time of a caesarean section.

 Description of Technique

Ovariectomy (OVE) is removal of the ovaries. Ovariohysterectomy (OVH, OHE) is removal of both the uterus and ovaries and is commonly referred to as a *spay* operation.

An appropriate preoperative evaluation that includes a physical examination and blood tests is usually recommended, even for elective procedures. Comprehensive laboratory tests are advisable in older cats to detect any problems that may present a risk for anesthesia and surgery. Other preoperative testing depends on the presence of underlying diseases.

The conventional manner of performing a sterilization procedure requires an incision into the abdomen that is long enough to allow the reproductive organs to be found. The incision is significantly longer for removal of a diseased or enlarged uterus, compared with a healthy, nonpregnant uterus. Rarely, a veterinarian may recommend making incisions on both flanks (behind the last rib) when performing an OVE.

Preparation of Animal

Your veterinarian will instruct you to withhold food and sometimes water for a certain period of time, depending on the anesthesia to be used for the surgery.

Potential Complications

Most cats do well after surgery, with no or minimal complications.

- Minor complications include licking at the incision, development of inflammation or a small pocket of fluid (seroma) beneath the skin at the incision, and premature loss of external skin sutures.
- Hemorrhage after surgery is more common in larger, obese cats and is more of a concern if it originates from the uterine vessels.
- As is possible with all abdominal incisions, a breakdown of the abdominal wall with herniation of abdominal contents can occur, albeit rarely.
- Delayed complications of removing only the ovaries include a return of heat cycles and infection of the uterus (pyometra), especially if removal of ovarian tissue was incomplete.
- If the ovaries and the uterus were both removed, the small portion of the uterus left behind may become infected at a later date. This complication is referred to as *stump pyometra*, and it is sometimes associated with incomplete removal of ovarian tissue at the time of the original sterilization procedure.

🐾 **Postoperative/Follow-up Care**

In many instances, the sterilization procedure is uncomplicated and the cat may be discharged from the veterinary hospital on the same day, often with appropriate pain management. When an OVH is performed in cats at risk for bleeding or with serious underlying uterine disease, continued hospitalization may be recommended so the animal can be monitored and appropriate therapy delivered.

The cat should be kept quiet for 10-14 days or longer, according to your veterinarian's instructions. Limiting the animal's activity (no running, rough playing, or jumping) helps minimize the chance of breakdown of the abdominal incision. If possible, the cat should be kept inside in a clean, dry environment until the incisions have healed.

No recheck visits may be needed if external sutures were not used. In other cases, recheck visits are scheduled based on the reason for the sterilization procedure. Notify your veterinarian if any bleeding or persistent oozing occurs at the incision, if the cat continues to lick or traumatize the incision, if any swelling develops under the incision, or if the incision starts to open.

SPECIAL INSTRUCTIONS:

Sterilization of Female Dogs

Ronald M. Bright, DVM, MS, DACVS

Purpose of Procedure

Elective sterilization is done primarily to prevent estrus (heat) cycles and unwanted pregnancies and offspring. This goal is accomplished by removing the ovaries, alone or in combination with removal of the uterus.

Sterilization also prevents or dramatically reduces the incidence of mammary (breast) tumors:

- If sterilization is done before 6 months of age, the risk of mammary gland tumors is almost completely eliminated.
- Some decrease in tumor development still occurs if the surgery is done before the fourth estrus or 2½ years of age.
- Sterilization is also done in the intact bitch after mammary tumors are removed, so that it is easier to detect new tumors.

Ovariohysterectomy is the treatment of choice for uterine diseases such as pyometra (uterine infection), metritis, cystic changes, rupture or twisting (torsion) of the uterus, and tumors involving the uterus. Vaginal prolapse, uterine prolapse, and some hormonal (endocrine) problems, such as diabetes mellitus, may benefit from a sterilization procedure. Pregnancy termination is another indication for sterilization. Some bitches are sterilized at the time of a caesarean section.

Description of Technique

Ovariectomy (OVE) is removal of the ovaries. Ovariohysterectomy (OVH, OHE) is removal of both the uterus and ovaries and is commonly referred to as a *spay* operation.

An appropriate preoperative evaluation that includes a physical examination and blood tests is usually recommended, even for elective procedures. Comprehensive laboratory tests are advisable in older dogs to detect any problems that may present a risk for anesthesia and surgery. Other preoperative testing depends on the presence of underlying diseases.

The conventional manner of performing a sterilization procedure requires an incision into the abdomen that is long enough to allow the reproductive organs to be found. The incision is significantly longer for removal of a diseased or enlarged uterus, compared with a healthy, nonpregnant uterus. Rarely, a veterinarian may recommend making incisions on both flanks (behind the last rib) when performing an OVE.

Preparation of Animal

Your veterinarian will instruct you to withhold food and sometimes water for a certain period of time, depending on the anesthesia to be used for the surgery.

Potential Complications

Most dogs do well after surgery, with no or minimal complications.

- Minor complications include licking at the incision, inflammation or formation of a small pocket of fluid (seroma) or blood (hematoma) beneath the skin at the incision, and premature loss of external skin sutures.
- Hemorrhage after surgery is more common in large, obese dogs and in dogs that are in heat. Bleeding is also more likely in older bitches that have underlying blood clotting disorders and in some breeds with a higher incidence of inherited clotting disorders, such as von Willebrand disease in the Doberman pinscher.
- As is possible with all abdominal incisions, a breakdown of the abdominal wall with herniation of abdominal contents can occur, albeit rarely.
- Delayed complications of removing only the ovaries include a return of heat cycles and infection of the uterus, especially if removal of ovarian tissue was incomplete.
- If the ovaries and the uterus were both removed, the small portion of the uterus left behind may become infected at a later date. This complication is referred to as *stump pyometra*, and it is sometimes associated with incomplete removal of ovarian tissue at the time of the original sterilization procedure.

Postoperative/Follow-up Care

In many instances, the sterilization procedure is uncomplicated and the dog may be discharged from the veterinary hospital on the same day, often with appropriate pain management. When an OVH is performed in dogs at risk for bleeding or with serious underlying uterine disease, continued hospitalization may be recommended so the animal can be monitored and appropriate therapy delivered.

The dog should be kept quiet for 10-14 days or longer, according to your veterinarian's instructions. Limiting the animal's activity (no running, stair-climbing, or jumping) helps minimize the chance of breakdown of the abdominal incision. If possible, the dog should be kept inside in a clean, dry environment until the incision has healed.

No recheck visits may be needed if external sutures were not used. In other cases, recheck visits are scheduled based on the reason for the sterilization procedure. Notify your veterinarian if any bleeding or persistent oozing occurs at the incision, if the dog continues to lick or traumatize the incision, if any swelling develops under the incision, or if the incision starts to open.

SPECIAL INSTRUCTIONS:

Subcutaneous Fluid Administration

Cathy E. Langston, DVM, DACVIM (Small Animal)

Purpose of Procedure

The most common reason for subcutaneous (SC, SQ) fluid treatment at home is for treatment of kidney disease. When the kidneys are unable to make concentrated urine, fluid loss from the body is increased. Although some animals drink enough to compensate, other animals do not drink enough and become dehydrated. SQ fluid therapy helps prevent or treat the dehydration and also helps the kidneys flush more waste products from the body. SQ fluids are most often administered on a chronic basis to cats. They can be administered to dogs and other small animals for various other reasons.

✚ Description of Technique

The supplies needed to perform SQ fluid therapy at home include an intravenous (IV) fluid bag, an IV tubing administration set, and needles. The equipment is set up as follows:

- Take out the administration set (tubing). The flow of fluid through the tubing is controlled by a pinch clamp (usually blue or green) and a roller clamp (usually white). The roller clamp is used for adjusting flow rates in incremental steps. Initially, close both clamps.
- Tear off the plastic outer wrap and remove the fluid bag, holding it with the tab or plug up. To attach the tubing to the bag, pull off the tab or plug, remove the cap from the spiked portion of the tubing, and insert the spike all the way into the fluid bag.
- Invert the bag so that the plug is at the bottom. Hold the bag up and squeeze it so that about one quarter of the clear chamber beneath the spike fills with fluid. While holding the bag up, open the clamps to allow the fluid to fill the tubing. Take the cap off the free end of the tubing. When fluid begins to flow out of the tubing, close the clamp. If there are air bubbles in the tubing, let the fluid run out until the bubbles are gone.
- Twist the cap off the needle, and place the needle over the free end of the tubing.

To administer the fluid, do the following:

- Find a quiet spot. Placing your cat or other small animal in a box or carrier with an open top may help keep it still. If you have a squirmy pet, you may need someone to hold your pet while you administer the fluids.
- Grasp the skin on the back of the animal's neck between the shoulders and gently pull it up. Any area where there is loose skin is fine to use; the best area is the front half of the animal.
- Remove the needle cover and insert the needle under the skin. Hold the needle parallel to the ground or at a 45-degree angle. If the needle comes out the other side of the skin, pull back a little. If fluid leaks out as you give it, the needle has gone through to the other side and needs to be repositioned.
- Hang the bag up on a hook or hold it well above the animal. Open the clamp to start the flow. The bag can be squeezed, or the fluid can be allowed to drip by gravity. Continue until the prescribed dose has been given.
- A lump will gradually develop under the animal's skin where the fluid enters; it will slowly disappear over the next few hours. The fluid may settle lower over the shoulders because of gravity.

After giving the fluids, close the clamp, pull the needle out of the skin, and replace the needle cover. If fluid leaks out after you remove the needle, do not be alarmed. Simply pinch the leaking spot briefly.

Use a new needle for each administration. Place used needles in a puncture-proof container, and return them to the veterinary hospital for disposal.

Dosage

The frequency and amount of fluid needed are dependent on a number of factors, such as the size of your pet and the severity of its disease. Fluid bags generally hold 250, 500, or 1000 milliliters (mL). The bags are marked with numbers; when the fluid level drops from one number to the next, 100 mL has been administered. Although the measurements are not precise, they are accurate enough for SQ fluid treatments. Monitoring your pet's condition with blood tests helps to determine the effectiveness of the SQ fluid therapy and provides guidance on the need for changes in the dosage.

SPECIAL INSTRUCTIONS:

Total Hip Arthroplasty

Mark C. Rochat, DVM, MS, DACVS

Purpose of Procedure

The purpose of a total hip arthroplasty (THA) is to replace the natural hip with an artificial hip prosthesis. THA is done only if no other alternatives exist for restoring the function of the natural hip.

Description of Technique

THA is a complex, technically demanding surgical procedure that involves placing an artificial plastic cup in the pelvis and an artificial metal stem and ball in the femur (thigh bone). The cup and stem are held in place in the bone by bone cement or by subsequent growth of bone into the prosthesis. Either approach, in the hands of a capable surgeon, can result in excellent function that lasts for the life of the dog. Although THA is usually done in large- or giant-breed dogs, it can also be performed in small dogs.

Preparation of Animal

It is critical that the dog be thoroughly evaluated prior to THA to identify and resolve other orthopedic and neurologic conditions and any sources of potential contamination, such as urinary tract infection. Obesity is another common problem in dogs examined for THA. Weight reduction may ease hip pain and dysfunction enough that THA is not required. Weight loss also decreases the risk of complications associated with THA, even if lameness persists after weight loss. The evaluation process usually involves complete physical, orthopedic, and neurologic examinations; preoperative laboratory (blood and urine) tests; and radiographs (x-rays) of the hip. Preoperative evaluation and surgery are usually performed by a specialist in veterinary orthopedic surgery.

Potential Complications

Although they are relatively uncommon, early complications of THA include infection, dislocation of the new hip joint, nerve injury, and fracture of the thigh bone. Other complications, such as loosening or breakage of the prosthesis, can occur years after THA.

Postoperative/Follow-up Care

It is critical that the dog be kept confined to a cage and walked on a short leash for 8 weeks after surgery, with a sling placed beneath the back legs for support. Strict restriction of activity is necessary to prevent dislocation of the prosthesis while the soft tissues (muscles, tendons) around the joint are healing. Generally, the sling support is stopped after 4 weeks and other exercise restrictions continue for another month. After the surgical site has fully healed, the dog is allowed unrestricted activity.

SPECIAL INSTRUCTIONS:

Transfusion Therapy in Cats

Kristi S. Lively, DVM, DABVP

Purpose of Procedure

Transfusion therapy replaces components of the blood that are needed to maintain vital functions. It involves the delivery of one or more substances, usually through an intravenous (IV) catheter. These substances may include whole blood (all components of blood), red blood cells only, platelets (involved in clotting), or plasma (the clear, liquid part of blood). The type of transfusion recommended depends on the underlying disease or condition being treated:

- Plasma transfusions may be recommended for protein-losing diseases of the kidneys or intestinal tract, liver disease, clotting factor deficiencies, burns, or inflammatory diseases.
- Adequate numbers of platelets are required for the blood to clot. Although they often are not available, platelet transfusions may be recommended when platelet counts become very low.
- Red blood cells deliver oxygen throughout the body. When a cat is severely anemic (low red blood cell count), oxygen delivery is decreased. Severe anemia may be treated with a transfusion of whole blood or packed (concentrated) red blood cells. In cases of sudden blood loss, such as trauma, a single transfusion may be needed to stabilize the patient while the bleeding is being treated. Chronic conditions, such as infections, cancer, or autoimmune diseases, may require repeated transfusions until the underlying disease can be controlled.

Description of Technique

Transfusions are given only when necessary and under close supervision, because the possibility exists for transfusion reactions. A *cross-match test* is usually performed to make sure the material to be transfused is compatible with the animal's own blood and to minimize reactions. Cats have three blood types: A, B, and AB. Most cats are type A, but blood type varies by breed and country of origin. All type B cats have naturally occurring antibodies to A and AB blood types. Therefore, blood typing and cross-matching is usually performed before a transfusion, if time allows.

In the United States, more than 99% of domestic cats are type A. Certain breeds, such as the Abyssinian, Himalayan, British shorthair, Persian, Scottish fold, Devon Rex, Birman, and Somali, have a higher incidence of type B. These breeds are at greater risk for incompatibility with transfused blood. Transfusion reactions in cats result in rapid destruction of the transfused cells.

Patients receiving transfusions often are already hospitalized because of the severity of their underlying disease, and hospitalization is required for administration of the transfusion and to monitor for signs of a reaction.

Preparation of Animal

An IV catheter is inserted, and the cat may be premedicated with the antihistamine drug, diphenhydramine (*Benadryl*), to help minimize reactions. The volume of material to be transfused is calculated based on the cat's weight and the amount of red blood cells, platelets, protein, or other factors needed. Blood or plasma products may be commercially prepared and stored in a refrigerator or freezer or freshly obtained from a donor.

The transfusion is administered over several hours, with repeated monitoring of vital signs. In kittens with tiny veins, some blood products may be given through a catheter inserted into the bone marrow (center cavity of the bone) of the major bone in the rear leg.

Potential Complications

The most serious risk with transfusions is an acute reaction. For red blood cell transfusions, the recipient may suddenly destroy the donated red cells. This type of reaction can further compromise an already critical patient and often manifests as fever, welts, shock, and vomiting. If these signs occur, the transfusion is discontinued, and the cat is stabilized with other IV fluids and steroid injections. If the cat cannot be transfused because of reactions or if red cells are unavailable, synthetic oxygen-carrying products such as *Oxyglobin* may be an alternative treatment option.

Other rare complications include infection from contaminated blood products and blood circulatory overload from transfusion of an excessive volume of material. Donor cats are usually screened for contagious diseases such as hemobartonellosis, feline leukemia virus, and feline immunodeficiency virus.

Follow-up Care

For blood transfusions, the red blood count is monitored during and after the transfusion to assess whether it is increasing adequately. For chronic conditions, the count may be monitored for weeks to months. Transfused red blood cells have a shorter life span than a patient's own cells. Repeated transfusions may be needed if the red blood cell count falls below acceptable levels. When plasma transfusions are administered, various laboratory tests may be recommended to monitor response to the transfusion and to assess resolution of the underlying disease.

SPECIAL INSTRUCTIONS:

Transfusion Therapy in Dogs

Kristi S. Lively, DVM, DABVP

 Purpose of Procedure

Transfusion therapy is utilized to replace components of the blood that are needed to maintain vital functions. It involves the delivery of one or more substances, usually through an intravenous (IV) catheter. These substances may include whole blood (all components of blood), red blood cells only, platelets (involved in clotting), or plasma (the clear, liquid part of blood). The type of transfusion recommended depends on the underlying disease or condition being treated:

- Plasma transfusions may be recommended for protein-losing diseases of the kidneys or intestinal tract, liver disease, clotting factor deficiencies, burns, or inflammatory diseases.
- Adequate numbers of platelets are required for the blood to clot. Although they often are not available, platelet transfusions may be recommended when platelet counts become very low.
- Red blood cells deliver oxygen throughout the body. When a dog is severely anemic (low red blood cell count), oxygen delivery is decreased. Severe anemia can be life-threatening and may be treated with a transfusion of whole blood or packed (concentrated) red blood cells. In cases of sudden blood loss, such as trauma, a single transfusion may be needed to stabilize the patient while the bleeding is being treated. Chronic conditions, such as infections, cancer, or autoimmune diseases, may require repeated transfusions until the underlying disease can be controlled.

 Description of Technique

Transfusions are given only when necessary and under close supervision, because the possibility exists for transfusion reactions. A *cross-match test* is usually performed to make sure the material to be transfused is compatible with the animal's own blood and to minimize reactions. Dogs have three common blood types, and blood typing tests are sometimes recommended to determine which type your pet has.

Because reactions are very rare the first time a transfusion is done (especially in emergency situations when there is not enough time for cross matching), it is acceptable to immediately start a transfusion in a dog that has not received one before. Patients receiving transfusions often are already hospitalized because of the severity of their underlying disease, and hospitalization is required for administration of the transfusion and to monitor for signs of a reaction.

Preparation of Animal

An IV catheter is inserted, and the dog may be premedicated with the antihistamine diphenhydramine (*Benadryl*) to help minimize reactions. The volume of material to be transfused is calculated based on the dog's weight and the amount of red blood cells, platelets, protein, or other factors needed. Blood or plasma products may be commercially prepared and stored in a refrigerator or freezer or freshly obtained from a donor.

The transfusion is administered over several hours, with intermittent monitoring of the dog's vital signs. In puppies with tiny veins, some blood products may be given through a catheter inserted into the bone marrow (center cavity of the bone) of the major bone in the rear leg.

Potential Complications

The most serious risk with transfusions is an acute reaction. For red blood cell transfusions, this means rapid destruction of the donated red cells by the recipient dog. This type of reaction can further compromise an already critical patient, and it often manifests as fever, welts, shock, and vomiting. If these signs occur, the transfusion is discontinued, and the dog is stabilized with other IV fluids and steroid injections. If the dog cannot be transfused because of reactions or if red cells are unavailable, synthetic oxygen-carrying products such as *Oxyglobin* may be an alternative treatment option.

Other rare complications include infection from contaminated blood products and blood circulatory overload from transfusion of an excessive volume of material. Donor dogs are usually screened for contagious diseases such as heartworm disease, babesiosis, ehrlichiosis, Lyme disease, and Rocky Mountain spotted fever.

 Follow-up Care

For blood transfusions, the red blood count is monitored during and after the transfusion to assess whether it is increasing adequately. For chronic conditions, the count may be monitored for weeks to months. Transfused red blood cells have a shorter life span than a patient's own red cells. Repeated transfusions may be needed if the red blood cell count falls below acceptable levels. When plasma transfusions are administered, various laboratory tests may be recommended to monitor response to the transfusion and to assess resolution of the underlying disease.

SPECIAL INSTRUCTIONS:

Triple Pelvic Osteotomy for Hip Dysplasia

Mark C. Rochat, DVM, MS, DACVS

 Purpose of Procedure

The purpose of a triple pelvic osteotomy (TPO) is to reorient the acetabulum (socket part of the hip joint) so that the femoral head (ball part of the hip joint) sits more firmly in the joint and is less likely to subluxate (slide in and out) with normal activity. This procedure is best used for treating hip dysplasia in dogs that are still actively growing, have normal bone structure within the hip, have no osteoarthritis in the hip, and are lame from the hip dysplasia. Performing a TPO in a dog that does not meet these strict criteria is a judgment call that is best made by the veterinary surgeon performing the TPO.

✚ **Description of Technique**

A TPO involves making three cuts (osteotomies) in the pelvis—one in the pubis (floor of the pelvis), one behind the hip joint through the side of the pelvis (ischiatic table), and one in front of the hip joint through the front part of the pelvis (ilium). After all three osteotomies have been made, the hip joint and surrounding bone are rotated downward, and the osteotomy in the ilium is secured with a special bone plate and screws.

Preparation of Animal

An orthopedic examination and radiographs (x-rays) are performed to evaluate the dog's hips and determine whether the dog is a good candidate for the procedure. The initial orthopedic examination is done while the dog is awake; it is then repeated and x-rays are taken while the dog is anesthetized. Preoperative laboratory tests are commonly recommended to identify anesthetic risks. Your dog may be referred to a veterinary surgery specialist for evaluation of the hip and performance of the surgery.

Potential Complications

TPO is a technically demanding procedure. Numerous complications can occur but are rare in the hands of a properly trained surgeon. Complications include infection, nerve damage, severe bleeding, and failure of the bone plate and screws to maintain the acetabulum in its newly rotated position. Failure to properly confine the dog after surgery until the osteotomies have healed can also result in failure of the procedure.

 Postoperative/Follow-up Care

The dog is usually confined to a crate until the osteotomies have healed, generally about 6-9 weeks. X-rays are taken every 4-6 weeks to evaluate the progress of healing. Rehabilitation exercises and physical therapy can speed the recovery process and the extent to which the dog improves.

SPECIAL INSTRUCTIONS:

Urine Protein Assays in Dogs

Cathy E. Langston, DVM, DACVIM (Small Animal)

Purpose of Procedure

Normally there is very little protein in the urine, but certain conditions can cause abnormally high amounts (*proteinuria*). When a certain part of the kidney (the glomerulus) is damaged, large amounts of protein can leak into the urine, a condition called *glomerulonephritis* or *protein-losing nephropathy*. Many other conditions and diseases in the body, including bladder infections, can also cause proteinuria. When protein is detected in the urine, it is important to determine whether it is from glomerular damage or from one of these other causes.

Description of Test

Several assays are available to test for protein in the urine, including urinalysis, urine protein/creatinine ratio, and detection of microalbuminuria.

Urinalysis is a standard part of patient assessment in many situations, including preanesthetic screening and screening of geriatric animals. Urinalysis includes determination of urine specific gravity (a measure of urine concentration), use of a urine dipstick that evaluates several substances, and microscopic examination of urine sediment to look for crystals, blood cells, and bacteria.

One of the components of the dipstick test is a rough assessment of protein. The dipstick may indicate a negative, trace, 1+, 2+, or 3+ protein level present in the urine. Because these values are only approximate, a more specific measurement of protein in the urine, such as a urine protein/creatinine ratio, is usually recommended if the dipstick level is 1+ or higher. A number of factors can cause the dipstick to be positive when protein is not actually present.

The *urine protein/creatinine ratio* actually measures the amount of protein in the urine instead of providing an estimate. Because more protein is acceptable in more concentrated urine, the test also measures the amount of creatinine in the urine. If the protein/creatinine ratio is abnormally high, investigation for the underlying cause is recommended.

The *microalbuminuria* test is a relatively new test that detects very small quantities of albumin protein in the urine. This test is more sensitive than the standard urinalysis and is not always accurate in cats. If the test shows a low positive value, a recheck is usually recommended in 1-2 months to determine whether the amount of protein is increasing. If the test result is medium to highly positive, investigation for the underlying cause is recommended.

Preparation of Animal

Urine samples can be collected by several methods. Sometimes the owner is asked to bring in a urine sample from home. The best method for collecting urine from a male dog is to collect it in a clean container as the dog is urinating. Allow the dog to start urinating first, before collecting the urine sample, and make sure that hair is not in the way of the urine stream. This method can also be used for some female dogs, although it may be easier to use a flat container (such as a pie plate). For dogs that are paper trained, the "wee-wee pad" can be turned upside down so that the plastic side is up, and the urine can be collected from the plastic surface. Refrigerate the urine sample until it can be transported to your veterinarian.

Urine may also be obtained by your veterinarian directly from the dog's bladder using a needle (cystocentesis). This procedure is no more invasive than drawing a blood sample, but it does require the patient to lie on its back or side very briefly.

Alternatively, a urinary catheter can be passed into the bladder to obtain a urine sample. Catheterization is usually a simple procedure in male dogs. Catheterization is more difficult in female dogs, often requires sedation or anesthesia, and is not commonly used for simple urine collection.

Potential Complications

Occasionally a little blood may be detected in the urine (microscopically) after collection of a urine sample by cystocentesis. A small risk of a bladder infection is associated with passage of a urinary catheter.

SPECIAL INSTRUCTIONS:

SECTION 2

Cardiovascular System

Section Editor: Rebecca E. Gompf, DVM, MS, DACVIM (Cardiology)

Arrhythmogenic Right Ventricular/Cardiomyopathy
  in Boxers
Arterial Thromboembolism, Peripheral
Atrial Fibrillation
Atrial Premature Contractions and Tachycardia
Atrioventricular Valve Degeneration in Dogs
Cardiac Tumors
Cardiopulmonary Resuscitation
Congestive Heart Failure in Dogs, Left-Sided
Congestive Heart Failure in Dogs, Right-Sided
Dilated Cardiomyopathy in Cats
Dilated Cardiomyopathy in Dogs
Endocarditis
Heartworm Disease in Cats
Heartworm Disease in Dogs
Hypertrophic Cardiomyopathy in Cats
Occult Cardiomyopathy in Doberman Pinschers

Patent Ductus Arteriosus
Pericardial Effusion
Peritoneopericardial Diaphragmatic Hernia
Persistent Right Aortic Arch
Pulmonary Hypertension
Pulmonic Stenosis
Second- and Third-Degree Heart Block
Sick Sinus Syndrome and Atrial Standstill
Sinus Arrhythmia
Sinus Bradycardia
Subaortic Stenosis
Systemic Hypertension
Tetralogy of Fallot
Tricuspid and Mitral Valve Dysplasia
Ventricular and Atrial Septal Defects
Ventricular Fibrillation and Cardiac Arrest
Ventricular Premature Contractions and Tachycardia

Arrhythmogenic Right Ventricular/ Cardiomyopathy in Boxers

Rebecca E. Gompf, DVM, MS, DACVIM (Cardiology)

BASIC INFORMATION

Description

Boxer cardiomyopathy is a disease of the heart muscle of boxers. The condition causes abnormal heart rhythms (arrhythmias) that arise in the right ventricle, the large chamber on the right side of the heart. Because many people confuse this problem with dilated cardiomyopathy, the disease has been given a new name, *arrhythmogenic right ventricular cardiomyopathy* (ARVC).

Causes

The heart muscle cells of affected boxers, mainly in the right ventricle, are replaced by fatty or fibrofatty scar tissue. Sometimes these abnormal changes occur in the left ventricle also. These changes cause arrhythmias, such as ventricular premature contractions (VPCs) and ventricular tachycardia (VT). (See the handout on **Ventricular Premature Contractions and Tachycardia**.) The overall heart size and function are normal in these dogs. Later in the disease, however, some dogs develop dilated cardiomyopathy. (See also the handout on **Dilated Cardiomyopathy in Dogs**.)

ARVC runs in families of boxers, and a genetic basis for the heart changes is proposed, although the exact genes that cause this defect have not yet been identified.

Clinical Signs

Most boxers with ARVC are clinically normal and show signs only when the arrhythmias are severe. Sometimes arrhythmias are found on routine physical examination or when an electrocardiogram (ECG) is run as a screening test. Some dogs have fainting episodes or die suddenly from severe ventricular arrhythmias. Arrhythmias can develop at any age in these dogs.

Diagnostic Tests

In boxers with a family history of sudden death or ARVC, an ECG or Holter monitoring is often done yearly. (See handout on **Electrocardiography**.) The exact age at which screening ECGs and Holter monitoring should be done is often based on the dog's family history.

If VPCs are detected and confirmed by ECG, the diagnosis of ARVC is made by eliminating all other causes of these arrhythmias. Since many problems can cause VPCs, extensive testing must be done to rule out other diseases. Chest and abdominal x-rays and laboratory tests (including thyroid tests and possibly titers for tick-borne diseases and others) are often recommended. An echocardiogram (heart ultrasound) is done to rule out other heart diseases.

TREATMENT AND FOLLOW-UP

Treatment Options

If fainting episodes, VT, or severe VPCs are present, hospitalization is often needed to treat the arrhythmias with injectable medications. The more severe the arrhythmia, the higher the possibility of sudden death.

Once the heart rhythm is stabilized, several different drugs or drug combinations can be used orally. Not every drug works in every dog, so changes may be needed in therapy to control the ventricular arrhythmia.

- Oral drugs that may be used for the arrhythmias caused by ARVC include sotalol, mexiletine, and a combination of mexiletine and atenolol.
- If these medications do not control the arrhythmia, then a combination of mexiletine and sotalol may be tried.
- Amiodarone may be used as a last resort and often requires referral to a veterinary specialist for its administration.

Side effects of antiarrhythmic drugs include lethargy, anorexia, vomiting, and diarrhea. The last three effects are more common with mexiletine. Occasionally these drugs can make the arrhythmia worse, so that the dog must be switched to another medication. Amiodarone has multiple side effects, including liver damage with elevated liver tests, decreased white blood cell counts, and damage to the thyroid gland.

Follow-up Care

Affected boxers require frequent ECGs until their VT or VPCs are controlled. Ideally, a Holter monitor is applied to dogs with non–life-threatening arrhythmias to document the frequency of the arrhythmias prior to treatment. Then another Holter recording is done after the drug has reached adequate blood levels to judge how effective it is in controlling the abnormal beats. Affected dogs require antiarrhythmic therapy for the rest of their lives.

Prognosis

Boxers whose arrhythmias are well controlled with medications can live a long time. No drug is 100% effective in preventing sudden death, however. Animals on medication can still die suddenly. The better the arrhythmia is controlled, the less likely it is for sudden death to occur. Holter monitors provide the best way to evaluate how well the medication is controlling the arrhythmias.

Because this problem has a genetic basis and runs in families, it is wise not to breed dogs that have ARVC.

SPECIAL INSTRUCTIONS:

Arterial Thromboembolism, Peripheral

Rebecca E. Gompf, DVM, MS, DACVIM (Cardiology)

BASIC INFORMATION

Description

Arterial thromboembolism occurs when a blood clot lodges in an artery. The place where the blood clot comes to rest depends on the size of the clot and the size of the artery. Most blood clots are small and lodge in smaller arteries. The clots can cause strokes if they cut off blood to certain areas of the brain. Clots can cause damage and eventual failure of any organ in the body. In cats, the clots usually lodge in a front leg or at the termination of the aorta where it divides into arteries that supply the rear legs. This disease occurs most often in cats; it is uncommon in dogs.

Causes

Dogs can develop clots secondary to kidney diseases, Cushing's disease (excessive levels of circulating steroid hormones), infections of the left heart valves (bacterial endocarditis), and other conditions that affect clotting. Cats usually develop clots in the left atrium, the small chamber on the left side of the heart, when it becomes dilated from hypertrophic (HCM) or dilated (DCM) cardiomyopathy or other diseases of the heart muscle. Cats have sticky platelets, and clots may form if there is decreased blood flow in the big left atrium. Pieces of the clot can break off and travel in the bloodstream to other areas, especially to the end of the aorta.

Clinical Signs

Signs of the underlying diseases are usually present but can be subtle in cats. The first sign of a problem may be sudden paralysis of a front leg or both rear legs. If the incident is recent, the animal may be crying in pain. The affected limbs are cold and limp, with blue nail beds. Muscles in the affected legs may feel hard.

Diagnostic Tests

Numerous tests are required to find the underlying cause of the problem and to assess the extent of damage from the clot. Laboratory tests, chest x-rays, and an echocardiogram (heart ultrasound) are commonly performed. Abdominal x-rays and a Doppler ultrasound study of the aorta may also be recommended to assess other organs and the extent of the clot. Additional tests may be needed based on the results of initial procedures.

TREATMENT AND FOLLOW-UP

Treatment Options

Hospitalization is usually required for initial testing and therapy. Supportive care is started, with pain medications, sedatives, and intravenous (IV) fluids. Manual expression of the bladder and physical therapy for paralyzed legs are often needed. Specific treatments are given for the underlying disease.

Medications to break down the clot are rarely used in dogs and cats; they are often ineffective, perhaps because they must be given within a few hours of the arterial obstruction, and the event is not often witnessed in animals. Streptokinase and tissue plasminogen activator (TPA) are used in people, and both drugs have been used in cats, but with varying impact on survival. They have been used only infrequently in dogs, and there is little information about their effects.

Medications are started to prevent the clot from getting bigger and to try to prevent future clots. Injectable heparin is commonly used during hospitalization. Clopidogrel (*Plavix*) may be given orally in cats.

After discharge from the hospital, home care may involve the following:

- Medications for the underlying problem that caused the initial clot
- Supportive care, including physical therapy and possible bladder expression
- Medications to prevent additional clot formation, such as warfarin and aspirin in cats and dogs, and clopidogrel in cats

Follow-up Care

Frequent, often weekly, monitoring of the underlying problem and effects of the clots (such as kidney dysfunction) are usually needed. Repeated blood clotting tests are needed if warfarin is used. After a few weeks, the frequency of rechecks may be modified, depending on the response to treatment.

Prognosis

Animals with blood clots in the legs have a guarded prognosis. If there is no return of blood flow to the rear legs within a couple of days, prognosis is very poor, and it is unlikely the animal will recover function of the legs. Future clots are likely to develop if the underlying problem cannot be controlled or the preventive medications do not work.

Overall prognosis also depends on the underlying heart disease. In cats, each form of cardiomyopathy has a different prognosis; however, the formation of clots always makes the prognosis much worse. In dogs, some underlying diseases are easier to treat than others, so prognosis depends on the disease that is causing the clots.

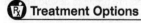
SPECIAL INSTRUCTIONS:

Atrial Fibrillation

Rebecca E. Gompf, DVM, MS, DACVIM (Cardiology)

BASIC INFORMATION

Description

Atrial fibrillation (AF) is an abnormal heart rhythm caused by rapid, irregular contractions of the upper chambers (atria) of the heart. Because the heart is beating faster and more irregularly than normal, it does not fill or pump blood properly. Failure to pump blood normally can result in fluid accumulation in the lungs, chest, or abdomen and can lead to weakness and heart failure.

Causes

The most common cause of AF is advanced heart disease, with enlargement of one or both atria. Advanced heart diseases in dogs may include degeneration and leakage of heart valves, diseases of heart muscle (cardiomyopathy), and certain congenital heart deformities.

AF can occur spontaneously for unknown reasons (idiopathic) in giant-breed dogs such as the Great Dane and Irish wolfhound. Occasionally the administration of narcotics has caused AF in large dogs.

Clinical Signs

Clinical signs of both heart disease and AF are usually present. Weakness and inability to exercise are common. Fainting episodes may occur, especially with exertion. Cats are often less active than usual. Breathing may be faster and labored, and coughing may be noted.

Giant-breed dogs usually have no symptoms at first, and the AF may be detected only when an irregular rhythm is heard with a stethoscope and an electrocardiogram (ECG) is performed. Some of these dogs eventually develop signs of heart disease.

Diagnostic Tests

An ECG is needed to confirm the presence of AF. Additional tests, such as chest x-rays and an echocardiogram (heart ultrasound), are then done to search for the underlying cause. Any fluid removed from the chest or abdomen may be sent for analysis. Laboratory tests are usually recommended to rule out other diseases that cause similar signs.

TREATMENT AND FOLLOW-UP

Treatment Options

Treatment is initially directed at any underlying heart disease or heart failure and may include drugs to increase contractility (such as pimobendan) or decrease fluid retention (diuretics).

Then medications such as the following are started to bring the heart rate down to a more normal range.

- Digoxin (a form of digitalis) increases the heart's ability to contract and helps to slow the heart rate. It may be used in combination with other drugs (diltiazem, beta-blockers) to achieve the best control of heart rate. Side effects such as decreased appetite, vomiting, diarrhea, and other arrhythmias often limit it use. Cats do not tolerate digoxin well.
- Diltiazem is a calcium channel blocker commonly used to decrease heart rate in animals with AF. It also decreases the heart's ability to contract, so it is not started until heart failure is controlled in dogs. In cats it may be used right away, because their underlying heart disease usually does not affect contraction. Side effects include depression, decreased appetite, worsening of heart failure, constipation (cats), and very slow heart rates.
- Multiple beta-blockers (atenolol, metoprolol, propranolol, carvedilol) are used in dogs, but in cats atenolol is used most commonly. These drugs slow the heart rate and also decrease contractions. Side effects include very slow heart rates, weakness, depression, low blood pressure, and worsening of heart failure.
- Giant breeds of dogs with spontaneous AF are usually started on a beta-blocker to control their heart rate. In some cases, a procedure called *electrical cardioversion* may be performed with the animal under anesthesia to try and convert the AF back to a normal sinus rhythm. Although the rate of conversion is good, recurrences are common.

Follow-up Care

Once medications are started, ECGs are periodically repeated to monitor heart rate and make adjustments in medications. A Holter monitor, which is a 24-hour continuous monitor, may be recommended to ensure that the heart rate stays within an acceptable range during normal activities. Chest x-rays, echocardiograms, abdominal x-rays, and laboratory tests may be repeated until the animal is stable and then periodically, especially in giant-breed dogs, to monitor for any signs of significant heart disease or in any animal if signs of heart failure develop.

Prognosis

Dogs with advanced heart disease and AF may live 3-12 months, depending on the type and severity of their heart disease. Cats live an average of 3-6 months. Affected cats are prone to develop blood clots in their left atrium, so they are usually placed on blood thinners such as aspirin or clopidogrel (anticoagulation therapy). Giant-breed dogs with idiopathic AF can live for years; however, their AF can progress to serious heart disease (dilated cardiomyopathy).

SPECIAL INSTRUCTIONS:

Atrial Premature Contractions and Tachycardia

Rebecca E. Gompf, DVM, MS, DACVIM (Cardiology)

BASIC INFORMATION

Description

The normal heartbeat originates in the small upper chambers of the heart, the atria. When the atria become irritated, irregular, premature beats called *atrial premature contractions* (APCs) may be generated, and the heart may beat faster than usual (tachycardia). Atrial tachycardia (AT) is a sequence of four or more APCs, usually occurring at a fast rate. As the number of abnormal beats increases and the heart rate becomes higher, the heart may not fill and pump blood properly.

Causes

The most common cause is heart disease that results in enlargement of one or both atria. The stretching of the atria causes abnormal beats to occur. These arrhythmias can also arise with other problems in the body, such as bruising of heart muscle after blunt trauma (such as being hit by a car), or liver or kidney failure.

Clinical Signs

No clinical signs occur if only sporadic, infrequent APCs are present. Frequent APCs may lead to an inability to exercise, increased rate and effort of breathing, and coughing. AT can cause weakness and possibly fainting. Fainting due to AT can be hard to tell from seizures.

Diagnostic Tests

An electrocardiogram (ECG) is needed to confirm the presence of APCs or AT. If these abnormal rhythms are not present all the time, continuous ECG monitoring may be recommended. Such monitoring can be done in the hospital or with a 24-hour, continuous Holter monitor or an event monitor that the animal wears at home.

Because APCs and AT are usually associated with heart disease and other systemic problems, additional tests are often recommended. Such tests may include laboratory tests, chest x-rays, an echocardiogram (heart ultrasound), an abdominal ultrasound study, and other tests. Any fluid in the chest or abdomen may be removed and sent for analysis.

TREATMENT AND FOLLOW-UP

Treatment Options

Treatment is initially directed at any heart disease present. If the overall heart rate is close to normal and no signs are present, then the APCs or AT may not be treated. If the heart rate is too fast, medications (alone or in combinations) are used to slow it down and may include the following:

- Digoxin (a form of digitalis) increases the heart's ability to contract and helps to slow the heart rate. It may be used in combination with other drugs (diltiazem, beta-blockers) to achieve the best control of heart rate. Side effects such as decreased appetite, vomiting, diarrhea, and other arrhythmias often limit it use. Cats do not tolerate digoxin well.
- Diltiazem is a calcium channel blocker commonly used to decrease heart rate in affected animals. It also decreases the heart's ability to contract, so it is not started until heart failure is controlled in dogs. In cats it may be used right away, because their underlying heart disease usually does not affect contraction. Side effects include depression, decreased appetite, worsening of heart failure, constipation (cats), and very slow heart rates.
- Multiple beta-blockers (atenolol, metoprolol, propranolol, carvedilol) are used in dogs, but in cats atenolol is used most commonly. These drugs slow the heart rate and also decrease contractions. Side effects include very slow heart rates, weakness, depression, low blood pressure, and worsening of heart failure.

If other diseases are causing the APCs, then those diseases are usually treated first, and the arrhythmia is monitored with ECGs. If the APCs do not resolve and AT occurs, they are treated as outlined earlier.

Follow-up Care

Once medications are started, ECGs are periodically repeated to monitor heart rate and make adjustments in medications. A Holter monitor may be used to make sure the heart rate stays within an acceptable range during normal activity. If the patient is started on medications, periodic laboratory tests may be recommended to check kidney function and monitor resolution of other diseases. Chest x-rays and echocardiograms may be repeated if heart disease is present.

Prognosis

Prognosis depends on the underlying disease that is causing the APCs or AT. Each disease has its own prognosis, and some are better than others. The more severe atrial arrhythmias are usually indicators of advanced heart disease.

SPECIAL INSTRUCTIONS:

Atrioventricular Valve Degeneration in Dogs

Rebecca E. Gompf, DVM, MS, DACVIM (Cardiology)

BASIC INFORMATION

Description

The left atrioventricular (AV) or mitral valve lies between the left atrium and the left ventricle. The right AV or tricuspid valve lies between the right atrium and ventricle. These valves keep blood from flowing backward into the atria when the heart contracts.

As these valves age, deposits occur and they become scarred (myxomatous degeneration), which causes them to leak when the heart pumps. As a result, the heart is less efficient in pumping blood and slowly enlarges. If the leakage is minor, the heart usually compensates, but as the leakage worsens, heart failure can develop. The mitral valve is most commonly affected and mitral degeneration may eventually lead to left-sided heart failure.

Causes

The cause of the myxomatous degeneration is unknown. AV valvular disease is the most common heart disease in dogs. It most commonly affects small to medium-sized breeds, especially the papillon, poodle, Chihuahua, dachshund, and Cavalier King Charles spaniel.

AV valvular disease is common in older dogs. The disease tends to develop at a younger age and progresses more rapidly in male dogs than in females. Genetic factors play a role in this disease, but other conditions (level of exercise, obesity, diet) may influence the severity of the problem.

Clinical Signs

The leaking valve often causes a heart murmur that can be detected on a routine physical examination before signs occur. The first clinical sign is usually coughing that is triggered by excitement or exercise. As the left heart enlarges, signs of heart failure may develop, such as more severe coughing, restlessness and pacing at night, inability to exercise normally, and rapid, labored breathing.

Dogs that go into right heart failure may also cough, but more often they tire while exercising, lose weight and muscle mass, and develop fluid in their abdomen. Eventually fluid also builds up in the chest, and they have trouble breathing.

Diagnostic Tests

Heart murmurs are often graded in severity based on how loud they are. Low-grade murmurs require monitoring over the course of the dog's life. If the murmur changes rapidly or reach a more severe grade, if the dog develops clinical signs, or if irregular heart rhythms are detected, then tests may be done to evaluate the heart and other organs, such as:

- Chest and possibly abdominal x-rays
- Echocardiogram (heart ultrasound)
- Electrocardiogram (ECG), especially if an irregular rhythm is detected
- Laboratory tests

Some dogs that are in severe distress from left heart failure require stabilization before testing is done.

TREATMENT AND FOLLOW-UP

Treatment Options

Treatment is usually started after clinical signs develop, because no drugs have yet been found that stop progression of this disease. Dogs with mild signs may be treated on an outpatient basis, but more severely ill dogs require hospitalization. A number of drugs are available for stabilizing heart failure, including injectable diuretics (such as furosemide) to decrease fluid in the lungs, vasodilators (such as nitroglycerine ointment, nitroprusside, or hydralazine) that decrease the heart's workload, and oxygen therapy. Some fluid may be drained from the chest cavity or abdomen.

After heart failure is stabilized, long-term oral medications are started. Some of these drugs may also be used in dogs with mild clinical signs.

- Furosemide may be continued indefinitely and may be combined with other diuretics, such as spironolactone.
- Angiotensin-converting enzyme (ACE) inhibitors, such as enalapril, benazepril, or ramipril, may be used to improve the quality of the dog's life and help reduce fluid retention.
- Pimobendan is a newer drug that helps relieve the workload of the heart and improves the heart's contractions. It is reserved for dogs in heart failure.
- Other drugs (digoxin, beta-blockers, calcium channel blockers) may be started for high heart rates associated with abnormal rhythms such as atrial fibrillation.

In addition to drug therapy, dogs with heart failure should not be fed salty foods, and low-salt diets may be used to limit salt intake. Although strenuous exercise is avoided, mild to moderate exercise may be done based on guidelines from your veterinarian.

Follow-up Care

Dogs with no clinical signs are commonly monitored with physical examinations every 6-12 months and yearly chest x-rays. If your dog develops problems breathing, notify your veterinarian immediately. Intensive monitoring is needed during hospitalization for heart failure. Following discharge, periodic recheck visits and testing are needed for the rest of the dog's life.

Prognosis

Dogs with asymptomatic disease may live for years without developing clinical problems. The more severe the leak in the valve and the bigger the left atrium, the more likely it is that the dog will develop heart failure. The average survival time for dogs with heart failure is 8-10 months, but every dog varies in how it responds to treatment. Dogs with other diseases, such as kidney failure, tend to do poorly.

Cavalier King Charles spaniels and other small dogs that develop AV valve degeneration before 5 years of age should not be used for breeding.

SPECIAL INSTRUCTIONS:

Cardiac Tumors

Rebecca E. Gompf, DVM, MS, DACVIM (Cardiology)

BASIC INFORMATION
Description
Cardiac tumors arise from heart tissues (primary tumors) or metastasize to the heart from another location (secondary tumors). These tumors can interfere with normal heart function or cause bleeding into the pericardial sac (the sac around the heart). Decreased heart function may result in poor circulation and heart failure.

Causes
Primary tumors of the heart include hemangiosarcoma, heart base tumors, mesothelioma, rhabdomyosarcoma, fibrosarcoma, and lymphosarcoma. These tumors can also originate from other areas and metastasize to the heart. The cause of these tumors is unknown.

Hemangiosarcomas are highly malignant tumors of blood vessels. They often invade the wall of the right atrium—the small, upper chamber of the right heart. The tumor destroys the wall of the atrium and may bleed into the pericardial sac, causing pericardial effusion. (See also the handout on **Pericardial Effusion**.) Golden retrievers and German shepherd dogs are prone to develop hemangiosarcoma. Primary cardiac hemangiosarcoma has been reported in only one cat.

Heart base tumors form from structures close to the heart. They are slow growing and may cause no problems until they interfere with the blood supply to the pericardial sac. Although they are the second most common cardiac tumor in dogs, they are 10 times less common than hemangiosarcomas. The English bulldog, boxer, and Boston terrier breeds develop these tumors most frequently, usually between 6 and 15 years of age. These tumors are occasionally found in cats.

Mesotheliomas are small tumors that spread over the pericardial sac and chest wall. They can cause pericardial effusion that is lethal to dogs, but they are rare in cats. Lymphosarcomas, rhabdomyosarcomas, and fibrosarcomas occur in both dogs and cats. They often invade the wall of the heart, which decreases its ability to contract. They can also cause the heart valves to leak, in which the end result is heart failure.

Clinical Signs
Most animals with significant effusion have a sudden onset of lethargy, weakness, and collapse. Trouble breathing occurs in about half of affected dogs, and 23% have abdominal swelling. Loss of appetite, vomiting, or coughing may be noted. Signs associated with cancer in other organs may be present.

Diagnostic Tests
X-rays of the chest and abdomen are usually recommended. If an enlarged heart is seen on the x-rays, an echocardiogram (heart ultrasound) and an electrocardiogram (ECG) are done to differentiate pericardial effusion from other cardiac diseases. The echocardiogram also helps identify the presence of a tumor and its effects on the heart.

Laboratory tests and an abdominal ultrasound are often done to look for tumors in other organs and to evaluate their systemic effects. Some of these tests may be delayed until fluid has been removed from the pericardial sac and the animal is stable. Fluid may be submitted for analysis. Additional tests may also be indicated.

TREATMENT AND FOLLOW-UP

Treatment Options
If pericardial effusion is causing symptoms, it is removed by pericardiocentesis, which involves insertion of a catheter into the pericardial sac to drain the fluid. Removal of fluid helps prevent sudden death from cardiac tamponade, which is caused by poor filling of the heart due to severe fluid pressure.

Dogs with right atrial hemangiosarcoma are difficult to treat. Pericardiocentesis provides temporary relief, but the effusion returns in a short time. Surgical removal of the tumor and chemotherapy may be attempted in some cases. Dogs with heart base tumors benefit from removal of the pericardial sac, because these tumors grow very slowly. Treatment of other tumors depends on the tumor type and may involve removal of the pericardial sac and chemotherapy.

Follow-up Care
The frequency of recheck visits and repeated testing is determined by the treatment protocols chosen. Dogs with heart base tumors whose pericardial sacs are removed may only need to be rechecked every 3-6 months.

Prognosis
Dogs with right atrial hemangiosarcoma have a median survival time of 56 days (range, 0-229 days). Pericardial mesothelioma also carries a grave prognosis. Prognosis is better for heart base tumors; average survival time is 730 days after removal of the pericardial sac or 42 days if no surgery is performed.

Dogs with cardiac lymphosarcoma that is stage III or higher have a poor prognosis for remission and survival. In a study of 12 dogs treated with removal of the pericardial sac and chemotherapy, the median survival time was 41 days. Three dogs did live 328 days or longer, so not all of them did poorly.

SPECIAL INSTRUCTIONS:

Cardiopulmonary Resuscitation

Rebecca E. Gompf, DVM, MS, DACVIM (Cardiology)

BASIC INFORMATION

Description

Cardiopulmonary resuscitation (CPR) is a group of procedures that are done to try to revive an animal whose heart has gone into ventricular fibrillation (heart is just vibrating, not beating) or has totally stopped (cardiac arrest). Once the heart stops beating normally, the animal also stops breathing (respiratory arrest); sometimes breathing stops first.

The first step in CPR is placement of a tube into the animal's throat, so that artificial respiration (assisted breathing) can be done. At the same time, chest compressions are started in an attempt to circulate blood throughout the body, and an intravenous catheter is inserted so that drugs can be given to help stimulate the heart. An electrical shock (defibrillation) may be applied to stop the fibrillation and stimulate the heart to beat normally. In extreme cases, your veterinarian may decide to open the animal's chest and squeeze the heart by hand so that blood begins to circulate. When the chest is open, drugs can be administered directly into the heart.

Causes

Many factors can cause the heart to stop or go into ventricular fibrillation, including serious diseases, certain drugs, drowning, electrocution, being struck by a car, certain toxins, and general anesthesia, among others.

Clinical Signs

An animal that has gone into cardiac arrest will suddenly collapse and stop breathing. The animal may also become rigid or have muscle twitching. A few gasps of breath may be seen, but there is no continuous breathing.

Diagnostic Tests

Listening to your animal's heart with a stethoscope will identify that the heart is not beating. A lack of breathing may also be noted. CPR is started immediately, and an electrocardiogram (ECG) is performed to determine what heart rhythm is present.

Laboratory tests may be run throughout CPR to monitor the response to the procedures. If your animal is successfully resuscitated, then numerous laboratory tests, chest and abdominal x-rays, and other tests may be recommended to determine why your animal went into cardiac arrest and its effects on other organs.

TREATMENT AND FOLLOW-UP

Treatment Options

If CPR is successful, additional therapy is usually needed for the underlying cause of the arrest and is based on results of additional tests. Hospitalization is often required for several days following CPR so that the animal can be stabilized and treated.

Successful CPR is difficult to perform on animals that are not hospitalized. Some owners have been able to revive their animals by breathing for them when the animal has suffered only respiratory arrest. If the heart stops, then multiple individuals are needed, working as a team, to perform CPR successfully.

Follow-up Care

Follow-up visits and monitoring are based on the underlying problem and how much damage was done to other organs before effective heartbeats were re-established.

Prognosis

Animals that experience only respiratory arrest have a better chance of being successfully resuscitated than if their heart also stops. Following cardiac arrest, the survival rate for dogs is only 4%, and for cats it is only 2%. These rates are low because most affected animals have serious underlying medical problems that cannot be easily corrected. In addition, most animals that have arrested once will have another cardiac arrest within a short time.

People who experience a cardiac arrest have about a 30% chance of being resuscitated successfully, but fewer than 20% of those individuals ever leave the hospital, because they also have serious underlying medical problems. The most successful CPR outcomes occur in people who have suffered drug overdoses, electrocution, or drowning.

Fictional television programs have given people the wrong expectations with respect to successful CPR. In most television shows, the person who has arrested is saved and leaves the hospital at the end of the show healthy and happy. This is not a realistic depiction of CPR in animals, because most do not survive a cardiac arrest.

Because the success rate of CPR is low in seriously ill animals, consider discussing with your veterinarian what you would like to have done if your animal arrests. You may elect not to have CPR performed on your animal if the underlying disease is extremely serious. This is always a difficult decision to make and a very personal one. Your veterinarian can give you the information that you need to make a wise, informed decision on whether you want CPR performed if your animal goes into cardiac arrest while hospitalized.

SPECIAL INSTRUCTIONS:

Congestive Heart Failure in Dogs, Left-Sided

Rebecca E. Gompf, DVM, MS, DACVIM (Cardiology)

BASIC INFORMATION

Description

Left heart failure occurs when the left side of the heart is no longer working properly and cannot pump blood effectively to the body. Blood accumulates in the lungs and interferes with the ability of oxygen to enter the bloodstream. If left heart failure is not treated or if your dog does not respond to treatment, then death may occur from this accumulation of blood.

Causes

A number of diseases can cause left heart failure in dogs (see also the handouts on each of these conditions):

- Atrioventricular valve degeneration of the left atrioventricular (mitral) valve
- Bacterial endocarditis, an infection of either the aortic or the mitral valve
- Dilated cardiomyopathy, a disease of heart muscle in large-breed dogs that results in a big, flabby heart
- Congenital heart defects, particularly a patent ductus arteriosus (PDA) and sometimes a ventricular septal defect or mitral valve dysplasia
- Systemic hypertension (high blood pressure), an uncommon cause

Clinical Signs

Dogs with left heart failure cannot exercise; they cough when lying down, and they may get up and pace after lying down. As signs worsen, they eventually start breathing faster (more than 50 times per minute) and with more effort. A loud heart murmur that can be heard with a stethoscope is a common finding on physical examination.

Diagnostic Tests

Dogs in severe distress may require stabilization before many tests can be performed to evaluate the heart and other organs that depend on normal heart function. Tests may include the following:

- Chest and possibly abdominal x-rays
- Echocardiogram (heart ultrasound)
- Electrocardiogram (ECG), especially if an irregular rhythm is detected
- Laboratory tests

TREATMENT AND FOLLOW-UP

Treatment Options

If the dog has moderate to severe left heart failure, it may be hospitalized for stabilization with injectable diuretics (such as furosemide), vasodilator drugs (such as nitroglycerin ointment, hydralazine, or sodium nitroprusside), and oxygen therapy. If the dog has mild heart failure, it may be managed on an outpatient basis. Dogs with left heart failure are very fragile and need aggressive treatment, with as little stress as possible. Once the dog is stable and breathing is improved, long-term oral medications are started, such as the following:

- Furosemide (*Lasix*) diuretic is usually continued indefinitely and may be combined with other diuretics, such as spironolactone. Dosages are adjusted to the lowest ones that keep the dog out of heart failure.
- Angiotensin-converting enzyme (ACE) inhibitors, such as enalapril, benazepril, or ramipril, may be used to improve the quality of your dog's life and help reduce fluid retention by the body. Their effects are not immediate, but they exert modest positive effects over weeks to months.
- Pimobendan is a newer drug that acts as a vasodilator to relieve the workload of the heart and to increase the force of contractions. Pimobendan is commonly used with other medications, such as diuretics and ACE inhibitors.
- Digoxin is used in some dogs that have moderate to severe heart failure and very fast heart rates secondary to abnormal rhythms, such as atrial fibrillation.
- Beta-blockers, such as carvedilol, are being investigated to determine whether they can improve the quality of life in dogs with atrioventricular valve degeneration. Beta-blockers are also used to slow the heart rate secondary to atrial fibrillation.
- Occasionally, other classes of drugs, such as calcium channel blockers, may be needed to control the high heart rate caused by atrial fibrillation.

In addition to drug therapy, dogs with heart failure should not be fed salty foods, and low-salt diets may be used to limit salt intake. Although strenuous exercise should be avoided, mild exercise may be done based on guidelines from your veterinarian.

Follow-up Care

Intensive monitoring is often needed during hospitalization. Laboratory tests, chest x-rays, and other tests are often repeated until the dog is stable. Follow-up visits are usually scheduled within 7-14 days after discharge. Recheck visits may include chest x-rays and laboratory tests. The interval between visits and further testing depends on the underlying disease and how your dog responds to medications. Periodic monitoring is needed for the life of your dog. Notify your veterinarian if any signs of heart failure return while the dog is on therapy.

Prognosis

Dogs with left-sided heart failure can live from days to years, with the prognosis depending on the cause and severity of the heart failure.

SPECIAL INSTRUCTIONS:

Congestive Heart Failure in Dogs, Right-Sided

Rebecca E. Gompf, DVM, MS, DACVIM (Cardiology)

BASIC INFORMATION

Description

Right heart failure occurs when the right side of the heart is no longer working properly and cannot pump blood effectively to the lungs and left heart. Fluid accumulates in the abdomen and the chest. Eventually, if right heart failure is not treated, breathing is affected and death may occur.

Causes

A number of diseases can cause right heart failure in dogs (see also the handouts on each of these conditions):
* Atrioventricular valve degeneration of the right (tricuspid) valve
* Dilated cardiomyopathy, mainly in large- and giant-breed dogs
* Chronic heartworm disease
* Some congenital heart defects, such as tricuspid dysplasia, ventricular septal defect, and atrial septal defect

A disease that can mimic right heart failure is pericardial effusion. If a large amount of fluid builds up in the pericardial sac around the heart, the right heart does not fill properly, and fluid may accumulate in the abdomen.

Clinical Signs

Dogs with right heart failure cannot exercise. They develop abdominal distention and loss of muscle mass, which can be so severe that the back bones and ribs become prominent. When the abdomen is full of fluid, the dog may not be comfortable lying down and may breathe faster (more than 50 times per minute), with increased effort.

Diagnostic Tests

Dogs in severe distress often require stabilization before many tests can be performed to evaluate the heart and other organs that depend on normal heart function. Tests may include the following:
* Chest and abdominal x-rays
* Echocardiogram (heart ultrasound)
* Electrocardiogram (ECG), especially if an irregular rhythm is detected
* Laboratory tests, including a heartworm test

TREATMENT AND FOLLOW-UP

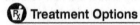 Treatment Options

If there is a significant amount of fluid in the chest, it is usually removed so that the dog can breathe easier. Fluid may also be removed from the abdomen and from the pericardial sac to make the dog more comfortable.

Dogs with moderate to severe right heart failure may be hospitalized for stabilization with injectable diuretics (such as furosemide) and oxygen therapy. Once the dog is stable, oral medications are started. Which medications are chosen depends on the disease causing the right heart failure. Choices include the following:

* Furosemide (*Lasix*) diuretic is usually continued indefinitely and may be combined with other diuretics, such as spironolactone (especially to keep fluid levels low). Dosages are adjusted to the lowest ones that keep the dog out of heart failure.
* Angiotensin-converting enzyme (ACE) inhibitors, such as enalapril, benazepril, or ramipril, may be used to improve the quality of your dog's life and help reduce fluid retention by the body. Their effects are not immediate, but they exert modest positive effects over weeks to months.
* Pimobendan is a newer drug that acts as a vasodilator to relieve the workload of the heart and to increase the force of contractions of the heart. Pimobendan is commonly used with other medications, such as diuretics and ACE inhibitors.
* Digoxin is used in some dogs that have moderate to severe heart failure and very fast heart rates secondary to abnormal rhythms, such as atrial fibrillation.
* Beta-blockers, such as carvedilol, are being investigated to determine whether they can improve the quality of life in dogs with heart disease. Beta-blockers are also used to slow the heart rate secondary to atrial fibrillation.
* Occasionally, other classes of drugs, such as calcium channel blockers, may be needed to control high heart rates caused by atrial fibrillation.

In addition to drug therapy, dogs with heart failure should not be fed salty foods, and low-salt diets may be used to limit salt intake. Although strenuous exercise should be avoided, mild exercise may be done based on guidelines from your veterinarian. If heartworm disease is present, it will be treated once the right heart failure is stable.

Follow-up Care

Intensive monitoring is often needed during hospitalization. Follow-up visits are usually scheduled within 7-14 days after discharge. Recheck visits may include chest x-rays, laboratory tests, and ECGs. The interval between visits and further testing depends on the underlying disease and how your dog responds to medications. Periodic monitoring is needed for the life of your dog. Notify your veterinarian if any signs of heart failure return while the dog is on therapy.

Prognosis

Most dogs with right heart failure have an average life span of 6-12 months; however, survival time is dependent on the underlying cause.

SPECIAL INSTRUCTIONS:

Dilated Cardiomyopathy in Cats

Rebecca E. Gompf, DVM, MS, DACVIM (Cardiology)

BASIC INFORMATION

Description

Dilated cardiomyopathy (DCM) is a disease in which the heart muscle becomes flabby and weak and the heart chambers dilate. The heart cannot effectively pump blood to the body, so the cat lacks energy and fluid may accumulate in the lungs, chest cavity, or both. As the heart dilates, the valvular openings between the chambers of the heart enlarge and the valves begin to leak, which adds an additional burden on the heart. Abnormal heart rhythms (arrhythmias) are also common, especially atrial fibrillation and ventricular arrhythmias.

Causes

Taurine deficiency can cause a reversible type of DCM in cats. Taurine is an essential amino acid that must be supplied in the food of cats. Commercial cat foods are supplemented with taurine, so taurine-deficient DCM is uncommon unless the cat is on a vegetarian diet, is fed exclusively dog food or a single kind of canned cat food, or has a medical problem that interferes with absorption of taurine from the intestinal tract.

Idiopathic DCM occasionally occurs in cats, which means the cause is unknown.

Clinical Signs

Signs often develop suddenly in cats with DCM. Some of the early signs may be exercise intolerance, weakness, decreased appetite, and cold feet. Increased rate and effort of breathing (faster than 50 times per minute) may be the first sign noted by the owner. If a blood clot becomes lodged in one of the front legs or in both rear legs, those legs will be paralyzed and cold, with blue foot pads. Your cat also may also be in pain if the clot happened recently.

Diagnostic Tests

Cats in severe distress often require stabilization before many tests can be performed to evaluate the heart and other organs (that depend on normal heart function). Tests may include the following:

- Chest x-rays
- Echocardiogram (heart ultrasound)
- Electrocardiogram (ECG), especially if an irregular rhythm is detected
- Laboratory tests to assess the kidneys, liver, blood electrolytes, and taurine level
- Analysis of fluid removed from the chest
- Possibly abdominal x-rays and ultrasound studies

TREATMENT AND FOLLOW-UP

Treatment Options

If moderate to severe heart failure is present, the cat is often hospitalized for stabilization with injectable diuretics (such as furosemide), oxygen therapy, removal of fluid from the chest, and other measures. After the cat is stable, oral medications are started and may include the following:

- Furosemide (*Lasix*) diuretic is usually continued indefinitely and may be combined with other diuretics.
- Angiotensin-converting enzyme (ACE) inhibitors, such as enalapril, benazepril, or ramipril, may be used to improve the quality of your cat's life and help reduce fluid retention in the body.
- Pimobendan is a newer drug that acts as a vasodilator to relieve the workload of the heart and to increase the force of contractions of the heart. It is not yet approved for use in cats but shows promise.
- Digoxin is used in some cats with moderate to severe heart failure and very fast heart rates secondary to abnormal rhythms, such as atrial fibrillation. Cats with DCM do not tolerate digoxin very well.
- Beta-blockers and calcium channel blockers are used to slow fast heart rates secondary to atrial fibrillation. They can cause weakness and worsen in heart failure, so they are used cautiously.
- Ventricular arrhythmias are often treated with atenolol and sometimes sotalol, which are beta-blockers.

Cats with heart failure should not be fed salty foods, and low-salt diets may be used to limit their salt intake. Some cats do not like to eat low-salt diets, however. All cats with DCM are started on taurine supplementation, because some cats with normal taurine blood levels respond to taurine supplementation. If the left atrium is enlarged, medications may be started to prevent blood clots from forming. Baby aspirin has been used for many years for this purpose, and clopidogrel (*Plavix*) may also be beneficial.

Follow-up Care

Cats with heart failure are usually re-evaluated 7-14 days after discharge from the hospital. Chest x-rays, laboratory tests, and an ECG are often repeated. Echocardiograms may be done every 2-3 months, and recheck visits are needed for the life of the cat.

Prognosis

Cats with taurine-deficiency cardiomyopathy have a good prognosis if they survive the first several weeks after being treated for heart failure. Cats with idiopathic DCM have a grave prognosis, with survival times of several weeks to months.

SPECIAL INSTRUCTIONS:

Dilated Cardiomyopathy in Dogs

Rebecca E. Gompf, DVM, MS, DACVIM (Cardiology)

BASIC INFORMATION

Description

Dilated cardiomyopathy (DCM) is a disease in which the heart muscle becomes flabby and weak and the heart chambers dilate. The heart cannot effectively pump blood to the body, so the animal lacks energy and fluid accumulates in the lungs, abdomen, or both.

As the heart dilates, the valvular openings between the chambers of the heart enlarge, and the valves begin to leak, which adds an additional burden on the heart. Abnormal heart rhythms (arrhythmias) are also common, especially atrial fibrillation and ventricular arrhythmias.

Causes

DCM is more common in large and giant breeds of dogs and in the American cocker spaniel. In most cases, no exact cause is found (idiopathic), but the disease is inherited as an autosomal dominant characteristic in certain families of boxers and Doberman pinschers.

Nutritional deficiencies of taurine and L-carnitine may cause DCM in American cocker spaniels. Taurine deficiency may also cause DCM in the golden retriever and Newfoundland. Less common causes of secondary cardiomyopathy include myocarditis (an inflammation of heart muscle), hormonal problems (hypothyroidism, hypoadrenocorticism, hyperthyroidism), and high doses of the chemotherapeutic drug doxorubicin.

Clinical Signs

Signs often develop suddenly in dogs with DCM. Some of the first signs are exercise intolerance, weakness, and cold feet. Coughing, loss of appetite, and increased rate and effort of breathing may occur. Abdominal distention with fluid and loss of muscle mass may be noted.

Diagnostic Tests

Dogs in severe distress often require stabilization before many tests can be performed to evaluate the heart and other organs that depend on normal heart function. Tests may include the following:
• Chest and abdominal x-rays
• Echocardiogram (heart ultrasound)
• Electrocardiogram (ECG), especially if an irregular rhythm is detected
• Laboratory tests, including hormonal assays, analysis of abdominal fluid, and possibly taurine levels

TREATMENT AND FOLLOW-UP

Treatment Options

If moderate to severe heart failure is present, the dog is often hospitalized for stabilization with injectable diuretics (such as furo-

semide), oxygen therapy, removal of fluid from the chest and abdomen, and other measures. After the dog is stable, oral medications are started and may include the following:
• Furosemide (*Lasix*) diuretic is usually continued indefinitely and may be combined with other diuretics, such as spironolactone (especially to keep fluid levels low).
• Angiotensin-converting enzyme (ACE) inhibitors, such as enalapril, benazepril, or ramipril, may be used to improve the quality of your dog's life and help reduce fluid retention by the body.
• Pimobendan is a newer drug that acts as a vasodilator to relieve the workload of the heart and to increase the force of contractions of the heart. Pimobendan is commonly used with other medications, such as diuretics and ACE inhibitors.
• Digoxin is used in some dogs that have moderate to severe heart failure and very fast heart rates secondary to abnormal rhythms, such as atrial fibrillation.
• Beta-blockers, such as carvedilol, are being investigated to determine whether they can improve the quality of life in dogs with DCM. Beta-blockers and calcium channel blockers are also used to slow a very fast heart rate secondary to atrial fibrillation.
• Ventricular arrhythmias are often treated with mexiletine, mexiletine plus atenolol, sotalol, or sometimes amiodarone.

Dogs with heart failure should not be fed salty foods, and low-salt diets may be used to limit salt intake. If your dog has taurine deficiency, taurine supplements will be started. Fish oils are sometimes used. Any underlying diseases are also addressed, and DCM may resolve once the disease is treated.

Follow-up Care

Follow-up visits are usually scheduled within 7-14 days after discharge. Recheck visits may include chest x-rays, laboratory tests, and ECGs. The interval between visits and further testing depends on the underlying disease and how your dog responds to medications. Periodic monitoring is needed for the life of your dog.

Prognosis

In secondary DCM, if an underlying cause (such as taurine deficiency) is identified and treated, prognosis is good. Some of these dogs are cured or remain asymptomatic for years. In dogs with primary DCM, prognosis is variable. Dobermans and boxers typically live only a few weeks to months. Other breeds may survive up to 1 year or longer. Prognosis is worse in dogs with atrial fibrillation, congestive heart failure, or poorly controlled ventricular arrhythmias.

SPECIAL INSTRUCTIONS:

Endocarditis

Rebecca E. Gompf, DVM, MS, DACVIM (Cardiology)

BASIC INFORMATION
Description
Endocarditis is an infection of one of the heart valves. The infection is usually by bacteria that have traveled in the bloodstream from somewhere else in the body. The bacteria attach to the valve and destroy it, which causes the valve to leak. When a valve leaks, blood flows backward in the heart.

The two most commonly affected valves are the mitral and aortic valves. The mitral valve lies between the left atrium and the left ventricle. The aortic valve lies between the aorta and the left ventricle. If either of these valves leaks, the left ventricle must handle a bigger volume of blood, so it enlarges. For a while, the ventricle can manage the extra blood, but eventually it fails and signs of left-sided heart failure occur.

Causes
Endocarditis is uncommon in dogs and rare in cats. Bacteria from infections of the spine, prostate, lungs, bladder and kidney, skin, teeth and gums, and long-term intravenous catheters may infect the heart valves. Some dogs with congenital heart defects, such as subaortic stenosis, have such abnormal flow in their hearts that their heart valves are damaged and are more prone to endocarditis. If an animal's immune system is depressed by disease or chronic use of steroids, it may also be more prone to endocarditis.

Many different bacteria cause endocarditis; some more commonly than others. Occasionally fungal organisms can infect valves, but most endocarditis is associated with bacteria.

🪟 Clinical Signs
Bacterial endocarditis is more common in large-breed dogs that are middle-aged or older. The first signs are often of an infection in some other part of the body. Lameness, swollen joints, lethargy, decreased appetite, respiratory problems, weakness, and collapse may occur with endocarditis. Your dog may also have a fever. Signs of heart failure (coughing and labored, difficult breathing) do not develop until the problem is very advanced.

🩺 Diagnostic Tests
If your veterinarian discovers a new heart murmur in your dog and signs of an infection are present, then bacterial endocarditis may be considered. Laboratory tests and bacterial cultures are often done to look for infection. Blood may also be submitted to test for *Bartonella* or other bacteria. Chest and abdominal x-rays may be recommended.

An echocardiogram (heart ultrasound) checks the heart valves for signs of infection and leakage. Multiple blood cultures may also be done to try and isolate circulating bacteria. If your dog is lame and has swollen joints, x-rays may be taken, and joint taps, with retrieval of fluid for analysis and culture, may also be considered.

TREATMENT AND FOLLOW-UP

℞ Treatment Options
Antibiotics are used long term (for at least 3-4 months) in most dogs with bacterial endocarditis. Ideally, the antibiotics are given intravenously for the first 1-2 weeks; this often requires daily visits to the veterinary clinic or prolonged hospitalization. The bacteria are protected on the valve leaflets by thickened tissue (vegetations), so prolonged therapy is needed. The goal is to stop the bacteria from further damaging the valves and prevent them from leaking, or prevent any leakage from worsening.

If your dog has moderate to severe left heart failure, it may be hospitalized for stabilization. Dogs with left heart failure are very fragile and need aggressive treatment, with as little stress as possible. (See also the handout on **Congestive Heart Failure in Dogs, Left-Sided**.)

🐾 Follow-up Care
Blood cultures are often repeated 2-3 weeks after starting antibiotics and again 1-2 weeks after stopping antibiotics. An echocardiogram may be repeated 1-2 weeks after starting therapy, 4 weeks into therapy, and 2-3 weeks after stopping antibiotics. If the infection was caused by *Bartonella* bacteria, a blood titer may be repeated 1 month after starting antibiotics. Dogs in heart failure often require more intensive monitoring, with frequent recheck visits, chest x-rays, and laboratory tests until they are stable.

Dogs that are at increased risk for bacterial endocarditis may be started on prophylactic antibiotics at the time of surgery or a dental procedure. At-risk dogs may also be treated more aggressively if they develop infections elsewhere in their body.

Prognosis
Prognosis is very poor for dogs with bacterial endocarditis of the aortic valve, with survival time as low as 3 days. Bacterial endocarditis of the mitral valve has an average survival time of 476 days. Dogs with bacterial endocarditis usually die of left heart failure or die suddenly from embolic disease if pieces of the infection break off and lodge in other organs.

SPECIAL INSTRUCTIONS:

Heartworm Disease in Cats

Rebecca E. Gompf, DVM, MS, DACVIM (Cardiology)

BASIC INFORMATION

Description

Heartworms (HWs) are parasites (*Dirofilaria immitis*) that live primarily in the lungs of dogs and wild canines; however, domestic and wild cats are also susceptible. Mosquitoes spread the HWs from dogs to cats. The changes caused by HWs in the lungs of cats are different from the problems they cause in dogs.

Causes

HWs are found in most parts of the world and in every state of the United States. HWs molt in mosquitoes to their infective form and are spread to cats when mosquitoes are present. Once a cat is bitten by an infected mosquito, the HWs molt again and travel to the lungs, where they develop into adults. Since the cat is not the natural host of HWs, some of the immature worms die and irritate the lungs, about 2½ to 5 months after the cat is infected. Some cats have clinical signs from this lung irritation.

About 6 months after the cat is infected, a few HWs mature to adults, but they live only 1-3 years. Adult HWs release substances that irritate the lungs and other organs of the body. The death of HWs can cause sudden lung injury. Unlike in the dog, HW disease in the cat is only a respiratory problem and does not affect the heart.

Some of the adult females may produce larvae (microfilariae), but they do not survive long in the cat, and their death can also irritate the lungs or other tissues. Because cats rarely have circulating microfilariae, cats do not serve as a source of HW infection for other animals.

Clinical Signs

Affected cats may be asymptomatic and may not be tested routinely for HWs. Signs of HW disease include coughing; intermittent heavy, labored breathing; sporadic vomiting; weight loss; and lethargy. Occasionally, sudden death occurs from the death of HWs and blockage of the arteries in the lungs (pulmonary embolism).

Diagnostic Tests

Commonly recommended tests include chest x-rays, routine laboratory tests, and tests for both HW proteins (antigens) and HW antibodies. If the HW antigen test is positive, then your cat has or recently had adult HWs. Because of the low number of HWs in most cats, this test can be falsely negative. If the HW antibody test is positive, your cat was exposed to HWs but may not have any adults present. Because the diagnosis of HW disease can be difficult in cats, an echocardiogram (heart ultrasound), and a radiologic contrast study of the lungs may be done to detect any HWs and rule out other causes of lung disease.

TREATMENT AND FOLLOW-UP

Treatment Options

Treating adult HWs with melarsomine (*Immiticide*) is rarely done in cats, because the death of adult HWs can be fatal to the cat if too many HWs die at once. One dose of *Immiticide* typically kills 30% of the HWs, which may cause no problems; however, the safety of *Immiticide* has not been proven in the cat. The cat's lungs cannot handle more than 1-2 HWs dying at once, so if large numbers of HWs die at the same time, they could kill the cat.

Surgical removal of adult HWs has had only limited success, so most often the recommendation is to treat the cat's symptoms and allow the adult HWs to die naturally (which may take 1-3 years). A steroid, prednisolone, may be used to decrease lung irritation and reduce vomiting. Because of its side effects, it is used for only a short time and discontinued after the symptoms are controlled. Bronchodilators, such as theophylline, help relieve respiratory signs. Antileukotriene drugs have been used for life-threatening respiratory crises, which are rare in cats.

Because cats do not have circulating microfilariae, they do not require therapy for them. HW-preventive medications, such as ivermectin, milbemycin oxime, or selamectin, are usually given so the cat does not become reinfected. It is rare for cats to have a reaction to any of these drugs. Preventive medications are often recommended for uninfected cats, especially in areas with a high incidence of HW disease in dogs.

Follow-up Care

Periodic monitoring (laboratory tests, chest x-rays) is needed, especially for cats with respiratory problems. Once your cat is stable, chest x-rays may be done every few months until the problem resolves.

Prognosis

The majority of cats do well with symptomatic treatment. A few cats continue to have chronic respiratory disease even after the HWs have died. Occasionally, a cat has several HWs die at once, which can result in sudden death. Unfortunately, sudden death cannot be prevented in these cats.

SPECIAL INSTRUCTIONS:

Heartworm Disease in Dogs

Rebecca E. Gompf, DVM, MS, DACVIM (Cardiology)

BASIC INFORMATION

Description

Heartworms (HWs) are parasites that live in the arteries of the lungs (pulmonary arteries) of dogs and wild canines. HWs cause elevated pressure in the pulmonary arteries (pulmonary hypertension), which increases the workload of the right side of the heart. If HWs persist (they can live 5-7 years), the right heart eventually fails. HWs also cause inflammation in the lungs.

Causes

HWs (*Dirofilaria immitis*) are found in most parts of the world and in every state of the United States. Domestic dogs, as well as wolves, foxes, and coyotes, serve as the primary hosts. HWs also occur in cats (domestic and wild), ferrets, and California sea lions.

HWs are spread from an infected animal to other animals by mosquitoes. HWs molt in the mosquitoes to their infective form and are then passed on to the dog. HW disease is only spread when mosquitoes are present. Adult female HWs produce larvae (microfilariae) that migrate throughout the body. The microfilariae are picked up by the mosquitoes when they feed on the dog, molt in the mosquitoes, and then are spread to other animals.

Physiologic Effects

Once a dog is bitten by an infected mosquito, the HW organisms molt and travel to the lungs, where they develop into adults. It takes about 6 months from the time the dog is bitten until the HWs are mature in the pulmonary arteries. Adult female HWs produce a substance that irritates the arteries of the lungs. The physical presence of HWs also injures the lining of the arteries, which causes the arteries to become thickened and stiff. As adult HWs die, they become lodged in the smaller pulmonary arteries, which contributes to the overall problem.

Some dogs are bitten by many infected mosquitoes at one time, especially in areas where there are large numbers of infected mosquitoes. As a result, many HWs become adults at the same time. If there is no room for all of them in the pulmonary arteries, the HWs will live in the heart and the large vein (posterior vena cava) that carries blood back to the heart from the abdomen. The presence of HWs in the vena cava is called *caval syndrome*. A large mass of adult HWs in the vena cava alters blood flow and damages red blood cells. If HWs are not removed from the vena cava within a short time, the dog usually dies.

Migration of the microfilariae throughout the dog's body sometimes causes inflammation in other organs, such as the kidneys and skin. The microfilariae may also contribute to changes in the lungs that result in pulmonary hypertension.

Clinical Signs

Most dogs with HW disease have no signs, and the disease is detected by routine HW blood tests. The more athletic and active the dog, the earlier signs are seen. The first signs are often lethargy, decreased activity, and coughing. As the disease worsens, breathing rate (more than 50 breaths per minute) and effort increase. Some dogs have fainting episodes when stressed. With advanced disease and right heart failure, fluid may build up in the abdomen, and weight loss may occur.

If large numbers of adult HWs obstruct blood flow in the vena cava, lethargy, weakness, loss of appetite, and fever may occur. The membranes in the mouth may be pale or yellow (jaundiced) from red blood cell destruction and anemia.

Diagnostic Tests

Two blood tests can be run to diagnose HW disease in your dog. A Knott's test looks for microfilariae in the blood. Because some dogs have no circulating microfilariae or are on HW-preventive drugs that kill microfilariae, an occult (ELISA) HW blood test may be needed to detect antigens (proteins) given off by the adult female HWs. The occult (ELISA) HW test is the most common screening test used, but both tests may be done in a dog that has received no preventive medications in the past (such as stray dogs).

If a dog is positive for HWs, chest x-rays are done to look for lung and heart changes. An echocardiogram (heart ultrasound) is done in dogs with right heart failure to rule out other causes of heart failure and to assess the heart. Echocardiography is also done when caval syndrome is suspected.

Prior to treatment, routine laboratory tests are usually recommended. If other problems, such as liver or kidney disease, are found, they are treated first, because the drug used to kill adult HWs can adversely affect the kidneys and liver.

Continued

Heartworm Disease in Dogs—*cont'd*

Rebecca E. Gompf, DVM, MS, DACVIM (Cardiology)

TREATMENT AND FOLLOW-UP

℞ Treatment Options

If right heart failure, kidney disease, or liver disease is present, it is treated before treatment for adult heartworms (HWs) is started. No single drug treats all stages of HW disease. Adult HWs are killed by adulticide drugs, such as melarsomine (*Immiticide*). Two dosing schedules are available:

- In one schedule, two intramuscular (IM) doses of melarsomine are given 24 hours apart. This regimen kills 90-95% of adult HWs, usually within 2-3 weeks.
- Dogs with right heart failure or x-ray changes in their lungs are treated with split doses. This method kills fewer HWs with each injection, which decreases the risk of worsening lung problems or causing acute death. With this schedule one dose of melarsomine is given IM. The dog is rested for 4-6 weeks, and then two doses of melarsomine are given 24 hours apart.

Ivermectin is an HW-preventive drug that can slowly kill some of the adult HWs if given for at least 18 months. Dogs that are not confined have an increased risk of pulmonary embolism and sudden breathing problems with this method, so it is used only for dogs with other medical problems that make use of melarsomine risky.

Circulating microfilariae may be treated before or after adulticide therapy, depending on the time of year and the presence of other diseases. Either ivermectin (at high doses) or milbemycin is used. If large numbers of microfilariae die, a shock-like syndrome can occur 2-8 hours after the drugs are given. The dog may be hospitalized for 12-24 hours of observation.

Once the adult HWs and microfilariae are treated, HW-preventive drugs are started. Several drugs are available that prevent adult HWs from developing after a dog is bitten by an infected mosquito. Ivermectin (*Heartgard*) is safe in all breeds of dogs, including collies and Shetland sheepdogs at the preventive dose. If ivermectin is given at high doses, it can cause death in collies and other susceptible dogs.

Ivermectin, milbemycin, and selamectin are given monthly. Moxidectin is an injectable HW-preventive that lasts for 6 months. Moxidectin should not be given to animals that are debilitated or have other medical problems. Daily preventive drugs, such as diethylcarbamazine, are no longer recommended.

Shock from caval syndrome is treated aggressively with intravenous fluids and supportive care. Once the dog is stable, the adult HWs are removed surgically. A bacterium (*Wolbachia*) that lives in the reproductive tract of female HWs has been discovered, but its role in HW disease is unknown. Further research is needed to determine whether treating the bacteria with tetracycline before giving adulticides will result in less reaction to the death of HWs.

🐾 Follow-up Care

When adult HWs die, they break up and lodge in the smaller pulmonary arteries (embolism). If the dog has no or few lung changes on x-rays and no symptoms, the dead HWs may cause no significant problems. All dogs receiving melarsomine *must* be kept quiet for 6 weeks to lessen the risk of acute death from pulmonary embolism. Recheck visits are often scheduled during this 6-week period. Notify your veterinarian if any coughing (especially with blood) or breathing problems develop after adulticide therapy. Occasionally, even with the best care and rest, a dog will die when the adult HWs die.

Four to six months after adult HWs are treated, a blood test is done to determine whether all the adults were killed. A few dogs may remain positive and require repeated adulticide treatment. After successful HW treatment, preventive therapy is often given year round or at least during the mosquito season. An annual or biannual occult (ELISA) HW test is done to ensure that the preventive is working.

Prognosis

Dogs that are asymptomatic have a very good prognosis. Occasionally a healthy dog will die when the adult HWs die, but this is uncommon if the animal's exercise is restricted for 4-6 weeks after adulticide therapy. Dogs with liver or kidney problems have a guarded (uncertain) prognosis if the problems persist, because melarsomine may cause an adverse reaction in these patients.

Dogs with lung changes on their x-rays have a more guarded prognosis. Some of these dogs return to normal activity after being treated, but athletic dogs may not be able to perform as well. Dogs with right heart failure have a poor prognosis, because their significant lung changes may not reverse after HW disease is treated. They may improve with therapy but will require medication for the rest of their lives.

SPECIAL INSTRUCTIONS:

Hypertrophic Cardiomyopathy in Cats

Rebecca E. Gompf, DVM, MS, DACVIM (Cardiology)

BASIC INFORMATION

Description

Hypertrophic cardiomyopathy (HCM) is a heart disease caused by thickening of the walls of the left ventricle, which decreases the space available for the blood. Blood accumulates in the left atrium, causing it to dilate. Eventually blood accumulates in the lungs, left ventricular filling diminishes, and left-sided heart failure occurs.

Retained blood in the left atrium may form clots that can break off and travel to other areas of the body. Outflow of blood from the left ventricle can also be obstructed (obstructive HCM), which makes it harder to pump blood to the rest of the body.

Causes

The cause of HCM is unknown (idiopathic) in many cases. It is a genetic disease in the Maine coon cat, American shorthair, and ragdoll breeds. HCM may also be genetic in the Norwegian forest cat, Turkish van, Scottish fold, British shorthair, and Devon Rex.

HCM can also occur secondary to hyperthyroidism, hypertension (high blood pressure), or aortic stenosis (a congenital heart defect). Males develop HCM more often than females.

Clinical Signs

HCM is commonly detected before heart failure develops, because 80% of affected cats have heart murmurs that are heard on a routine physical examination. An abnormal heart rhythm (arrhythmia) or an extra heart sound (gallop rhythm) may also be heard. HCM comes in all different degrees of severity. Milder forms may progress and worsen, or may stay static for years.

Early signs, such as lethargy and exercise intolerance, are often missed. The first signs noticed may be increased breathing rate (faster than 50 times per minute) and effort of breathing. If a clot lodges in a blood vessel to a front leg or to the rear legs, the affected legs will be paralyzed, with cold, blue foot pads. At the onset, this condition is also very painful.

Diagnostic Tests

Tests that may be recommended after a heart murmur is detected include chest x-rays, an echocardiogram (heart ultrasound), blood pressure measurements, and thyroid hormone levels (in cats older than 5 years of age). Other laboratory tests to check the kidneys and other organs may be done in cats with heart failure and blood clots. If an arrhythmia is present, an electrocardiogram (ECG) is indicated.

Blood tests can be performed for the gene that causes HCM in Maine coon cats and ragdolls.

TREATMENT AND FOLLOW-UP

Treatment Options

No drug is known to prevent the progression of HCM, so asymptomatic cats may not be treated unless they have significant outflow obstruction or significant ventricular hypertrophy, enlargement of the atrium, and faster than normal heart rates. These cats may be treated with atenolol or diltiazem. Asymptomatic cats with HCM secondary to hypertension or hyperthyroidism may need no medication for their HCM if the primary disease is successfully treated.

Cats in heart failure often require hospitalization for stabilization with oxygen therapy, injectable diuretics (furosemide), and nitroglycerin ointment treatment. If a significant amount of fluid is present in the chest, it may be manually removed. Once heart failure is stabilized, the cat is often switched to oral furosemide and either atenolol (a beta-blocker) or diltiazem (a calcium channel blocker). These latter drugs keep the heart rate low so that the left side of the heart has adequate time to fill.

If the left atrium is enlarged, medications may be started to prevent blood clots from forming. Baby aspirin has been used for many years, and clopidogrel (*Plavix*) may also be beneficial.

An angiotensin-converting enzyme (ACE) inhibitor, such as enalapril, benazepril, or ramipril, may also be recommended to reduce the amount of fluid retained by the body, especially in animals with left heart failure.

Follow-up Care

Cats with asymptomatic HCM and no left atrial enlargement are usually rechecked initially every 4-6 months (with repeated echocardiograms), then annually if they remain stable. Mildly affected cats on therapy may be rechecked more often, depending on the medication used. Cats with left heart failure are rechecked frequently, with chest x-rays and laboratory tests, with the frequency determine by the cat's response to therapy.

Cats with secondary HCM often have echocardiograms repeated 4-6 months after treatment of their underlying problem to ensure that the HCM is regressing. Cats with murmurs and normal echocardiograms may be monitored with yearly echocardiograms.

Prognosis

Cats with left heart failure may survive 1 year or longer if response to initial therapy is good. Cats with advanced HCM usually die from heart and kidney failure. Cats with thrombosis have a very poor prognosis. Asymptomatic cats may survive for years if their disease remains stable.

SPECIAL INSTRUCTIONS:

Occult Cardiomyopathy in Doberman Pinschers

Rebecca E. Gompf, DVM, MS, DACVIM (Cardiology)

BASIC INFORMATION
Description

Occult cardiomyopathy (OC) is a slowly progressive heart muscle disease that results in abnormal heart rhythms (arrhythmias) in Doberman pinschers. Because it causes arrhythmias, often ventricular premature contractions (VPCs) and ventricular tachycardia (VT), it is also called *arrhythmogenic cardiomyopathy*. Dobermans with OC may have no clinical signs for long periods, which is why the disease is referred to as *occult*. Eventually the dog develops arrhythmias and, later, dilated cardiomyopathy.

Causes

OC runs in families of Dobermans, so a genetic factor is involved. It can be traced back to the original seven sires of Doberman lines in the United States, three of which died suddenly when they were middle-aged. The exact gene or genes causing OC have not yet been identified, but it may be an autosomal dominant characteristic.

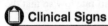 Clinical Signs

OC can start as early as 9-12 months of age, but most dogs are between 2-4 years old. By 6 years of age, about 50% of Dobermans have OC. Most dogs with OC have no symptoms. Their arrhythmias may be detected on a routine physical examination or on a screening electrocardiogram (ECG) or Holter monitor study.

Dogs with more frequent VPCs or VT may have fainting episodes (syncope). About 30% of affected dogs die suddenly, without prior symptoms. Older dogs may have exercise intolerance.

Diagnostic Tests

Since OC is very prevalent in Dobermans, annual screening of adult dogs often starts at 2-3 years of age, and may include a 24-hour Holter monitor and echocardiogram (heart ultrasound) study. The likelihood of finding VPCs, VT, or echocardiographic changes increases as the dog ages. Once arrhythmias have been found, the only way to diagnose OC is to rule out all other causes of ventricular arrhythmias. Routine laboratory tests, chest and abdominal x-rays, thyroid hormone tests, an echocardiogram, and possibly other tests may be recommended.

TREATMENT AND FOLLOW-UP

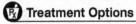 Treatment Options

If VT, severe VPCs, or fainting episodes are occurring, it may be necessary to hospitalize your dog for treatment with intravenous drugs. The more severe the arrhythmia, the greater the chance of sudden death. Once your dog's heart rhythm has been stabilized,

it can be managed on an outpatient basis with the use of several different drugs, alone or in combination. Not every drug works in every dog, so sometimes a dog must be switched from one drug to another to control the ventricular arrhythmias.

- Oral drugs that are used for controlling ventricular arrhythmias caused by OC include the combination of mexiletine and atenolol, mexiletine and carvedilol, sotalol, or mexiletine alone.
- If these medications do not control the arrhythmia, then a combination of mexiletine and sotalol may be tried.
- Amiodarone is used as a last resort and often requires referral to a veterinary specialist for its administration.

Side effects of antiarrhythmic drugs include lethargy, anorexia, vomiting, and diarrhea. The last three effects are more common with mexiletine. Occasionally, antiarrhythmic drugs can make the arrhythmia worse, so that the dog must be switched to another medication. Amiodarone has multiple side effects, including liver damage, decreased white blood cell counts, and damage to the thyroid gland.

Follow-up Care

Affected Dobermans require frequent ECGs until their VT or VPCs are controlled. Ideally, a Holter monitor is applied to dogs with non–life-threatening arrhythmias to document the frequency of the arrhythmias prior to treatment. Another Holter recording is done after the drug has reached adequate blood levels, to judge how effective it is in controlling the abnormal beats. Affected dogs require antiarrhythmic therapy for the rest of their lives. Echocardiograms may be done every 6-12 months to monitor for evidence of dilated cardiomyopathy, which can follow OC.

Prognosis

Dobermans with infrequent VPCs that are feeling well usually develop changes on their echocardiograms within 1 year. Within 2 years, their VPCs and heart changes often get worse, and 30-50% of these dogs may die suddenly.

Dobermans with severe VPCs or VT that are well controlled with medication can live up to 1 year or longer. No drug is 100% effective in preventing sudden death. The better the arrhythmia is controlled, the less likely it is that sudden death will occur. Holter monitors provide the best way to evaluate how well the medications are controlling the arrhythmias.

If dilated cardiomyopathy develops, the dog's life span is only weeks to months (average, 3-4 months). Because OC has a genetic basis and runs in families, it is wise not to breed dogs that have the problem.

SPECIAL INSTRUCTIONS:

Patent Ductus Arteriosus

Rebecca E. Gompf, DVM, MS, DACVIM (Cardiology)

BASIC INFORMATION

Description

Patent ductus arteriosus (PDA) is a congenital heart defect. Prior to birth, all mammals have a blood vessel (ductus arteriosus) that connects the two main arteries leaving the heart, the aorta and the pulmonary artery (to the lungs). The ductus arteriosus allows the blood to go from the pulmonary artery into the aorta, bypassing the lungs, because the fetus is not breathing yet.

After the animal is born and starts to breath on its own, the ductus arteriosus normally closes. In 2 or 3 of every 1000 dogs, it does not close and is called a *PDA*. In these animals, some of the blood flows from the aorta through the PDA into the pulmonary artery and the lungs, then back to the left side of the heart. This extra blood flow overloads the left heart and eventually causes left heart failure.

Causes

The ductus may not close because the muscle that causes the sides to contract, collapse, and fuse is lacking. In many breeds of dogs this defect may be inherited, so affected dogs should not be used for breeding. PDA is one of the most common congenital defects found in dogs. It is uncommon in cats.

Clinical Signs

Most puppies with PDA have no signs, and the murmur caused by the PDA is discovered when the puppies are examined by a veterinarian. Occasionally a puppy has such a large PDA that it dies before weaning. If left heart failure occurs, breathing rate and effort are increased. Coughing, lethargy, and failure to gain weight may also be noted.

Diagnostic Tests

If your veterinarian discovers a murmur suspicious for PDA, chest x-rays and an echocardiogram (heart ultrasound) will be done to confirm the diagnosis and to determine the size of the left heart and how well it is functioning. Blood tests may be done prior to anesthesia.

TREATMENT AND FOLLOW-UP

Treatment Options

If the animal is in heart failure or has an abnormal heart rhythm (atrial fibrillation), treatment is required prior to anesthesia and surgical correction. If the heart has not been affected much by the PDA, surgery may be delayed until the pup is larger and has completed all of the puppy vaccinations. Closure of the PDA is usually done by a specialist in veterinary surgery or cardiology.

Surgically tying the PDA closed is the oldest method of treatment. It is used in puppies that are too small to be catheterized or that have a PDA with a shape not easily closed by other methods. Surgery involves opening the left side of the chest under general anesthesia.

Less invasive methods of closing PDAs also require anesthesia and insertion of a catheter into the heart. Coils or a special plug (*Amplatzer*) may be placed in the opening of the PDA to occlude (block) it. These methods require the presence of veins and arteries large enough to accommodate the special catheters used for these procedures.

Follow-up Care

Following open-chest surgery, the animal is usually hospitalized for a few days and then must be kept quiet until the incision heals. Sutures can be removed in 10-14 days by your veterinarian.

Following closure by coils or an Amplatzer plug, the animal must also be kept quiet for a few days to allow the rear leg vessels, where the catheter was inserted, to heal. If sutures were placed in the rear leg, they are removed in 10-14 days.

If the animal was in heart failure prior to PDA closure, medications may be continued long term, and periodic monitoring is required. If heart failure was not present, most dogs need no further monitoring once their sutures are removed.

Prognosis

Prognosis is excellent in dogs that are not in heart failure and do not have atrial fibrillation. Success rates with surgery or catheter occlusion are 90-95%. Most of these dogs have a normal life span and few complications. Complications of surgery include death, which usually occurs when the PDA ruptures while being dissected. Occasionally, ligatures can slip and break after surgery, which necessitates a second procedure; this tends to occur in older dogs.

Complications of coil placement include dislodgement and movement of the coils into the lungs. Occasionally, the coils do not close the PDA completely, which may or may not cause future problems.

Complications of Amplatzer occlusion are uncommon, but some PDAs cannot be closed by them. With any catheter procedure, swelling may develop at the site where the catheter was inserted into the leg.

SPECIAL INSTRUCTIONS:

Pericardial Effusion

Rebecca E. Gompf, DVM, MS, DACVIM (Cardiology)

BASIC INFORMATION

Description

Pericardial effusion is an abnormal accumulation of fluid in the sac around the heart (pericardial sac). A small amount of fluid is always present in the sac, but when an abnormal amount accumulates, the fluid puts pressure on the walls of the heart and keeps the heart from filling properly. Since the heart cannot fill properly, blood backs up, causing signs of heart failure. Severe pressure and lack of filling of the heart is called *cardiac tamponade* and can cause acute death. Pericardial effusion is more common in dogs than in cats.

Causes

In up to 19-23% of dogs the cause is unknown (idiopathic). Tumors, such as hemangiosarcoma, are the most frequent cause. Hemangiosarcoma is a highly malignant tumor that can involve the wall of the right atrium and bleed into the pericardial sac. Golden retrievers and German shepherd dogs are predisposed to hemangiosarcomas.

Heart base tumors form from structures near the heart. They may eventually interfere with the blood supply to the pericardial sac and result in effusion. They are 10 times less common than hemangiosarcomas. The English bulldog, boxer, and Boston terrier are prone to these tumors.

Bacterial infections are uncommon causes and usually arise after penetration of the pericardial sac by a foreign body, via trauma or migration into the chest (such as grass awns). Systemic fungal infections and feline infectious peritonitis virus (in cats) are rare causes.

Clinical Signs

Most animals with significant effusion have a sudden onset of lethargy, weakness, and collapse. Trouble breathing occurs in about half of affected dogs, and 23% have abdominal swelling. Loss of appetite, vomiting, or coughing may be noted. Other signs of an underlying disease may also be present.

Diagnostic Tests

Pericardial effusion may only be suspected when x-rays of the chest show an enlarged heart. An echocardiogram (heart ultrasound) and an electrocardiogram (ECG) may be recommended to differentiate pericardial effusion from other cardiac diseases. Laboratory tests, abdominal x-rays, and an abdominal ultrasound study are often done to look for a cause and to identify any tumors in other organs. Some of these tests may be delayed until fluid is removed from the pericardial sac and the animal is stable. Often, the fluid is submitted for analysis. Additional tests may also be indicated.

TREATMENT AND FOLLOW-UP

Treatment Options

If the effusion is causing symptoms, it is removed by pericardiocentesis, which involves insertion of a catheter into the pericardial sac to drain the fluid. Dogs with idiopathic effusions usually improve markedly after removal of the fluid; however, the effusion usually recurs in 1-2 months. Removal of the pericardial sac may be considered, especially if the effusion recurs. The sac may be removed by open-chest surgery or by thoracoscopy (in which an endoscope passed through small holes in the chest).

Dogs with right atrial hemangiosarcomas are difficult to treat. Pericardiocentesis may provide temporary relief, but the fluid returns within a short time. Surgical removal of the tumor and chemotherapy may be attempted in some cases. Dogs with heart base tumors benefit from removal of the pericardial sac, because these tumors are very slow growing. Treatment of other tumors depends on the tumor type.

Dogs with bacterial infections in the pericardial sac must undergo surgery to remove the sac, followed by chest drains, flushing, and antibiotics. No effective treatment exists for feline infectious peritonitis, but removal of the effusion may temporarily make the cat more comfortable. Appropriate treatments for underlying heart or systemic diseases are also started.

Follow-up Care

Animals with idiopathic effusion that are treated only with pericardiocentesis are often monitored with monthly echocardiograms for several months, then periodically for 1 year. Periodic rechecks are also done for months following removal of the pericardial sac. The frequency of visits for animals with hemangiosarcoma or other tumors is determined by the treatment protocols. Dogs with bacterial infections need intensive monitoring for several months.

Prognosis

Dogs with hemangiosarcomas have an average survival time of 56 days (range, 0 to 229 days). Following surgery to remove the pericardial sac, the average survival time for dogs with heart base tumors is 730 days; without surgery, it is only 42 days. Dogs with idiopathic effusions that do not have the sac removed have a high rate of recurrence within 1-2 months and a high incidence of death from cardiac tamponade. Dogs with idiopathic pericardial effusion that have their pericardial sacs removed soon after the effusion first occurs are often cured.

SPECIAL INSTRUCTIONS:

Peritoneopericardial Diaphragmatic Hernia

Rebecca E. Gompf, DVM, MS, DACVIM (Cardiology)

BASIC INFORMATION

Description

Peritoneopericardial diaphragmatic hernia (PPDH) is a congenital heart defect that is present at birth. Animals with PPDH have a hole in their diaphragm (the muscle that separates the chest from the abdomen) and a hole in the sac around their heart (pericardial sac). The pericardial sac is fused or attached to the diaphragm, creating a sort of tunnel that allows organs from the abdomen to move into the sac around the heart.

Causes

PPDH is uncommon in cats and dogs, but Persian cats and Weimaraner dogs may be predisposed to them. It is not known why this congenital defect occurs. PPDH is not caused by trauma.

Clinical Signs

Many animals with PPDH have no clinical signs, because the abdominal organs easily slip in and out of the pericardial sac and cause no problems. PPDH may be discovered only when your animal has chest or abdominal x-rays taken for another problem.

Some animals have intermittent vomiting, lack of appetite, weight loss, and diarrhea. These signs may be related to movement of the stomach or intestines into the pericardial sac. Other animals develop a cough or rapid or labored breathing. If the liver or other organs enter the pericardial sac, it can restrict the space available for the lungs and adversely affect breathing. The heart's ability to fill with blood can also be affected by the organs in the pericardial sac, especially if a lobe of liver twists or strangulates (blocking the veins to the liver), which causes fluid to form in the pericardial sac. In these cases, heart failure may develop.

Diagnostic Tests

PPDH is diagnosed by taking chest and abdominal x-rays and identifying stomach, intestines, or liver in the pericardial sac. A barium study, which is a series of x-rays taken after barium is swallowed, may be recommended to positively identify the presence of abdominal organs in the pericardial sac. An echocardiogram may also be done to assess the amount of fluid in the pericardial sac and the effects of pericardial fluid and organs on the heart. An abdominal ultrasound study helps verify that some organs are missing in the abdomen.

TREATMENT AND FOLLOW-UP

Treatment Options

The only effective treatment for PPDH is surgery. Surgery is recommended for all animals with clinical signs from the PPDH and for young animals even if they do not have clinical signs. In older animals, adhesions between the herniated organs and the pericardium may make the surgery more complicated. If the older animal is symptomatic; however, surgery is still the best option. If the older animal is having no symptoms, the PPDH may be monitored and surgically corrected if any problems begin to develop.

Follow-up Care

After surgery, keep your animal quiet until the sutures are removed at 10-14 days. Older, asymptomatic animals with PPDH that do not have surgery are usually rechecked at least every 6 months. Notify your veterinarian if your animal becomes lethargic, stops eating, develops vomiting or diarrhea, or has any problems breathing.

Prognosis

The survival rate after PPDH surgery is high, and the lifespan of affected animals is usually normal after successful repair of the PPDH. The percentage of animals with asymptomatic PPDH that become symptomatic over time is unknown.

SPECIAL INSTRUCTIONS:

Persistent Right Aortic Arch

Rebecca E. Gompf, DVM, MS, DACVIM (Cardiology)

BASIC INFORMATION

Description

A persistent right aortic arch (PRAA) is a congenital heart defect that is present at birth. When the heart is developing in the fetus, certain structures are supposed to grow while others disappear. The aorta is the main artery that takes blood from the left side of the heart and to the body. Two different structures in the fetus can develop to become the aorta: the right and left aortic arches. Normally, the left aortic arch forms the aorta, and the right aortic arch disappears prior to birth. If the right aortic arch persists and forms the aorta, blood flow is normal but the aorta and some of its nearby vessels can affect the esophagus (the tube that connects the mouth to the stomach). The esophagus becomes trapped between the aorta, the base of the heart, and the ductus arteriosus (a connection between the aorta and the pulmonary artery to the lungs).

A PRAA does not usually cause a problem until the puppy or kitten starts to eat solid foods. The solid food cannot pass through the esophagus where it is trapped by the blood vessels. Food accumulates in the esophagus in front of the heart and causes the esophagus to stretch. Food is regurgitated and can be inhaled into the lungs.

Causes

Why the right aortic arch forms the aorta instead of the left aortic arch in these animals is unknown. PRAA is an uncommon defect in puppies or kittens.

🔲 Clinical Signs

As soon as the puppy or kitten starts to eat solid foods, the food does not stay down. Undigested food may be regurgitated immediately after eating and may be tubular in shape. If the inability to swallow solid food persists long enough, the puppy or kitten does not gain weight and does not develop well. Pneumonia occurs if the puppy or kitten aspirates food into its lungs. Pneumonia often causes a fever, depression, coughing, and increased rate and effort of breathing. If the pneumonia is untreated, the animal may die quickly.

🔳 Diagnostic Tests

Chest and abdominal x-rays are usually recommended in puppies and kittens with clinical signs, to check for a dilated esophagus and evidence of pneumonia. Laboratory tests may also be done if pneumonia or infection is suspected.

A procedure called an *esophagram* may be done, in which the animal swallows food mixed with barium to outline the esophagus and identify the location of the narrowing of the esophagus. Sometimes the esophagram is done under fluoroscopy (a video x-ray procedure) so that the motility of the esophagus can also be evaluated.

If another congenital heart defect is suspected in addition to the PRAA, then an echocardiogram (heart ultrasound) with Doppler capabilities may be done. These latter tests may require referral of your pet to a veterinary specialist.

TREATMENT AND FOLLOW-UP

💊 Treatment Options

The only treatment for PRAA is surgical dissection and removal of the ductus arteriosus to free up the esophagus. If the ductus is patent (contains blood), then it is also tied off (ligated). If the patient has pneumonia, the pneumonia must be treated first and the animal stabilized before surgery can be done.

🐾 Follow-up Care

Follow-up x-rays are needed to monitor the treatment response of the pneumonia and to monitor the esophagus after surgery. The frequency and timing of recheck appointments depend on the success of the surgery and whether any regurgitation or aspiration pneumonia persists.

Prognosis

The sooner the surgery is done in these young animals, the fewer problems the puppy or kitten will have afterward. However, once the esophagus is stretched, it rarely returns completely to normal, so these animals continue to have some problems with regurgitation and must be fed with their heads elevated. They may also have periodic episodes of aspiration pneumonia, so they must be watched closely. Notify your veterinarian if any signs of pneumonia occur.

SPECIAL INSTRUCTIONS:

Pulmonary Hypertension

Rebecca E. Gompf, DVM, MS, DACVIM (Cardiology)

BASIC INFORMATION

Description

Pulmonary hypertension (PH) is increased pressure in the arteries of the lungs (pulmonary arteries). The increased pressure makes the right side of the heart work harder than normal, which causes it to enlarge. Eventually, the right heart can fail. In addition, less blood is pumped to the left side of the heart, which decreases blood flow to the body.

Causes

Many different diseases can result in PH. Some of these diseases develop rapidly, such as clots that lodge in the smaller pulmonary arteries and obstruct blood flow (pulmonary embolism). As a result of this blockage, more blood is forced to other areas in the lungs, resulting in generalized PH.

Other acute respiratory diseases, such as severe pneumonia, can cause vessels in the affected area of the lungs to constrict and direct blood elsewhere, which also results in PH. Surgical removal of a lung lobe because of torsion (twisting) or tumors, or any other disease that affects large areas of the lungs, can cause a sudden increase in pulmonary pressure.

Most causes of PH are chronic, not acute, diseases. Chronic lung diseases, such as bronchitis, bronchiectasis, emphysema, tumors, allergies, and heartworm disease, cause changes either directly or indirectly in the pulmonary vessels. Some of these diseases cause constriction of vessels, whereas others damage the vessels directly. Certain congenital heart diseases can also cause PH.

The end result of PH is restricted or absent blood flow in the affected arteries. The right heart must pump against a higher pressure gradient, which can eventually cause it to fail. With advanced PH, the chronic changes in the pulmonary arteries decrease the amount of blood that is exposed to oxygen in the lungs, so inadequate amounts of oxygen are taken in.

Clinical Signs

The clinical signs depend on the underlying cause. Most animals with advanced lung disease and PH have coughing and rapid breathing. They are not able to exercise normally, because they do not take in enough oxygen. Some animals suddenly develop trouble breathing. If the dog has right heart failure, its abdomen may be distended with fluid. Cats in right heart failure may develop fluid in their chests, which makes it more difficult for them to breathe.

Diagnostic Tests

Animals with respiratory distress must be stabilized before diagnostic tests are performed. Chest x-rays, blood tests, a urinalysis, and heartworm tests are usually done after the animal is stable. An echocardiogram (heart ultrasound) is performed to document the presence of PH and to determine the severity of the right heart involvement. Other tests may be considered, depending on the results of the initial tests.

TREATMENT AND FOLLOW-UP

Rx Treatment Options

Animals with respiratory distress are treated with oxygen, as described in the handout on **Oxygen Therapy**. Some animals may need sedation or need to have their breathing assisted with a ventilator (which requires anesthesia). The cause of the PH must be identified and treated, if possible. The animal may require treatment with multiple drugs to control the underlying problem.

Sildenafil (*Viagra*) can successfully reduce PH in some cases, especially if the primary cause of the PH can be treated and controlled. Sildenafil may cause weakness from low blood pressure (hypotension), but this is uncommon.

Follow-up Care

Patients with an underlying severe respiratory disease usually need frequent follow-up visits. Chest x-rays, laboratory tests, and other tests may be repeated based on the underlying disease.

Prognosis

Prognosis depends on the cause of the PH and how well the animal responds to therapy. PH is a serious condition, and if the underlying problem continues to worsen, so will the PH. The animal will eventually die from the progression of PH. In some cases PH can be reversed, but only if the underlying cause can be cured or very well controlled.

SPECIAL INSTRUCTIONS:

Pulmonic Stenosis

Rebecca E. Gompf, DVM, MS, DACVIM (Cardiology)

BASIC INFORMATION
Description
Pulmonic stenosis (PS) is a congenital heart defect that is present at birth. Stenosis or narrowing may involve the area under the pulmonic valve (subvalvular pulmonic stenosis), which is the valve between the right side of the heart and the pulmonary artery that goes to the lungs. The narrowing may also involve the valve itself (valvular stenosis), if the valve leaflets are fused and do not open normally. The stenosis may occur in the pulmonary artery above the valve (supravalvular stenosis). The most common type of PS is valvular. Occasionally, animals have stenosis at two or three locations.

Stenosis makes it harder for the right heart to pump blood into the lungs; therefore, the right heart becomes thick. As less oxygen reaches the thickened heart muscle, abnormal rhythms (arrhythmias) can occur that result in sudden death. If the tricuspid valve (the valve between the two chambers of the right heart) is abnormal, it may leak (tricuspid regurgitation), which increases the chance that the animal will go into right heart failure.

Causes
PS is common in small-breed dogs and is occasionally found in large-breed dogs. It is rare in cats. Certain breeds are predisposed, such as the English bulldog, Airedale terrier, beagle, Boykin spaniel, boxer, Chihuahua, cocker spaniel, mastiff, Samoyed, schnauzers, and West Highland white terrier. PS can occur spontaneously for unknown reasons.

Clinical Signs
Most dogs with PS have no signs but may have a murmur detected on physical examination. If the PS is severe, the dog may have exercise intolerance, fatigue, and fainting episodes. If right heart failure is present, the abdomen may be distended with fluid. Up to 30% of dogs with PS die suddenly.

Diagnostic Tests
Once a murmur that may be from PS is discovered, further tests are done to confirm the diagnosis and determine the severity of the problem. Chest x-rays and echocardiography (heart ultrasound) with Doppler capabilities are usually performed and may involve referral to a cardiology specialist.

TREATMENT AND FOLLOW-UP

Treatment Options
Dogs with mild PS often require no treatment but may be monitored long term to make sure the problem does not progress. Dogs with valvular PS that is moderate to severe may be referred to a specialist for balloon dilation to open up the valve. Balloon dilation does not cure the problem but will decrease the severity of the PS (often by about 50%) and extend the dog's life. Prior to balloon dilation, a cardiac catheterization is done to make sure that the dog does not have abnormal heart (coronary) arteries. These occur mainly in English bulldogs and, if present, make balloon dilation dangerous.

Surgery may be considered if valvular PS cannot be dilated or if the PS is subvalvular or supravalvular. Surgery can involve removing the valve, applying a patch graft, or possibly inserting a stent (tube) into the narrowed area of the pulmonary artery. These procedures are usually done by veterinary specialists.

Dogs with severe PS and a very thick right heart may not be candidates for either balloon dilation or surgery but may be treated medically with atenolol (to protect the heart). Atenolol may also be started in dogs with moderate to severe PS after successful dilation. Atenolol is continued for life and produces few side effects.

Follow-up Care
Echocardiograms are usually rechecked in animals with mild PS every 3-6 months. If PS worsens, therapy may be considered. After 1 year of age, dogs with mild PS may only need an echocardiogram if signs of exercise intolerance or lethargy develop or the murmur gets louder.

Following balloon dilation, echocardiograms are done 3-6 months later and then yearly. An echocardiogram is commonly repeated after surgical correction once the incision has healed and then yearly.

Prognosis
Dogs with mild PS may live more than 8 years, almost a normal life span. Dogs with very severe PS may survive only a couple of years, and sudden death is more common with severe PS.

Complications of balloon dilation are uncommon, but there is a slight risk that the balloon could break and rupture a vessel. Complications of surgery depend on the surgical procedure done. If the right heart is very thick, the chance of surviving surgery is slim.

Because PS can be inherited, affected animals should not be bred. Female dogs with moderate to severe PS are prone to dying in the last trimester of pregnancy because of the extra blood volume that occurs with pregnancy.

SPECIAL INSTRUCTIONS:

Second- and Third-Degree Heart Block

Rebecca E. Gompf, DVM, MS, DACVIM (Cardiology)

BASIC INFORMATION
Description

Second-degree heart block occurs when *some* of the impulses that arise in the small chambers of the heart (atria) are blocked from entering the lower chambers (ventricles). As a result, the heart rhythm pauses, and the ventricles do not contract. If these pauses are frequent, less blood is pumped by the heart, and the animal cannot exercise and may faint.

With third-degree heart block, *none* of the impulses reach the ventricles; the blockage is complete. The ventricles may take over and produce a heartbeat by themselves, but the heart rate is very slow and the heart does respond when the animal becomes active (so it may faint).

Causes

The cause of these heart blocks may not be found. Second-degree block can arise from increased vagal tone due to irritation of the vagus nerve. Occasionally, high potassium levels (hyperkalemia) can cause heart block, and the block is reversible once the hyperkalemia is treated. Certain heart medications (beta-blockers, calcium channel blockers, digoxin) can slow conduction between the atria and ventricles, and second-degree block can result.

If second-degree block is advanced or if complete block is present, then a major problem exists in the conduction system of the heart. Tumors, infections of the heart valves, and Lyme disease may all cause these advanced heart blocks. Most of the time, however, the cause is never found.

Clinical Signs

Animals with occasional second-degree block often have no signs. If another disease is causing hyperkalemia, signs of that disease are present. Drugs that interfere with conduction in the heart may also cause vomiting, diarrhea, and a lack of appetite.

Animals with advanced second-degree block or complete block are not able to exercise and are lethargic. They may also faint when stressed.

Diagnostic Tests

An electrocardiogram (ECG) is needed to diagnosis these abnormal rhythms. If the ECG is normal and the animal is having fainting episodes, then a 24-hour continuous ECG (Holter monitor) or a 2-week intermittent ECG (event monitor) may be needed to document the cause of the fainting.

Animals with second-degree block may undergo an atropine challenge test to determine whether the block will disappear. If it does disappear, then additional tests are usually performed to identify why the animal has increased vagal tone. Causes of increased vagal tone include diseases of the respiratory, digestive, and neurologic systems.

If the second-degree block is advanced or does not disappear with atropine, or if third-degree block is present, then additional tests may be recommended, such as laboratory tests, chest and abdominal x-rays, and an echocardiogram (heart ultrasound).

TREATMENT AND FOLLOW-UP
Treatment Options

If second-degree block disappears with the atropine challenge test, no further therapy may be required except for treatment of the underlying cause. If episodes of second-degree block are frequent and cause signs, then drugs such as propantheline bromide, albuterol, terbutaline, or theophylline may be tried. Response to these drugs is unpredictable, and side effects include anxiety, excessive panting, decreased appetite, vomiting, diarrhea, and constipation. If the drugs do not help the clinical signs, then insertion of a pacemaker may be necessary.

Animals with third-degree block do not respond to atropine challenge tests or to any of the oral medications listed above. These animals always require insertion of a pacemaker.

Follow-up Care

If the animal responds to the atropine challenge test and the underlying disease resolves with treatment, no further follow-up may be needed. Periodic ECGs may be done to ensure that the second-degree block has not recurred. Animals with second-degree block whose clinical signs respond to oral therapy usually have monthly recheck visits and ECGs to make sure the problem is not advancing to third-degree block.

Animals that receive pacemakers usually have a follow-up visit with the cardiologist at 1 and 3 months. After the pacemaker has received its final adjustments, you will be asked to monitor the heart rate weekly and to have your veterinarian run ECGs every 3 months.

Prognosis

Animals whose second-degree block disappears after an atropine challenge test or following resolution of their underlying disease have an excellent prognosis. Animals with advanced second-degree or complete heart block require pacemaker implantation. Placement of a pacemaker usually results in years of additional life for the patient. The pacemakers that are implanted in dogs and cats have a battery life of about 5 years and are usually replaced after that time.

SPECIAL INSTRUCTIONS:

Sick Sinus Syndrome and Atrial Standstill

Rebecca E. Gompf, DVM, MS, DACVIM (Cardiology)

BASIC INFORMATION

Description

Sick sinus syndrome is a condition in which pauses occur in the heart rate and the heart does not beat. These pauses can be so long that the animal collapses or faints. Very fast heart rates may follow the pauses or occur at other times, and they also result in fainting. *Atrial standstill* occurs when the small chambers of the heart (atria) are not beating at all, which results in a slower than normal heart rate.

Causes

Sick sinus syndrome has been reported in the miniature schnauzer, American cocker spaniel, West Highland white terrier, dachshund, and other small breeds. With this syndrome, the normal pacemaker in the heart does not fire, the backup system does not work, and other areas of the heart that can usually generate a heartbeat do not. During the long pauses, no heart contractions occur, so blood is not pumped to the body and the animal collapses. These pauses may initially be infrequent but tend to increase in frequency with time. The reason the conduction system stops working has not been identified.

Atrial standstill can be caused by increased potassium levels in the body due to problems with the adrenal gland (hypoaldosteronism, Addison's disease), a urethral obstruction, or a blood clot to the rear legs in cats. With extremely high potassium levels (hyperkalemia), the whole heart stops. Atrial standstill can also arise from diseases of the atria, such as tumors. It can occur with a scapulohumeral muscular dystrophy of English springer spaniels.

Clinical Signs

Most affected animals cannot exercise normally and have fainting episodes that increase in frequency over time. Animals with hyperkalemia will have signs of their underlying disease. English springer spaniels with scapulohumeral muscular dystrophy and atrial standstill are young dogs that cannot exercise well; they often have fainting episodes and other muscle problems that limit their mobility.

Diagnostic Tests

An electrocardiogram (ECG) is needed to diagnose these abnormal rhythms. Dogs with fainting episodes may also need to wear a Holter monitor, which is a 24-hour continuous ECG, to document whether their fainting is caused by a slow or a fast heart rhythm or by another disease. An atropine challenge test may be done in dogs with sick sinus syndrome to determine whether it will cause the heart rate to speed up and the pauses to disappear.

Other laboratory tests, chest and abdominal x-rays, and possibly an echocardiogram (heart ultrasound) may be recommended to look for any underlying diseases and to rule out other disorders that can cause similar clinical signs.

TREATMENT AND FOLLOW-UP

Treatment Options

Some cases of sick sinus syndrome may be managed for a period of time on drugs that increase the heart rate (similar to atropine). Examples include propantheline bromide, albuterol, terbutaline, and theophylline. Even dogs that do not respond to an atropine challenge test may respond to these drugs for awhile. Side effects of these drugs include anxiety, excessive panting, lack of appetite, vomiting, diarrhea, and constipation.

If these drugs do not work or stop working, your pet may be referred to a veterinary specialist for insertion of a pacemaker. Pacemakers stabilize the heart and prevent the pauses from occurring. Additional drugs (beta-blockers or calcium channel blockers) may be needed for periods of fast heart rates.

Atrial standstill caused by other diseases usually improves or resolves once the underlying problem is treated. English springer spaniels and dogs with atrial standstill from heart problems require a pacemaker to stabilize their heart rate.

Follow-up Care

When sick sinus syndrome is treated with medications, ECGs are initially done at least monthly. If any additional fainting episodes occur, ECGs are done more frequently. Other monitoring is based on the underlying disease.

Following implantation of a pacemaker, recheck visits are usually scheduled at 1 and 3 months. After the pacemaker has received its final adjustments, you will be asked to monitor the heart rate weekly and to have your veterinarian run ECGs about every 3 months.

Prognosis

Animals with sick sinus syndrome that have fainting episodes eventually need a pacemaker, because medications rarely provide good long-term results. Animals with atrial standstill have an excellent prognosis if their underlying problem can be corrected. Dogs with atrial standstill from heart disease have a guarded prognosis and will require a pacemaker. Placement of a pacemaker usually results in years of additional life for the patient. Pacemakers typically have a battery life of about 5 years and are usually replaced after that time.

SPECIAL INSTRUCTIONS:

Sinus Arrhythmia

Rebecca E. Gompf, DVM, MS, DACVIM (Cardiology)

BASIC INFORMATION

Description

Dogs can have several different (yet normal) rhythms to their heartbeats. Cats, however, should always have a very regular heartbeat, just as people do. When the heart rate is very regular, there is no variation in the time between beats, and the rhythm originates in the usual place in the heart (sinus node), the rhythm is called a *sinus rhythm*. The heart rate can speed up with exercise or slow down with sleep, but the time between beats at a given rate does not vary.

The word *arrhythmia* refers to an irregular heartbeat. Dogs and cats with a sinus arrhythmia have times when their heart beats faster and times when it beats slower. In contrast to a normal sinus rhythm, there is a variation in the time between the heartbeats.

Causes

The most common cause of sinus arrhythmia in the dog is increased vagal tone. The vagus nerve supplies many different areas of the body and can be stimulated when a disease occurs in any of these body systems. The most common diseases that increase vagal tone are gastrointestinal, respiratory, neurologic, and eye diseases. Heart disease is a very uncommon cause of sinus arrhythmia in the dog.

When the vagal nerve is stimulated, it causes variation in the time between heartbeats. This variation in time may be associated with breathing, or it may have no distinct pattern. If no pattern is detected, it is difficult to tell whether the rhythm is a sinus arrhythmia or a more pathologic (serious or dangerous) arrhythmia. Not being able to differentiate between sinus arrhythmia and a pathologic arrhythmia is of concern to your pet's veterinarian.

Increased vagal tone can occur in cats from the same diseases as in dogs, but sinus arrhythmia caused by increased vagal tone is very uncommon in cats. Sinus arrhythmia in the cat usually indicates that an underlying heart disease is present.

Clinical Signs

Dogs with a sinus arrhythmia often have no clinical signs from the arrhythmia itself, but they may have signs of an underlying disease. On physical examination, your veterinarian may detect a random pattern of heartbeats that indicates an abnormal rhythm and problems in one or more of the body systems that affect vagal tone.

Cats with a sinus arrhythmia may have signs of heart disease. They may be quieter than usual and lack the energy to exercise. Breathing may be faster and harder than usual. Some cats with heart disease also cough.

Diagnostic Tests

The only test that can tell a sinus arrhythmia from another, more pathologic rhythm is an electrocardiogram (ECG). The sinus arrhythmia is easily differentiated from other rhythms with this very simple test. If a sinus arrhythmia is detected on the ECG, further testing may or may not be indicated. Depending on the clinical signs, laboratory tests and chest and abdominal x-rays may be recommended, as well as an echocardiogram (heart ultrasound) in cats.

TREATMENT AND FOLLOW-UP

Treatment Options

Since a sinus arrhythmia causes no clinical problems in dogs, no treatment is required. The underlying problem causing the sinus arrhythmia may require treatment; however. In cats, no specific treatment is usually administered for the sinus arrhythmia, but therapy is started for the underlying heart disease.

Follow-up Care

Your dog or cat may need additional ECGs to monitor the sinus arrhythmia if it has a very erratic rhythm. Periodically repeating the ECG is the only way to make sure another, more pathologic rhythm is not present. Other follow-up visits, monitoring, and testing may be required, depending on the cause of the sinus arrhythmia or the underlying disease.

Prognosis

Prognosis is excellent in dogs, because a sinus arrhythmia causes no clinical problems. Prognosis in cats depends on the severity and type of underlying heart disease present.

SPECIAL INSTRUCTIONS:

Sinus Bradycardia

Rebecca E. Gompf, DVM, MS, DACVIM (Cardiology)

BASIC INFORMATION

Description

Bradycardia is a heart rate that is slower than normal for the size of the animal and for the activity being performed. If the slow heartbeat originates from the normal location (sinus node) in the heart, it is called a *sinus bradycardia*. The rhythm of the slow heart rate may be regular or irregular.

Dogs' heart rates can fall as low as 20 beats per minute if they are sound asleep, and cats' heart rates are also reduced during sleep. More active and physically fit animals also have slower resting heart rates. Heart rates are usually higher in smaller and younger animals. Your veterinarian will take these factors into consideration when determining whether your animal's heart rate is too slow.

Causes

The most common cause of sinus bradycardia is increased vagal tone. The vagus nerve can be stimulated by gastrointestinal, respiratory, neurologic, and eye diseases, as well as head trauma. Other diseases that can cause sinus bradycardia include hypothyroidism (low thyroid hormone levels), low body temperature, and increased blood potassium levels from various conditions. Certain drugs (narcotics, beta-blockers, calcium channel blockers, digoxin) can also cause sinus bradycardia.

Occasionally sinus bradycardia is associated with underlying heart diseases, such as problems in the conduction system of the heart, advanced heart failure, or other heart problems.

Clinical Signs

Most animals have no clinical signs from the sinus bradycardia but have signs of their underlying disease. Occasionally dogs show weakness, exercise intolerance, or fainting. Cats may be quieter than usual. Some animals have signs of heart disease, such as lethargy, decreased appetite, increased breathing rate and effort, or coughing. On physical examination, the animal's heart rate is slower than normal.

Diagnostic Tests

An electrocardiogram (ECG) will reveal whether your animal has a sinus bradycardia or a more pathologic abnormal rhythm (arrhythmia). Once a diagnosis of sinus bradycardia is made, an atropine challenge test may be done to determine whether increased vagal tone is the cause. The test is positive if the bradycardia disappears (heart rate speeds up) after atropine is given. If it is positive, further tests may be recommended based on the clinical signs.

If the test is negative, then more tests are usually performed to look for a cause. These may include routine laboratory tests, hormonal assays, and chest and abdominal x-rays. If heart disease is detected, an echocardiogram (heart ultrasound) is usually recommended.

TREATMENT AND FOLLOW-UP

Treatment Options

Often, if the sinus bradycardia disappears with the atropine challenge test, further therapy for the slow rate is not needed. However, treatment of the underlying cause of the sinus bradycardia is usually required.

If the sinus bradycardia is causing clinical signs and does not disappear with atropine, certain drugs (such as propantheline bromide, albuterol, terbutaline, or theophylline) may be tried. These drugs may or may not work to speed up the heart rate. Side effects include erratic results, anxiety, excessive panting, decreased appetite, vomiting, diarrhea, and constipation. If the drugs do not help and the animal is having signs from the slow rate, referral may be recommended to a veterinary specialist for possible insertion of a pacemaker.

Follow-up Care

Repeated ECGs are used to monitor the animal's heart rate and response to therapy. A Holter monitor, which is a 24-hour, continuous ECG recording device, may be recommended in some patients to make sure that the heart rate increases adequately during routine activities.

If a pacemaker is implanted, then monthly ECGs are usually done by your veterinarian, and recheck visits with the specialist are scheduled at 3, 6, and 12 months during the first year to make any necessary adjustments.

Prognosis

Since sinus bradycardia usually develops from diseases that increase vagal tone, the prognosis depends on what disease is present and how the animal responds to therapy. If the sinus bradycardia is not causing problems in these cases, the prognosis is excellent.

If the sinus bradycardia requires either medical therapy or placement of a pacemaker, prognosis depends on the response to the therapy. Medical management of patients with clinical signs from the bradycardia may be successful for only 6-12 months, after which a pacemaker may be needed. Prognosis after pacemaker implantation is excellent, with most animals living years longer. Eventually, however, heart function may worsen or the animal may develop other cardiac diseases that affect the prognosis.

SPECIAL INSTRUCTIONS:

Subaortic Stenosis

Rebecca E. Gompf, DVM, MS, DACVIM (Cardiology)

BASIC INFORMATION
Description
Subaortic stenosis (SAS) is a congenital heart defect that is usually present at birth. Stenosis is a narrowing of the area below the aortic valve, which is the valve that sits between the left side of the heart and the aorta. The stenosis is caused by a fibrous ring of tissue that forms below the valve. The severity of the stenosis depends on the amount of fibrous tissue in the ring. The less tissue that develops, the less severe the SAS and the later problems are likely to occur. The more tissue present, the more severe the defect and the earlier it can be detected.

The fibrous ring in SAS causes the left side of the heart to work harder to pump blood through the narrowed area. As a result, the left heart becomes thickened (hypertrophied). When less oxygen reaches the thickened heart muscle, abnormal rhythms (arrhythmias) can occur that may lead to sudden death. Occasionally, stenosis can arise if the aortic valve does not form properly and is stiff.

Causes
SAS can occur spontaneously in any dog for unknown reasons. It is rare in cats. SAS is an inherited problem in some large-breed dogs, such as the boxer, bull terrier, German shepherd dog, golden retriever, Great Dane, mastiff, Newfoundland, Rottweiler, and Samoyed. English bulldogs may also have a genetic predisposition to SAS.

Clinical Signs
Most dogs with SAS have no clinical signs. In some dogs, a murmur may be detected when the puppy is very young; in others, a murmur is not detected until the dog is about 1 year of age. Therefore, it is important to screen all dogs of breeds that are genetically predisposed to SAS after 1 year of age.

Dogs with severe SAS may experience exercise intolerance or lethargy, fainting episodes, or sudden death. A few dogs have an increased rate and effort of breathing from left heart failure.

Diagnostic Tests
If a murmur has been detected that could be from SAS, further tests are usually needed. Chest x-rays are commonly done to rule out other congenital heart defects. Echocardiography (heart ultrasound) with Doppler capabilities is usually needed to diagnose the problem and determine its severity. Severe and moderate SAS may be detected with routine echocardiography equipment; however, referral to a veterinary specialist may be recommended if mild SAS is suspected.

TREATMENT AND FOLLOW-UP
Treatment Options
Dogs with mild SAS often require no treatment. In dogs with moderate to severe SAS, balloon dilation may be considered, but the long-term results from balloon dilation are no usually better than with medical management. Most of these dogs are started on atenolol, a beta-blocker drug that helps the heart. The side effects of atenolol are rare and usually temporary; however, if any exercise intolerance or decreased appetite occurs, notify your veterinarian.

Dogs with SAS are at a higher risk for infection of the aortic valve than healthy dogs, so they may be given antibiotics when surgery, teeth cleaning, or tooth extractions are performed or if any wounds occur.

Follow-up Care
For puppies with mild SAS, an echocardiogram is often repeated at 1 year of age. If SAS worsens during the first year, medication may be started. For dogs with moderate to severe SAS that have been started on atenolol, electrocardiograms (ECGs) are often done every 3-6 months in an attempt to detect any arrhythmias that could cause sudden death. Medications may be added or adjusted if an abnormal heart rhythm is detected. Yearly echocardiograms are also typically done in these dogs to evaluate how well the left heart is working.

Prognosis
Dogs with mild SAS often have close to normal life spans. Occasionally, a dog with mild SAS dies suddenly, but this is uncommon. The more severe the SAS, the shorter the life span. Dogs with very severe SAS may live only 1-2 years; however, some of these dogs survive up to 4 years with atenolol therapy. Dogs with severe SAS tend to die suddenly from arrhythmias, but a few develop left heart failure that can be stabilized for awhile with medications.

Any dog with SAS, even if it is mild, should not be used for breeding. In some large-breed dogs, such as the Newfoundland, 50% of the litter can inherit the defect from an affected parent.

SPECIAL INSTRUCTIONS:

Systemic Hypertension

Rebecca E. Gompf, DVM, MS, DACVIM (Cardiology)

BASIC INFORMATION

Description

Systemic hypertension (SH) is elevated blood pressure (BP), defined as a systolic BP greater than 180 mm Hg or a diastolic BP greater than 95 mm Hg. In dogs and cats pressure is measured with a BP cuff in a manner similar to that in people, but special equipment must be used to detect blood flow in their tiny arteries. SH can cause damage to the kidneys, eyes, heart, and other organs.

Causes

In both dogs and cats, SH can be associated with chronic kidney disease or be idiopathic, which means that a primary cause cannot be found. In dogs, hyperadrenocorticism (Cushing's disease) and a tumor of the adrenal gland (pheochromocytoma) can cause SH. In cats, hyperthyroidism is a cause. Hypertension is a rare complication of some medications.

Clinical Signs

SH does not cause any clinical signs until a serious problem occurs. In some animals, the first sign is detachment of the retinas of the eyes, with sudden blindness. Other sign of the underlying disease may be present. (See also the handouts on **Hyperadrenocorticism in Dogs, Hyperthyroidism in Cats, Chronic Kidney Disease in Dogs,** and **Chronic Kidney Disease in Cats.**) Dogs with pheochromocytoma have vague symptoms that may include lethargy and weakness. A few animals with chronic SH develop left-sided heart failure and show signs of exercise intolerance, increased respiratory rate and effort, and coughing.

Diagnostic Tests

Hypertension is confirmed by repeated BP measurements. Once the diagnosis is established, further tests are needed to find the underlying cause. These may include routine laboratory and urine tests, thyroid tests (in cats), chest x-rays, and cortisol tests (in dogs). Abdominal x-rays and ultrasound studies may also be recommended. An echocardiogram (heart ultrasound) is often done in animals with signs of heart failure or with murmurs detected on physical examination. A diagnosis of idiopathic hypertension is reached only if all other test results are normal.

TREATMENT AND FOLLOW-UP

Treatment Options

Treatment is indicated in all affected animals to prevent further damage to various organs from the hypertension. The goal is to reduce the systolic BP to less than 160 mm Hg. Hypertension in most cats responds well to oral amlodipine given once or twice daily. The dosage and frequency are determined by repeated BP measurements. Amlodipine rarely causes side effects, but a few cats can become weak if hypotension (low BP) develops. Notify your veterinarian if your cat seems lethargic after starting the drug. If the amlodipine does not work, it may be replaced or combined with an angiotensin-converting enzyme (ACE) inhibitor. Occasionally, beta-blocker drugs are used, alone or in combination with other drugs.

Dogs are similar to people in that no single drug works all the time in every dog. Dogs may need a combination of amlodipine and an ACE inhibitor to control their SH. A few dogs may have beta-blockers added to their therapy. In dogs with SH that is refractory to the most common therapies, hydralazine can be tried. All these drugs can cause hypotension, so notify your veterinarian if your dog acts weak after starting them. Hydralazine also causes vomiting and diarrhea in about half of treated dogs, so it is not well tolerated. Research is being done to find other drugs that may control SH in dogs.

If a cause of the SH is found, then it is also treated. If the underlying cause can be cured (such as hyperthyroidism) or controlled (such as hyperadrenocorticism), then the SH may eventually disappear, and antihypertensive drugs may be discontinued.

Follow-up Care

BP is commonly monitored every 7-14 days until normal, after which it is measured every few months for awhile. If the hypertension remains well controlled, BP monitoring may eventually be decreased to every 6 months. The frequency of follow-up visits also depends on the underlying disease and what is required to treat that disease.

Prognosis

Patients with idiopathic SH have a good prognosis if the SH can be controlled with medication. Prognosis is variable in patients whose SH is associated with other diseases, depending on their severity. If the animal has gone acutely blind from detached retinas, the retinas can reattach if the SH is diagnosed early and treated aggressively and quickly. It is rare that cats regain sight, even with the adequate therapy; however, some dogs may regain vision.

SPECIAL INSTRUCTIONS:

Tetralogy of Fallot

Rebecca E. Gompf, DVM, MS, DACVIM (Cardiology)

BASIC INFORMATION
Description
Tetralogy of Fallot is a congenital heart defect that is present at birth. It arises from three primary, spontaneous defects and a fourth defect that results from the other three. The three main defects are *pulmonic stenosis,* which is a narrowing of the pulmonary artery, which travels from the right side of the heart to the lungs; an *overriding aorta,* in which the aorta is too large and drains blood from both the right and left sides of the heart; and a *ventricular septal defect,* which is a hole between the two large chambers of the heart. The fourth defect is *thickening of the right ventricle,* which arises from the need to generate more energy to push blood into the aorta through the narrowed pulmonary artery.

Cause
Tetralogy of Fallot is inherited in some breeds, but the inheritance pattern is not well understood. Exposure of a pregnant animal to certain toxins, infections, or drugs can theoretically affect heart development and allow a tetralogy of Fallot to occur.

Tetralogy of Fallot occurs because the two main vessels leaving the heart, the aorta and the pulmonary artery, do not divide equally during the heart's development. As a result, the aorta is too large and the pulmonary artery is too small. Since the aorta is too big, it has an opening into both of the ventricles (larger chambers) of the heart, and unoxygenated blood from the right heart mixes with oxygenated blood from the left heart. This mixing of blood causes the gums to be blue, hence the term "blue baby." Because the pulmonary artery is narrow, less blood reaches the lungs to be oxygenated, which also contributes to the lack of oxygen entering the body. The severity of the pulmonic stenosis determines the degree to which an animal is clinically affected.

Clinical Signs
Animals with tetralogy of Fallot are smaller than their littermates, and some remain stunted. They also cannot keep up with their littermates when they play and run. Eventually the animal may have fainting episodes and rapid breathing from the lack of oxygen. On physical examination, a heart murmur may be heard, and the membranes in the mouth and around the eyes appear bluish.

Diagnostic Tests
Chest x-rays are commonly performed if a heart murmur is detected. An echocardiogram (heart ultrasound) with Doppler capabilities usually confirms the diagnosis and the severity of the problem. Because many veterinarians do not have the Doppler equipment, your pet may be referred to a veterinary specialist for the procedure. Laboratory tests may be recommended to evaluate the body's response to the decreased oxygen levels.

TREATMENT AND FOLLOW-UP
Treatment Options
Animals with tetralogy of Fallot are treated medically. Children with this condition undergo complete repair via open heart surgery, but dogs and cats do not tolerate being on a heart bypass machine long enough to do a total repair of their defects. Some surgeries have been tried to shunt extra blood through the lungs, but these are not routinely done in animals. In some cases, the pulmonic stenosis may be treated by balloon dilation, to increase the amount of blood going to the lungs and thereby reduce the animal's symptoms.

Two types of medical treatment may be used. When the body senses that less oxygen is being delivered to the tissues, it starts making more red blood cells. If too many red blood cells circulate in the bloodstream, the blood thickens like sludge, and seizures can arise from blood clots and strokes. In these patients, blood is periodically removed (phlebotomy) to lower the number of red blood cells. Some animals may also be given a drug (hydroxyurea) that decreases the amount of red blood cells produced.

Follow-up Care
Animals with tetralogy of Fallot are monitored frequently to make sure their red blood cell count does not become too high. The older the animal, the more frequently it must be checked.

Prognosis
Animals with a sedentary lifestyle may tolerate this problem and live for 5 years or longer. However, most animals develop serious signs at 1-2 years and die suddenly between 1 and 5 years of age from blood clots, sludging of the blood, abnormal heart rhythms, or chronic lack of oxygen in the body.

Because this congenital heart defect may be inherited, these animals should not be bred. Females with tetralogy of Fallot are likely to die during the last trimester of pregnancy because of the increased demands put on their hearts from the developing fetuses.

SPECIAL INSTRUCTIONS:

Tricuspid and Mitral Valve Dysplasia

Rebecca E. Gompf, DVM, MS, DACVIM (Cardiology)

BASIC INFORMATION

Description

The mitral valve is the valve between the two chambers on the left side of the heart, and the tricuspid valve separates the two chambers on the right side of the heart. Valves function to keep blood flowing in one direction through the heart and to the lungs and body. Dysplasia is malformation of the valve that results in stiffness and decreased ability to open properly, leakage, or both. Dysplasia is a congenital defect that is present at birth.

When dysplasia causes the valves to leak, blood flows in the wrong direction. This increases the workload of the heart and makes the affected side dilate. Eventually right- or left-sided heart failure may occur. If the valve is also stiff and does not open adequately, the large chamber (ventricle) on the affected side of the heart does not fill properly with blood. This also contributes to heart failure.

Causes

Most of these defects are spontaneous and occur randomly. They may be inherited in some breeds, such as the Labrador retriever, bull terrier, German shepherd dog, golden retriever, Great Dane, mastiff, Newfoundland, Old English sheepdog, Rottweiler, and Weimaraner. They have also been reported in cats.

Clinical Signs

Most puppies and kittens have no signs, but a murmur may be discovered on physical examination. If the dog or cat is older, signs of heart failure may be present. With mitral dysplasia, most animals are normal until they develop signs of left heart failure by 6-9 months of age. Exercise intolerance, lethargy, labored breathing, increased respiratory rate, and coughing may be noted.

Animals with mild tricuspid dysplasia may never develop signs. Animals with more severe tricuspid dysplasia are often normal until their right atrium enlarges and develops an abnormal heart rhythm called *atrial fibrillation*. This often occurs between 4 and 7 years of age. Once atrial fibrillation is present, exercise intolerance, lethargy, and abdominal fluid may develop. Cats may develop fluid in their chest and have trouble breathing.

If the animal has a second congenital heart defect, such as an atrial septal defect, fatigue and bluish discoloration of the gums may be noted.

Diagnostic Tests

If a heart murmur is discovered, chest x-rays and an echocardiogram (heart ultrasound) with Doppler capabilities are often needed to identify the exact defect and determine its severity. An electrocardiogram (ECG) is done if an arrhythmia is detected.

TREATMENT AND FOLLOW-UP

Treatment Options

Treatment is usually given to animals that are in heart failure. Once left or right heart failure develops, the following medications may be started:

- An angiotensin-converting enzyme (ACE) inhibitor, such as enalapril or benazepril, helps control fluid accumulation and improves the function of the failing heart. The main side effect is weakness from hypotension (low blood pressure).
- Diuretics, such as furosemide or thiazides, are used to decrease fluid accumulation in the lungs or other parts of the body and may be combined with spironolactone (another diuretic). Side effects include dehydration and electrolyte abnormalities. These drugs also increase water consumption and urine output, so provide plenty of water at all times.
- Pimobendan increases the heart's ability to pump blood and may improve the animal's quality of life. Most dogs and cats tolerate this drug very well, but watch for any decrease in appetite, vomiting, or diarrhea.
- If the animal is in atrial fibrillation, digoxin may be used alone or combined with a beta-blocker, or a calcium channel blocker (diltiazem) may be used to slow the heart rate.

If the dysplastic valve is stiff and does not open properly, your animal may be referred to a specialist for possible balloon dilation. In the United States, surgery to repair or replace these valves can be done at only a few veterinary specialty facilities.

Follow-up Care

Yearly echocardiograms are often recommended for animals with mild dysplasia to monitor their heart function and any changes in the heart. More frequent monitoring and testing are needed for animals in heart failure. (See also the handouts on **Congestive Heart Failure**.)

Prognosis

Animals with mitral valve dysplasia usually develop left heart failure before 6-9 months of age and rarely survive past 1 year even with therapy. Animals with mild tricuspid dysplasia typically have no problems, but dogs with more advanced tricuspid dysplasia may develop atrial fibrillation between 4 and 7 years of age. Once atrial fibrillation develops, right heart failure eventually occurs. With medical management, these dogs usually live an additional 6-12 months.

SPECIAL INSTRUCTIONS:

Ventricular and Atrial Septal Defects

Rebecca E. Gompf, DVM, MS, DACVIM (Cardiology)

BASIC INFORMATION

Description

Ventricular and atrial septal defects are congenital heart deformities that are present at birth. An atrial septal defect (ASD) is a hole in the membrane between the atria, the two smaller chambers of the heart. An ASD can be any size and can be located in different parts of the membrane.

A ventricular septal defect (VSD) is a hole in the septum, the tissue that separates the two larger chambers of the heart (the ventricles). Most VSDs are small and are located just below the aortic valve.

Causes

Some breeds of dog develop ASDs and VSDs because defective genes cause the holes to form while the heart is developing. If a pregnant dog is exposed to certain toxins, infections, or drugs while the puppies' hearts are developing, then ASD or VSD could also occur. Most of the time, the cause of the VSD and ASD is not known.

Clinical Signs

Most ASDs are small and do not cause much of a problem and may not produce a murmur. They may be discovered as an incidental finding when your dog has an echocardiogram (heart ultrasound) for another reason. If the ASD is large or is associated with other congenital heart defects, signs of right- or left-sided heart failure may be present. These signs include increased rate and effort of breathing, possibly coughing, and exercise intolerance. Cats are more prone to large ASDs associated with other congenital defects and are more likely to have signs of heart failure.

Most VSDs are small but cause loud murmurs that are detected on a physical examination. Most dogs and cats with small VSDs never have clinical signs; however, if the VSD is large or is associated with other congenital heart defects, the dog or cat can develop signs of left or right heart failure.

Diagnostic Tests

If your animal has a murmur typical of an ASD or VSD, your veterinarian may recommend chest x-rays followed by echocardiography with Doppler capabilities. Not all veterinarians have the equipment needed to perform this last test, so you may be referred to a veterinary specialist for the procedure. These tests usually confirm the diagnosis and determine the size of the ASD or VSD.

If an abnormal heart rhythm (arrhythmia) is detected, an electrocardiogram (ECG) may be done. If the ASD or VSD needs to be repaired via surgery or catheter occlusion, then laboratory tests are often done prior to anesthesia. A cardiac catheterization procedure is also usually performed prior to repair of the defect.

TREATMENT AND FOLLOW-UP

Treatment Options

Small ASDs and VSDs usually are not corrected, because they do not commonly shorten an animal's life span. If the ASD or VSD is large and has resulted in heart failure, the heart failure is treated with diuretics (furosemide), vasodilators (enalapril), and an agent that improves heart contractions (pimobendan). Other drugs may be needed to control any arrhythmias that are present.

Surgical repair of large ASDs or VSDs is usually done at specialized facilities that can perform open-heart procedures on dogs. Only a few such facilities exist in the United States. The dogs must also be large enough to undergo heart bypass surgery.

Some of the larger ASDs and VSDs can be closed with an Amplatzer device that is placed via a cardiac catheter. This treatment option also requires referral to a veterinary cardiologist who can perform the procedure.

Follow-up Care

Yearly x-rays are commonly done in dogs and cats with ASD or VSD to evaluate heart size and to monitor the lungs for signs of heart failure. Notify your veterinarian immediately if any of the clinical signs of heart failure develop.

Prognosis

Animals with a small ASD or VSD often do well and have a normal life span, with no complications. The bigger the hole in the heart, the more likely it is that heart failure will develop, and the younger the animal will be when that failure occurs. Animals with heart failure can often be successfully managed with medications for months or possibly 1 year.

Because ASDs and VSDs are inherited in some breeds, animals with these defects should not be bred, in order to prevent the spread of this problem. A female with a large ASD or VSD is also likely to go into heart failure during the last trimester of pregnancy because of the increased volume of blood her body must handle due to the developing fetuses.

SPECIAL INSTRUCTIONS:

Ventricular Fibrillation and Cardiac Arrest

Rebecca E. Gompf, DVM, MS, DACVIM (Cardiology)

BASIC INFORMATION

Description

Ventricular fibrillation is spasm or vibration of the heart, with no effective heartbeats. It may arise when a ventricular premature contraction (VPC) falls on the beat before it, causing the heart's electrical conduction system to malfunction. As a result, the heart does not contract effectively, and blood is not pumped to the body. In a short time, the heart stops. Cardiac arrest occurs when ventricular fibrillation starts and the pumping of blood stops.

Causes

Problems in the body that cause the ventricles of the heart to become irritated can result in VPCs and ventricular tachycardia. These abnormal rhythms (arrhythmias) can lead to ventricular fibrillation. Examples of such problems include being hit by a car (bruising of the heart), gastric dilation, surgery, pancreatitis, hyperthyroidism (cats), serious infections (sepsis), severe changes in the body's electrolytes (potassium, calcium, magnesium), tumors, and drugs (digoxin, antiarrhythmic drugs, opioids, tricyclic antidepressants).

Other potential causes include decreased blood volume (from bleeding or dehydration), decreased oxygenation of the blood (from respiratory or cardiac problems), decreased blood glucose levels, hypothermia, elevated blood potassium levels, drugs, head trauma, fluid in the sac around the heart, air in the chest, blood clots, and many others.

Heart diseases can also be a cause. Unlike people, dogs and cats rarely have "heart attacks" in which the blood supply to an area of heart muscle is cut off and the heart muscle dies. In animals, ventricular fibrillation and cardiac arrest are more likely to occur with diseases such as dilated cardiomyopathy in big dogs, congenital heart diseases (subaortic or pulmonic stenosis), or advanced valvular disease in small dogs.

Clinical Signs

Signs of underlying disease or fainting episodes may be present in some animals. Other animals have no signs of an abnormal heart rhythm until they suddenly die from ventricular fibrillation. In these cases, the animal initially collapses, becomes unresponsive, and stops breathing. No heartbeat can be felt through the chest wall, and no pulses can be felt in the neck or rear legs.

Diagnostic Tests

An animal that has gone into cardiac and respiratory arrest needs immediate emergency care and resuscitation. (See the handout on Cardiopulmonary Resuscitation.) An electrocardiogram (ECG) is needed to confirm that the heart is in ventricular fibrillation. All other tests are postponed until after successful resuscitation has occurred.

An animal that is successfully resuscitated requires numerous diagnostic procedures to search for a cause and evaluate the effects of the arrest, including laboratory tests, chest and abdominal x-rays, and an echocardiogram (heart ultrasound). Further testing is based on the test results.

TREATMENT AND FOLLOW-UP

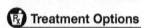 Treatment Options

The only treatment for ventricular fibrillation and cardiac arrest is cardiopulmonary resuscitation (CPR) done by a veterinary team. You can attempt to breathe for your animal through its mouth and do chest compressions, but these are rarely successful. If you find the animal collapsed, seek immediate veterinary care. If CPR is successful, additional therapy is started based on the cause of the cardiac arrest. The animal will remain hospitalized for further treatment and observation.

Follow-up Care

If the animal survives, the type and frequency of follow-up visits depend on the underlying cause of the cardiac arrest and the treatment required.

Prognosis

Prognosis is very poor for an animal that has suffered cardiac arrest from ventricular fibrillation. Even if the arrest occurs in a veterinary hospital, *very few* patients are successfully resuscitated and live to leave the hospital.

About 30% of people who are observed to have a cardiac arrest in the hospital are successfully resuscitated. Of that 30%, only about 10% ever leave the hospital. The most successful resuscitations are usually those done on humans who have suffered a drug overdose, drowning, or electrocution. In animals, the rate of successful resuscitation is much lower.

Prognosis also depends on the cause of the cardiac arrest and how well that problem can be treated. Animals that arrest once tend to arrest again within a short period of time unless the underlying cause is treated successfully. Cats that suffer a cardiac arrest may be blind for 1-3 weeks from lack of oxygen to the brain, but some will recover their eyesight.

SPECIAL INSTRUCTIONS:

Ventricular Premature Contractions and Tachycardia

Rebecca E. Gompf, DVM, MS, DACVIM (Cardiology)

BASIC INFORMATION
Description

Ventricular premature contractions (VPCs) are beats that originate from the large chambers of the heart (ventricles). They occur before the heart has time to fill adequately and alter the pattern of the heartbeat, which can decrease the ability of the heart to pump blood effectively.

Ventricular tachycardia (VT) arises when three or more VPCs occur in a row. The longer and faster the VT, the more the pumping effectiveness of the heart is affected, and the less blood is received by the body. If one of the abnormal beats occurs at the wrong time, it can stop the heart and the animal dies.

A few VPCs can occur daily in normal dogs and cats, but if VPCs become frequent and arise from multiple places in the ventricles, then serious problems can develop.

Causes

Problems in the body that cause the ventricles to become irritated can generate these abnormal heart rhythms (arrhythmias). Examples include being hit by a car (bruising of the heart), gastric dilation, surgery, pancreatitis, hyperthyroidism (in cats), serious infections (sepsis), severe changes in the body's electrolytes (potassium, calcium, magnesium), tumors, and drugs (digoxin, antiarrhythmic drugs, opioids, tricyclic antidepressants). Sometimes the cause cannot be found.

Heart diseases can also cause these arrhythmias. Dilated cardiomyopathy in big dogs, congenital heart diseases (such as subaortic or pulmonic stenosis), and advanced valvular disease in small dogs can result in ventricular arrhythmias. Doberman pinschers, boxers, and German shepherd dogs can develop these arrhythmias as a part of heart diseases specific to their breed.

Clinical Signs

Signs are mainly related to the underlying disease, especially if the VPCs are infrequent. If the VPCs are frequent, fast, and constant (VT), then the animal may experience weakness, fainting episodes, intermittent rapid breathing, or sudden death. In boxers, fainting during exercise, stress, or excitement may be the only sign.

Diagnostic Tests

An electrocardiogram (ECG) is necessary to diagnose these arrhythmias. If an animal is having fainting episodes and the ECG is normal, then a 24-hour Holter monitor or an event monitor may be needed to document the frequency and severity of the arrhythmia. (See the handout on **Electrocardiography**.) Once VPCs or VT is diagnosed, extensive testing is done to find the cause.

Laboratory tests, chest and abdominal x-rays, and an echocardiogram (heart ultrasound) are usually done first. Depending on their results, further tests may be necessary.

TREATMENT AND FOLLOW-UP
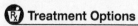 Treatment Options

Whether the VPCs or VT are treated depends on the frequency of the beats (single, infrequent beats are not treated); the rate at which they are occurring (VT is treated); the appearance of the beats (the more bizarre and closer to other beats, the more likely they are to be treated); and the animal's symptoms (fainting animals are treated). Boxers, Doberman pinschers, and German shepherd dogs with VPCs are treated, because sudden death can occur in these breeds.

Dogs with serious arrhythmias must be hospitalized and treated with intravenous lidocaine to stabilize the heart rhythm. Life-threatening ventricular arrhythmias are less common in cats, and hospitalization is primarily needed to treat the underlying problem rather than the arrhythmia.

Once the heart rhythm has been stabilized, several different drugs may be used orally. Sometimes the dog must be switched from one drug to another to control the arrhythmia. Ideally, Holter monitoring is done before and during therapy to evaluate the drug's effectiveness. Oral drugs used in dogs include sotalol, mexiletine, mexiletine-atenolol combinations, and sotalol-mexiletine combinations. Amiodarone is used as a last resort (because of its multiple side effects) and requires referral to a veterinary specialist for its administration. Cats may be given atenolol or sotalol.

Follow-up Care

Frequent ECGs and, ideally, Holter monitoring are performed to assess the response to treatment. The duration of the therapy depends on the underlying problem. If the underlying disease process cannot be cured, the animal often remains on antiarrhythmic therapy indefinitely. Boxers, Doberman pinschers, and German shepherd dogs are usually treated for the rest of their lives.

Prognosis

If the underlying disease is curable, prognosis is excellent, because ventricular arrhythmias usually disappear once the disease is gone. With chronic diseases, prognosis depends on how well the arrhythmia can be controlled. No drug can prevent sudden death in all cases. Affected boxers may do well for more than a year with controlled arrhythmias, but Dobermans may eventually develop dilated cardiomyopathy. Arrhythmias in German shepherd dogs can be hard to control, so their prognosis is more guarded.

SPECIAL INSTRUCTIONS:

SECTION 3

Respiratory System

Section Editor: Ronald M. Bright, DVM, MS, DACVS

Acute Respiratory Distress Syndrome
Allergic Bronchitis in Cats
Allergic Bronchitis in Dogs
Brachycephalic Syndrome
Bronchitis, Acute
Bronchitis, Chronic
Bullous Lung Disease
Diaphragmatic Hernia
Flail Chest
Laryngeal Collapse in Dogs
Laryngeal Paralysis
Laryngeal and Tracheal Neoplasia
Laryngitis and Tracheitis
Lung Lobe Torsion
Lung Tumors

Mediastinal Masses
Nasal and Nasopharyngeal Polyps in Cats
Nasal Tumors, Malignant
Pleural Effusion
Pneumonia, Aspiration
Pneumonia, Bacterial
Pneumonia, Fungal
Pneumothorax
Pulmonary Contusions
Pulmonary Edema
Rhinitis and Sinusitis in Cats
Rhinitis and Sinusitis in Dogs
Tracheal Collapse in Dogs
Tracheal Obstruction
Tracheal Trauma

Acute Respiratory Distress Syndrome

Ronald M. Bright, DVM, MS, DACVS

BASIC INFORMATION

Description

Acute respiratory distress syndrome (ARDS) is a life-threatening form of respiratory failure that results in severe compromise of the animal's ability to take in oxygen. It is associated with a high rate of death.

Following some precipitating event, the blood vessels of the lungs leak fluid into the air spaces of the lungs. This leakage of fluid induces an inflammatory response, which produces microscopic membranes and scarring within the tiny air spaces (alveoli). The available space and surface area for oxygen exchange decrease dramatically. Why this syndrome occurs is poorly understood.

Causes

ARDS often arises after some sort of lung injury or insult, such as:

- Inhalation or aspiration of stomach contents, pneumonia
- Overwhelming systemic infection
- Shock
- Pancreatitis
- Drug reaction or overdose
- Multiple transfusions
- Major trauma or surgery

Clinical Signs

Acute onset of severe respiratory distress is the major sign. Severe distress can occur within hours after the onset of another serious disease (most common), or it can be delayed for several days.

Panting and open-mouth breathing, increased heart rate, anxiety and agitation, and cyanosis (blue gums from lack of oxygen) may be seen. Sometimes wheezes and crackling sounds, especially on expiration (while breathing out), are heard with a stethoscope.

Diagnostic Tests

ARDS may be suspected in any seriously ill animal that develops acute respiratory distress. X-rays of the chest may demonstrate a classic pattern in all lobes of the lungs. Other tests, such as echocardiography (heart ultrasound) and laboratory tests, are often needed to rule out other causes of respiratory distress.

Catheterization and measurement of pressures within major blood vessels can confirm ARDS but requires specialized equipment. Evaluation of fluid taken from the airways in ARDS patients shows a high protein content, which can help confirm the diagnosis.

TREATMENT AND FOLLOW-UP

Treatment Options

Oxygen therapy is necessary and may require unconventional methods of administration. Routine methods of oxygen supplementation (see the handout on **Oxygen Therapy**) may be inadequate in ARDS patients. If blood oxygen levels fail to rise with the use of routine methods, the animal may be anesthetized or heavily sedated, intubated, and placed on a mechanical ventilator; oxygen may then be piped into the lungs under positive pressure. The need for mechanical ventilation and intensive care may necessitate referral of your pet to a veterinary specialty center.

Intravenous fluids must be given carefully, because fluid readily leaves the circulation and moves into the lungs during ARDS. Diuretics may be used to remove excess water from the lungs; these drugs are usually helpful in the initial few days but are of no benefit later in the course. Corticosteroids may be tried, but their benefit is poorly defined. Treatment of the underlying or precipitating condition is also very important.

Follow-up Care

Intensive, continuous monitoring of respiratory rate and effort, blood oxygen levels, heart rate and rhythm, blood pressures, urine output, and other parameters is needed. Laboratory tests and chest x-rays are commonly repeated every 24-48 hours until the animal is stable.

Prognosis

Prognosis for ARDS is guarded (uncertain) to poor. Many animals die from the condition.

SPECIAL INSTRUCTIONS:

Allergic Bronchitis in Cats

Ronald M. Bright, DVM, MS, DACVS

BASIC INFORMATION

Description

Feline allergic bronchitis is inflammation of the lower airways (primarily bronchi). The inflammation is often complicated by narrowing of the airways (bronchoconstriction), which can greatly reduce the intake of oxygen.

Allergic bronchitis has two forms. The acute form (sudden onset, less that 3 months' duration) is associated with reversible inflammatory changes and is also referred to as *feline asthma*. The chronic form (long-term, often intermittent signs) is associated with irreversible airway damage. It can eventually lead to emphysema, a debilitating disease that results from enlargement and dysfunction of the smallest airways in the lungs.

Causes

The acute form may be triggered by a hyperactive immune response to environmental irritants such as dust (including dust from kitty litter), molds, or smoke. In most cases, the specific inciting cause (allergen) is never identified. Mycoplasmal bacterial infections can trigger this disease in some cats.

Clinical Signs

Most cats are young to middle-aged when they are first affected. The cat usually appears healthy and has no systemic signs of illness. Wheezing and coughing are common signs. The cough can be mistaken for retching associated with hairballs. If signs are mild and intermittent, the cat may be normal between episodes.

Occasionally, episodes of breathing difficulty may progress to become severe and life-threatening. The cat may sit hunched over with the neck extended, trying to take in air. Panting and drooling may be noted. The gums may become blue (cyanotic) from inadequate intake of oxygen. Severe episodes may result in collapse and shock.

Diagnostic Tests

A tentative diagnosis may be made from the history and physical examination findings. Physical examination sometimes reveals severe respiratory distress, a "barrel-shaped chest" (from air being trapped within the lungs), and lung sounds that are typical for this condition. Many diagnostic tests are delayed in severely compromised cats until they are stable.

X-rays may or may not reveal changes compatible with allergic bronchitis but help to rule out other causes of coughing. Laboratory tests may be normal or may show evidence of an allergic response or secondary infection. Examination of airway secretions obtained by a tracheal wash or bronchoscopy often identifies inflammation and elevated numbers of white blood cells. The presence of eosinophils helps confirm the diagnosis. Bacterial culture and tests for heartworm and other parasites are often recommended.

TREATMENT AND FOLLOW-UP

Treatment Options

Cats in severe respiratory stress require hospitalization and intensive therapy with oxygen supplementation; injectable, rapid-acting corticosteroids; bronchodilators; and intravenous fluids. Once the cat becomes stable, long-term management is mandatory to control inflammation and prevent or minimize recurrence of the signs.

Long-term therapy includes continuation of steroids, which are given in tablet form or via an inhaler.

- High doses of steroids are used initially, then slowly decreased after the signs abate to the lowest dose that controls the disease. Abruptly decreasing or stopping the steroids may cause severe signs to recur.
- Injectable medications may be considered for cats that do not tolerate inhalant therapy or cannot be given oral medications. Injectable medications are often repeated every 2-8 weeks.
- Although the injectable form is convenient, it is not considered the best choice because of a higher risk for side effects. Some possible side effects are urinary tract infections, diabetes mellitus, and the development of refractory allergic bronchitis.

Cyclosporine may be substituted for corticosteroids in those cats that develop resistance to steroids or require large doses of steroids to control the signs. Cyclosporine blood levels must be adjusted to ideal therapeutic levels, so weekly blood tests are often needed until the target level is reached, and then periodically.

Bronchodilators such as albuterol, theophylline, or terbutaline are frequently given as tablets or via metered-dose inhalers. An antihistamine, cyproheptadine, may also be added. Efforts to reduce potential irritants and allergens in the cat's environment are also very important.

Follow-up Care

Cats with severe signs often require intensive monitoring and hospitalization for several days. Recheck visits are scheduled after discharge. Most cats require periodic monitoring and adjustment of medications for the rest of their lives. Repeated testing may be needed in cats that do not respond to therapy or have recurrent signs.

Prognosis

Most cats respond favorably to therapy, with good control of the clinical signs. Long-term therapy is usually necessary, and occasional relapses are common. If the disease is not controlled, the development of progressive, irreversible changes in the airways and lungs is likely.

SPECIAL INSTRUCTIONS:

Allergic Bronchitis in Dogs

Ronald M. Bright, DVM, MS, DACVS

BASIC INFORMATION

Description

Allergic bronchitis is inflammation of the lower respiratory tract (bronchi) that results from exposure to some type of allergen that is inhaled or carried in the blood. The inflammation may also affect the trachea (windpipe).

Causes

Immunologic stimulation occurs, often from common environmental allergens such as:

* Dusts and molds
* Cigarette smoke
* Aerosol sprays
* Dust and grain mites

Parasites (heartworms) and fungal infections can also cause a hypersensitivity reaction in the airways.

Clinical Signs

Allergic bronchitis most often affects young to middle-aged dogs. It may be more common in obese dogs. Cough is a consistent sign. The cough is usually dry and nonproductive. It may be aggravated by exposure to cold temperatures, exercise, and pressure placed on the trachea or chest. Sometimes respiratory distress occurs, with wheezing and increased effort on expiration (breathing out).

Diagnostic Tests

Routine laboratory, heartworm, and fecal tests, as well as chest x-rays are often recommended to investigate potential causes of a cough. Chest x-rays may be normal or show findings consistent with bronchitis.

Analysis of secretions taken from the trachea and bronchus during a transtracheal wash may reveal a type of white blood cell, the eosinophil. Eosinophils are commonly present with allergic and parasitic diseases and occasionally are seen with fungal infections. The secretions may also be cultured for bacteria. Bronchoscopy, which involves the passage of a fiberoptic scope into the airway, may help eliminate parasites, foreign bodies, a collapsing trachea, or tumors as potential causes of the cough.

If allergic disease is suspected or confirmed, it is important to search for potential allergens in the household. Allergy skin or blood tests may be recommended in some cases. Blood tests for fungal infections may also be considered.

TREATMENT AND FOLLOW-UP

Treatment Options

Antibiotics are administered if a secondary bacterial infection is present. If a fungal disease is present, antifungal drugs are indicated. (See the handouts on **Fungal Pneumonia** and the specific fungal disease involved.) Corticosteroids are usually administered at high doses for 14 days, then slowly tapered. Bronchodilator drugs may be recommended if increased expiratory effort and wheezing are present. Steroids and bronchodilators may be given in oral form or through an inhaler, or both.

Humidification of the environment may help to decrease inflammation and improve clearance of secretions. If an allergen can be identified, it should be avoided or eliminated from the environment. Weight reduction is beneficial in some dogs. Some refractory cases, such as cases of chronic bronchitis or atopic (allergic) dermatitis, may require additional therapy.

Follow-up Care

Initially, close monitoring is needed to evaluate response to treatment and make alterations in medications to ensure that the signs are controlled. The goal of therapy is to aggressively treat the airway inflammation so that a chronic bronchitis does not develop. Notify your veterinarian if any signs recur, because acute relapses may develop that require adjustment of the medications.

Prognosis

Prognosis is often good with the following three measures:

* Removal of the offending allergens from the environment
* Strict compliance with giving medications as prescribed by your veterinarian
* Institution of a strict weight reduction program for obese dogs

SPECIAL INSTRUCTIONS:

Brachycephalic Syndrome

Ronald M. Bright, DVM, MS, DACVS

BASIC INFORMATION

Description

Brachycephalic syndrome occurs when anatomic and acquired abnormalities of one or several structures located in the upper respiratory tract result in partial airway obstruction. The abnormalities make it difficult for the animal to take in air, and progressive breathing problems develop. The syndrome affects primarily the flat-faced, short-nosed breeds of dogs (brachycephalics), which explains its name. Commonly affected breeds include the English bulldog, French bulldog, Boston terrier, pug, Pekingese, shih tzu, boxer, and occasionally other breeds. Rarely, it occurs in brachycephalic cats, such as the Himalayan and the Persian.

Causes

Signs of upper airway obstruction arise from one or a combination of the following conditions:

- Small openings of the nostrils (stenotic nares)
- Elongation of the soft palate
- Eversion or prolapse of laryngeal saccules of the voice box into the tracheal airway
- Underdeveloped, narrowed trachea (primarily in the English bulldog)
- Excessive soft tissue within the throat area that obstructs the airway

Enlarged and inflamed tonsils sometimes contribute to airway obstruction.

Clinical Signs

Because breathing is affected, increased noises are heard from the nose and throat, usually on inspiration (breathing in). Many dogs gag or cough, and some occasionally vomit. Panting is common. When the animal is relaxed or sleeping, loud snoring often occurs.

Some dogs have so much trouble breathing that their tongues and gums turn blue and they become overheated. Engaging in any exercise can cause the dog to collapse. Many affected dogs are obese.

Diagnostic Tests

The presence of these clinical signs in a short-faced breed may allow a tentative diagnosis. Checking for an elongated soft palate, everted saccules, collapse of the larynx, or other problems involving the larynx (such as laryngeal paralysis or the presence of a mass obstructing the opening of the larynx) can be done accurately only with the animal under heavy sedation or briefly anesthetized. Other abnormalities may be diagnosed during an oral examination.

X-rays of the chest help define any additional problems of the trachea (narrowed diameter, collapse) or lungs, as well as the presence of a hiatal hernia, which can accompany this airway problem.

TREATMENT AND FOLLOW-UP

Treatment Options

Emergency therapy may be necessary in a severely compromised animal. Sedation, oxygen therapy, lowering of the body temperature (if the animal is overheated) may all be needed, and possibly a temporary tracheostomy until corrective surgery can be done.

Conservative management in nonemergency cases includes weight loss, exercise restriction, and avoiding situations that may precipitate the respiratory problems (such as excitement or exposure to increased ambient temperatures). Conservative management must usually be followed (in a timely fashion) by surgical correction of the abnormalities to prevent worsening of the problem and development of secondary changes such as collapse of the larynx. In some dogs, esophageal problems, such as hiatal hernia, also require treatment.

Shortening of the soft palate, widening of the nasal openings, and correction of secondary changes in the laryngeal area are done ideally while the animal is young (6-18 months of age) to ensure a better outcome and to prevent any catastrophic respiratory event. Steroids may be given prior to surgery to prevent excessive swelling of the tissues in the throat after surgery. Other drugs may be given to prevent aspiration pneumonia postoperatively.

In high-risk patients (especially English bulldogs), a temporary tracheostomy may be done at the time of surgery and left in place for 24-48 hours postoperatively. This allows time for postoperative swelling to resolve and the airway opening to enlarge. If moderate to severe laryngeal collapse is present, a permanent tracheostomy that bypasses the larynx and provides a permanent opening in the trachea (windpipe) may be necessary.

Follow-up Care

After surgery, very close monitoring is required. Aspiration pneumonia is a serious problem that can occur, and x-rays may be recommended to monitor for this condition. Gagging and coughing are common after surgery and may last for several days. Food is generally withheld for at least 18-24 hours after surgery. Water intake is unrestricted.

Prognosis

Prognosis without surgery is poor, because respiratory distress often worsens over time and may become life-threatening. Most dogs recover from surgery with immediate improvement in their respiratory signs.

SPECIAL INSTRUCTIONS:

Bronchitis, Acute

Ronald M. Bright, DVM, MS, DACVS

BASIC INFORMATION

Description

Acute bronchitis is the sudden onset of inflammation or irritation of the small airways (bronchioles) and medium-sized airways (bronchi) in the lungs. It is usually short-lived and associated with coughing.

Causes

There are many different causes of acute bronchitis, including the following:

- Bacterial or viral infections
- Parasites
- Inhaled foreign bodies
- Irritation from smoke, dust, fumes, or other substances
- A tumor that has grown large enough to put pressure on the bronchus
- Allergies

Clinical Signs

The cough is either dry and hacking or has a moist-sounding component. A moist cough is often associated with mucus production. A dry hacking cough is typical of a virus infection, whereas a moist-sounding cough is more common with a bacterial infection. A cough that is often confused with bronchitis is the "goose-honking" dry cough associated with tracheal collapse in toy breeds of dogs. Sometimes the affected dog is systemically ill, especially if the lungs are also involved.

Diagnostic Tests

Diagnosis of acute bronchitis is largely dependent on the presence of compatible clinical signs and physical examination findings. X-rays of the lungs are not often helpful in confirming the diagnosis but can demonstrate pneumonia that may accompany the bronchitis and can rule out other problems in the chest. Laboratory tests may show an elevated white blood cell count in animals with bacterial infections but may be normal in other cases.

Analysis of secretions taken from the trachea and bronchus during a transtracheal wash can help determine a specific cause. Culturing of the secretions may demonstrate bacteria in some cases. Bronchoscopy, which involves the passage of a fiberoptic scope into the airway, may demonstrate parasitic lesions, a foreign body, a collapsing trachea, or possibly a tumor.

Determining the underlying cause of acute bronchitis can be difficult because there are so many potential causes and the disease is often short lived.

TREATMENT AND FOLLOW-UP

Treatment Options

If an inciting cause can be found and eliminated, the bronchitis usually resolves quickly and spontaneously. If an infection is diagnosed, antibiotics are usually needed. When a foreign body is suspected, bronchoscopy can often be used to retrieve it. Removing the animal from irritants, such as smoke or dust, may allow spontaneous recovery.

Symptomatic treatment may also be tried. Sometimes placing a humidifier near the animal while it is confined in a small space can be helpful. If the cough is the dry hacking type and there is no evidence of a bacterial infection, then cough suppressants may be recommended. If breathing is affected and wheezing is noticed, bronchodilator drugs may be helpful. In some cases, a short-term course of corticosteroids may be warranted.

Follow-up Care

If the cause is identified and specific therapy is instituted, the clinical signs usually resolve. Failure to eliminate the cause and any delay in starting therapy may allow the condition to progress to chronic bronchitis. Recheck visits may be scheduled to monitor response to treatment. Notify your veterinarian if any signs persist or return.

Prognosis

Aggressive treatment of acute bronchitis usually results in complete recovery, especially if the underlying cause is not serious.

SPECIAL INSTRUCTIONS:

Bronchitis, Chronic
Ronald M. Bright, DVM, MS, DACVS

BASIC INFORMATION
Description
Chronic bronchitis is inflammation or irritation of the small airways (bronchioles) and medium-sized airways (bronchi) in the lungs that lasts for longer than 2 months. Chronic bronchitis is associated with a cough that may persist indefinitely, because the cause may never be identified. Pathologic changes (damage from the inflammation) to the airways are irreversible in most cases.

Causes
Usually, the cause is not determined. Chronic bronchitis may be related to inhaled irritants (smoke, dust, fumes), allergies, or chronic infections. In rare cases, it is caused by a congenital abnormality of the airways (primary ciliary dyskinesia) that prevents them from clearing inhaled substances. Pneumonia and tumors do not often cause bronchitis alone; they usually also involve the lungs.

Clinical Signs
Most dogs with chronic bronchitis are middle-aged or older small-breed dogs that are overweight. A chronic, persistent, moist or dry cough is the main sign. Generally the dog's overall health is good. Exercise intolerance may be noted in some dogs. Episodes or spasms of coughing and difficulty breathing may be noted in some instances. Signs may worsen with excitement, stress, exposure to irritants in the air, and secondary infections.

Diagnostic Tests
The diagnosis is often made by excluding other potential causes of chronic coughing, such as heart disease, tumors, pneumonia, collapsing trachea, and other airway problems. X-rays of the lungs may reveal certain changes consistent with a chronic bronchitis. X-rays are also helpful in ruling out other causes of coughing. Laboratory tests may be recommended to look for evidence of infections, allergies, and other conditions.

Analysis of secretions taken from the trachea and bronchi during a transtracheal wash may help determine a cause. Culturing of the secretions may demonstrate bacteria associated with chronic infections of the respiratory tract, such as mycoplasmosis. Bronchoscopy, which involves the passage of a fiberoptic scope into the airway, may help eliminate parasites, foreign bodies, a collapsing trachea,

or tumors as potential causes. Other tests may be recommended to rule out other diseases that can cause a chronic cough.

TREATMENT AND FOLLOW-UP
Treatment Options
Because the cause is not often identified, symptomatic treatment is usually begun. If a cause is found, therapy is also directed at the cause. Potential therapies include the following:
• Obese dogs benefit greatly from a weight-reduction plan.
• Environmental irritants, such as smoke, dust, heat, and low humidity, should be eliminated.
• Humidifiers can be used intermittently while the dog is confined to a small space.
• Antibiotics are used if an infection is suspected or confirmed.
• Cough suppressants may be recommended if no infection is present.
• Drugs used to dilate the bronchioles may help reduce some clinical signs, such as exercise intolerance, breathing difficulty, or wheezing.
• A short course of corticosteroids can be helpful in some cases to decrease the amount of inflammation in the airways; however, they are used cautiously and in situations where the bronchitis is not complicated by respiratory infection, heart disease, or infection elsewhere in the body.

Follow-up Care
Lifelong therapy is usually required to control or minimize the clinical signs. If the disease is not treated adequately, the inflammation usually worsens, so recheck visits and repeated x-rays and testing may be needed to monitor response to therapy. Repeat testing may also be needed if signs flare up and do not respond to the usual therapy. Notify your veterinarian if any signs recur or worsen.

Prognosis
Complete recovery from chronic bronchitis is not a realistic goal, and owners should be prepared for lifelong therapy for their affected pet. Adequate, consistent therapy allows many affected animals to have a good quality of life. It is important that owners comply with prescribed therapies. If an infection is part of the disease, it usually responds to antibiotics, but they may need to be administered for some time.

SPECIAL INSTRUCTIONS:

Bullous Lung Disease

Ronald M. Bright, DVM, MS, DACVS

BASIC INFORMATION

Description

Bullous lung disease is the formation of contained or confined pockets of air and fluid in one or more portions of the lungs. These pockets ultimately form cysts (bullae) that are air-filled and surrounded by normal lung tissue.

When bullous lesions rupture, air escapes into the chest cavity (pneumothorax), which decreases the ability of the lungs to expand. The presence of a large number of cysts within the lungs may also affect normal lung function.

Causes

Bullous cysts can be congenital (present at birth), but most often they are acquired lesions. Inflammation, emphysema, trauma, and unknown factors (idiopathic) can result in their formation. Sometimes a lung fluke (parasite), *Paragonimus kellicotti,* forms inflammatory lesions that become air-filled cysts. Bullae may develop when air enters the central portion of an abscess or tumor in the lung. Large, deep-chested breeds of dogs, such as sight hounds, are predisposed to idiopathic bullous lung disease.

Clinical Signs

Some affected animals have a history of chronic bronchitis, prior chest trauma, or other lung diseases. Significant leakage of air into the chest cavity can cause severe respiratory distress, with increased respiratory rate and effort, cyanosis (blue gums from lack of oxygen), and collapse. Occasionally, bullae are found as incidental lesions on chest x-rays, and the animal has no clinical signs.

Diagnostic Tests

Routine laboratory tests and chest x-rays are often recommended to investigate potential causes of the respiratory distress. Chest x-rays may show one or more air-filled cystic structures in the lungs. Free air in the chest and lung collapse are indicative of pneumothorax. Animals in severe distress often require therapy, such as removal of the free air, before x-rays and other tests can be performed.

If fluid is also present in the chest cavity, it may be withdrawn and analyzed. Sometimes fluke eggs may be found when the fluid is examined microscopically. Direct aspiration of a bulla with a needle is not recommended, because it can lead to significant escape of air from the cyst and pneumothorax.

TREATMENT AND FOLLOW-UP

Treatment Options

Pneumothorax is usually treated as an emergency, with aspiration of air via a syringe and needle (thoracentesis). If air accumulates quickly after withdrawal of large amounts by thoracentesis, insertion of a chest tube is necessary to allow more effective evacuation of the air. If air continues to leak or large amounts of air accumulate, the chest tube may be hooked to a continuous suction device.

Some cystic lesions heal spontaneously after several days. As the bullae scar over, the leakage of air begins to subside. If the pneumothorax does not resolve within 48-72 hours or if evacuation efforts do not keep up with leakage of air, open chest surgery is done. It is usually necessary to enter the chest cavity through the sternum (breast bone), so that lung lobes on both sides of the chest can be inspected for bullae. A portion of a lung lobe or an entire lobe (containing one or several bullae) may need to be removed. In instances in which multiple, intact cysts are present throughout the lungs, the surfaces of the lungs may be rubbed with a rough piece of surgical gauze so that they subsequently stick to the lining of the chest wall (pleurodesis). Pleurodesis is an attempt to obliterate the space into which air can escape if a bulla ruptures in the future.

Follow-up Care

Careful monitoring of respiration, heart rate, blood pressure, lung sounds, color of the gums, and blood oxygen levels is done after surgery. Chest tubes usually remain in place until all air leakage stops. The chest tubes must be carefully monitored to ensure that they are working well and that no air is leaking around or into the tube and back into the chest.

X-rays are repeated to monitor the presence or absence of air in the chest. Most animals remain in the hospital at least 24 hours after chest tube removal, so that they can be closely monitored. The incision is usually rechecked and sutures removed 10-14 days after surgery. X-rays may be obtained again at that time.

Prognosis

It is possible for more bullae to form in different areas of the lung in the future, so x-rays are periodically taken to monitor for their development. If bullae are found on x-rays in the future, no treatment may be recommended unless pneumothorax recurs. One in every eight animals develops a recurrence of a pneumothorax after surgical treatment.

SPECIAL INSTRUCTIONS:

Diaphragmatic Hernia

Ronald M. Bright, DVM, MS, DACVS

BASIC INFORMATION

Description

The diaphragm is the muscle that separates the abdominal cavity and its contents from the chest cavity. A hernia is a disruption of this muscle that allows movement of abdominal organs into the chest cavity. Diaphragmatic hernias may be congenital or acquired. (See the handout on **Peritoneopericardial Diaphragmatic Hernias** for a discussion of congenital hernias.) This handout discusses acquired diaphragmatic hernias, which usually result from trauma.

Causes

Traumatic diaphragmatic hernias can arise from any type of blunt trauma to the abdomen, including an automobile accident, being kicked, or jumping or falling from a high elevation. The last condition is a common cause in cats.

🗎 Clinical Signs

Traumatic diaphragmatic hernias are more commonly seen in animals younger than 2 years of age. The hernia can be discovered within hours or up to several years after the incident. Most of the clinical signs are caused when various abdominal organs are displaced into the chest cavity and cause collapse of the lungs or when the production of fluid further impairs lung expansion. Approximately 40% of animals with a traumatic hernia have some degree of breathing difficulty, ranging from panting to open-mouth breathing.

If the trauma is severe, many animals are in shock and have concurrent injuries, such as fractured ribs, bruising within the lungs, or bleeding from abdominal organs such as the spleen or liver. The gums may be pale or cyanotic (blue from lack of oxygen) in an animal with severe respiratory compromise and/or shock. Occasionally, an affected animal becomes jaundiced or develops a dilated (bloated) stomach that moves into the chest cavity and compresses the lungs.

🐾 Diagnostic Tests

The inciting traumatic event may or may not be witnessed, but a history of trauma may help the veterinarian in formulating a tentative diagnosis. Listening to the chest cavity with a stethoscope may reveal sounds that indicate the presence of fluid and organs in the chest cavity and damage to the lungs.

X-rays often demonstrate a loss of the outline of the diaphragm, the presence of organs and fluid in the chest cavity, and a decreased number of organs in the abdominal cavity. Sometimes a liquid contrast material (a dye that shows up white on x-rays) is injected into the abdominal cavity and x-rays taken shortly afterward show this material in the chest cavity, which indicates a hole in the diaphragm. Barium is sometimes given orally to help demonstrate that the stomach and/or small intestines have moved into the chest.

Fluid in the chest sometimes decreases the accuracy of x-rays, and in this instance ultrasonography is very helpful to clearly delineate a herniation. In rare cases, advanced imaging with computed tomography (CT scan) or magnetic resonance imaging (MRI) may be necessary to define the hernia. Laboratory tests are often recommended to assess the effects of trauma and the hernia on other organs.

TREATMENT AND FOLLOW-UP

℞ Treatment Options

Surgery is the only viable option for correcting a diaphragmatic hernia. The objective of surgery is to return the abdominal organs to the abdominal cavity, inspect the organs of the chest cavity for signs of trauma, and repair the rent in the diaphragm.

The approach for repairing the hernia is usually through the abdomen. If the hernia is thought to be chronic or long-standing, adhesions may have formed that make the surgical correction more challenging. A median sternotomy, which involves splitting the breast bone, may be required for some chronic hernias to improve exposure of the chest cavity.

🐾 Follow-up Care

Postoperative monitoring of cardiac and respiratory function is important. Bleeding (from adhesions broken down during replacement of organs into the abdomen) can result in severe anemia and possibly shock. A chest tube is left in place at the end of the surgery to monitor and remove any air (pneumothorax) or blood (hemothorax) that collects within the chest cavity. Oxygen is often administered in the immediate postoperative period. Accumulation of fluid in the lungs (pulmonary edema) may be a postoperative problem, especially in cats, that requires medical therapy.

Prognosis

Surgical complications are relatively rare, and prognosis is generally good, especially for hernias that have not been present for a long time. If the animal survives the first 24 hours after surgery, the prognosis improves. Older cats and those animals with other serious injuries are more likely to die after hernia repair.

SPECIAL INSTRUCTIONS:

Flail Chest

Ronald M. Bright, DVM, MS, DACVS

BASIC INFORMATION
Description and Cause

Flail chest arises with trauma and occurs when several contiguous ribs are broken in such a way that a segment of the chest wall moves in and out independent of the movement of the remaining normal rib cage. The fractured segment of ribs moves paradoxically, meaning that it moves inward on inspiration (breathing in) and outward on expiration (breathing out), which is opposite to normal chest cage movement.

For this paradoxical movement to occur, a certain amount of damage to soft tissues (muscles, tendons) must also be present. The degree of trauma responsible for multiple rib fractures usually results in damage to the underlying lung tissue.

Clinical Signs

Because of damage to the lungs, difficulty breathing, panting, cyanosis (blue gums caused by lack of oxygen), and open-mouth breathing may occur. Paradoxical movement of a segment of the thorax is always seen. Pain is usually present over the traumatized area, and the animal is often reluctant to move. Other signs of trauma may also be present.

Diagnostic Tests

A preliminary diagnosis may be made based on a history of trauma and the typical clinical findings. Abnormal lung sounds are often heard through a stethoscope. Chest x-rays confirm multiple rib fractures and other lung or chest cavity abnormalities.

TREATMENT AND FOLLOW-UP

Treatment Options

The first objective of emergency care is to ensure adequate intake of oxygen and to treat the animal for shock, often with intravenous fluid therapy and oxygen supplementation. Pain management is very important and is usually accomplished by administration of narcotics and a local anesthetic nerve block during the first several days after injury.

A soft-padded bandage is usually applied around the chest, and the animal may be placed with the affected side down to prevent excessive movement of the flailed segment. An external splint is sometimes used, with sutures being placed around the middle of the fractured ribs and tied to the splint to stabilize the segment. Rarely, the ribs are stabilized with an open surgical approach, using orthopedic fixation devices such as pins. In animals with severe, crushing injuries, the entire fractured segment may be removed and the chest wall reconstructed with a muscle flap or synthetic mesh.

Follow-up Care

Continuous, close monitoring of cardiovascular and respiratory functions (particularly blood oxygen levels) is needed until the animal is stable. The animal may be hospitalized in a 24- hour veterinary facility during this time. Chest x-rays are usually repeated on a daily basis for a few days to evaluate any accompanying lung problems.

Prognosis

Prognosis for recovery from the trauma that produced the flail chest is primarily based on the severity of underlying lung damage and how well it responds to therapy. Cats have a poorer prognosis with multiple rib injuries than with a single fracture. If lung damage is not too severe, recovery can be expected in 10-14 days. Movement of the flail segment usually decreases within that same time period.

SPECIAL INSTRUCTIONS:

Laryngeal Collapse in Dogs

Ronald M. Bright, DVM, MS, DACVS

BASIC INFORMATION

Description

Laryngeal collapse is also referred to *aryepiglottic collapse* or *corniculate collapse*. This condition arises when the cartilages of the larynx (voice box) become weak and lose their structural rigidity. It almost always leads to severe inspiratory distress (difficulty breathing air in). Laryngeal collapse usually occurs in dogs older than 2 years of age, but it may develop earlier in dogs with severe upper airway obstruction from other causes. (See also the handout on **Brachycephalic Syndrome**.)

Causes

Most often, the condition results from chronic airway obstruction related to brachycephalic syndrome. Fatigue of the cartilages that surround the laryngeal opening occurs because of the chronic negative pressures produced by the increased effort needed to take in air. Rarely, the condition can arise from direct trauma to the cartilages.

Clinical Signs

Noisy breathing and difficulty breathing have usually been present for years. A sudden worsening of respiratory distress may occur in dogs with various components of brachycephalic syndrome. Cyanosis (blue color of the tongue or gums caused by lack of oxygen), gagging, choking, vomiting, and restlessness are often seen. Labored, open-mouth breathing; retraction of the lips (indicating great effort is being made to breathe); panting; and elevated body temperature from exaggerated breathing effort may all occur. In severe cases, the animal may collapse and possibly die before therapy can be started.

Diagnostic Tests

A tentative diagnosis is often based on a history of chronic breathing problems in certain breeds. Diagnosis is confirmed by examination of the larynx (laryngoscopy) under anesthesia. X-rays of the chest help define any additional problems of the trachea (narrowed diameter, collapse) or lungs, as well as the presence of a hiatal hernia, which can accompany chronic airway problems.

TREATMENT AND FOLLOW-UP

Treatment Options

Emergency treatment of dogs with acute respiratory distress usually consists of oxygen therapy, sedation, and administration of anti-inflammatory drugs. If these measures are unsuccessful, a temporary tracheostomy may be needed to stabilize the dog until corrective surgery is done.

If the laryngeal collapse is mild, treatment consists of surgical correction of the underlying cause of the problem, such as shortening of an elongated soft palate, enlargment of the external openings of the nose, or removal of any excessive, obstructive tissues within the throat area. In instances of moderate to severe laryngeal collapse, a portion of one of the collapsed cartilages may be surgically removed via an oral approach (through the mouth). In severe cases or if signs persist after surgical therapy, a permanent tracheostomy may be required.

Follow-up Care

Close, continuous monitoring for airway obstruction is required after recovery from surgery. In some animals, a temporary tracheostomy is needed for several days until postoperative swelling subsides. Aspiration pneumonia is a serious problem that may occur.

Following a permanent tracheostomy, it is critical that the new opening be kept clean and that the trachea remain clear of mucus and blood. Postoperative care and monitoring often requires 4-5 days of hospitalization before it is safe to discharge the animal.

- The opening will decrease in size over several months to approximately 30-40% of the original size.
- The dog should not be allowed to engage in swimming, and harnesses (rather than collars) are preferred for restraint.
- The hair around the new opening must be kept short.
- Secretions around the opening sometimes irritate the skin, which can be treated with petrolatum or zinc oxide ointments for a short time.
- In some breeds (pugs, English bulldogs), a significant amount of skin around the new opening must be removed to prevent the excessive skin folds from obstructing the new opening. Overlapping skin folds may also become a problem months to years later and require additional surgery.
- In extremely cold environments or in dusty conditions, a lightweight scarf or wrap should be placed over the opening.
- Most dogs can no longer bark (vocalize).

Prognosis

In mild cases, surgical correction of the elongated soft palate, narrow nasal openings, or redundant tissue around the larynx results in a favorable outcome. In some instances, correction of the underlying abnormalities or partial removal of one of the laryngeal cartilages does not provide enough relief, and a permanent tracheostomy is needed.

Dogs with a permanent tracheostomy can develop life-threatening problems immediately after surgery if a mucus plug or blood clot forms within the trachea. Most dogs that survive the first 5-7 days do well, with few short- or long-term problems. Owners must be very committed to keeping the tracheostomy clean and dry.

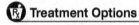

SPECIAL INSTRUCTIONS:

Laryngeal Paralysis

Russell W. Fugazzi, DVM

BASIC INFORMATION

Description

Laryngeal paralysis is inadequate opening of the larynx due to weakness or paralysis of the vocal folds. The disease ranges widely in severity. It can be an inherited (rare) or an acquired disease.

Although many dogs can develop the condition, most are large-breed dogs, such as the Labrador retriever, golden retriever, Afghan, Irish setter, and others.

Affected dogs are usually 9½ years of age or older, and males are affected two to four times more frequently than females. Cats rarely develop the condition.

Causes

The congenital, inherited form is seen in young dogs (usually less than 1 year of age). It occurs mostly in the Bouvier des Flandres, bull terrier, Siberian husky, and Dalmatian. The cause of the acquired form is not often known, so the condition may be called *idiopathic laryngeal paralysis*.

In these cases, it is possible that the muscle responsible for opening the larynx is diseased, or a problem may arise with the nerves that supply this muscle. The muscle eventually shrinks or atrophies. Damage to the laryngeal nerve can be a cause of laryngeal paralysis and may be associated with cancer in the neck area, damage from blunt trauma or bite wounds, and injury acquired during surgery of the neck. Hypothyroidism (low thyroid hormone levels) is present in some affected dogs.

Clinical Signs

Voice change, exercise intolerance, difficulty and noisy breathing, and panting are common signs. The dog produces a raspy, hoarse sound while breathing, especially on expiration (breathing air out). Coughing, gagging, retching, and vomiting may occur. Restlessness and anxiety may be noted.

Sometimes no obvious signs are present at rest, but the dog becomes symptomatic after exercise, excitement, or exposure to warm temperatures. The breathing rate increases rapidly when the dog becomes active, and body temperature may rise. The dog may collapse, and the gums may be blue (cyanotic) if the dog does not take in adequate oxygen.

Diagnostic Tests

A tentative diagnosis may be made based on compatible signs in an older, large dog. Definitive diagnosis is made by direct visualization of the cartilages of the voice box, which are supposed to move outwardly (abduct) on inspiration (while breathing air in). Minimal or complete lack of movement is diagnostic. The vocal cords often fall into the laryngeal opening of the airway on inspiration instead of moving away from the opening.

Other tests may be recommended to search for an underlying cause or accompanying conditions. Such tests may include x-rays or an ultrasound of the neck, thyroid tests, and other preoperative laboratory tests.

TREATMENT AND FOLLOW-UP

Treatment Options

In an emergency situation in which the animal has become stressed and overheated and is in respiratory distress, intensive care with oxygen therapy, sedation, intravenous fluids, and procedures to cool the animal may be necessary. A temporary tracheostomy may be considered in some cases. Once the animal is stable, surgery is often needed to open the airway.

The mainstay of therapy for moderate to severe cases is surgery. Several different surgical techniques may be used. One of the more popular surgical procedures (tie-back technique) consists of permanently pulling one of the laryngeal cartilages out of the airway with suture so that the size of the laryngeal opening is substantially increased.

Mildly affected dogs may benefit from temporary sedation, followed by avoidance of stressful situations and a sedentary lifestyle. The condition often worsens over time, however. Any underlying or ancillary conditions are also treated. Thyroid supplements are started in hypothyroid dogs, but even with appropriate treatment, the laryngeal paralysis remains.

Follow-up Care

A serious potential postoperative complication is aspiration pneumonia, although the incidence is relatively low. The dog may remain hospitalized for 1-2 days after surgery for close monitoring. Water is introduced first. A soft cough is common after drinking, but excessive coughing may indicate aspiration pneumonia. Food is commonly withheld for at least 12-24 hours, depending on how the animal handles water.

Occasionally, a fluid-filled swelling (seroma) develops near the surgical incision within 2-3 days, but it usually resolve spontaneously within 10-14 days. A voice change occurs with some surgical procedures. Following recovery, notify your veterinarian if coughing increases, noisy breathing or other signs return, or activity decreases.

Prognosis

Mildly affected animals may do well (and not need surgery) if clinical signs do not progress.

Most dogs that have the tie-back surgery (almost 90%) experience good results, with improved breathing and increased exercise tolerance. Some hunting and athletic dogs can resume their activities at their previous level of performance.

SPECIAL INSTRUCTIONS:

Laryngeal and Tracheal Neoplasia

Ronald M. Bright, DVM, MS, DACVS

BASIC INFORMATION
Description and Causes
Laryngeal and tracheal tumors are uncommon in dogs and cats. Two benign tumors, osteochondroma of the trachea and oncocytoma (rhabdomyoma) of the larynx, are found in younger dogs. Lymphosarcoma may occur in cats or dogs of any age. Most other tumors occur in older animals; in general, these tumors are more likely to be malignant and locally invasive to surrounding tissues. Examples include the squamous cell carcinoma, adenocarcinoma, fibrosarcoma, mast cell tumor, osteosarcoma, melanoma, plasmacytoma, and chondrosarcoma.

Clinical Signs
With laryngeal tumors, a voice change, swallowing problems, coughing, and difficulty breathing are common. Tracheal masses most often result in difficulty breathing, especially on inspiration (breathing air in). Coughing, noisy breathing, cyanosis (blue gums caused by lack of oxygen), and exercise intolerance can also be associated with obstructive tumors of the trachea.

Diagnostic Tests
Certain changes on the physical examination are suspicious for a laryngeal or tracheal inflammation or tumor, including the following:
- Abnormal respiratory sounds may be auscultated (heard) with a stethoscope.
- Musical or wheezing noises may be heard over the trachea.
- Pressing on the trachea easily elicits a cough from increased sensitivity of the tracheal lining.
- Many tracheal tumors can be palpated (felt), whereas most laryngeal tumors cannot.
- Lymph nodes in the neck may be enlarged with a malignant laryngeal tumor and occasionally with a tracheal tumor.

Further testing is usually needed to confirm the presence of a mass. Routine laboratory tests and chest x-rays may be done to look for evidence of inflammation or tumors elsewhere and to rule out other diseases that cause similar signs. Bronchoscopy (examination of the airway with a fiberoptic viewing scope) often confirms

the presence of a mass, helps define the extent of the tumor, and allows tissue to be obtained for a biopsy. A biopsy and microscopic analysis are needed to determine the tumor type.

TREATMENT AND FOLLOW-UP
Treatment Options
Some laryngeal tumors (oncocytoma) can be surgically removed, although laryngeal function may be impaired. More malignant laryngeal tumors require aggressive surgery (partial or complete removal of the larynx) followed by a permanent tracheostomy. Removal of a portion of the tumor in an attempt to preserve laryngeal function is an option when follow-up chemotherapy is possible (such as with lymphoma or mast cell tumors).

If a tumor is attached to the trachea by a narrow stalk, it may be possible to remove it at the time of bronchoscopy. For larger, broader-based tumors, the mass and a portion of the trachea must often be removed surgically. The greatest amount of trachea that can be removed is eight cartilage rings in length. Most infiltrative tumors require follow-up chemotherapy or radiotherapy because complete removal is not possible at the time of surgery. Chemotherapy, often combined with surgery, is the preferred treatment for some tumors, including lymphoma, mast cell tumors, and plasmacytomas.

Follow-up Care
These patients require intensive postoperative monitoring, because breathing problems are common. Corticosteroids may be recommended to decrease swelling and inflammation while chemotherapy or radiation therapy is proceeding. A temporary or permanent tracheostomy may be required if respiratory problems are severe. Follow-up examinations, repeated laboratory tests, and chest x-rays are often recommended on a regular basis during therapy.
Prognosis
Prognosis for laryngeal oncocytoma is good. Osteochondromas are also associated with a good prognosis if the tumor can be completely removed. Most other laryngeal tumors carry a guarded (uncertain) to poor prognosis. Malignant tumors of the trachea respond variably to therapy and carry a poor prognosis.

SPECIAL INSTRUCTIONS:

Laryngitis and Tracheitis

Ronald M. Bright, DVM, MS, DACVS

BASIC INFORMATION
Description
The terms *laryngitis* and *tracheitis* refer to inflammation of the larynx (voice box) and the trachea (windpipe), respectively. Because they are located close to each other, the larynx and trachea may become inflamed at the same time; this is called *laryngotracheitis*. These conditions may develop acutely (suddenly) or be chronic in nature.

Causes
Laryngotracheitis can be caused by a variety of agent or events, such as the following:
- Primary causes include certain viruses, such as canine distemper and the viruses involved in kennel cough in the dog, and calicivirus and herpesvirus in the cat.
- Inflammation can develop from smoke inhalation, regurgitation, or aspiration of material originating in the esophagus or stomach.
- Placement of an endotracheal tube for anesthetic purposes can irritate the lining of the trachea or larynx.
- Trauma of any kind (blunt, penetrating) can be a cause.
- Some parasitic diseases can cause a tracheitis, especially in younger dogs.

Clinical Signs
A dry cough is commonly noted and may persist despite antibiotic therapy, because often the underlying cause is not bacterial. It is common with laryngitis for other portions of the upper airway (trachea, bronchi, nasal cavity) to be inflamed, so nasal discharge and other signs may be present. Difficulty swallowing and voice changes occasionally accompany laryngitis. If the larynx becomes swollen, breathing may become noisy and difficult, resulting in exercise intolerance. With tracheitis, the windpipe may be so sensitive that any pressure from a collar or excitement may induce a cough.

Diagnostic Tests
Laryngotracheitis may be suspected based on signs of upper respiratory inflammation. The history or presence of other clinical signs may provide clues as to the origin of the inflammation. For example, recent exposure to other dogs may indicate a viral cause, and a history of exposure to smoke may indicate an irritant-induced inflammation. Other tests that may be recommended include the following:
- A fecal examination may reveal parasites or their eggs.
- Chest and neck x-rays may be done to look for signs of pneumonia and other causes of coughing.

- Bronchoscopy (examination of the airway with a fiberoptic viewing scope) or a tracheal wash may be done in chronic cases to obtain material for microscopic examination.
- Laryngoscopy (examination of the larynx) may be recommended if masses or an obstruction is suspected. A biopsy of abnormal tissue may be helpful in making a diagnosis.

TREATMENT AND FOLLOW-UP
Treatment Options
Eliminating exposure to smoke and noxious fumes helps resolve irritant tracheitis. Dogs with this form of tracheitis may also benefit from inhalation of steroid medications. Parasitic tracheitis is usually treated with a combination of drugs and institution of preventive measures.

Acute laryngitis is usually self-limited, but medications that reduce coughing may be helpful. Dogs with either laryngitis or tracheitis often benefit from use of a harness instead of a collar and from rest in a calm, quiet environment.

Most cases of mild trauma resolve with time. Antibiotics may be used for penetrating injuries, and anti-inflammatory medications may also be considered. In cases of severe trauma to the larynx, a temporary tracheostomy may be necessary. Reconstructive surgery may be needed if severe anatomic malalignment of laryngeal or tracheal cartilages has occurred. When surgical reconstruction is not possible, a permanent tracheostomy may be considered.

Surgery may also be considered if a mass is present or if laryngeal swelling obstructs the windpipe.

Follow-up Care
Follow-up visits are often helpful to monitor resolution of clinical signs, and chest x-rays may be repeated. If signs persist and become chronic, further testing may be recommended. When inflammation of the trachea is severe, a narrowing of the trachea (stricture) may occur weeks to months later, so notify your veterinarian if any signs return or if any breathing difficulties are noted. Animals with marked inflammation of the airway must also be kept cool, because their usual cooling method (panting) may be compromised.

Prognosis
Prognosis is good for most forms of acute laryngotracheitis. Mild cases usually respond well to time and therapy. Resolution of signs is likely after removal of noxious irritants from the environment. Prognosis with laryngeal or tracheal trauma depends on the severity of the damage and the degree of any obstruction of the airway.

SPECIAL INSTRUCTIONS:

Lung Lobe Torsion
Ronald M. Bright, DVM, MS, DACVS

BASIC INFORMATION
Description
Lung lobe torsion is the twisting of a portion (lobe) of the lungs around its blood vessels and bronchus (the airway that leads from the windpipe into the lung). Some lung lobes are more mobile (moveable) than others, which predisposes them to torsion.

Causes
Deep-chested, large-breed dogs are prone to lung lobe torsion for unknown reasons (idiopathic). Any animal that develops fluid within the chest cavity may develop a torsion, because the lung lobe may "float" on the fluid and twist on its long axis. Trauma and thoracic surgery may also be causes.

Clinical Signs
The onset of signs is usually sudden and may include rapid and difficult breathing, coughing with or without the production of blood, and shock and collapse (in severely affected animals). Lethargy and fever are also common. Other signs of an underlying cause may also be present.

Although most cases of lung lobe torsion produce sudden, serious signs, some animals with this condition exist for days or weeks with signs limited to coughing, fever, and decreased appetite.

Diagnostic Tests
Lung lobe torsion may be suspected in large, deep-chested dogs with respiratory signs, especially if evidence of fluid in the chest is found on physical examination. Routine laboratory tests and chest x-rays are often recommended to investigate potential causes of the respiratory signs. Chest x-rays are helpful to identify free fluid in the chest and may show changes compatible with lung lobe torsion. Fluid aspirated from the chest (thoracentesis) is often bloody. The fluid sample is commonly sent for microscopic analysis and culture to rule out other diseases, such as cancer or other conditions that can produce fluid in the chest.

Bronchoscopy, which involves the passage of a fiberoptic scope into the airway, is sometimes necessary to confirm that the bronchus is twisted as it enters the lobe of lung. Bronchoscopy also helps eliminate foreign bodies, other forms of pneumonia, and tumors as potential causes. Other tests may be recommended to rule out other diseases that can cause fluid in the chest and similar x-ray changes.

TREATMENT AND FOLLOW-UP
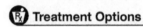 Treatment Options
Initial therapy involves measures to stabilize the animal and improve breathing. Supportive care may include fluid therapy, oxygen supplementation, and possibly antibiotics. If there is fluid in the chest, it is often removed to allow the animal to breathe easier. Once the animal is stable, surgery is needed to remove the affected lung lobe. Any underlying conditions are also treated.

Follow-up Care
Following open-chest surgery (thoracotomy) and lung lobe removal (lobectomy), a chest tube is usually left in place for 24-48 hours. Monitoring of vital signs, such as respiratory rate, heart rate and rhythm, oxygen levels in the blood, body temperature, and blood pressure (when available) is critical following surgery.

The lung lobe removed should be submitted for pathologic analysis to be certain that no additional diseases, such as cancer, are present.

Prognosis
Removal of the affected lung lobe is curative, so the prognosis is good for idiopathic cases. Prognosis for patients with underlying diseases is dependent on the ability to successfully manage those conditions after lobectomy for the torsion.

SPECIAL INSTRUCTIONS:

Lung Tumors

Ronald M. Bright, DVM, MS, DACVS

BASIC INFORMATION
Description
Tumors involving the lungs comprise approximately 1.2% of all tumors affecting the dog, and 0.5% of those affecting the cat. Lung tumors can arise from lung tissue (primary tumors), or they can spread to the lungs (metastasize) from a tumor arising in another organ (secondary tumors). Most tumors of the lung are secondary. Lung tumors can occur as single or multiple masses, and they can involve one or several lobes. Older animals are most commonly affected, although younger dogs (1-6 years old) can develop tumors such as lymphomatoid granulomatosis.

Causes
Most tumors are malignant, and carcinoma is the most common type. Benign tumors are rare. It appears that large dogs, especially boxers and Bernese Mountain dogs are at increased risk for lung tumors. It is possible that passive cigarette smoke and genetic factors influence the development of lung tumors.

Clinical Signs
Approximately 25% of dogs with lung tumors have no clinical signs. Coughing and panting, with or without some degree of respiratory distress, are common. Exercise intolerance may be observed. Dogs with more advanced disease may have decreased appetite, lethargy, and weight loss. Fever may be detected if a secondary bacterial infection is also present. Lung tumors can be associated with swelling of some or all of the legs, leading to lameness. (See also the handout on **Hypertrophic Osteopathy in Dogs.**)

Diagnostic Tests
Routine laboratory tests may be recommended to investigate the clinical signs. Lung masses may be found incidentally when x-rays of the chest are taken for some other reason. Routine chest x-rays usually reveal masses in the chest if they are a significant size. If a lung tumor is suspected, three views of the chest are often necessary to identify and confirm the location of the masses. X-rays may also reveal fluid in the chest cavity and enlargement of the lymph nodes in the chest. If fluid is present, some of it may be aspirated for microscopic analysis and culture.

A definitive diagnosis of lung tumor requires biopsy of the mass. Depending on the location within the chest, biopsy may be done through the chest wall with ultrasound guidance; by retrieval of a fluid or tissue sample from the bronchus via bronchoscopy (passage of a fiberoptic viewing scope into the lower airways with the animal under general anesthesia); or by open-chest surgery. Occasionally, analysis of fluid from the chest reveals tumor cells.

Additional tests may be recommended to rule out other diseases that can cause similar signs or to search for tumors elsewhere in the body. A thorough search of the rest of the body is very important, because many lung tumors have metastasized from tumors elsewhere.

TREATMENT AND FOLLOW-UP
Treatment Options
Surgical removal of the tumor by lobectomy is the treatment of choice for solitary tumors, especially if they are believed to be primary lung tumors. Other lung lobes that are accessible at the time of surgery are also examined for any involvement. Enlarged lymph nodes in the chest may be removed for biopsy to determine whether the tumor has spread. Because many primary lung tumors are malignant, surgery may be followed by chemotherapy.

For secondary tumors, treatment options depend on the type and location of the primary tumor. Chemotherapy may be tried to decrease the size metastatic tumors in the lungs.

Follow-up Care
Following open-chest surgery, the animal is usually hospitalized for several days. A chest tube placed at the end of surgery is used to monitor for any air or fluid production. After discharge from the hospital, your pet must be strictly confined for several weeks. The timing of recheck visits is usually determined by the postoperative treatments chosen. Follow-up x-rays are often taken at 3- to 6-month intervals after removal of primary tumors to monitor for any recurrence. Follow-up x-rays may be taken more often to monitor response to chemotherapy.

Prognosis
The most important factors in determining prognosis are the tumor type and whether it has spread to other lung lobes or to the lymph nodes. Dogs with a small, primary lung lobe tumor and no metastases have the best prognosis, with survival times that can be greater than 1 year. Even dogs with a large, single lung lobe masses (if removed successfully) can have survival times of greater than 6 months. In cats, 75% have a poor prognosis, because most tumors of the lungs are inoperable at the time of diagnosis. Prognosis is grave for animals with metastatic lung tumors.

SPECIAL INSTRUCTIONS:

Mediastinal Masses

Ronald M. Bright, DVM, MS, DACVS

BASIC INFORMATION

Description

The mediastinum is an enclosed space in the center of the chest between the lung lobes. The anterior or cranial mediastinum is the space in front of the heart. The cranial mediastinum contains a number of important structures, such as blood vessels, the trachea, lymph nodes, the esophagus, and the thymus. A mass within the mediastinum can arise from any tissue occupying that space and can include tumors, cysts, blood clots, and granulomas (inflammatory nodules or masses).

Causes

Tumors can originate from any tissue within the mediastinum; they can arise from surrounding tissue such as the lungs; or occasionally they may spread to the mediastinum from tumors in a distant organ outside the chest. Examples of tumors include the following:

- Lymphosarcoma is more commonly seen in cats. Rarely (3%), it involves only the anterior mediastinum, but more often it is part of a generalized disease. Young Siamese cats appear to be predisposed to mediastinal lymphoma.
- The most common tumor of the thymus is the thymoma. Thymomas may be well defined and benign or invasive and malignant. The German shepherd dog is predisposed to thymomas.
- Other tumors include a heart base tumor (chemodectoma), tumors of misplaced thyroid and parathyroid tissue, histiocytic tumors, and others.

Benign cysts can arise from embryonic tissue in the mediastinum. Noncancerous lymph node enlargement can occur with bacterial or fungal infections or inflammation. Esophageal tumors and granulomas may also occur in the mediastinum.

Clinical Signs

Many clinical signs are associated with the underlying disease or are vague (lack of appetite, lethargy, weight loss). Small masses cause no signs. Respiratory signs (coughing, difficulty breathing, panting, noisy breathing) or gastrointestinal signs (difficulty swallowing, excessive salivation, regurgitation) may be present, depending on which tissue is involved. Swelling of the head, the neck, or the front of the chest can occur if the mass puts pressure on the great blood vessels.

Thymomas may be associated with myasthenia gravis and may cause signs of megaesophagus (regurgitation, aspiration pneumonia) or muscle weakness. Increased drinking and urinating may occur if the mass has secondary effects on the kidneys or on blood calcium levels.

Diagnostic Tests

X-rays of the chest are helpful to delineate masses in the mediastinum, as well as the effects these masses have on surrounding organs, such as elevation of the trachea, displacement of the lungs or heart, or collapse of a lung lobe. Other potential findings on x-rays include fluid within the mediastinum or chest, enlargement of the lymph nodes, and megaesophagus.

Contrast x-ray studies may be recommended if esophageal disease is suspected. Ultrasonography can help to define the size of the mass and whether it invades other tissues; it can also guide the collection of tissue or fluid samples for analysis. Additional laboratory tests, x-rays, and advanced imaging techniques may also be recommended to better define the cause and search for tumors elsewhere in the body.

TREATMENT AND FOLLOW-UP

Treatment Options

Treatment depends on the type of mass present and its tissue of origin. Lymphoma is best treated with chemotherapy. Surgical removal may be tried for benign tumors of the thymus and other structures of the mediastinum. Some cystic structures can be drained to alleviate the clinical signs, but if the cyst recurs, then surgical removal may be the best option. Radiation therapy may be considered for tumors that cannot be removed with surgery.

Additional measures may be needed for the secondary effects that some tumors cause, such as elevated calcium levels and myasthenia gravis. (See also the handouts on **Cancer-Associated Hypercalcemia** and **Myasthenia Gravis**.)

Follow-up Care

Following open-chest surgery, the animal is usually hospitalized for several days. Hemorrhage is a major concern postoperatively, because surgery in the mediastinum is done near numerous large blood vessels. A chest tube is inserted at the end of surgery and is used to monitor for air or fluid in the chest. Dogs with esophageal problems are closely monitored for regurgitation and subsequent aspiration pneumonia. Follow-up chest x-rays of the mediastinum are indicated in some instances.

Prognosis

Thymomas that are completely excised, unless there are concurrent esophageal problems, have a good long-term prognosis. Prognosis for other tumors treated with surgery is dependent on the type of tumor and whether it is invading surrounding tissue. Prognosis for tumors treated with chemotherapy varies. Benign processes such as cysts, abscesses, and foreign bodies within the mediastinum generally carry a good prognosis.

SPECIAL INSTRUCTIONS:

Nasal and Nasopharyngeal Polyps in Cats

Ronald M. Bright, DVM, MS, DACVS

BASIC INFORMATION

Polyps are the most common disease involving the nose and throat of cats. They are small, benign masses that can obstruct the back of the nasal passages where they enter into the back of the mouth (nasopharynx). Polyps may also grow into the ear canal via the auditory (eustachian) tube, which connects the nasopharynx with the middle ear.

Causes

These polyps probably arise from chronic inflammation of the upper respiratory tissues. Bacterial and viral infections may contribution to their formation.

Clinical Signs

Rough-sounding, noisy breathing can be heard from the throat area in cats with nasopharyngeal polyps. Difficulty breathing, increased nasal sounds on inspiration (while breathing air in), sneezing, and nasal discharge are common with nasal polyps. Polyps in the external ear canal may be associated with discharge from one or both ears. Head shaking and chronic ear infections are also common. Sometimes signs of middle ear disease occur, such as loss of balance. Middle ear polyps may also cause signs of Horner's syndrome, namely prolapse of the third eyelid over part of the eye and a small pupil in the same eye.

Diagnostic Tests

Polyps may be suspected based on clinical signs such as airway noises, nasal discharge, chronic ear discharge, and recurrent ear infections. Occasionally, your veterinarian may feel (palpate) a mass in the pharynx and possibly above the soft palate. Ear examination may reveal a mass deep within the ear canal. X-rays or advanced imaging of the head and neck area may locate a mass within the throat, middle ear, nasal cavity, or a combination of these locations. Endoscopy (passage of a flexible fiberoptic instrument) of the nasal cavity may reveal polyps. In some cases, the mass is discovered only with surgical exploration. Biopsy and histopathology are require to confirm the diagnosis.

TREATMENT AND FOLLOW-UP

Treatment Options

Surgical removal of the polyp or polyps is the only option that provides a chance for a cure. Removal of a polyp within the throat area usually involves gentle traction (pulling) on the base of the stalk of the polyp, so that the entire mass can be removed. Extension into the middle ear requires opening the middle ear surgically, which is termed a *ventral bulla osteotomy*. Polyps deep in the ear canal can usually be removed with this same procedure.

Follow-up Care

Anti-inflammatory drugs are helpful postoperatively, along with pain medications. Surgery on the middle ear (ventral bulla osteotomy) usually injures the nerve that causes Horner's syndrome, so clinical signs of that syndrome may develop after surgery. The facial nerve also lies in this area, so facial paralysis may occur. Incoordination or a lack of balance may also be noted after surgery. All surgery-related signs usually resolve within 1-6 weeks.

Prognosis

The chance of recurrence of polyps is decreased greatly when the entire polyp is removed from the middle ear. Resolution of signs can approach 90% in these cases. Recurrences are more likely when bulla osteotomy is not performed.

SPECIAL INSTRUCTIONS:

Nasal Tumors, Malignant

Ronald M. Bright, DVM, MS, DACVS

BASIC INFORMATION

Description

Tumors of the nasal cavity and nearby sinuses account for approximately 1-2% of tumors in dogs and 1-5% in cats. In dogs, most nasal tumors occur in large-breed dogs older than 8 years of age. Most nasal tumors are malignant (cancerous).

Causes

The cause of these tumors is unknown. Numerous types can occur, including primary tumors that arise from tissues within the nasal cavity (adenocarcinoma, squamous cell carcinoma) and sinuses, and secondary tumors that invade the nose (osteosarcoma, lymphoma, fibrosarcoma, melanoma, and others).

Clinical Signs

Most signs are very subtle initially, and the tumor can be present in the nasal cavity or sinuses for months before any abnormalities are seen. At first, nasal discharge is usually clear or pink-tinged; then it often becomes yellow-green or mixed with blood. The discharge usually comes from one side of the nose early in the course but is seen from both nostrils once the tumor invades the septum (tissue that separates the nose into two cavities). Intermittent nose bleeds may occur.

Advanced tumors cause distortion of the facial bones, the eyes, and the bone overlying the frontal sinuses of the forehead. As the tumor grows, it may also distort the hard palate and other structures in the mouth. Discharge from one or both eyes may be seen. Open-mouth, noisy breathing is common if the nasal cavity is obstructed. Invasion of the bone that lies between the nasal cavity and the brain may result in neurologic signs.

Diagnostic Tests

Tumors may be suspected in animals with chronic nasal discharge unresponsive to symptomatic therapy. X-rays of the head may demonstrate changes in the nasal cavity or sinuses that are compatible with a tumor, but they do not provide a definitive diagnosis. Occasionally, chronic inflammation and infection can lead to similar radiographic signs. Computed tomography (CT scan) or magnetic resonance imaging (MRI) may be recommended.

Microscopic analysis of material aggressively flushed from the nasal cavity following infusion of saline provides a diagnosis in fewer than 50% of cases. Rhinoscopy (examination of the nasal cavity with a fiberoptic viewing scope) allows direct visualization and biopsy of some tumors. Definitive diagnosis and determination of tumor type requires a biopsy.

Additional tests, such as laboratory tests and chest x-rays, may be recommended to rule out other nasal diseases that cause similar signs and to ensure that cancer is not present in other organs.

TREATMENT AND FOLLOW-UP

Treatment Options

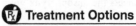

Radiation therapy alone can control some nasal tumors in the dog and cat, depending on their location and extent. Surgery, alone or prior to radiation therapy, has not been proven to be superior to radiotherapy alone. In some cases, the best results are obtained by surgery that is done after radiation therapy has shrunk the tumor. Radioactive implants have been used in dogs after surgery with limited success. When surgery is done, the incision usually is made along the bridge of the nose and may extend into the frontal sinuses.

Chemotherapy is not very effective in most tumors except for lymphosarcoma. The chemotherapeutic drug cisplatin can help alleviate some signs related to nasal tumors, such as nasal discharge, sneezing, and nose bleeds, for varying periods of time. A vaccine has been developed against melanomas in dogs.

Follow-up Care

Facial appearance changes somewhat following surgery of the nasal cavity; however, cosmetic results are generally good. It is common for nasal discharge to be present for several days after surgery.

Radiation therapy can have some acute side effects, including skin irritation, eye inflammation, oral discomfort, hair loss, and inflammation of the nasal cavity. Longer-term complications of radiation therapy include retinal damage and cataract formation with blindness in one or more eyes; skin ulceration on the face; brain damage; and death of bones of the skull that were in the radiation field. Chronic inflammation of the nasal cavity and bone damage are more common when radiation therapy is combined with surgery (compared with radiation alone).

Prognosis

Prognosis is variable with nasal tumors. In dogs, the 2-year survival rate with radiotherapy followed by surgery is 69%, compared to 44% with radiation alone. Radiation and cisplatin therapy produces an average survival time of 474 days. In cats, typical survival time ranges from 13 to 20 months with radiation therapy alone. Cats with lymphosarcoma respond best to chemotherapy.

Spread of most nasal tumors to other tissues (lymph nodes, lungs) is rare, but with increased survival times it may become more of a concern in the future.

SPECIAL INSTRUCTIONS:

Pleural Effusion

Ronald M. Bright, DVM, MS, DACVS

BASIC INFORMATION

Description

Pleural effusion is an abnormal accumulation of fluid within the chest cavity in the space between the lungs and the chest wall (pleural space). Depending on the volume, fluid collection can compromise respiratory function.

Causes

A variety of conditions can cause pleural effusion, including the following:

- Infection (bacterial or fungal) within the chest cavity
- Heart failure
- Penetrating foreign bodies that enter the chest cavity via the chest wall, respiratory tract, or esophagus
- Infection with feline infectious peritonitis (FIP) virus (cats)
- Heartworm disease (mainly dogs)
- Primary lung tumors and tumors of other structures in the chest
- Leakage of chyle (a milky white fluid containing white blood cells) from the major lymphatic duct
- Bleeding from trauma, a clotting defect, or surgery

Other, less common causes of pleural effusion include decreased protein levels in the blood, a blood clot in a major vessel in the chest (thromboembolism), torsion (twisting) of a lung lobe, pancreatitis, congenital cysts, and diaphragmatic hernias (often from trauma).

Clinical Signs

How severely the animal is affected is largely dependent on how much fluid is present. As fluid collects, it eventually diminishes the lungs' ability to expand. Increased respiratory effort (panting, open-mouth breathing), decreased activity, cyanosis (blue gums caused by lack of oxygen), coughing, and lethargy may occur. With chronic conditions, weight loss, decreased appetite, and coughing are common. Signs of recent trauma may be present with diaphragmatic hernia and bleeding into the chest.

Diagnostic Tests

Sometimes abnormal sounds or muffling of the heart and lung sounds is detected with a stethoscope. A fever suggests the possibility of an inflammatory, infectious, or tumor-related problem.

Pleural effusion is usually discovered on chest x-rays. Animals that are in respiratory distress may have a chest tap to remove air or fluid so that breathing improves before x-rays are taken. Fluid removed from the chest is sent for analysis and culture. Additional laboratory tests are helpful in characterizing the type of fluid present. Some types of fluid are more likely with certain causes.

Other tests that may be recommended to search for an underlying cause include routine laboratory tests, x-rays of the abdomen, ultrasound studies of the chest and abdomen, an echocardiogram (heart ultrasound), and tests for various infectious agents.

TREATMENT AND FOLLOW-UP

Treatment Options

Treatment consists initially of removing the fluid from the chest cavity to help alleviate breathing problems. If fluid accumulation continues, a chest tube may be inserted in one or both sides of the chest. The chest tubes may be attached to a low-pressure drainage system to allow constant drainage of fluid when it is accumulating at a rapid rate.

Once the type of fluid and the underlying cause are identified, treatment is designed specifically for that problem. For example, when treating pyothorax (pus in the chest from a bacterial infection), chest tubes are often used to flush infected material out of the chest cavity with saline, and antibiotics are administered. If heart failure is present, appropriate medications are given. Some pleural effusions require surgical intervention. Examples include removal of tumors and foreign bodies, correction of problems related to the abnormal accumulation of chyle (chylothorax), and removal of the sac around the heart if pericardial fluid is the source. (See the handout on **Pericardial Effusion**.)

If fluid analysis reveals a tumor, surgery or chemotherapy or both may be indicated. In some instances, the chemotherapeutic agent is injected directly into the chest cavity for the best results.

Follow-up Care

Intensive monitoring is needed both before and after surgery. Respiratory rate, heart rate, blood oxygen levels, body temperature, and continued production of fluid are monitored. Following open-chest surgery, the animal is usually hospitalized for several days. A chest tube is placed at the end of surgery to monitor for any air or fluid production. After discharge from the hospital, your pet must be strictly confined for several weeks. The timing of recheck visits is usually determined by the postoperative treatments chosen for the specific underlying condition.

Prognosis

Prognosis depends on the cause of the pleural effusion and its response to treatment. Some causes of pleural effusion (such as diaphragmatic hernia and lung lobe torsion) are often cured by surgery. Other causes (such as heart failure and low protein levels) may be controlled with medications for variable periods of time. Pleural effusion from lung, heart, or chest cavity tumors has a grave prognosis.

SPECIAL INSTRUCTIONS:

Pneumonia, Aspiration

Ronald M. Bright, DVM, MS, DACVS

BASIC INFORMATION
Description
Aspiration pneumonia results from the inhalation of liquid, food, or bacteria into the respiratory tract (lungs). Most often the onset is rapid, but sometimes the signs are chronic and insidious.

Causes
Material that is aspirated usually originates in the stomach or esophagus. Under normal circumstances, opening and closing of the larynx and pharynx are coordinated so that liquids and foodstuffs do not pass into the airway. Any disorder that increases reflux of stomach contents into the esophagus or alters normal laryngeal-pharyngeal function can potentially result in aspiration pneumonia.

Swallowing disorders or inability of the larynx to close during swallowing are two common neurologic or muscular problems that can lead to aspiration. Dilation of the esophagus (megaesophagus), secondary regurgitation, and aspiration during vomiting are other potential causes. Animals that are under general anesthesia, recumbent (lying on their side) for prolonged periods, profoundly depressed, or comatose are predisposed to aspiration.

Attempts to force animals to take pills, food, or liquid can sometimes overwhelm the protective reflexes of the larynx and result in aspiration pneumonia. Accidental passage of a stomach tube or administration of barium and other substances into the airway can also cause pneumonia.

Clinical Signs
Usually, sudden onset of coughing, panting, difficulty breathing, and fever is noted. Cyanosis (blue gums caused by lack of oxygen) may accompany these signs. Affected animals are depressed and may not eat. Progressive respiratory impairment can occur and can be life-threatening.

Diagnostic Tests
The history and sudden onset of signs may be suspicious for aspiration pneumonia. Routine laboratory tests and chest x-rays are often recommended to investigate potential causes of a cough or respiratory distress. Chest x-rays may show lungs changes consistent with aspiration pneumonia. Animals in severe distress often require therapy before other tests can be performed.

In animals that are stable, analysis of secretions taken from the trachea and bronchus by transtracheal wash may help confirm the cause. Culturing of the secretions may demonstrate bacteria. Bronchoscopy, which involves passage of a fiberoptic scope into the airway, may help eliminate parasites, foreign bodies, other forms of pneumonia, and tumors as potential causes. Other tests may be recommended to rule out other diseases that can cause coughing and similar x-ray changes, and to search for an underlying cause.

TREATMENT AND FOLLOW-UP
Treatment Options
Most affected animals require hospitalization for aggressive therapy. In severe cases, treatment for shock, supplemental oxygen, and mechanical ventilation (if available) may be needed. Bronchodilator drugs may decrease spasms in the lower respiratory tract. Antibiotics are often given, either before or after culture results are known.

Nebulization using a humidifier may be tried in some cases. Chest coupage, which is gentle but forceful thumping on the rib cage, may help loosen secretions in the respiratory tract. An important goal of therapy is to identify any predisposing conditions and correct them so that further aspiration is prevented.

In some cases, lung changes become so severe and chronic that surgical removal of the diseased lung is necessary.

Follow-up Care
Intensive, continuous monitoring of respiratory function is usually needed while the animal is hospitalized. Repeated chest x-rays are an excellent way to evaluate response to therapy and are usually obtained every 24-48 hours. After the animal is stable and discharged from the hospital, chest x-rays are often taken again in 5-7 days. Laboratory tests may be performed every 2-3 days to monitor changes caused by inflammation and infection.

Antibiotics are continued at home by the owner. One of the reasons for treatment failure is noncompliance by owners; that is, failure to administer the medications as directed. Other reasons include continued aspiration and inadequate control of the underlying cause.

Notify your veterinarian if signs persist or worsen, because failure to improve on therapy may indicate further progression and development of irreversible changes in the lungs.

Prognosis
When aspiration pneumonia is recognized and treated early, most animals make a complete recovery. If the underlying condition cannot be treated successfully, aspiration pneumonia is not likely to resolve. Aspiration pneumonia that involves a large portion of both lungs or aspiration of particularly toxic material can be fatal.

SPECIAL INSTRUCTIONS:

Pneumonia, Bacterial

Ronald M. Bright, DVM, MS, DACVS

BASIC INFORMATION

Description

Bacterial pneumonia is inflammation of the lungs that is caused by or associated with a bacterial infection. When a single lung lobe is involved, it is referred to as *lobar pneumonia*. Bronchopneumonia is inflammation of both the lower airways (bronchi) and the lungs.

Causes

Most cases of bacterial pneumonia develop secondary to some other underlying disease or condition:

- Bronchitis can progress to pneumonia.
- Some congenital diseases (such as ciliary dyskinesia) predispose dogs of certain breeds to pneumonia, but these are rare.
- Cases of viral or fungal pneumonia may develop secondary bacterial infections.
- Areas of aspiration pneumonia may become infected.
- Penetrating foreign bodies in the lung may introduce bacteria.
- Drug therapy and certain diseases (diabetes mellitus, adrenal gland hyperfunction) that suppress an animal's natural immune system make it vulnerable to bacterial pneumonia.
- Animals that lie on their side for prolonged periods because of some disease process or anesthesia are predisposed to partial collapse of the lungs, and these areas can then become infected.
- Trauma and cancer of the lungs can be followed by bacterial invasion.

Clinical Signs

A productive cough (coughing up phlegm) and nasal discharge are common signs. Rate and effort of breathing may be increased, and wheezing may be heard. The animal may be lethargic and unable to exercise. Fever, weight loss, and decreased appetite may occur.

Diagnostic Tests

Be sure to give your veterinarian details as to travel history, prior illnesses, and prior vaccinations of your pet, because they may provide insight into the possible causes of pneumonia. For example, a history of chronic airway disease, regurgitation, or a recent anesthetic event may be important in solving the diagnosis. Certain characteristic lung sounds (crackles) and sometimes an expiratory (while breathing out) wheeze may be heard with a stethoscope on physical examination.

Routine laboratory tests and chest x-rays are often recommended to investigate potential causes of a cough or respiratory distress. Chest x-rays may show lungs changes consistent with bacterial pneumonia. Animals in severe distress may require therapy before other tests are performed.

In animals that are stable, analysis of secretions taken from the trachea and bronchi by transtracheal wash may help confirm the cause. Culturing of the secretions usually demonstrates bacteria. Bronchoscopy, which involves passage of a fiberoptic scope into the airway, may help eliminate parasites, foreign bodies, other forms of pneumonia, and tumors as potential causes. Lung biopsies are rarely done but are sometimes considered.

Other tests may be recommended to rule out other diseases that can cause coughing and similar x-ray changes, and to search for an underlying or contributing cause.

TREATMENT AND FOLLOW-UP

Treatment Options

Antibiotics are the primary therapy and are usually chosen based on results of bacterial culture and antibiotic sensitivity testing. Oxygen supplementation is warranted for more severe cases. Bronchodilators sometimes help improve breathing problems.

Keeping the animal well hydrated with fluid therapy and humidifying the environment are often helpful. Affected animals may also benefit from frequent walks to prevent them from lying in one position for long periods. Chest coupage, which is gentle but forceful thumping on the rib cage, may help loosen secretions in the respiratory tract.

An important goal of therapy is to identify any predisposing conditions and correct them. In some cases, lung changes become so severe and chronic that surgical removal of the diseased lung is necessary.

Follow-up Care

Intensive, continuous monitoring of respiratory function is usually needed while the animal is hospitalized. Repeated chest x-rays are an excellent way to evaluate response to therapy and are usually done every 24-48 hours. After the animal is stable and discharged from the hospital, chest x-rays are often taken again in 5-7 days. Laboratory tests may be performed every few days to monitor changes caused by inflammation and infection.

Notify your veterinarian if signs persist or worsen, because failure to improve on therapy may indicate the need to change antibiotics or the development of complications such as a lung lobe abscess, spread of the infection to other parts of the body (sepsis), or irreversible lung lobe changes. Failure to improve also may be a sign that an underlying cause (such as regurgitation or diabetes) is not being effectively managed.

Prognosis

Most cases of bacterial pneumonia resolve with appropriate use of antibiotics, assuming that the underlying cause is also successfully managed. Unresponsive animals may become systemically ill and may not respond even to intensive therapy in the hospital.

SPECIAL INSTRUCTIONS:

Pneumonia, Fungal

Ronald M. Bright, DVM, MS, DACVS

BASIC INFORMATION

Description

Fungal pneumonia is caused by fungal (mycotic) organisms and is often part of a widespread systemic fungal infection.

Causes

Several fungal organisms can cause pneumonia, including *Coccidioides immitis, Blastomyces dermatitidis, Histoplasma capsulatum, Cryptococcus neoformans* (most common in cats), and *Aspergillus flavus.*

Clinical Signs

Signs are often indistinguishable from those of other types of pneumonia. Nasal discharge is often seen with lung involvement. Systemic signs are common and include weight loss, fever, lameness, and enlarged lymph nodes. Eye lesions and central nervous system (neurologic) signs can also occur. (See also the specific handouts for the various fungal diseases.)

Diagnostic Tests

Routine laboratory tests and chest x-rays are often recommended to investigate potential causes of respiratory signs. Chest x-rays may show lung changes consistent with fungal pneumonia. In contrast to other forms of pneumonia, the diagnosis is usually made by identification of the fungal agent on aspirates or biopsies of other tissues or from positive blood tests. Occasionally the diagnosis is made only when samples of exudates are obtained from the lower respiratory tract using bronchoscopy. Cultures of exudates can be attempted, but the organisms often do not grow.

TREATMENT AND FOLLOW-UP

Treatment Options

Antifungal drugs are indicated and must often be continued for weeks to months to effect a cure. Other supportive care for the pneumonia may be started, such as hospitalization for oxygen supplementation, fluid therapy, nebulization, and physiotherapy.

Follow-up Care

Fungal pneumonia requires close monitoring, especially early in the course of treatment. With severe pneumonias, death of the fungi (which occurs soon after therapy is started) can create a significant amount of inflammation in the lungs. Notify your veterinarian immediately if respiratory signs worsen, especially during the first week that antifungal drugs are administered. Once the pneumonia starts to resolve, the animal usually begins to feel better. Chest x-rays are periodically repeated to monitor progress and response to therapy.

Prognosis

Many cases resolve as the systemic fungal infection improves. Severe fungal pneumonia has a guarded (uncertain) prognosis, however, because death can occur early in the treatment and long-term therapy is necessary to provide the best chance of recovery. Recurrence is a possibility, even after apparent resolution of the infection.

SPECIAL INSTRUCTIONS:

Pneumothorax

Ronald M. Bright, DVM, MS, DACVS

BASIC INFORMATION

Description

Pneumothorax is the accumulation of air in the pleural space, the space between the lungs and the wall of the chest cavity. As air accumulates in the chest, the lungs collapse and the ability to take in oxygen is severely compromised. A severe, life-threatening form of pneumothorax, called *tension pneumothorax*, can arise when a large volume air accumulates within the closed chest cavity.

Causes

Pneumothorax can spontaneously occur as a result of some underlying disease, or it can arise with trauma. Trauma from an automobile accident, falling from a height, or any form of blunt trauma can result in pneumothorax. Penetrating wounds (such as bullet or bite wounds) allow atmospheric air to enter the chest, and air may also leak from a ruptured esophagus.

Certain diseases of the lungs, such as blebs or cysts, infections and abscesses, heartworm disease, and certain types of lung parasites, may allow air to escape into the pleural space. Certain diagnostic procedures can inadvertently cause a pneumothorax; these include insertion of a needle into the chest cavity to obtain a sample of tissue or fluid, problems with gas anesthesia or mechanical ventilation, and certain surgical procedures of the chest, spine, and abdomen.

Clinical Signs

Rapid, shallow breathing and decreased activity are common signs. If pneumothorax becomes severe (often seen with tension pneumothorax), respiratory distress develops, with open-mouth breathing, standing with the elbows held out to the side and the head extended, cyanosis (blue gums) from lack of oxygen or pale gums (from shock), and collapse.

Diagnostic Tests

Evidence of trauma may be present in some animals, such as bruising, lacerations, fractures, and crackling sounds under the skin (from collection of air). Physical examination findings may include reduced lung sounds in the top part of the chest (heard with a stethoscope), muffled heart sounds, and abnormal sounds when the chest wall is thumped with the fingers. Animals in distress that were recently traumatized may have a chest tap performed to test for the presence of air and to remove some air so that breathing improves.

The presence of air can also be confirmed with chest x-rays. Other possible radiographic findings include rib fractures, bruising of the lungs (pulmonary contusion), esophageal foreign body, diaphragmatic hernia, and lung abscesses, bullae, or tumors. Further tests may be needed to search for the cause of the pneumothorax if trauma has not occurred. Laboratory tests may be recommended to assess the effects on other organs in the body.

TREATMENT AND FOLLOW-UP

Treatment Option

Treatment consists initially of removing air from the chest cavity to help alleviate breathing problems and treating any other acute injuries. Air may be initially removed with a needle and syringe (thoracentesis). If air accumulation continues, a chest tube may be inserted in one or both sides of the chest cavity. The chest tube may be attached to a low-pressure drainage system to allow constant evacuation of air when it is accumulating at a rapid rate. Additional therapy may include administration of oxygen, intravenous fluids, and medications for shock and pain.

Once the animal is stabilized and the underlying cause has been identified, treatment is designed specifically for that problem. For example, open wounds in the chest wall are covered immediately with a sterile dressing, air is withdrawn, and surgical exploration and closure of the wound is done after the animal is stable.

Follow-up Care

Careful monitoring of respiration, heart rate, blood pressure, lung sounds, color of the gums, and blood oxygen levels is often needed for a few days. Chest tubes usually remain in place until all air accumulation stops or for at least 24 hours after surgery (if open-chest surgery was performed). The chest tubes must be carefully monitored to ensure that they are working well and that no air is leaking around or into the tube and back into the chest.

X-rays are repeated to monitor resolution of air in the chest. Most animals remain in the hospital at least 24 hours after chest tube removal, so that they can be closely monitored.

Prognosis

Mild pneumothorax resulting from blunt trauma can often be treated successfully via thoracentesis followed by cage rest. More severe pneumothorax or pneumothorax from a penetrating injury can often be successfully resolved with chest tubes and closure of the wound. Other causes of pneumothorax have a guarded (uncertain) prognosis unless the underlying cause can be identified and successfully corrected.

SPECIAL INSTRUCTIONS:

Pulmonary Contusions

Ronald M. Bright, DVM, MS, DACVS

BASIC INFORMATION
Description and Causes
A pulmonary contusion is a form of bruise that occurs from bleeding within the lungs. The collection of blood deep within lung tissue usually results from blunt trauma to the chest, and it can occur even if there is no outward evidence of trauma.

Clinical Signs

With mild or localized pulmonary contusions, no visible respiratory signs may be present. Acute onset of panting and some degree of respiratory distress are common with moderate to severe contusions. External signs of trauma may be seen around the chest or elsewhere on the body. Sometimes other clinical signs produced by the blunt trauma can overshadow those associated with mild to moderate pulmonary contusions.

Diagnostic Tests

A known history of trauma combined with finding abnormal lung sounds on the physical examination may allow a tentative diagnosis. X-rays of the lungs often show characteristic changes of pulmonary contusions. Other abnormalities may also be seen on the x-rays, such as broken ribs, fluid or air (or both) in the chest cavity, and collapse of one or several lung lobes. Other x-rays and laboratory tests may be recommended depending on the extent of the injuries.

TREATMENT AND FOLLOW-UP

Treatment Options

Most animals with pulmonary contusions are hospitalized for therapy and monitoring. Depending on the degree of respiratory compromise, supplemental oxygen may be needed. (See the handout on **Oxygen Therapy**.) No specific therapy exists for pulmonary contusions, and treatment usually involves oxygen therapy, supportive care, rest, and treatment of other trauma-related problems. Bronchodilator drugs may be helpful in some cases.

Fluid therapy is often administered to animals in shock. When pulmonary contusions are suspected, the rate of fluid therapy must be carefully monitored, because overly aggressive therapy can make the contusions worse, especially in cats. To help decrease the amount of fluid that escapes into the lungs associated with the contusion, a transfusion of plasma, blood, or synthetic starch (colloid agent) may be considered.

Corticosteroids may be administered, but this must be done soon after the traumatic event or they may be of little benefit. Antibiotics are often given to animals with severe contusions or open wounds on the body to minimize the potential for secondary bacterial pneumonia. Good nursing care and medications to relieve pain and distress are also important.

Follow-up Care

Animals with moderate to severe pulmonary contusions require intensive monitoring for several days. Chest x-rays are often repeated every 24 hours to monitor resolution of the contusions. X-ray changes often worsen during the first 24 hours following the injury and may take several days to improve.

Other vital signs, such as respiratory rate, heart rate, and blood oxygen levels, are also commonly monitored. If respiratory signs worsen despite treatment, the animal may placed on a mechanical ventilator for a short period of time, if one is available. Other monitoring and follow-up testing depends on the presence of other trauma-related injuries.

Prognosis
Animals with mild pulmonary contusions have a good prognosis if their other injuries can be successfully treated. Prognosis is poor for animals with severe contusions or contusions complicated by other serious injuries to the chest or body.

SPECIAL INSTRUCTIONS:

Pulmonary Edema

Ronald M. Bright, DVM, MS, DACVS

BASIC INFORMATION

Description

Pulmonary edema is the accumulation of fluid within the lungs. The amount and severity of the edema can range from mild to life-threatening. Pulmonary edema can arise from heart disease (cardiogenic) or from other, noncardiogenic causes.

Causes

Heart disease is one of the most common causes. Numerous other conditions can cause pulmonary edema, including widespread systemic infections (sepsis), decreased circulating levels of proteins in the blood (hypoproteinemia) from a variety of diseases, pancreatitis, acute kidney failure, pulmonary embolism, aspiration pneumonia, and cancer. Smoke inhalation, snake evenomation, chest trauma, severe upper airway obstruction, head trauma, seizures, electric cord injury, and electrocution are also potential causes. Excessive administration of intravenous fluids and adverse effects of certain drugs can also cause pulmonary edema, especially in animals compromised from other diseases or illnesses.

Clinical Signs

The type and severity of the clinical signs correspond directly with the severity of the pulmonary edema. With mild edema, a moist cough, lethargy, exercise intolerance, and restlessness may be noted. A sudden onset of panting, coughing, and cyanosis (blue gums from lack of oxygen) can occur with severe edema. Most animals exhibit exaggerated efforts to breathe, sometimes with the elbows held away from the body and the neck stretched out. Coughing or retching may produce a blood-tinged fluid.

On physical examination, abnormal lung sounds are often heard through a stethoscope; abnormal heart sounds or rhythms are often heard if heart disease is the primary problem. Other abnormalities may be discovered on the physical examination, depending on the underlying cause.

Diagnostic Tests

The presence of pulmonary edema is often suspected based on the history, clinical signs, and physical examination findings. These findings may also point to an underlying cause of the edema. Pulmonary edema can usually be confirmed from characteristic abnormalities seen on chest x-rays. Chest x-rays may also provide evidence of heart or other diseases that can cause pulmonary edema.

Because so many conditions can cause pulmonary edema, numerous tests are often needed to determine the underlying cause. Testing may be delayed, however, because animals with severe edema must be treated and stabilized first. Routine laboratory (blood and urine) tests, abdominal x-rays and/or ultrasound studies, an electrocardiogram (ECG), an echocardiogram (heart ultrasound), and others may be recommended to search for the underlying cause.

TREATMENT AND FOLLOW-UP

Treatment Options

Animals with severe signs usually require hospitalization and intensive care. It is important to minimize stress in animals with labored breathing. Affected animals may require supplemental oxygen given through a nasal cannula, face mask, or oxygen cage. (See also the handout on **Oxygen Therapy**.) Diuretics are given to remove fluid from the lungs. Diuretics may initially be given by injection, then switched to oral forms once the edema improves. Bronchodilator drugs are often helpful. Specific treatment for the underlying cause is also instituted.

Follow-up Care

Close monitoring of both lung and heart functions is needed on a continuous or frequent basis early in the course of therapy. Chest x-rays are usually repeated every 24-48 hours to monitor the edema and the response to therapy. Monitoring of hydration status, urine output, body weight, and blood pressure (when available) is commonly done. Other monitoring tests, such as repeated ECGs and laboratory assays, are frequently required depending on the underlying cause.

Prognosis

Recovery from pulmonary edema relies on aggressive treatment of both the edema and any underlying cause of the problem. If the edema responds to therapy, then the short-term prognosis is good. Long-term prognosis is highly variable and depends on the underlying cause.

SPECIAL INSTRUCTIONS:

Rhinitis and Sinusitis in Cats

Ronald M. Bright, DVM, MS, DACVS

BASIC INFORMATION

Description

Rhinitis is inflammation of the nasal cavity, and sinusitis involves the sinuses. The inflammation can affect just one area or both (rhinosinusitis) and can be either acute or chronic.

Causes

Bacterial infection of the nose or sinuses seldom occurs as a primary disease. It is usually associated with viral, fungal, or parasitic diseases. A number of viral infections can infect kittens between 6 and 12 weeks of age. Cryptococcosis is the most common fungal cause of rhinosinusitis in the cat.

Allergic conditions rarely cause rhinosinusitis in the cat. Trauma to the nasal cavity or bones of the forehead over the sinuses is a potential cause. Rarely, blades of grass that are ingested may migrate into the nasal cavity, but other nasal foreign bodies are uncommon. Dental or gum disease may be associated with nasal infections. Sometimes the source of the inflammation is never identified (idiopathic).

Clinical Signs

Sneezing and nasal discharge are common. Sometimes gagging occurs from postnasal drainage. Acute onset of episodes of violent sneezing is often associated with inhalation of a foreign object. Chronic, periodic sneezing is associated with most other nasal diseases.

Discharge may be seen from one or both sides of the nose. The type of discharge sometimes helps determine the cause. For example, yellow-green discharge is common with viral, bacterial, or fungal infections, whereas a bloody discharge is more likely with trauma, foreign bodies, or a bleeding disorder.

Facial deformity can be seen with tumors, trauma, or secondary infections. A swelling below one of the eyes may indicate that a tooth root abscess has extended into the nasal cavity. Occasionally, discharge from one or both eyes may be seen. Open-mouth breathing may occur if one or both of the nasal cavities are obstructed.

Diagnostic Tests

A thorough examination of the head and mouth is usually done to identify any abnormalities in the bones, teeth, and nearby structures. Routine laboratory tests and special fungal assays may be recommended. Blood clotting tests may be done if the discharge is bloody.

X-rays are often helpful in detecting abnormalities within the nasal cavity and frontal sinuses, such as increased fluid density or destruction of the overlying bones or bony tissue. Advanced imaging with computed tomography (CT scan) or magnetic resonance imaging (MRI) is generally considered superior to x-rays for defining the extent of involvement.

Occasionally examination of cells in the nasal discharge is helpful, but usually a biopsy is necessary to obtain a diagnosis. Samples may be retrieved by forceful flushing of the nasal cavity with saline or by several biopsy techniques. Rhinoscopy (examination of the nose using a fiberoptic viewing scope) allows the veterinarian to directly examine the nasal cavity and obtain biopsy samples. Cultures may also be submitted for bacterial and fungal testing.

TREATMENT AND FOLLOW-UP

Treatment Options

Treatment of rhinitis or sinusitis depends on the underlying cause:
- When bacteria are identified by culturing methods, an appropriate antibiotic may be prescribed.
- Medical management of chronic, recurrent bacterial rhinosinusitis usually provides only temporarily relief, because clinical signs often return when therapy is stopped. In addition, chronic infections of the nasal cavity sometimes extend to the frontal sinuses. Because frontal sinus infections do not respond well to medical therapy, surgical removal of the lining of the frontal sinus, followed by insertion of fat into the sinus, may be necessary.
- Viral rhinitis is often self-limited and may run its course in several weeks. An exception is infection with herpesvirus, which can become chronic or recur throughout much of the cat's life. Antiviral medications may be tried in these cases. Secondary bacterial infection may require antibiotics.
- Fungal causes (cryptococcosis) are treated with systemic antifungal drugs.
- Any infected teeth are extracted.
- Tumors may require surgery.
- Displaced or badly injured pieces of bone (from trauma) may be removed.
- Foreign bodies can often be successfully removed using rhinoscopy, and antibiotics may be started afterward.

Follow-up Care

Many infections resolve within 2 weeks with therapy. Periodic recheck visits and repeated testing may be needed for signs that persist. Notify your veterinarian if any signs recur after treatment is stopped.

Prognosis

Chronic infections can be very difficult to treat successfully and may require an indefinite period of continuous or intermittent antibiotic or antiviral medications. If significant destruction of tissue is present, nasal discharge may persist indefinitely.

SPECIAL INSTRUCTIONS:

Rhinitis and Sinusitis in Dogs

Ronald M. Bright, DVM, MS, DACVS

BASIC INFORMATION

Description

Rhinitis is inflammation of the nasal cavity, and sinusitis involves the sinuses. The inflammation can affect just one area or both (rhinosinusitis) and can be either acute or chronic.

Causes

Bacterial infection of the nose or sinuses seldom occurs as a primary disease. It is usually associated with viral, fungal, or parasitic diseases. Distemper virus infection is seen mostly in young, unvaccinated dogs. Aspergillosis is the most common fungal cause of rhinosinusitis. Cryptococcosis can also occur in dogs; it may cause neurologic signs and may spread to other organs.

Allergic conditions can predispose dogs to chronic inflammation of the nasal cavity or sinuses. Trauma and exposure to foreign bodies are potential causes. Foreign bodies such as grass awns, sticks, or rocks may enter the nasal cavity via the nostrils or from the mouth. Tooth root abscesses may extend into the nasal cavity. Dental disease and tumors involving the nasal cavity or sinuses are often compounded by bacterial infection. Sometimes the source of the inflammation is never identified (idiopathic).

Clinical Signs

Sneezing and nasal discharge are common. Sometimes gagging occurs from postnasal drainage. Acute onset of episodes of violent sneezing is often associated with inhalation of a foreign object. Chronic, periodic sneezing is associated with most other nasal diseases.

Discharge may be seen from one or both sides of the nose. The type of discharge sometimes helps determine the cause. For example, yellow-green discharge is common with viral, bacterial, or fungal infections, whereas a bloody discharge is more likely with trauma, foreign bodies, or a bleeding disorder.

The opening of the nose can become ulcerated, especially with a chronic fungal infection. Facial deformity can be seen with tumors, trauma, or secondary infections. A swelling below one of the eyes may indicate that a tooth root abscess has extended into the nasal cavity. Occasionally, discharge from one or both eyes may be seen. Open-mouth breathing may occur if one or both of the nasal cavities are obstructed.

Diagnostic Tests

A thorough examination of the head and mouth is usually done to identify any abnormalities in the bones, teeth, and nearby structures. Routine laboratory tests and special fungal assays may be recommended. Blood clotting tests may be done if the discharge is bloody.

X-rays are often helpful in detecting abnormalities within the nasal cavity or frontal sinuses, such as increased fluid density or destruction of the overlying bones or bony tissue. Advanced imaging with computed tomography (CT scan) or magnetic resonance imaging (MRI) is generally considered superior to x-rays for defining the extent of involvement.

Occasionally examination of cells in the nasal discharge is helpful, but usually a biopsy is necessary to obtain a diagnosis. Samples may be retrieved by forceful flushing of the nasal cavity with saline or by several biopsy techniques. Rhinoscopy (examination of the nose using a fiberoptic viewing scope) allows the veterinarian to directly examine the nasal cavity and obtain biopsy samples. Cultures may also be submitted for bacterial and fungal testing.

TREATMENT AND FOLLOW-UP

Treatment Options

Treatment of rhinitis or sinusitis depends on the underlying cause and may involve the following:

- When bacteria are identified by culturing methods, an appropriate antibiotic may be prescribed.
- A viral rhinitis is often self-limited and usually runs its course in several weeks. Secondary bacterial infection may require antibiotics.
- Fungal infections are treated with antifungal drugs given systemically or through tubes inserted into the nose and frontal sinuses.
- Parasitic infections usually respond to drugs given orally or applied to the skin.
- Any infected teeth are extracted.
- Tumors may require surgery, alone or in combination with radiotherapy. (See the handout on **Nasal Tumors**.)
- Displaced or badly injured pieces of bone (from trauma) may be removed.
- Foreign bodies can often be successfully removed using rhinoscopy, and antibiotics may be started afterward.
- Allergic rhinitis may require drugs aimed at minimizing the inflammation associated with the allergy, such as antihistamines, oral and inhalant corticosteroids, certain antibiotics, or antifungal medications.

Follow-up Care

Many infections resolve within 2 weeks. Periodic recheck visits and repeated testing may be needed for signs that persist.

Prognosis

Some cases of rhinitis resolve quickly, but others do not respond to treatment well and become chronic. If significant destruction of nasal tissue is present, nasal discharge may persist indefinitely. Multiple treatments or prolonged treatment (months) may be necessary if the cause is a fungal infection.

SPECIAL INSTRUCTIONS:

Tracheal Collapse in Dogs

Ronald M. Bright, DVM, MS, DACVS

BASIC INFORMATION

Description

The cartilage rings of the trachea (windpipe) are shaped like the letter C, lying on its back. A small membrane covers the top of the ring. In some dogs, the tracheal cartilages lose their rigidity, and the membrane stretches. The rings collapse, the windpipe flattens, and mild to severe obstruction of the airway develops. Tracheal collapse occurs primarily in small-breed dogs, such as the miniature poodle, Yorkshire terrier, Pomeranian, and Chihuahua.

This is an acquired, not congenital, disease. Some dogs can start showing signs of tracheal collapse at a relatively young age, but it is usually a disease of older dogs. Tracheal collapse can occur in the neck region, within the chest, or in both locations.

Causes

The cause is not well understood, but proposed theories include genetic factors, nutritional influences, neurologic problems, and degeneration of the tracheal cartilages.

Clinical Signs

Abnormal respiratory noises, difficulty breathing, cyanosis (blue gums and tongue from lack of oxygen), exercise intolerance, and possibly fainting may occur. An intermittent "goose-honking" cough that has a sudden onset is a common sign. Applying pressure to the trachea often induces a cough.

Diagnostic Tests

Flattened cartilages may be detected when your veterinarian palpates (feels) the neck area. Chest x-rays demonstrate tracheal collapse in only 60% of affected patients, but they help rule out heart and other lung diseases as a cause of the signs. Video x-rays (fluoroscopy) show the movement of the trachea throughout the entire respiratory cycle and detect some cases of tracheal collapse that are missed on plain x-rays. Fluoroscopy is available at some referral institutions and veterinary hospitals.

The definitive diagnostic method is endoscopy (tracheobronchoscopy), which involves passage of a fiberoptic viewing scope into the trachea. This procedure demonstrates the degree and exact location of the collapse. Endoscopy also allows collection of samples for bacterial culture, as many affected dogs have a secondary infection. During the procedure, laryngeal function may also be evaluated, because 25-30% of dogs with tracheal collapse also have laryngeal paralysis. Tracheobronchoscopy has some inherent risks and is not performed in all patients with suspected tracheal collapse.

TREATMENT AND FOLLOW-UP

Treatment Options

Medical therapy usually is effective in dogs with mild collapse and signs. It often includes cough suppressants, drugs to dilate the bronchial tree, and antibiotics for secondary infections. Anti-inflammatory steroid medications (tablets or inhaler) may be used on a short-term basis to reduce inflammation of the lining of the trachea. Some dogs benefit from use of tranquilizers during periods of excitement that could result in severe respiratory distress.

Dogs with additional types of upper airway disease, such as laryngeal paralysis, may benefit from surgical correction of these disorders. Avoidance of high environmental temperatures and situations that induce excitement helps many of these patients. Obese dogs are placed on a weight-reduction diet.

Because of the inherent risks and potential complications related to tracheal surgery, most of these cases are managed medically whenever possible. Surgery is reserved for those dogs with severe collapse and little or no response to medical therapy or for those that become refractory to medications. If the collapse is at the very end of the trachea, where the bronchi of the lungs begin, it is usually considered unsuitable for any type of surgery.

The purpose of tracheal surgery is to support the tracheal cartilages and expand the tracheal diameter. Support of the tracheal cartilages can be accomplished by using prosthetic tracheal rings that are applied on the external surface of the windpipe. This type of surgery is usually limited to those dogs with collapse in the neck region. Placement of stents inside the trachea can be used to correct collapse of the trachea within the chest or the neck. The stents are usually inserted using endoscopy or fluoroscopy.

Follow-up Care

Close monitoring is required in the immediate postoperative period, so the dog may remain hospitalized. Because the placement of external tracheal rings is difficult and tedious, laryngeal paralysis may develop that requires another surgery (to treat the paralysis). Chronic coughing is associated with either surgery, but especially with stent placement. The coughing can often be managed with concurrent medical therapy.

Prognosis

Medical therapy can provide relief, in many cases for the life of the patient. When surgery is successful, it often reduces the clinical signs and improves the quality of the dog's life. The duration of the benefit from surgery is variable, because tracheal collapse is a progressive disease.

SPECIAL INSTRUCTIONS:

Tracheal Obstruction

Ronald M. Bright, DVM, MS, DACVS

BASIC INFORMATION

Description

Obstruction of the trachea (windpipe) is narrowing of the internal diameter of the trachea resulting from external or internal conditions. Obstruction of the trachea decreases the passage of air into and out of the lungs.

Causes

External conditions that can cause obstruction of the trachea include compression of the windpipe from a tumor, abscess, blood clot, or enlargement of a nearby structure (such as the esophagus). Tracheal narrowing can also result from blunt trauma, such as from a motor vehicle accident or fall.

Internal conditions include aspiration of foreign bodies or strictures (scarring) from a previous penetrating injury (dog bite, bullet wound, laceration), endotracheal intubation, or temporary tracheostomy. Internal obstruction can also be associated with tumors, abscesses, or scar tissue reaction to parasites. Rarely, dogs are born with narrowing of the trachea, which leads to subsequent obstruction.

Clinical Signs

Signs include exercise intolerance, noisy sounds while breathing, and panting. Difficulty breathing may induce restlessness, anxiety, and pawing at the face. Difficulty swallowing and halitosis (foul odor to the breath) may be noted in some cases. Coughing may occur, with or without the presence of blood. Cyanosis (blue gums from lack of oxygen), extreme respiratory distress, and collapse can occur in animals with near-total obstruction of the windpipe.

The signs may develop weeks after an injury or insult to the trachea if they are due to stricture and scar formation. Signs may be sudden in onset if they are associated with bleeding, foreign bodies, or certain forms of trauma.

Diagnostic Tests

Physical examination often reveals a sensitive trachea and high-pitched musical sounds as air moves within the trachea. If the obstruction is high in the neck, loud noises (stridor) may be heard during breathing. Other abnormalities may be detected in the neck.

In severely compromised animals, diagnostic tests may be delayed until the animal has been stabilized. X-rays of the neck and chest may show a foreign body within the trachea, a narrowed segment of the trachea, or a mass in or around the windpipe. Tracheoscopy (examination of the trachea through a fiberoptic viewing scope) is helpful in defining the cause of the problem and allows tissue or secretions to be obtained for microscopic analysis and bacterial culture. Chest x-rays and routine laboratory tests are useful in ruling out other causes of respiratory distress.

TREATMENT AND FOLLOW-UP

Treatment Options

Severely compromised animals require hospitalization and intensive care, with supplemental oxygen, fluid therapy, and treatment of shock. If conventional oxygen therapy (see handout on **Oxygen Therapy**) is inadequate, the animal may be anesthetized so that a temporary tracheostomy can be done (for obstructions high in the neck) or to allow passage of a small tube past the obstruction. Both procedures provide a way to deliver adequate oxygen to the lungs.

Once the animal is stable, specific therapy is instituted and may include the following:

* Tracheal foreign bodies are usually retrieved using a bronchoscope.
* Tracheal narrowing can be dilated in some instances with special balloon dilators, and occasionally the opening in the trachea can be made wider with laser therapy.
* In some cases of tracheal narrowing, the abnormal portion of the trachea is surgically removed, and the trachea is reconnected. As many as eight of the tracheal rings can be removed.
* When a tumor external to the trachea is suspected, further diagnostic studies, such as computed tomography (CT scan), may be indicated to better define the extent of the tumor and the feasibility of surgical removal of the mass.
* Tumors arising from inside the trachea may be partially removed with a bronchoscope. Further treatment, such as chemotherapy or surgery, is then pursued based on the tumor type.

Accompanying infections are treated with antibiotics. Other supportive care may include sedation, medications for pain, cough suppressants, and other measures.

Follow-up Care

Intensive monitoring is required both before and after bronchoscopy or surgery. Vital signs, such as respiratory rate, heart rate and rhythm, blood oxygen levels, and body temperature, are measured frequently. Following tracheal surgery, animals must be kept quiet and may remain on supplemental oxygen until swelling at the surgery site has subsided. Collars are replaced with a harness for a period of 3-4 weeks after surgery.

Prognosis

Many causes of tracheal obstruction are correctable and have a fair to good prognosis. Occasional coughing and gagging may persist because of chronic irritation of the trachea.

SPECIAL INSTRUCTIONS:

Tracheal Trauma

Ronald M. Bright, DVM, MS, DACVS

BASIC INFORMATION
Description and Causes

The trachea is the windpipe that carries air from the nose into the lungs. Tracheal trauma is usually associated with dog bites, penetrating neck injuries (such as gunshot or knife wounds), or blunt trauma from being hit by a car. Injury can be caused by accidental overinflation of the cuff on an endotracheal tube used to administer anesthesia or from administration of high air pressures through a mechanical ventilator. Surgical sites in the trachea (tracheotomy, tracheostomy) can fail or break down and produce many of the same signs as are seen with tracheal trauma.

Clinical Signs

Signs are not always noticed immediately and may be delayed for days or weeks until a portion of the trachea dies or scars. If the trachea is ruptured, air can escape into the tissues of the neck, resulting in air-filled spaces (subcutaneous emphysema) that cause swellings on the neck. These swellings are not painful. They are soft and may crackle or pop when compressed or squeezed. Air can also travel along the tissues down the neck and enter the chest cavity. Once in the chest, this air can cause varying degrees of lung collapse, leading to severe breathing problems, cyanosis (blue gums from lack of oxygen), and occasionally death.

With severe tracheal wounds that are accompanied by swelling in the surrounding tissues or bleeding into the windpipe, dramatic breathing problems may develop immediately. Difficulty breathing, sucking noises at the wound site, coughing of blood, weakness, and collapse may occur.

Diagnostic Tests

A tentative diagnosis is based on a history of recent or prior trauma to the trachea. Supportive evidence includes:

- Recent dental procedures, especially in cats, in which an endotracheal tube was used
- Obvious bite wounds or lacerations around the neck area
- Air accumulation under the skin in the neck area that may eventually extend all over the body
- X-rays demonstrating the presence of air under the skin and possibly within the chest

Endoscopy of the trachea, which involves passage of a flexible fiberoptic viewing scope, may be used to confirm the presence and location of the tracheal tear or puncture and to assess the extent of damage. This procedure requires general anesthesia, which can be tricky because it may not be possible to use an endotracheal tube. Your pet may be referred to a veterinary specialist for this procedure.

TREATMENT AND FOLLOW-UP

Treatment Options

If the trauma was blunt and no penetration of the trachea occurred, bandaging the neck, administering oxygen, and keeping the animal quiet in a cage for several days may resolve the problem. If the amount of air under the skin causes severe compression of the airway and tracheal collapse, needles may be inserted into the inflated tissue spaces to try and release some of the air.

In severe cases, when there is a lot of air leakage from the trachea and the animal's breathing is compromised, it is necessary to surgically explore the neck and repair the hole in the trachea. In some instances, the damage is so severe that removal of one or more tracheal rings is necessary. The trachea is then repaired and sewn back together. Surgery may also be used to explore the neck area for any other damage that may have occurred to the esophagus or nerves supplying the larynx.

Follow-up Care

In uncomplicated cases, air under the skin usually goes away within 7-10 days. It can take as long as 4-6 weeks for the air to resolve in some cases. If the air worsens or persists, then surgery to explore the neck area may be recommended. X-rays may be repeated to monitor resolution of the escaped air.

Prognosis

For trauma from penetrating wounds, early diagnosis and surgical correction often lead to good results, assuming there is limited damage to other structures. Taking a "wait and see" approach to severe tears involving the trachea can result in life-threatening respiratory problems, so surgery is often recommended in these cases.

Depending on the extent of the damage to the trachea and the type of surgery done, some degree of stricture (narrowing) of that portion of the trachea may occur during the healing process. Notify your veterinarian if any respiratory signs develop in the days to weeks after surgery.

SPECIAL INSTRUCTIONS:

SECTION 4

Neurologic System

Section Editor: Marc Kent, DVM, DACVIM (Small Animal and Neurology)

Atlantoaxial Subluxation in Dogs
Botulism
Brachial Plexus Avulsion
Brain Tumors
Canine Distemper Neurologic Disease
Caudal Cervical Spondylopathy (Wobbler Syndrome)
Caudal Occipital (Chiari-like) Malformation and
    Syringohydromyelia
Degenerative Myelopathy
Discospondylitis
Fibrocartilaginous Embolic Myelopathy
Granulomatous Meningoencephalitis and Necrotizing Encephalitis
Head Trauma
Hydrocephalus
Idiopathic Facial Nerve Paralysis
Idiopathic Peripheral Vestibular Disease
Idiopathic Trigeminal Neuropathy

Intervertebral Disc Disease
Ischemic Brain Injury (Stroke)
Lumbosacral Disease, Degenerative
Myasthenia Gravis
Peripheral Nerve Sheath Tumors
Polyradiculoneuritis in Dogs, Acute
Seizures: Causes and Diagnosis
Seizures: Idiopathic Epilepsy
Seizures: Treatment
Seizures: Treatment of Resistant Cases
Spinal Cord Trauma
Spinal Tumors
Spondylosis Deformans
Steroid-Responsive Meningeal Arteritis
Tick Paralysis
Tremor Syndrome

Atlantoaxial Subluxation in Dogs

A. Courtenay Freeman, DVM
Marc Kent, DVM, DACVIM (Small Animal and Neurology)
Simon R. Platt, BVM&S, MRCVS, DACVIM (Neurology), DECVN

BASIC INFORMATION

Description

The spine is made up of small bones called *vertebrae*, which surround and protect the spinal cord. The first and second vertebrae in the neck are called the *atlas* and the *axis*, respectively. These vertebrae form the atlantoaxial (AA) joint, which is connected by ligaments. The second vertebra in the neck has a bony, finger-like projection (the dens) that extends into the first vertebra and provides further stabilization of the two vertebrae. AA subluxation is a partial dislocation of the two vertebrae. It occurs when the connection between the first and second vertebrae is unstable, and it usually results in compression of the spinal cord.

Causes

Typically, AA subluxation arises from a developmental problem or birth defect. In affected dogs the dens is absent or deformed, which results in an unstable joint. Additionally, some of the supporting ligaments may not form properly. AA subluxation can also occur as a result of trauma and disruption of the connection between these two vertebrae.

This condition is more common in toy and small-breed dogs, such as the Chihuahua and the Yorkshire terrier. Because it is usually a developmental problem, affected animals are typically young (less than 2 years old); however, older dogs may develop clinical signs later in life, particularly after trauma to the neck.

Clinical Signs

Affected animals may have neck pain, an uncoordinated gait involving all four legs, and weakness. Clinical signs may develop after mild trauma, such as jumping or playing. The severity of clinical signs depends on the degree of spinal cord injury. Mild clinical signs include neck pain or an uncoordinated gait. More severely affected animals may be unable to walk. Severe spinal cord injury can affect the dog's ability to breathe and can even result in death.

Diagnostic Tests

AA subluxation may be suspected in young, toy breed dogs with compatible clinical signs. In many cases, a diagnosis can be made from x-rays of the neck that demonstrate an obvious dislocation of the vertebrae. X-rays must be obtained carefully to avoid further dislocation of the vertebrae. Magnetic resonance imaging (MRI) may be recommended to evaluate the spinal cord for compression and damage and to assess alignment of the vertebrae.

TREATMENT AND FOLLOW-UP

Treatment Options

Medical and surgical treatments exist for dogs with AA subluxation. Although medical therapy can be effective, surgery is the preferred treatment in most animals.

Surgical treatment involves alignment and stabilization (fusion) of this joint:

- Stabilizing the AA joint prevents further spinal cord injury and allows the spinal cord to recover.
- The AA joint is fused by the placement of orthopedic implants (often wires or screws) into the small bones and application of surgical cement.
- Strict cage confinement is necessary after surgical stabilization to allow proper joint fusion and recovery of the spinal cord.

Medical therapy involves placing a splint around the head and neck of the affected animal to immobilize the AA joint:

- The splint usually stays in place for at least 8 weeks and periodically must be replaced.
- The splint immobilizes the AA joint for enough time to allow scar tissue to form and also helps stabilize the joint.
- Because the scar tissue may not be strong enough to stabilize the joint, these animals may re-injure their spinal cord at a later date.
- Strict cage confinement is necessary while the splint is in place and for an additional 4 weeks after its removal.
- Activity is restricted to short, controlled walks (with the dog in a body harness) that allow the animal enough time to urinate and defecate. Many small patients find it difficult to walk with the splint in place.
- The dog cannot be allowed to run, jump, or play during the confinement period.

Follow-up Care

Animals with neck splints are often re-evaluated weekly, and the bandage or splint is changed. Follow-up visits are also needed frequently after surgery, and x-rays are usually done to evaluate healing 6-8 weeks after surgery. During the recovery period, notify your veterinarian immediately if any new neurologic signs develop or if previous ones recur or worsen.

Prognosis

Prognosis depends on the severity of the spinal cord injury and the treatment option pursued. Animals with mild clinical signs have a good prognosis. If clinical signs are severe, prognosis is variable and guarded (uncertain). Recurrence of signs is high with medical therapy, and surgical failure rates range from 10% to 40%.

SPECIAL INSTRUCTIONS:

Botulism

A. Courtenay Freeman, DVM
Marc Kent, DVM, DACVIM (Small Animal and Neurology)
Scott J. Schatzberg, DVM, PhD, DACVIM (Neurology)

BASIC INFORMATION

Description

Botulism is a rare disease that causes generalized weakness involving many of the nerves that activate the muscles of the body. Information travels down nerves to stimulate muscles to move (contract). This activation of muscles is mediated through a chemical called *acetylcholine*. Botulism blocks the release of acetylcholine from the nerve endings, which results in neurologic dysfunction and weakness.

Causes

Animals acquire botulism by ingesting the botulinum toxin, which is produced by a bacterial organism called *Clostridium botulinum*. This organism may be present in spoiled or rotting foods, garbage, and carrion.

Clinical Signs

After the animal eats spoiled, contaminated material, vomiting and diarrhea may occur prior to the onset of neurologic signs, which typically occurs 2-4 days after ingestion of the botulinum toxin. Affected animals usually develop hind leg weakness that is rapidly followed by front leg weakness. The animal has difficulty standing and walking. It may stand crouched and have a short-strided gait. Severely affected animals may not be able to stand, lift their heads up, or even move their legs. They may not be able to eat or drink because of weakness of the jaw and tongue muscles. Affected animals may not be able to bark or vocalize as a result of weakness of the muscles of the larynx. They may not be able to blink their eyes.

As a consequence of weakness of the muscles of the esophagus, it may become weakened and dilated (*megaesophagus*). Food and water may be regurgitated and can be inhaled (aspirated) into the lungs, leading to pneumonia. Signs of aspiration pneumonia include a cough, fever, and difficulty breathing. In severely affected animals, muscles involved in breathing, such as the diaphragm, may become weak, leading to respiratory failure and death.

Diagnostic Tests

A history of eating spoiled foods, garbage, or carrion and the presence of compatible clinical signs may cause an initial suspicion of botulism. Blood and feces can be tested for botulinum toxin; however, the toxin may not be detectable at the time clinical signs are occurring. Laboratory and other tests are needed to rule out diseases that cause similar signs. Chest x-rays may be recommended to look for pneumonia.

Specialized electrophysiologic procedures, such as electromyography and nerve stimulation testing, help to identify nerve dysfunction that supports the diagnosis. Sometimes the diagnosis can be made only after other diseases that cause similar clinical signs have been excluded.

TREATMENT AND FOLLOW-UP

Treatment Options

There is no specific treatment for botulism. Affected animals usually require hospitalization and intensive supportive care, such as intravenous fluids, during recovery. Medications may be given to stop vomiting and help the diarrhea. Affected animals require clean, dry, padded bedding and frequent changes in their position to prevent bedsores and pneumonia. Assistance is needed with urination and defecation and keeping the animal clean. If the muscles of the diaphragm are involved, the animal may be placed on a mechanical ventilator.

Animals that are able to eat and swallow can be fed with the head held up to prevent aspiration. Animals unable to eat may require insertion of a feeding tube and supplemental nutrition. The eyes may require lubrication if the animal cannot blink. Physical therapy exercises can be performed to prevent muscle wasting and encourage improved muscle tone. Any secondary problems that arise because of this disease also require specific treatment.

Follow-up Care

Recovery may be rapid in mild cases, but it can take weeks. After discharge from the hospital, continued nursing care is commonly needed at home. Recheck visits are often used to monitor the animal's progress and recovery.

Prognosis

Clinical signs usually improve gradually over 3-4 weeks. Most mildly affected animals return to normal. Prognosis is very poor (guarded) for animals with paralysis of the breathing muscles and aspiration pneumonia.

SPECIAL INSTRUCTIONS:

Brachial Plexus Avulsion

A. Courtenay Freeman, DVM
Marc Kent, DVM, DACVIM (Small Animal and Neurology)
Simon R. Platt, BVM&S, MRCVS, DACVIM (Neurology), DECVN

BASIC INFORMATION

Description

The brachial plexus is a group of nerves located in the arm-pit area, where the front leg joins the shoulder blade and the chest. The brachial plexus on each side includes the nerves that activate muscle movement and allow for sensation (feeling) in the leg. A brachial plexus avulsion occurs when these nerves are completely torn. Sometimes the nerves are only damaged or stretched.

Causes

Trauma is the most common cause of brachial plexus injuries, and automobile accidents are the most common cause of trauma. Damage to the brachial plexus can also occur from falls, gunshot wounds, and other injuries that stretch the front legs.

Clinical Signs

Clinical signs occur suddenly after the injury. Signs can vary depending on which nerves in the brachial plexus are damaged and the severity of the nerve damage.

*   Damage to the nerves in one portion of the brachial plexus leads to inability to move the shoulder or bend the elbow. In these cases, the animal may be able to straighten the elbow and, therefore, support weight and walk.
*   Damage to the nerves in another portion of the brachial plexus results in inability to support weight on the leg. The animal walks with the paw knuckled under and cannot bend the shoulder or elbow. Severe neurologic damage can result in loss of feeling in the leg.

A condition called *Horner's syndrome* can also occur following brachial plexus avulsion. Horner's syndrome affects the eye on the same side as the brachial plexus injury, resulting in a small pupil, a droopy upper eyelid, a raised third eyelid, and a sunken appearance to the eye. Vision is not affected.

Diagnostic Tests

The diagnosis of brachial plexus avulsion is usually made from the history and neurologic examination. Other body systems are also evaluated for damage from the trauma. Orthopedic injuries and damage to the heart and lungs may be present and require immediate attention. X-rays of the front legs, abdomen, and chest may be recommended to evaluate for other injuries.

Specialized tests such as electromyography (EMG) and nerve conduction studies can be performed to evaluate muscle and nerve function; however, changes in these tests may not develop for 7-10 days after the injury. These tests usually require referral to a veterinary neurologist, are performed with the use of general anesthesia, and rarely provide information about the potential return of limb function.

TREATMENT AND FOLLOW-UP

Treatment Options

There is no specific treatment for brachial plexus avulsion. If the nerves are only damaged and not torn, then recovery of function may be possible. Recovery can take weeks to months. During this time, it is important to prevent injuries to the affected leg caused by dragging of the toes. A foot protector or "bootie" may be recommended. Some severely affected animals may mutilate the affected leg, especially if they have lost sensation (feeling) in their toes. A drug called *gabapentin* may be tried to alleviate the "pins and needles" sensations that are associated with self-mutilation and foot chewing.

Physical therapy exercises may be recommended, such as massaging the muscles and moving the leg in a walking motion for a few minutes, several times a day. These exercises are essential to maintain muscle tone and prevent shrinkage of the muscles from disuse.

If the animal does not regain nerve function in the affected leg, amputation is usually recommended to prevent continued injury and self-mutilation.

Follow-up Care

Initially, frequent follow-up examinations are often needed to monitor for improvement and further damage to the leg. Once nerve function returns, or if the leg is amputated, long-term follow-up is not typically necessary.

Prognosis

Prognosis depends on the severity of nerve damage. Mildly damaged nerves can sometimes regenerate over time, but the process is very slow. Brachial plexus injuries that cause paralysis and loss of feeling have a poor prognosis for recovery. Injuries that result in complete brachial plexus avulsions are irreversible. In general, if there is no improvement in 2-4 weeks, amputation of the affected leg may be necessary. The maximum time in which recovery is still possible is approximately 3-4 months after the injury.

SPECIAL INSTRUCTIONS:

Brain Tumors

A. Courtenay Freeman, DVM
Marc Kent, DVM, DACVIM (Small Animal and Neurology)
Simon R. Platt, BVM&S, MRCVS, DACVIM (Neurology), DECVN

BASIC INFORMATION
Description

Brain tumors (sometimes called *neoplasms*) may affect both dogs and cats. They may be benign or malignant. These tumors may arise from brain tissue (called *primary tumors*), grow into the brain from nearby areas of the head (such as the skull), or spread to the brain from another site in the body (metastatic tumors). The latter two types are called *secondary tumors*.

Brain tumors occur more frequently in older dogs and cats; however, on rare occasions, young animals can be affected. Commonly affected breeds include the golden retriever, Labrador retriever, collie, Boston terrier, and boxer. The domestic shorthair is the cat most commonly affected.

Causes

The cause of most brain tumors is unknown, but several types of tumors exist:

- The most common brain tumor in dogs and cats is the meningoma, which develops from the tissue that covers the brain and spinal cord (the meninges).
- The most common tumors that develop from tissue within the brain are gliomas, which can be classified as astrocytomas or oligodendrogliomas.
- Sometimes, tumors form from cells lining the ventricles (cavities within the brain that are filled with cerebrospinal fluid). Examples of these tumors include choroid plexus tumors and ependymomas.

Secondary tumors that arise in the nose, sinuses, skull, ears, or eyes may invade the brain. Cancer in other areas of the body can spread (metastasize) to the brain.

Clinical Signs

Signs vary with the location and size of the tumor. Neurologic signs may develop gradually over weeks to months or arise suddenly. Common clinical signs include seizures, behavioral changes, loss of vision, and abnormalities in gait. As tumors enlarge the flow of cerebrospinal fluid (CSF) can become obstructed, causing signs of secondary hydrocephalus. (See also the handout on **Hydrocephalus**.)

Diagnostic Tests

A neurologic examination, laboratory tests, and x-rays are often recommended to rule out other diseases that produce similar signs and to search for tumors elsewhere in the body. Imaging of the brain via computed tomography (CT scan) or magnetic resonance imaging (MRI) usually reveals a mass in the brain suggestive of a tumor but may not provide a specific diagnosis. A brain biopsy may be required to confirm the diagnosis. Biopsy samples are sometimes obtained during surgery or by guiding a needle into the tumor during the CT scan.

A spinal tap and collection of CSF for analysis may be recommended to eliminate other brain diseases, such as inflammation, but this can be risky in some patients with elevated CSF pressure in the brain.

TREATMENT AND FOLLOW-UP

Treatment Options

Treatment options vary depending on the type and location of the tumor and the clinical signs produced. Surgery, radiation therapy, medical management, or a combination of these may be pursued.

Medications that may be administered include anticonvulsant drugs to control seizures and steroids to decrease inflammation and edema associated with the tumor. Although these medications do not affect the growth of the tumor, they can improve clinical signs and the animal's quality of life. Chemotherapy may be beneficial for certain brain tumors but has not been as successful as surgery or radiation therapy.

Surgery can be performed on tumors in certain regions of the brain. Because they arise from the tissue covering the brain, meningiomas are often amenable to surgery. Surgery may allow removal of most of the tumor and relieve clinical signs. Although most animals recover well from brain surgery, serious risks exist, including worsening of clinical signs and death.

Radiation therapy can be used for tumors that are inoperable or to destroy tumor cells left behind from surgery.

Follow-up Care

Frequent recheck visits are needed when therapy is initially started, to monitor for complications after surgery and to adjust medication dosages. Radiation therapy typically requires several weeks of treatment, followed by recheck visits about every 2 months. Continuous, long-term follow-up is needed for most patients with brain tumors.

Prognosis

Long-term prognosis for animals with a brain tumor is always very poor. Prognosis is affected by tumor type and location. Some cats with meningiomas may live 2-3 years after surgery, and dogs with meningiomas may survive for months or longer. It is not always possible to surgically remove the entire tumor in most dogs. Consequently, radiation therapy may be used after surgery to extend the survival time of affected animals. Without treatment, clinical signs in most animals worsen over several weeks. Most secondary tumors are cancerous, are very difficult to treat, and carry the worst prognosis.

SPECIAL INSTRUCTIONS:

Canine Distemper Neurologic Disease

A. Courtenay Freeman, DVM
Marc Kent, DVM, DACVIM (Small Animal and Neurology)
Scott J. Schatzberg, DVM, PhD, DACVIM (Neurology)

BASIC INFORMATION

Description

Canine distemper is a contagious viral infection of dogs that may cause respiratory, urogenital, gastrointestinal, ocular (eye), and central nervous system (brain and spinal cord) signs. The routine use of vaccines against canine distemper has greatly reduced the incidence of this disease in North America, but it still commonly occurs in many other parts of the world.

Causes

Canine distemper virus (CDV) is transmitted between dogs primarily through infected respiratory secretions. The virus multiplies within the lymph nodes (glands) of the head and throat. Infected white blood cells leave the lymph nodes and spread the infection throughout the body. Within 1 week, infection may involve the eyes, nose, intestinal and respiratory tracts, and the nervous system.

Unvaccinated puppies are most susceptible to CDV infection; however, older dogs may also become infected. The infection weakens (suppresses) the immune system, making the animal more susceptible to other diseases. Although vaccination is extremely effective for preventing CDV infection, occasionally animals become infected despite having been vaccinated.

Clinical Signs

Clinical signs are variable and depend on the strength of the dog's immune system. Vaccinated dogs with a strong immune system typically clear the virus and do not develop clinical signs. Dogs with a weak immune system, such as puppies, are often unable to fight off the infection and may develop severe clinical signs. Since it is not possible to determine the strength of a dog's immune system, care should be taken to prevent exposure of potentially susceptible dogs.

Some affected dogs only develop generalized (systemic) signs, whereas others have only nervous system signs. Initially, signs of a respiratory infection may occur, with severe ocular and nasal discharge, cough, and fever. The respiratory infection can progress to pneumonia in some animals. Additional signs include loss of appetite, vomiting, and diarrhea.

Nervous system signs include mental dullness, lethargy, unresponsiveness, disorientation, blindness, imbalance, and seizures. Affected dogs may stumble as they walk and some act as if they are in pain.

Telltale physical findings can indicate a previous infection, such as abnormal enamel on the teeth, thickened skin on the nose and footpads (hyperkeratosis), and involuntary, rhythmic jerking of one or more muscles (myoclonus). Typically, myoclonus is confined to a single limb. The muscles of the head can be affected, however, and the animal may rhythmically clench its teeth. Myoclonus may persist even when the animal is sleeping.

Diagnostic Tests

Routine laboratory tests are usually recommended to search for evidence of an infection and other organ involvement. CDV can cause a decrease in the white blood cell count. X-rays of the chest may reveal pneumonia.

Many tests can be used to diagnose CDV infection, but no single test is 100% diagnostic, so multiple tests are often needed. Samples that can be tested for CDV include the conjunctiva (tissue lining of the inside of the eyelids), skin biopsies, blood, cerebrospinal fluid (CSF, taken by spinal tap), and urine. Blood can also be tested for antibodies to CDV (canine distemper titer); however, this test can be difficult to interpret, because most animals produce antibodies after they are vaccinated.

Analysis of CSF may indicate evidence of inflammation in the nervous system of some dogs, but these changes are not specific for CDV infection and may not be seen in the early stages of the disease. Magnetic resonance imaging (MRI) can show multiple abnormal areas in the brain that are consistent with CDV infection.

TREATMENT AND FOLLOW-UP

Treatment Options

There is no specific treatment for distemper infection. Supportive care is important for animals that are systemically ill. Anticonvulsant medications may be given for seizures, but the seizures can be difficult to control. (See also the handout on **Canine Distemper Virus.**) Affected dogs must be kept isolated from other dogs, because the disease is contagious.

Follow-up Care

Many dogs require hospitalization for supportive care. Laboratory tests and x-rays may be repeated to monitor response to treatments. Recovery time can be prolonged, and recheck visits are often needed following discharge from the hospital. If the animal survives the acute infection, late-developing signs may still occur.

Prognosis

Prognosis is poor if the clinical signs are severe or worsen despite supportive care. CDV causes severe debilitation and death in many dogs; however, the disease is not fatal to all dogs. Dogs that develop neurologic signs have a worse prognosis. Neurologic signs, such as seizures, blindness, and myoclonus, may persist after recovery from infection. The disease is best prevented with appropriate vaccination.

SPECIAL INSTRUCTIONS:

Caudal Cervical Spondylopathy (Wobbler Syndrome)

A. Courtenay Freeman, DVM
Marc Kent, DVM, DACVIM (Small Animal and Neurology)
Scott J. Schatzberg, DVM, PhD, DACVIM (Neurology)

BASIC INFORMATION

Description

Caudal cervical spondylopathy (also called *cervical vertebral malformation-malarticulation* or *wobbler syndrome*) is a disorder that results in spinal cord compression due to instability of the spine. The spinal cord compression can be dynamic, which means the compression is worse when the neck is held in certain positions. The syndrome is most common in large- and giant-breed dogs.

Causes

Although the cause of wobbler syndrome is unknown, many factors may be involved. Compression may occur from bony malformation of the vertebrae, intervertebral disc herniation, or thickening of the supporting ligaments of the spine. The Doberman pinscher and Great Dane are the breeds most commonly affected. Great Danes are often affected before 2 years of age, whereas Dobermans are more commonly affected from 3-9 years of age.

Clinical Signs

Signs depend on the speed of onset, duration, and degree of compression. Signs may develop suddenly over a few days or slowly over weeks to months. Typically, all four legs are affected because the problem involves the neck region. Occasionally, signs begin in the hind legs, but over time the disease usually affects all four legs. Neurologic abnormalities depend on the severity of spinal cord compression:

- Mild compression may result in neck pain only.
- More severe compression causes an uncoordinated ("wobbly") gait in all four legs, crossing over of the legs when walking, toe scuffing, and weakness. The hind legs are often more affected than the front legs.
- As compression worsens, the animal may be unable to walk or may become paralyzed.

Diagnostic Tests

The syndrome initially is suspected based on the history and clinical signs. X-rays of the neck may show degenerative changes in the spine; however, they cannot demonstrate spinal cord compression. Advanced imaging of the spine, such as magnetic resonance imaging (MRI), computed tomography (CT scan), or myelography (x-rays taken after a dye is injected into the space around the spinal cord) is necessary for the diagnosis. MRI provides the most detailed evaluation of the spinal cord and spine. Images may be obtained with the neck held in several positions. Your veterinarian may also recommend laboratory tests to rule out diseases that cause similar signs.

TREATMENT AND FOLLOW-UP

Treatment Options

Conservative and surgical treatment options exist for dogs with wobbler syndrome. Conservative therapy is reserved for animals with pain and/or mild neurologic abnormalities and consists of exercise restriction, anti-inflammatory drugs, and pain medications.

- Exercise restriction involves strict confinement and limited leash walking, for the sake of urination and defecation only.
- Dogs should not be allowed to run, jump, or play during the period of confinement.
- Exercise restriction typically lasts 4-6 weeks and is followed by gradual return to normal activity over an additional month.
- Anti-inflammatory drugs, such as nonsteroidal anti-inflammatory medications or short-term corticosteroids, can be used, but they are not used together because of their combined side effects.

Surgery is often preferred for dogs with severe neurologic signs, such as moderate to severe incoordination, weakness, inability to walk, and paralysis, and for dogs with pain that is unresponsive to conservative treatment. Surgery may also be considered in dogs that have recurrent signs. Surgery may involve removal of herniated intervertebral disc material (common in the Doberman pinscher). It may also involve removal of various portions of the vertebrae that are compressing the spinal cord and spinal stabilization (fusion). Various techniques can be used to stabilize the spine. After surgery, conservative therapy is also usually started.

Follow-up Care

Initially, repeated neurologic examinations are often performed to monitor for improvement in clinical signs. These examinations can be performed daily if the dog is hospitalized or periodically during outpatient visits. Visits are often repeated every 1-2 weeks initially and then decreased to every 1-2 months if improvement is observed. Long-term follow-up is frequently needed. Notify your veterinarian if any signs worsen or recur.

Prognosis

Prognosis depends on the severity and duration of the clinical signs. Mildly affected dogs and dogs that have pain as the only clinical sign often respond well to conservative therapy. Many dogs with moderate to severe clinical signs improve after surgical therapy. Resolution of clinical signs may take weeks to months. Prognosis is worse for dogs with severe neurologic signs and for dogs with multiple areas of compression of the spinal cord. Dogs with severe clinical signs have a very poor (guarded) prognosis even with surgery. Clinical signs may recur in dogs managed both conservatively and surgically.

SPECIAL INSTRUCTIONS:

Caudal Occipital (Chiari-like) Malformation and Syringohydromyelia

A. Courtenay Freeman, DVM
Marc Kent, DVM, DACVIM (Small Animal and Neurology)
Simon R. Platt, BVM&S, MRCVS, DACVIM (Neurology), DECVN

BASIC INFORMATION

Description

The skull is made up of several flat bones that fuse together to encase and protect the brain. The bone of the back of the skull is called the *occipital bone*. Malformation or abnormal development of this bone compresses the back part of the brain, which is called the *cerebellum*. This compression causes the cerebellum to herniate (shift backward) and obstruct the hole in the skull where the brain joins the spinal cord. This hole is called the *foramen magnum*.

Obstruction of the foramen magnum alters the flow of cerebrospinal fluid (CSF). Normally, CSF is produced within the brain and flows around the brain and down the outside of the spinal cord. In caudal occipital or Chiari-like malformation, obstruction of CSF flow leads to the accumulation of fluid within the spinal cord. This fluid accumulation is referred to as *syringohydromyelia* (SHM).

The Cavalier King Charles spaniel is the most commonly affected breed of dog; however, other dogs, especially small-breed dogs, can also be affected.

Causes

Caudal occipital malformation is a congenital problem caused by abnormal development of the occipital bone of the skull. In the Cavalier King Charles spaniel, the condition may be inherited.

Clinical Signs

Onset of clinical signs may be sudden or may take several months to years to develop. Animals affected by this disease range from young to old.

Clinical signs often result from SHM and are related to spinal cord dysfunction. Signs include neck pain, weakness, incoordination, and muscle loss over the shoulders. Scoliosis (abnormal curvature of the spine) and twisting of the head can occur. Affected animals may excessively scratch at their head and neck, especially when excited. Facial muscle paralysis and imbalance are occasionally observed. Seizures have also occurred in some affected animals, but they may be unrelated to this malformation.

Diagnostic Tests

A neurologic examination, routine laboratory tests, and x-rays are often recommended to rule out other diseases that produce similar signs. Confirming the diagnosis usually requires magnetic resonance imaging (MRI). MRI can reveal distortion of the brain structures, obstruction of CSF flow at the foramen magnum, and the presence of SHM.

TREATMENT AND FOLLOW-UP

Treatment Options

Medical and surgical treatments exist. In most cases, medical therapy is pursued initially and is aimed at decreasing CSF production and providing pain relief. Corticosteroids can be used to reduce CSF production. Occasionally, diuretic drugs may also be needed. Pain medications, such as gabapentin or tramadol, may be used in animals that experience discomfort or painful episodes.

Surgical therapy involves enlarging the foramen magnum in an attempt to restore CSF flow. When the obstruction is relieved, the CSF does not continue to accumulate within the spinal cord. This surgery may not eliminate fluid that has already accumulated, so some clinical signs may not improve. Surgery is most often considered for dogs with severe signs or signs that worsen despite medical therapy.

Follow-up Care

Follow-up visits are scheduled frequently at first, to monitor the success of medical or surgical treatment. Recheck appointments may eventually be decreased to every 6 months if the animal responds to treatment and has no complications. A recheck MRI may be helpful to evaluate the success of treatment and to identify any progression of the disease.

Prognosis

Prognosis depends on the severity of clinical signs and the extent of structural damage to the brain and spinal cord. Many mildly affected dogs can be successfully treated with medical therapy. In some dogs clinical signs improve after surgery, but surgery is not always successful, and recurrence of signs is possible. In some dogs, surgery may halt worsening of the signs and allow medical therapy to be more effective.

SPECIAL INSTRUCTIONS:

Degenerative Myelopathy

A. Courtenay Freeman, DVM
Marc Kent, DVM, DACVIM (Small Animal and Neurology)
Scott J. Schatzberg, DVM, PhD, DACVIM (Neurology)

BASIC INFORMATION

Description

Degenerative myelopathy is a spinal cord condition that results in progressive hind leg weakness and incoordination. The spinal cord is composed of nerve cells and fibers (axons). Nerve impulses are transmitted along the axons of the spinal cord from the brain to the limbs, and vice versa. When portions of the spinal cord degenerate, nerve impulses are not properly transmitted in both directions. Consequently, the legs become weaker, and eventually the dog cannot voluntarily move them. Feeling in the legs is also affected. The degeneration involves primarily the spinal cord in the back region, so the hind limbs of the dog are predominantly affected.

Causes

The exact reason degenerative myelopathy develops is not well understood. An inherited (genetic) basis is suspected. The German shepherd dog is the most commonly affected breed, but any large-breed dog may develop the condition. Other breeds commonly affected include the boxer and Pembroke Welsh corgi. The myelopathy usually occurs in older dogs (older than 5 years).

Clinical Signs

Degenerative myelopathy causes a chronic, progressive, nonpainful hind leg weakness.

- Affected animals become uncoordinated (unsteady) in the hind legs, scuff or knuckle over on those toes, stumble, and have difficulty rising from a down position.
- Eventually, the disease worsens to the point where the dog can no longer walk and drags its hind legs.
- Loss of voluntary control of urination, fecal incontinence, and front leg weakness may occur late in the disease.

Diagnostic Tests

Currently, there is no definitive test for degenerative myelopathy. Routine laboratory tests may be recommended but are usually normal. A presumptive diagnosis can be made when advanced imaging studies reveal no abnormalities of the spinal cord or vertebral canal. In other words, advanced imaging rules out other diseases that can cause similar signs. The best imaging technique for this purpose is magnetic resonance imaging (MRI), but myelography (x-rays taken after insertion of a dye around the spinal cord) and computed tomography (CT scan) can also be used. Evaluation of cerebrospinal fluid (CSF) taken from a spinal tap may be normal, although sometimes the protein content of CSF is mildly increased.

A DNA test is available through the Orthopedic Foundation for Animals to look for the genetic mutation associated with this disease. The test identifies whether the dog is clear of the mutation, a carrier, or at risk for developing degenerative myelopathy. Unfortunately, definitive diagnosis can be made only by evaluating the spinal cord after death via an autopsy.

TREATMENT AND FOLLOW-UP

Treatment Options

Currently, no proven effective treatment exists for degenerative myelopathy. Treatment consists of nursing care and assisting movement in dogs that cannot walk well. Carts, similar to wheelchairs, are sometimes used to help weak or paralyzed dogs move around.

Follow-up Care

Animals are rechecked periodically to monitor the progression of disease. Urinary retention may predispose the dog to bladder infections, so periodic urinalyses may be recommended.

Prognosis

Long-term prognosis is very poor, because the disease progresses to paralysis over the course of 6 months to several years. Animals are usually euthanized when they become severely debilitated.

SPECIAL INSTRUCTIONS:

Discospondylitis

A. Courtenay Freeman, DVM
Marc Kent, DVM, DACVIM (Small Animal and Neurology)
Scott J. Schatzberg, DVM, PhD, DACVIM (Neurology)

BASIC INFORMATION

Description

Discospondylitis is an infection of the vertebrae and intervertebral disc spaces. The spine is made up of small bones called *vertebrae* that surround and protect the spinal cord. Between adjacent vertebrae there are discs (intervertebral discs) that act as cushions and provide strength and stability to the spine.

Discospondylitis occurs more commonly in young to middle-aged dogs and in medium to giant breeds, such as the Great Dane and the German shepherd dog. Male dogs are more commonly affected than females.

Causes

Infection occurs when a bacteria or fungus spreads to the disc space through the bloodstream from some other area in the body, such as the urinary tract, skin, heart valves, or mouth.

Staphylococcus species (Staph bacteria) are commonly responsible. Brucellosis causes the infection in a small percentage of dogs, especially breeding dogs. Brucellosis is also contagious to humans.

Clinical Signs

Affected dogs are often systemically ill and may have neurologic abnormalities. Signs of systemic illness include fever, decreased appetite, lethargy, weight loss, and depression. Other signs may be present, depending on the source of the infection.

Pain in the area of the spine may be the only clinical sign noted in some dogs. Neurologic signs vary with the degree and location of spinal cord compression or instability and may include weakness, uncoordinated gait, and paralysis.

Diagnostic Tests

A presumptive diagnosis is often made based on characteristic findings on x-rays of the spine. Routine laboratory tests (blood and urine) are usually performed to look for evidence of infection and to evaluate the dog's general health. Brucellosis testing is usually recommended. Bacterial cultures of urine, blood, or any other infected tissue may be done to try and isolate the organism responsible for the infection. X-rays of the chest, an abdominal ultrasound, and/or an echocardiogram (heart ultrasound) may be recommended to look for an underlying source of the infection.

Computed tomography (CT scan) and magnetic resonance imaging (MRI) may provide information that is not visible on plain x-rays and may help determine whether surgery is indicated. In some instances, a needle is passed into the infected intervertebral disc space during a CT scan for the purpose of obtaining material for bacterial culture.

TREATMENT AND FOLLOW-UP

Treatment Options

Treatment involves administration of antibiotics and pain medication, as well as cage rest:

- The infection is often treated with antibiotics for a minimum of 8 weeks. When possible, antibiotic therapy is based on bacterial culture results. If bacteria cannot be identified, then antibiotics are chosen that are effective against multiple types of bacteria.
- Because discospondylitis can be painful, pain medications are often used.
- Strict confinement is important during recovery, because infection of the intervertebral disc can cause spinal instability. Confinement involves cage rest, restriction of exercise, and leash walking only for urination and defecation.
- Improvement of signs associated with systemic illness (fever, lethargy) and pain is typically seen within the first week of treatment. If no improvement occurs, additional testing or treatment may be necessary.

Animals occasionally require surgery to remove material causing spinal cord compression and to stabilize the vertebral column. Surgery is usually done for animals with severe neurologic problems or pain that does respond to treatment.

Dogs that are positive for brucellosis present a dilemma with regard to treatment, because they may be contagious to other dogs and people. Contact your physician if there is a risk of human infection. (See the handouts on **Brucellosis** and **Infertility in Male Dogs**.)

Follow-up Care

X-rays may be recommended every 6-8 weeks to look for resolution of the infection. Laboratory and other tests may also be repeated, depending on the original source or location of the infection. Often x-rays show little change for months. Antibiotics are typically continued for a minimum of 8 weeks regardless of x-ray findings, and some affected animals require several months of antibiotic therapy.

Prognosis

Prognosis is good in animals that respond to treatment within the first week. Animals with mild neurologic signs also have a favorable prognosis. Bacterial infections usually respond better than fungal infections to treatment. Bacterial infections that are resistant to treatment, fungal infections, and the presence of brucellosis are associated with a worse prognosis. Animals with severe neurologic signs or spinal instability have a poor prognosis for full recovery; however, aggressive antibiotic therapy and surgery may allow a complete recovery even in animals with severe disease.

SPECIAL INSTRUCTIONS:

Fibrocartilaginous Embolic Myelopathy

A. Courtenay Freeman, DVM
Marc Kent, DVM, DACVIM (Small Animal and Neurology)
Simon R. Platt, BVM&S, MRCVS, DACVIM (Neurology), DECVN

BASIC INFORMATION

Description

The spinal cord needs a proper blood supply to maintain normal function. Any decrease in blood (ischemia) or loss of blood supply (infarction) to a region of the spinal cord causes spinal cord damage and neurologic abnormalities. Blood supply is usually lost when an obstruction (embolus) develops within a blood vessel supplying the spinal cord.

Between adjacent vertebrae are discs (intervertebral discs) composed of a fibrous outer portion (annulus fibrosis) and a gel-like center (nucleus pulposus). These discs act as cushions between vertebrae and provide strength and stability to the spine. Fibrocartilaginous embolic myelopathy (FCEM) occurs when microscopic pieces of an intervertebral disc lodge in the blood vessels that supply blood to the spinal cord. The end result is spinal cord ischemia or infarction.

Causes

The cause of FCEM is unknown. Medium- to large-breed dogs are more commonly affected; however, smaller dogs, such as the miniature schnauzer, Shetland sheepdog, and Yorkshire terrier, can also develop FECM. Rarely, FECM may occur in cats.

Clinical Signs

FCEM causes a sudden onset of neurologic abnormalities, which are dependent on the area of spinal cord affected. The condition is not typically painful; however, some animals cry out when the infarction occurs. Neurologic abnormalities do not usually progress or deteriorate from their initial severity and are usually worse on one side of the body or in one leg.

An uncoordinated gait suddenly develops that may involve all four legs, the legs on just one side of the body, or only the hind legs. The animals may be weak, scuff their feet, and cross their legs when walking. Severe injury to the spinal cord can result in paralysis and the inability to feel a painful stimulus applied to the toes.

Diagnostic Tests

FCEM is initially suspected in animals based on the history and neurologic examination findings. Routine laboratory tests and x-rays may be recommended to rule out other conditions that produce similar signs, but they are usually normal. Magnetic resonance imaging (MRI) is the best test available to diagnose FCEM and to rule out other conditions. Others tests, such as myelography (a series of x-rays taken after injecting a dye around the spinal cord) or computed tomography (CT scan), can be used to eliminate other conditions but are often normal in cases of FCEM. A spinal tap and evaluation of cerebrospinal fluid (CSF) may be recommended to help eliminate other neurologic diseases.

TREATMENT AND FOLLOW-UP

Treatment Options

No specific treatment exists for the spinal cord damage that develops during FCEM. Treatment involves supportive care and allowing time for the spinal cord to heal. Hospitalization is often required. Physical therapy, such as hydrotherapy, may be recommended during recovery. Supportive care is particularly important for paralyzed animals. These patients may develop urinary retention and bladder infections, urine-induced scalding of their skin, skin ulcers, and pneumonia if excellent nursing care is not provided.

Follow-up Care

While the animal is hospitalized, neurologic functions are reevaluated frequently. If the animal improves enough to be discharged, then periodic rechecks are usually done to evaluate signs of recovery. If the animal recovers the ability to walk and urinate on its own within the first 3 months, then long-term follow-up may not be necessary. If the animal does not regain the ability to walk or remains incontinent, frequent rechecks are necessary.

Prognosis

Prognosis depends on the severity of clinical signs. Many mild to moderately affected dogs improve over time. Recovery may take weeks to months, and some dogs do not return completely to normal. Residual neurologic problems can include inability to walk, weakness, and urinary or fecal incontinence. Any clinical signs remaining after 3-4 months are likely to be permanent. Prognosis is worse in animals that have severe spinal cord injury and do not (from the onset of FCEM) have the ability to feel a painful stimulus in the affected legs.

SPECIAL INSTRUCTIONS:

Granulomatous Meningoencephalitis and Necrotizing Encephalitis

A. Courtenay Freeman, DVM
Marc Kent, DVM, DACVIM (Small Animal and Neurology)
Scott J. Schatzberg, DVM, PhD, DACVIM (Neurology)

BASIC INFORMATION

Description

Granulomatous meningoencephalitis (GME) and necrotizing encephalitis (NE) are disorders that arise from inflammation of the brain and/or spinal cord and their coverings (the meninges). These diseases affect predominantly young, small-breed dogs.

Causes

Both GME and NE are presently considered to be autoimmune disorders, meaning that the body launches an abnormal attack against its own nervous system tissues. Potential triggers for the autoimmune attack may include infections and vaccinations. Genetics may also play a role in the development of GME and NE.

Although any breed of dog may be affected with GME, toy breeds are affected most often. Breeds commonly affected by NE include the pug, Maltese, Yorkshire terrier, Chihuahua, French bulldog, shih tzu, and Pomeranian.

Clinical Signs

Clinical signs are variable and relate to the area of the brain or spinal cord that is inflamed. Clinical signs often worsen rapidly and may include seizures, lethargy, circling, loss of balance, and decreased vision. Both GME and NE can be fatal, with or without aggressive therapy.

Diagnostic Tests

The breed and age of dog and the variety of neurologic signs may create an initial suspicion of GME or NE. A definitive diagnosis cannot be made without evaluation of brain tissue, which requires a biopsy. Because a brain biopsy is not practical in most dogs, information from other tests is valuable for establishing a presumptive diagnosis:

- Routine blood tests are often performed to evaluate the overall health of the affected dog and to eliminate other diseases.
- The key tests to establish a presumptive diagnosis are brain imaging, such as magnetic resonance imaging (MRI) and computed tomography (CT scan), and analysis of spinal fluid (CSF). MRI is the most sensitive method of brain imaging, but a CT scan may also be utilized. They often reveal areas of inflammation. Both GME and NE can affect any region of the brain, but they each have a tendency to involve particular areas, which may help tell them apart.
- Although CSF analysis may rarely be normal, it usually reveals elevated numbers of white blood cells and elevated protein levels. CSF analysis also helps to rule out other diseases (such as tumors and infections) that may affect the nervous system.

TREATMENT AND FOLLOW-UP

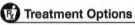

Treatment Options

Because GME and NE are caused by inflammation, treatment is initially directed at suppressing the inflammation with steroids. High doses are used initially; as the animal improves, the dosage may be lowered gradually over the course of months. The goal of therapy is to reduce the dosage to the minimal amount needed to control the clinical signs. Side effects of steroids include increased thirst, appetite, and urination. Animals may breathe heavily and pant excessively. Long-term side effects include a thin hair coat, poor wound healing, and muscle loss. Steroid therapy can also make the dog prone to infections of the skin and urinary tract. Notify your veterinarian if any of these side effects occur.

Affected dogs are often treated with additional immunosuppressive medications such as arabinoside-C (*Cytosar*), cyclosporine, or procarbazine. Arabinoside-C and procarbazine are chemotherapeutic drugs, so care must be taken to avoid human exposure to these medications. Dogs with seizures also may require anticonvulsant therapy. (See handout on **Seizures: Treatment**.)

Follow-up Care

Initially, rechecks are scheduled based on the severity of signs and the drugs used. More frequent visits may be necessary for dogs receiving arabinoside-C or procarbazine, because these drugs can have serious side effects, including decreased white blood cell counts, loss of appetite, vomiting, and diarrhea. Careful monitoring with frequent blood tests is indicated. Once the dog responds to therapy and the signs improve, treatment and recheck intervals may be extended.

Prognosis

GME and NE are difficult to cure, but clinical signs often are controllable with aggressive treatment. Treatment may decrease the severity of the clinical signs; however, some neurologic abnormalities may not completely resolve.

The long-term prognosis is guarded to poor, in that most dogs require lifelong treatment and some dogs do not respond even to aggressive therapy. Dogs that do respond to treatment can live for years with these diseases. Relapses may occur after an initial response to treatment, so notify your veterinarian if any clinical signs return. Without treatment, clinical signs usually worsen and can result in death within a few days to weeks.

SPECIAL INSTRUCTIONS:

Head Trauma

A. Courtenay Freeman, DVM
Marc Kent, DVM, DACVIM (Small Animal and Neurology)
Simon R. Platt, BVM&S, MRCVS, DACVIM (Neurology), DECVN

BASIC INFORMATION

Description

The skull is a bony case that protects the brain from injury. Trauma to the skull can result in brain injury. Any traumatic impact to the head may result in skull fractures, bleeding within the brain, or bruising of brain tissue (concussion/contusion). In addition to the direct injury, fluid buildup (edema) in brain tissue can develop, which worsens the brain damage. Because the brain is encased in the skull, it is trapped if it begins to swell. Swelling of the brain causes the pressure within the head to increase (elevated intracranial pressure). This increased pressure can lead to deterioration of clinical signs.

Causes

Head trauma most commonly occurs from automobile accidents. Other causes include falls, blows to the head, gunshot and bite wounds, and other types of accidents.

Clinical Signs

Clinical signs depend on the location and severity of brain damage. Common clinical signs include depression, seizures, circling, alteration in the size of the pupils of the eye, decreased vision, head tilt, falling to the side, an uncoordinated gait, and loss of consciousness (coma). Following automobile accidents, animals often have additional injuries to other areas of their bodies that may be life-threatening.

Diagnostic Tests

Diagnosis is based on a history of trauma and compatible clinical signs. If a traumatic event was not observed, injuries to other areas of the body may provide evidence of a traumatic insult. Thorough physical and neurologic examinations are usually performed. Routine blood tests, a urinalysis, and x-rays of the chest and abdomen are often needed to evaluate injuries to other areas of the body. X-rays of the head may reveal skull fractures, but they do not image or assess the brain.

Advanced imaging techniques such as magnetic resonance imaging (MRI) or computed tomography (CT scan) may be recommended to evaluate skull fractures and to identify bleeding, bruising, or inflammation of the brain. Careful evaluation of each animal is necessary prior to advanced imaging, because these procedures require general anesthesia, and anesthesia may need to be delayed until the animal is stable.

TREATMENT AND FOLLOW-UP

Treatment Options

Initial therapy is directed at stabilizing the animal's general condition and usually requires hospitalization. Other injuries must be addressed prior to treatment of the brain trauma, and measures must be taken to ensure normal blood pressure, hydration, and the ability to breathe properly. Many of the initial stabilizing treatments, such as intravenous fluid and oxygen therapy, have beneficial effects on the brain. Specific treatment for brain injury is usually aimed at decreasing intracranial pressure with diuretics and other drugs. Anticonvulsant therapy may be required if seizures develop after the trauma. Occasionally, surgery is required to treat a fracture of the skull or a blood clot in the brain, but surgery is usually delayed until after medical therapy has been attempted.

Follow-up Care

During hospitalization, affected animals are monitored frequently with serial neurologic examinations. Your veterinarian may refer your pet to a specialty center if round-the-clock monitoring and treatment are required. Once at home, frequent follow-up visits are usually needed to monitor neurologic signs and to assess recovery from other injuries. During the recovery period, notify your veterinarian immediately if any new neurologic signs develop or if previous ones recur or worsen. If the animal recovers and becomes normal again, long-term follow-up may not be necessary. Animals with persistent seizures require ongoing monitoring, as outlined in the handout on **Seizures: Treatment**.

Prognosis

Prognosis depends on the severity and location of the brain damage. The first 72 hours after the injury are critical. Most mildly affected animals will improve, and many regain normal neurologic function. Severe head trauma can result in death or long-term disability. Some animals develop seizures that require lifelong treatment.

SPECIAL INSTRUCTIONS:

Hydrocephalus

A. Courtenay Freeman, DVM
Marc Kent, DVM, DACVIM (Small Animal and Neurology)
Scott J. Schatzberg, DVM, PhD, DACVIM (Neurology)

BASIC INFORMATION
Description

Hydrocephalus occurs when there is an increased amount of cerebrospinal fluid (CSF) present within the brain. CSF is produced within specialized spaces or compartments of the brain called *ventricles*. This fluid flows through the ventricular system, around the brain, and eventually down the spinal cord. When the volume of CSF increases, the ventricles enlarge, and the fluid puts pressure on the surrounding brain tissue, which causes various neurologic problems.

Causes

The volume of CSF usually increases because of a blockage in the ventricular system (obstructive hydrocephalus), although the exact location of the obstruction is not often identified. Only rarely is an excessive amount of CSF produced. There are several potential causes of obstruction of CSF flow:

- Birth defects within the ventricular system can result in enlarged ventricles filled with CSF. This congenital form of hydrocephalus is most frequently seen in young, small-breed dogs such as the Chihuahua, Yorkshire terrier, Boston terrier, and Pekingese.
- Brain masses (usually tumors) can block the flow of CSF.
- Inflammation or infections in the brain may also prevent the flow of CSF.

Clinical Signs

Clinical signs are variable. Some animals have no clinical signs and lead normal, healthy lives, even with severe hydrocephalus. Mild clinical signs that can be seen with hydrocephalus include lethargy, depression, and behavioral changes. Some animals with hydrocephalus have difficulty with house training or learning commands. More severe clinical signs include seizures, blindness, and an uncoordinated gait.

With congenital hydrocephalus, the skull may be rounded or dome-shaped. A small opening in the top of the skull, called a *fontanelle*, may be felt under the skin in some animals.

Diagnostic Tests

Although the clinical signs and physical findings described are suggestive of hydrocephalus, special imaging the brain is required to confirm the diagnosis. Magnetic resonance imaging (MRI) allows detailed evaluation of brain tissue, ventricles, and CSF, and may also detect the underlying cause of hydrocephalus. Computed tomography (CT scan) also may be used to diagnose hydrocephalus. In young animals with a fontanelle, an ultrasound scan can be performed through the fontanelle to show the presence of dilated ventricles. CSF may be collected via a spinal tap to identify potential underlying causes of hydrocephalus, such as inflammation.

TREATMENT AND FOLLOW-UP
Treatment Options

Medical and surgical therapies exist for animals with clinical signs associated with hydrocephalus. In most cases, medical therapy is pursued initially, and surgery is reserved for cases that do not respond to medical treatment.

The goals of medical therapy are to treat the underlying cause (if possible) and to alleviate the clinical signs associated with hydrocephalus. Drugs such as steroids, acetazolamide, certain antacids called *proton pump inhibitors* (such as *Prilosec*), and diuretics can be used to decrease CSF production. Anticonvulsants may be used to control seizures. (See handout on **Seizures: Treatment**.)

Surgery involves the placement of a shunt (tube) that allows CSF to drain from the brain into the abdominal cavity. One end of the shunt is placed in the ventricular system of the brain and the other in the abdominal cavity. The tube is tunneled under the skin along the neck and back and is not visible. Not many veterinarians perform this surgery, so your pet may be referred to a specialist for an evaluation to determine whether it is a candidate for this surgery and for the actual surgery to be performed. Potential surgical complications include obstruction and infection of the shunt, which can result in return of the clinical signs.

Follow-up Care

In cases treated medically, animals are re-examined periodically to evaluate the effectiveness of therapy. Blood tests may be used to monitor animals treated with acetazolamide or diuretic therapy. After surgery, animals require frequent evaluations to ensure the success of the procedure. If no complications occur after the initial postoperative period, recheck visits may be decreased to every 6 months.

Prognosis

Prognosis depends on the severity of the clinical signs. Some animals live normal, healthy lives with this condition and do not require any treatment. Medical therapy often helps animals with mild signs. Surgery can improve clinical signs in some dogs; however, loss of brain tissue from fluid pressure may result in irreversible changes. In severely affected animals, clinical signs may not improve with treatment. Prognosis is guarded for patients with tumors blocking CSF flow. In animals with infection or inflammation, hydrocephalus may improve with proper treatment of the underlying condition.

SPECIAL INSTRUCTIONS:

Idiopathic Facial Nerve Paralysis

A. Courtenay Freeman, DVM
Marc Kent, DVM, DACVIM (Small Animal and Neurology)
Scott J. Schatzberg, DVM, PhD, DACVIM (Neurology)

BASIC INFORMATION

Description

The classic features of idiopathic facial nerve paralysis in dogs and cats include an inability to blink, drooping of the lips, and occasionally decreased tear production on the affected side.

The American cocker spaniel, Pembroke Welsh corgi, English setter, and domestic longhaired cats are predisposed to this disease. Any dog or cat can be affected, however. Twelve pairs of nerves (one on each side of the head) originate at the base of the brain and are responsible for certain neurologic functions of the head and face. These paired nerves are called the *cranial nerves,* and they are numbered I through XII. The seventh cranial nerve (VII) is the facial nerve, and it controls the muscles involved in facial expression, blinking, and tear production.

Causes

The term *idiopathic* indicates that the cause of the condition is unknown. Although some cases of facial nerve paralysis have an identifiable origin (such as diseases or surgery of the ear, tumors, metabolic disorders), in this disease the cause is not defined. All common causes of facial nerve paralysis must be ruled out in order to call it *idiopathic*.

Clinical Signs

Typically, a sudden weakness or paralysis occurs on one side of the face. If nerves on both sides of the head are affected, weakness is seen on both sides of the face. This weakness causes the ear and lips to droop. Animals may drop food or drool from the affected side of their mouth. Sensation (feeling) in the face is normal.

Because the facial nerve causes the eyelids to blink and controls the tear glands, affected animals may be unable to blink and may develop "dry eye" from a lack of tears on the affected side of the face. Dry eye may be associated with conjunctivitis

(redness), yellow-green discharge, and ulceration of the cornea. Vision remains normal.

Diagnostic Tests

Diagnosis is based on examination findings and the exclusion of other causes of facial nerve paralysis. Careful inspection of the ears is performed in affected animals. X-rays and advanced imaging of the ear canal and brain by computed tomography (CT scan) or magnetic resonance imaging (MRI) may be recommended in some animals. These tests are normal in animals with idiopathic facial paralysis. Dogs may also be tested for low thyroid function (hypothyroidism), which has been associated with facial nerve paralysis. Evaluation of tear production and other testing of the eyes may also be performed.

TREATMENT AND FOLLOW-UP

Treatment Options

There is no specific treatment for idiopathic facial nerve paralysis. Artificial tears may be applied to the eye on the affected side to prevent corneal ulcerations. If dry eye is present, additional medications may be recommended.

🐾 Follow-up Care

Initially, follow-up examinations may be done frequently to monitor for development of corneal ulcers. Notify your veterinarian if the eye on the affected side becomes red or squinty, if it has increased discharge, or if the cornea becomes cloudy, because these signs could indicate the presence of a corneal ulcer.

Prognosis

Prognosis for return of function is very poor in most cases. Most affected animals do not regain function of the facial nerve. If function returns, it may take weeks for an improvement to be detected. Sometimes only partial recovery occurs. A full recovery does occasionally happen.

SPECIAL INSTRUCTIONS:

Idiopathic Peripheral Vestibular Disease

A. Courtenay Freeman, DVM
Marc Kent, DVM, DACVIM (Small Animal and Neurology)
Scott J. Schatzberg, DVM, PhD, DACVIM (Neurology)

BASIC INFORMATION

Description

Idiopathic peripheral vestibular disease is a disorder that results in an acute loss of balance, head tilt, tendency to fall or circle in the same direction, and abnormal eye movements. Twelve pairs of nerves (one on each side of the head) originate at the base of the brain and are responsible for certain neurologic functions of the head and face. These paired nerves are called the *cranial nerves,* and they are numbered I through XII. The eighth cranial nerve (VIII) is the vestibulocochlear nerve, which is involved with the vestibular system and hearing. The vestibular system regulates balance, proper head position, and normal eye movements.

Anatomically, the vestibular system is divided into two portions—the peripheral and central vestibular systems. The peripheral vestibular system involves the vestibulocochlear nerve as it runs from receptors in the inner ear to the base of the brain. The central vestibular system is located in the base of the brain (brainstem). Regardless of the area affected, an abnormality of the vestibular system can result in clinical signs associated with imbalance or incoordination.

Idiopathic peripheral vestibular disease occurs in both dogs and cats. Affected dogs tend to be older (greater than 7 years of age). Sometimes the disease is referred to as *old dog* (or *geriatric*) *vestibular disease.* The disease occurs in cats of any age, but younger cats are more commonly affected. Feline idiopathic vestibular disease most commonly occurs in late July and August in the northeastern part of North America and tends to affect male, outdoor cats most often.

Causes

The term *idiopathic* indicates that the cause of a condition is unknown. Although some cases of vestibular dysfunction have an identifiable origin (such as autoimmune inflammation, infections of the inner ear and brainstem, stroke, tumors, metabolic and nutritional disorders, antibiotic toxicity), in this disease the cause is not defined. Common causes of vestibular dysfunction must be ruled out in order to call it *idiopathic.*

Clinical Signs

Onset of clinical signs is sudden, and severity can vary from mild to severe. The head is tilted to one side, making it look as if the animal is listening to the ground. Affected animals may have abnormal eye movements in which the eyes move rapidly side-to-side (*nystagmus*). The animal may stumble, fall, or circle to the same side as the head tilt. Walking and gait may be uncoordinated,

because balance is abnormal. Severely affected animals may continually roll over and be unable to walk. Some animals may be nauseated, refuse to eat, and vomit. Importantly, no additional neurologic abnormalities are seen with idiopathic peripheral vestibular disease.

Diagnostic Tests

Diagnosis is based on the history, physical and neurologic examination findings, and exclusion of other diseases that may produce similar clinical signs. Other causes of vestibular disease must be investigated before the diagnosis of idiopathic peripheral vestibular disease can be made. The neurologic examination helps the veterinarian determine whether the peripheral or central vestibular system is involved. Careful inspection of the ears (otoscopy) is usually performed. Routine laboratory tests and sometimes x-rays of the bony parts of the ears are recommended. Computed tomography (CT scan) or magnetic resonance imaging (MRI) of the inner ear and brain are normal in animals with idiopathic peripheral vestibular disease.

TREATMENT AND FOLLOW-UP

Treatment Options

There is no specific treatment for this disorder. Affected animals usually show signs of improvement within several days. Severely affected animals may initially require hospitalization to receive intravenous fluid therapy and antinausea drugs. Good nursing care is often required at home until the animal can walk normally. The animal may need assistance walking and may need to be hand fed if it is too uncoordinated to stand. Soft, padded bedding will help keep the animal comfortable while it is recovering.

Follow-up Care

Hospitalized animals are monitored with repeated neurologic examinations during the first few days until improvements are observed. Animals that are not hospitalized are usually re-evaluated after a few days to ensure that they are improving. Periodic recheck visits may be recommended until the animal has recovered. Complete recovery may take several weeks, and some animals may have a persistent head tilt. Long-term follow-up typically is not necessary once clinical signs have resolved.

Prognosis

Prognosis for recovery is excellent; however, a permanent head tilt may remain. Rarely, idiopathic vestibular disease can recur.

SPECIAL INSTRUCTIONS:

Idiopathic Trigeminal Neuropathy

A. Courtenay Freeman, DVM
Marc Kent, DVM, DACVIM (Small Animal and Neurology)
Scott J. Schatzberg, DVM, PhD, DACVIM (Neurology)

BASIC INFORMATION

Description

Trigeminal neuropathy is a disorder that affects the fifth or trigeminal nerve of the head and the muscles of the jaw. It has also been called *idiopathic bilateral mandibular nerve paralysis*. Twelve pairs of nerves (one on each side of the head) originate at the base of the brain and are responsible for certain neurologic functions of the head and face. These nerves are called *cranial nerves*, and they are numbered I through XII. The fifth cranial nerve (V) is the trigeminal nerve, and it is responsible for the muscles involved in chewing, as well as sensation (feeling) in the face.

Causes

The term *idiopathic* indicates that the cause of the condition is unknown. Although some cases of trigeminal nerve disease have an identifiable origin (such as infections, tumors, inflammation of the brain), in this disease the cause is not defined. It is speculated that either inflammation or an immune reaction may cause dysfunction and paralysis of the nerve. All common causes of trigeminal nerve dysfunction must be ruled out in order to call the condition *idiopathic*.

Clinical Signs

Trigeminal neuropathy results in paralysis of the muscles of the jaw. If both sides of the head are affected, the lower jaw (mandible) hangs open and the animal is unable to close the mouth. This appearance is referred to as a "dropped jaw." In most instances, the animal is unable to eat. Over time, the muscles on the top and sides of the head (cheek area) often shrink and the bones of the skull become more obvious. Some animals lose feeling on their face. When touched near their eye, they do not blink even though the eyelid muscles work well and they can blink voluntarily.

Rarely, affected animals also have other eye abnormalities, such as drooping of the upper eyelid, sinking of the eyeball, and movement of the third eyelid so that it partially covers the eye (Horner's syndrome). Vision remains normal.

Diagnostic Tests

Diagnosis is based on examination findings and exclusion of other diseases that affect the trigeminal nerve. Other potential causes must be investigated before a diagnosis of idiopathic trigeminal neuropathy can be made. A thorough physical examination, routine laboratory tests, and x-rays may be recommended to search for a cause. Advanced imaging of the brain by magnetic resonance imaging (MRI) or computed tomography (CT scan) may also be recommended to exclude other diseases.

TREATMENT AND FOLLOW-UP

Treatment Options

No specific treatment exists for trigeminal neuropathy; however, supportive care is very important. The animal may require assistance with eating and drinking, because it is unable to take in food and water on its own. Insertion of a feeding tube may be considered in some animals to provide adequate nutrition. If the animal does not blink often, lubricating ointments may be applied to the eyes.

Follow-up Care

Recheck visits are usually recommended periodically to monitor for improvement in clinical signs and to assess body weight and the nutritional status of the animal.

Prognosis

Prognosis for recovery from trigeminal neuropathy is good. Most animals regain nerve function in 2 to 4 weeks; however, a full recovery may take several months. Some animals recover only partially, and occasionally trigeminal nerve function does not return.

SPECIAL INSTRUCTIONS:

Intervertebral Disc Disease

A. Courtenay Freeman, DVM
Marc Kent, DVM, DACVIM (Small Animal and Neurology)
Simon R. Platt, BVM&S, MRCVS, DACVIM (Neurology), DECVN

BASIC INFORMATION

Description

Intervertebral disc disease (IVDD) is one of the most common spinal cord conditions in the dog. Cats are less commonly affected. The spine is composed of bones called *vertebrae*. The vertebrae form a canal that surrounds the spinal cord. Between adjacent vertebrae there are discs (intervertebral discs) composed of a fibrous outer portion (annulus fibrosis) and a gel-like center (nucleus pulposus). These discs act as cushions between vertebrae and provide strength and stability to the spine.

IVDD is a general term that refers to the condition in which the intervertebral disc protrudes from its normal anatomic location, usually as a result of degeneration of the disc. This herniation of the disc results in compression of the spinal cord.

Causes

Three types of IVDD occur in the dog:

- Type I arises with degeneration of the disc (primarily the nucleus pulposus) caused by loss of water content and calcification (mineralization). The nucleus pulposus may extrude out of the annulus fibrosis toward the spinal cord.
- In Type II, degeneration of the disc causes it to bulge or protrude into the spinal canal.
- Type III is a noncompressive herniation in which a small amount of disc material moves at high velocity into the spinal cord, resulting in spinal cord injury.

Clinical Signs

The age, breed, onset of clinical signs, and treatment options vary with the type of IVDD:

- Type I primarily affects young to middle-aged (3-6 years) dogs with short legs and long backs, such as the dachshund, Lhasa apso, shih tzu, beagle, cocker spaniel, and corgi. Onset of signs is typically sudden (acute).
- Type II primarily affects older, large-breed dogs such as the German shepherd dog and the Labrador retriever. Onset of clinical signs is often slow (chronic) and progressive over weeks to months.
- Dogs with type III IVDD have a sudden onset of clinical signs.

Neurologic signs are dependent on the location of disc herniation and the degree of spinal cord injury. Signs often occur in stages:

- Mild compression or injury may only cause pain.
- More severe compression or injury causes an uncoordinated (unsteady) gait, crossing over of the legs when walking, scuffing of the nails, and weakness (paresis).
- As the spinal cord injury worsens, the animal loses the ability to move the legs (paralysis) and may have difficulty urinating voluntarily.
- With the most severe injuries, affected animals are unable to feel a deep, painful stimulus applied to their toes.

Some dogs progress through these stages of neurologic dysfunction rapidly, whereas other dogs experience only pain. Because prognosis and treatment options vary with each level of neurologic dysfunction, it is important for affected animals to be examined by a veterinarian at the onset of clinical signs.

The degree of spinal cord compression does not always correlate well with the severity of the signs. Dogs with acute onset of signs may have severe neurologic problems despite mild compression of the spinal cord. In dogs with slow onset of signs, compression can be severe but only mild to moderate neurologic problems occur. Dogs with pain as the only sign can have severe compression of the spinal cord.

Compression of the spinal cord in the neck region causes signs in all four legs, whereas compression in the chest or back region causes signs in only the hind legs. Disc herniation can occur anywhere along the vertebral column; however, the thoracolumbar area (end of the chest and beginning of the back) is the site most commonly affected.

Diagnostic Tests

IVDD may be suspected based on history and neurologic findings; however, additional tests are required to confirm IVDD and allow appropriate treatment planning.

- X-rays may indicate IVDD, but they can be normal and do not provide enough information to plan surgical treatment.
- Myelography is an x-ray study that involves injecting a dye into the cerebrospinal fluid (CSF) that surrounds the spinal cord. This study can demonstrate spinal cord compression, but it is not specific for IVDD, and a swollen cord may hide the location of the disc herniation.
- Computed tomography (CT scan) can identify the site of disc herniation and can be combined with myelography.
- Magnetic resonance imaging (MRI) is the best imaging modality to evaluate the spinal cord and intervertebral discs, and it provides enough details to plan appropriate treatment.
- If surgical treatment is pursued, a myelogram, CT, or MRI is often needed, and all of these procedures require general anesthesia.

Continued

Intervertebral Disc Disease—*cont'd*

A. Courtenay Freeman, DVM
Marc Kent, DVM, DACVIM (Small Animal and Neurology)
Simon R. Platt, BVM&S, MRCVS, DACVIM (Neurology), DECVN

TREATMENT AND FOLLOW-UP

Treatment Options

Treatment of intervertebral disc disease (IVDD) consists of conservative and surgical therapies. The degree and duration of the neurologic signs are important factors when deciding among treatment options.

Conservative therapy can be tried in dogs if mild pain and incoordination are the sole clinical signs; that is, the dog can walk but with an unsteady gait (ataxia). Dogs with Type III IVDD may also be treated conservatively, because often little to no compression of the spinal cord is present. Conservative therapy consists of exercise restriction, anti-inflammatory drugs, and pain medications.

- Exercise restriction involves strict confinement and limited leash walking (only for the purpose of urinating and defecating). Dogs should not be allowed to run, jump, or play during their confinement. Exercise restriction typically lasts 4-6 weeks and is followed by a gradual return to normal activity over an additional month.
- Anti-inflammatory drugs, such as nonsteroidal anti-inflammatory or steroid medications, can be used. These two classes of drugs are not used together because of their combined side effects.
- Pain medications may be used to alleviate discomfort.

Surgical therapy is usually chosen in dogs with severe neurologic problems, such as moderate to severe incoordination, weakness, inability to walk, paralysis, or pain that is unresponsive to medications. Surgery is also considered in dogs whose signs recur.

- Surgery involves the removal of herniated, compressive disc material followed by exercise restriction as outlined for conservative therapy.
- Surgery may require removal of a portion of the vertebra at the site of compression to provide access to the spinal canal.
- After removal of the bone, the disc material is delicately removed from within the spinal canal to relieve spinal cord compression.
- Postoperatively, the animal is strictly confined for 4-6 weeks. Manual emptying of the bladder may be needed if the dog cannot urinate voluntarily. Good nursing care is important until the dog can walk well by itself. Pain and anti-inflammatory medications may also be used after surgery.

- It is critical to monitor for any decline in neurologic function or pain during the recovery period. Notify your veterinarian if any signs recur.

Follow-up Care

Recovery time varies depending on the onset (acute versus chronic) and severity of the clinical signs. Typically, time to recovery for dogs treated with surgery is 1-2 weeks. Severely affected dogs may require months to regain function of their legs and bladder; however, dogs treated conservatively may also require 1-2 weeks to regain function. Some severely affected dogs do not regain the ability to walk again, and some have persistent urinary incontinence. Carts (similar to wheelchairs) have been developed to assist dogs that are unable to walk. Maximal improvement occurs in the majority of dogs by 3 months after the initial injury to the spinal cord. Further improvement after this time is unlikely. Periodic rechecks are often needed throughout this period.

Prognosis

Most dogs with only mild to moderate pain or mild neurologic signs return to normal function with conservative therapy. Prognosis for more severely affected dogs treated with conservative therapy is poor. Dogs that are managed with surgery have a good prognosis for return to normal function even if they initially have moderate to severe neurologic signs. As long as the dog can still perceive a painful stimulus applied to the affected legs, and even if the legs are paralyzed, there is a reasonably good chance that normal function will be regained with surgery.

The prognosis is very poor (guarded) for dogs that are paralyzed and unable to perceive a painful stimulus in their legs. If treated surgically within the first 24 hours after onset of paralysis, dogs unable to perceive deep pain have a 50% chance of regaining the ability to walk. If left untreated for longer than 48 hours, these dogs have a grave prognosis for regaining the ability to walk and for having control of their bladder.

Recurrence of clinical signs suggestive of another intervertebral disc herniation can happen in some dogs. Recurrence is most likely within 2 years after the first episode and tends to occur more often in dogs that were managed conservatively.

SPECIAL INSTRUCTIONS:

Ischemic Brain Injury (Stroke)

A. Courtenay Freeman, DVM
Marc Kent, DVM, DACVIM (Small Animal and Neurology)
Simon R. Platt, BVM&S, MRCVS, DACVIM (Neurology), DECVN

BASIC INFORMATION

Description

The brain needs oxygen and nutrients such as glucose (sugar) to provide energy for its normal functions. Oxygen and nutrients are delivered to the brain through the blood. If the blood supply is disrupted, the brain is deprived of oxygen and nutrients, which results in neurologic dysfunction. Decreased oxygen delivery to the brain is referred to as *ischemia*. An obstruction in a blood vessel with loss of blood supply to an area of the brain is called an *infarction*. In people, an infarction is called a *stroke*. Ischemic brain injury is an uncommon event in animals; it occurs more frequently in dogs than in cats.

Causes

In most dogs, the reason for the infarction is unknown. Infarctions can occur secondary to a blood clot (thromboembolus), bacterial infection, inflammation, or invasion of blood vessels by cancer cells. Rarely, animals can develop atherosclerosis, similar to people; cholesterol and fat accumulate in the blood vessel wall, obstructing normal flow. Dogs with low thyroid hormone levels or increased fat in their blood are more prone to atherosclerosis. Other disorders that may be associated with infarctions include high blood pressure (hypertension), Cushing's disease (excessive steroid production by the adrenal glands), sugar diabetes, and kidney disease.

Disruption of the blood supply to the brain can also occur from rupture of a blood vessel and subsequent bleeding. Hemorrhage into the brain can occur with cancer or disorders that decrease the ability to form blood clots (such as anticoagulant drug treatment, certain rodent poisons, and hemophilia).

Clinical Signs

Clinical signs depend on the location of brain injury. Onset of signs is typically very sudden, and usually one side of the body is more affected than the other. Neurologic abnormalities do not often worsen with time unless edema (fluid buildup) forms in or around the damaged brain tissue or bleeding into the brain continues. Examples of common clinical signs include abnormal behavior, head tilt or turning, blindness in one eye, and seizures (less common).

Diagnostic Tests

Ischemic brain injury may be suspected based on the history and clinical signs. A presumptive diagnosis can be made with magnetic resonance imaging (MRI) or computed tomography (CT scan) of the brain. MRI is the best method for evaluating the brain for characteristics that are compatible with an ischemic infarction or hemorrhage.

Additional diagnostic tests are needed to rule out other neurologic diseases that produce similar signs and to identify the underlying cause. Routine blood tests, a urinalysis, measurement of blood pressure, and blood clotting tests may all be recommended. In certain cases, evaluation of thyroid function may be done because low function (hypothyroidism) can lead to atherosclerosis and infarctions. A spinal tap and cerebrospinal fluid (CSF) analysis may be indicated to look for inflammation or infection. X-rays and an abdominal ultrasound may be recommended if cancer is suspected.

TREATMENT AND FOLLOW-UP

Treatment Options

There are no specific treatments for this type of brain injury. Affected animals are often given supportive care, such as intravenous fluid therapy, to ensure that they are adequately hydrated. If indicated, medications may be started to control hypertension, seizures, or brain edema. Continuous monitoring of neurologic function is performed while the animal is hospitalized. If an underlying condition is identified, treatment is directed at that disease process. Most animals show gradual improvement over days to weeks.

Follow-up Care

Follow-up visits are done frequently at first, to monitor the animal's progress, and then tapered to every few weeks to months. Laboratory tests and blood pressure measurements may be repeated to monitor resolution or control of any underlying disease. If improvement is seen in brain function, neurologic examinations may eventually be decreased to every 6 months. During the recovery period, notify your veterinarian immediately if any new neurologic signs develop or if previous ones recur or worsen.

Prognosis

Prognosis varies with the severity of neurologic damage and dysfunction. With mild damage, prognosis is generally good, because most animals regain normal neurologic function. Prognosis also depends on the underlying cause of the ischemic injury. Residual signs such as blindness and altered gait or movement are possible. Maximal recovery is usually seen within 3 months. Recurrence is possible, especially in those animals with an underlying disease process that cannot be well controlled.

SPECIAL INSTRUCTIONS:

Lumbosacral Disease, Degenerative

A. Courtenay Freeman, DVM
Marc Kent, DVM, DACVIM (Small Animal and Neurology)
Simon R. Platt, BVM&S, MRCVS, DACVIM (Neurology), DECVN

BASIC INFORMATION

Description

Degenerative lumbosacral disease is a neurologic disorder involving the joint between the last (seventh) lumbar (L7) vertebra in the lower back and the sacrum. The sacrum is the bone that lies between the lumbar vertebrae and the tail bones and is attached to the pelvis.

Causes

The lumbosacral area is a complex joint that surrounds the spinal cord within the pelvic region, provides mobility to the lower back, and attaches the vertebral column to the pelvis. The following parts of this complex joint are involved in the disease process:

• Degeneration of the intervertebral disc at L7 leads to protrusion (bulging) of the disc into the spinal canal. (See also the handout on **Intervertebral Disc Disease**.)
• The vertebral processes overlying the top of the vertebral canal in this area degenerate and develop arthritis.
• The ligaments surrounding this area become thickened.
• The joint may become unstable and even subluxate (partially dislocate).

The end result of these degenerative changes is compression (squeezing) of the spinal nerves that go to the hind legs, rear end, tail, bladder, colon, and rectum. Older to middle-aged, large-breed dogs are most commonly affected, particularly the German shepherd dog.

Clinical Signs

Pain over the lumbosacral region (pelvic region, base of the tail) is the most common sign. Other signs include a reluctance to jump, climb stairs, or rise from a lying position. Hind leg weakness, a crouched stance, paralysis of the tail, and urinary and fecal incontinence may also occur. The degree of pain and neurologic signs varies with the severity of the compression.

Diagnostic Tests

The condition may be suspected in a dog of a typical breed and age with compatible neurologic examination findings. However, clinical signs are not very specific for degenerative lumbosacral disease. Other diseases, such as vertebral malformation, infection, trauma, and cancer, can cause similar neurologic findings. Some orthopedic conditions of the hind legs, such as arthritis of the hips (hip dysplasia), can also mimic the disease.

X-rays are often performed. They help to rule out orthopedic problems but rarely provide a definitive diagnosis of lumbosacral degeneration. Computed tomography (CT scan) offers more detailed images of the L7 disc space and can also demonstrate compression of the spinal nerves within the spinal canal. Magnetic resonance imaging (MRI) provides the best detailed evaluation of the spinal nerves, intervertebral disc, and vertebrae in this area. Other tests may be recommended to rule out diseases that cause similar clinical signs.

TREATMENT AND FOLLOW-UP

Treatment Options

Treatment options involve conservative and surgical therapies. Conservative therapy is often pursued if pain is the only clinical sign. Surgical therapy is often used in dogs with more severe neurologic signs, such as hind leg weakness, bladder and bowel incontinence, and tail paralysis. Dogs that do not respond to conservative therapy may also need surgery.

Conservative therapy consists of exercise restriction, anti-inflammatory drugs, and medications to relieve pain:

• Exercise restriction involves strict confinement and limited leash walking (for urinary and fecal elimination only).
• Dogs should not be allowed to run, jump, or play during this period of confinement.
• Exercise restriction typically lasts 4-6 weeks and is followed by a gradual return to normal activity over an additional month.
• Anti-inflammatory drugs, such as nonsteroidal anti-inflammatory or steroid medications, can be used. These two classes of drugs are not used together because of their combined side effects.

When surgery is done, the goal is to eliminate compression of the spinal nerves:

• Surgery involves opening the vertebral canal over the site of compression, which is called a *dorsal laminectomy*.
• Compression is relieved by removal of the herniated intervertebral disc.
• Occasionally, the lumbosacral joint is stabilized (fused) after the decompression.

Follow-up Care

Recovery time varies depending on the severity of the clinical signs. Time to recovery following surgery is 1-2 weeks, but severely affected dogs may require months for full improvement. Maximal improvement occurs by 3-4 months. Periodic rechecks are often needed throughout this period.

Prognosis

Prognosis depends on the degree of neurologic signs. Dogs with pain as the sole clinical sign typically respond well to conservative therapy. Most dogs treated surgically also improve. The outcome in dogs with severe neurologic problems (such as severe hind leg weakness or fecal and urinary incontinence) is less predictable. The most common long-term complication of lumbosacral degeneration is recurrence of clinical signs, so notify your veterinarian if any signs worsen or reappear.

SPECIAL INSTRUCTIONS:

Myasthenia Gravis

A. Courtenay Freeman, DVM
Marc Kent, DVM, DACVIM (Small Animal and Neurology)
Scott J. Schatzberg, DVM, PhD, DACVIM (Neurology)

BASIC INFORMATION

Description

Myasthenia gravis (MG) is a neurologic condition that is caused by abnormal transmission of information (impulses) from nerves to muscles resulting from a chemical blockage at the nerve endings. MG causes variable degrees of muscle weakness.

Causes

MG occurs in both congenital and acquired forms, with the acquired form being more common. Congenital MG arises from a defect in the muscle receptor at the nerve ending that is present at birth. It occurs in the Jack Russell terrier, English springer spaniel, and smooth fox terrier.

In acquired MG, the body's immune system produces antibodies (autoimmune disease) that block the chemical reaction at the nerve ending. Consequently, a muscle contraction cannot be generated, and muscle weakness develops. In most instances, the inciting cause of acquired MG is not identified; however, certain cancers, such as thymoma, can cause MG.

Clinical Signs

Three forms of MG are recognized, and each may produce different clinical signs:

• *Focal MG* causes muscle weakness in only one area, such as the esophagus. A weak esophagus becomes dilated (megaesophagus) and does not transfer food to the stomach well. Pneumonia can occur from regurgitation and inhalation (aspiration) of food into the lungs. Difficulty breathing, coughing, decreased appetite, lethargy, fever, and regurgitation are common signs. Focal MG may also involve the muscles of the face, back of the mouth, and larynx, causing decreased ability to blink, swallow food and water, or bark.

• *Generalized MG* involves all the muscles in the body. Affected animals become tired when walking and often can only walk a few steps before needing to rest. As they fatigue, their gait becomes short and choppy. The dog may be reluctant to move at all or may sit or lie down after a few steps. Following a rest, the gait may briefly return to normal. Generalized MG may also affect the esophagus.

• *Fulminant MG* is the most severe form and causes sudden onset of generalized weakness, with inability to walk. These dogs usually also have megaesophagus and frequently regurgitate. They may be so weak that they cannot breathe normally.

Diagnostic Tests

Acquired MG may be suspected based on the history and clinical signs. A definitive diagnosis is made with a blood test that identifies antibodies against the receptor on muscles that binds the chemical acetylcholine. A Tensilon test can be considered while results of the antibody titer are awaited. It involves giving the drug, edrophonium chloride (*Tensilon*), to determine whether it will temporarily improve the signs of weakness. Not all dogs with MG respond to this drug, and sometimes the test is positive in animals without MG.

Other laboratory tests are often recommended to rule out other diseases that can cause muscle weakness. Chest x-rays may be done to look for megaesophagus, pneumonia, and other problems, such as a thymoma. Electrocardiograms and other tests may be recommended to rule out heart disease as a source of the weakness.

Congenital MG is suspected in young animals that show weakness from birth. Definitive diagnosis requires a muscle biopsy.

TREATMENT AND FOLLOW-UP

Treatment Options

Drugs are given that increase the amount of acetylcholine in the nerve ending so that muscle strength is increased. Pyridostigmine bromide (*Mestinon*) may be given orally, or neostigmine bromide (*Prostigmin*) may be injected in dogs that cannot swallow. Sometimes steroids or other immune suppressive drugs are given in an attempt to stop the production of antibodies, but these are used cautiously in dogs with pneumonia.

Aspiration pneumonia is treated with antibiotics for several weeks. Animals with megaesophagus may require insertion of feeding tubes or feeding from an elevated position to decrease regurgitation. (See also the handout on **Megaesophagus**.) Severely affected dogs often require hospitalization and supportive care. Frequent medication adjustments may be needed at the start of treatment. Treatment for other underlying problems (thymoma) may also be started.

Follow-up Care

Frequent recheck visits are needed to evaluate response to treatment and adjust medications. Long-term follow-up is also required. Laboratory tests and x-rays may be repeated periodically.

Prognosis

Prognosis is good for animals that are mildly affected and show rapid improvement with initial treatment. Although many animals with acquired MG completely recover, some do not respond to therapy. Other dogs improve but signs recur during times of stress, such as after vaccination or surgery. Resolution of the disease is documented by a normal antibody titer and physical examination. Dogs with severe aspiration pneumonia, fulminant MG, congenital MG, or thymoma, have a worse prognosis and may not survive.

SPECIAL INSTRUCTIONS:

Peripheral Nerve Sheath Tumors

A. Courtenay Freeman, DVM
Marc Kent, DVM, DACVIM (Small Animal and Neurology)
Simon R. Platt, BVM&S, MRCVS, DACVIM (Neurology), DECVN

BASIC INFORMATION

Description

Nerves travel from the brain and spinal cord to various parts of the body. Some nerves are involved in muscle movements (motor nerves), whereas others (sensory nerves) are involved in transmitting information such as touch, temperature, pain, and position sense of the legs. Nerves referred to as *peripheral nerves* are located outside the brain and spinal cord.

Nerves are surrounded by supporting cells that protect and insulate them. Tumors (cancers) that develop from these cells are called *peripheral nerve sheath tumors* (PNSTs). These tumors usually grow along the nerve but do not typically spread to other sites in the body.

Causes

This type of cancer most commonly occurs in dogs; however, cats can also develop PNSTs. Affected animals are typically middle-aged to older. The cause of these tumors is unknown.

Clinical Signs

Clinical signs depend on the nerve involved. Usually a chronic, progressive lameness of one leg develops, although a sudden onset of lameness is sometime seen. Early in the disease, pain or muscle loss (atrophy) may be the only clinical sign. These tumors affect a front leg most often but can occur in a hind leg. As the tumor grows, the animal may be unable to use the leg, and adjacent nerves may be affected. If the cancer develops close to the spinal cord and grows into the spinal canal, weakness and an uncoordinated gait can occur in other legs.

PNSTs can also affect the nerves of the head and face. There are 12 pairs of these *cranial nerves*, and they are numbered I through XII. The fifth cranial nerve (V) is the one most commonly affected. It activates the muscles involved in chewing and transmits information on sensation (feeling) in the face. A PNST of this nerve causes shrinkage (atrophy) of the muscles on the top and side of the head. Consequently, the bony prominences of the skull may become more conspicuous. Other signs (such as inability to blink) may occur if the tumor arises in one of the other cranial nerves.

Diagnostic Tests

Because these tumors are not as common as other condition that can cause lameness, especially orthopedic problems, investigation of affected animals first by x-rays and laboratory tests is usually done. A PNST may be suspected if these tests are normal, the signs continue to worsen despite symptomatic medications, and the neurologic examination reveals a weak limb with atrophy of the muscles.

Establishing a diagnosis requires imaging studies, of which magnetic resonance imaging (MRI) is the best. MRI can identify which individual nerve is affected, may also show the extent of involvement of the nerve, and can determine whether the tumor has invaded the spinal cord. Other diagnostic imaging studies, such as ultrasound studies, computed tomography (CT scan), and myelography, can also be used to evaluate affected animals.

A definitive diagnosis is obtained through biopsy of the tumor. X-rays of the chest are usually performed to look for spread of the cancer (metastasis).

TREATMENT AND FOLLOW-UP

Treatment Options

Treatment may involve surgery to remove the tumor, which is often accomplished by amputation of the affected leg. If the cancer extends into the spinal canal, spinal surgery may be recommended. If the tumor cannot be completely removed or if surgery cannot be performed, radiation therapy may be recommended. If none of these treatments are pursued, then medications may be considered to keep the animal comfortable and mobile for as long as possible (palliative therapy).

Follow-up Care

Follow-up visits are needed to monitor progression of disease and response to treatment. Long-term monitoring is also required, because this tumor is difficult to remove or kill.

Prognosis

Prognosis depends on the location and severity of changes caused by tumor and the treatment chosen. The closer the tumor is to the spinal cord, the worse the prognosis. Animals with tumors close to the spinal cord may live only a few months, whereas those with tumors outside the cord may live up to 1 year. Affected animals are rarely cured with surgery unless the tumor arises far down on the leg and can be completely removed with amputation. Postoperative radiation therapy may improve the prognosis for animals with tumors close to the spinal cord.

SPECIAL INSTRUCTIONS:

Polyradiculoneuritis in Dogs, Acute

A. Courtenay Freeman, DVM
Marc Kent, DVM, DACVIM (Small Animal and Neurology)
Scott J. Schatzberg, DVM, PhD, DACVIM (Neurology)

BASIC INFORMATION
Description
Acute polyradiculoneuritis is an inflammation that develops suddenly when the body's immune system attacks the nerves. It results in generalized weakness and paralysis.

After leaving the spinal cord, spinal nerves join together to form the nerves that travel to peripheral (distant) areas of the body. Some nerves activate the muscles and are called *motor nerves.* Other nerves relay information on touch, temperature, pain, and sense of position of the legs and are called *sensory nerves.* In acute polyradiculoneuritis, autoimmune inflammation usually affects the motor nerves, resulting in weakness that may progress to complete paralysis. A similar condition, called *Guillain-Barré syndrome,* occurs in people.

Causes
In most dogs, the cause of acute polyradiculoneuritis is never identified. Some dogs develop the disease 7-10 days after fighting with raccoons, hence the name *coonhound paralysis.* In these dogs, the disease is caused by a reaction to the saliva of the raccoon. Rarely, the disease occurs after vaccination or an infection.

Clinical Signs
Clinical signs typically occur very suddenly (acutely). The primary sign is weakness, with the hind legs affected first. Signs usually progress rapidly over 1-2 days to also involve the front legs. Affected dogs may walk with a crouched, short-strided gait. They become tired quickly with any activity.

Paralysis of all four legs can occur within 2-5 days after the onset of clinical signs. Severely affected animals may not be able to stand, lift their heads, or move their legs. Decreased muscle tone in the legs is common, and over time the muscles may actually shrink (atrophy).

Rarely, the nerves of the head are involved, with decreased blinking and other signs. In severely affected animals, the muscles of the diaphragm may be affected. These dogs are unable to breathe on their own and require mechanical ventilation to survive. Some dogs appear to be in pain or very sensitive to touch and may cry out. These signs occur with inflammation of the sensory nerves.

Diagnostic Tests
A tentative diagnosis may be made from the history and clinical examination findings. Routine laboratory tests are usually recommended to search for an underlying illness. X-rays may be performed to look for pneumonia, which can occur from the animal lying on its side and inhaling (aspirating) food or stomach contents. Other tests may be needed to rule out other diseases that cause similar signs. A definitive diagnosis is difficult to establish, because there is no single test that can be performed for this disease.

A biopsy of peripheral nerves may reveal evidence of inflammation in some instances, but spinal nerve biopsies are difficult to obtain and are rarely done. Analysis of cerebrospinal fluid (CSF) obtained through a spinal tap may reveal evidence of inflammation, such as elevated protein content. Specialized electrophysiologic testing procedures, such as electromyography and nerve stimulation testing, help to identify nerve dysfunction that supports the diagnosis. Often the diagnosis is made by excluding other diseases that cause similar clinical signs.

TREATMENT AND FOLLOW-UP
Treatment Options
There is no specific treatment for acute polyradiculoneuritis. Supportive care is needed while the nerves try to recover. Physical therapy exercises can be performed to prevent muscle wasting and encourage improved muscle tone. Affected dogs require clean, dry, padded bedding and frequent changes in their position to prevent bedsores and pneumonia. Assistance is needed with urination and defecation and keeping the animal clean. If the muscles of the diaphragm are involved, the dog may need to be placed on a ventilator.

The eyes may require lubrication if the dog cannot blink, and assistance may be needed with eating and drinking. Supplemental nutrition may also be recommended. Many dogs require hospitalization for intensive care when they are paralyzed. Any secondary problems that arise because of this disease also require specific treatment.

Follow-up Care
Severely affected animals are often hospitalized for an extended period. Once they are discharged, frequent follow-up visits are needed during the recovery period. Continued nursing care may be required at home. Long-term follow-up may not be necessary in dogs that make a full recovery.

Prognosis
Most dogs will recover, but full recovery may take several weeks to months, depending on the severity of weakness. Prognosis is worst for dogs that have difficulty breathing or aspiration pneumonia.

SPECIAL INSTRUCTIONS:

Seizures: Causes and Diagnosis

A. Courtenay Freeman, DVM
Marc Kent, DVM, DACVIM (Small Animal and Neurology)
Simon R. Platt, BVM&S, MRCVS, DACVIM (Neurology), DECVN

BASIC INFORMATION

Description

Seizures (also called *convulsions* or *fits*) are sudden neurologic events that cause changes in consciousness and involuntary movements. Seizures have many manifestations, but the clinical signs are usually the same each time. The duration of a seizure ranges from a few seconds to several minutes. Seizures are classified as *generalized* (involving all of the body, also known as *grand mal*) or *partial* (involving just one area of the body).

Causes

Seizures can be classified by cause into three categories: those caused by structural brain disorders (such as tumors), those arising from metabolic problems and toxins that affect brain function, and those in which an underlying disorder cannot be identified (idiopathic epilepsy). (See the handout on **Seizures: Idiopathic Epilepsy**.)

Structural brain disorders that can cause seizures include congenital birth defects (such as hydrocephalus), brain tumors, traumatic brain injuries, inflammatory diseases, infections, vascular strokes, and degenerative brain diseases. Metabolic disorders associated with seizures include severe liver and kidney disease, imbalances of blood sodium or calcium, low blood sugar, high blood pressure, and hormonal disorders. A variety of toxins can cause seizures.

The age and breed, neurologic examination findings, and a description of the seizure are important when determining the underlying cause.

🗋 Clinical Signs

During a generalized seizure, the animal is often unconscious and unresponsive. It may fall or lie down. The legs are often rigidly stretched out or drawn up toward the body. The limbs may jerk or paddle as if running (*tonic/clonic* movements). Chewing motions, excessive salivation, urination, or defecation may occur.

During a partial seizure, jerking or twitching movements of a single limb may be seen, the head may turn to a one side, or one or both sides of the face may twitch. Repeated blinking of one or both eyes, chewing movements, and salivation may occur. Disorientation, unresponsiveness, excessive barking, unprovoked aggression, or excessive licking or biting at the air (referred to as fly biting) may also occur.

Some animals have abnormal behaviors prior to seizures, which are referred to as *preictal behaviors.* Examples include hiding, restlessness, hyperactivity, and attention seeking. Sometimes, owners can predict the onset of a seizure based on these behaviors. Some animals also have abnormal behaviors immediately after a seizure, which are referred to as *postictal behaviors.* Examples include restlessness, panting, hyperactivity, thirst, and hunger. Some animals become quiet and sleep. Others appear blind and bump into objects or seem fearful and growl or bite when approached. The postictal period ranges from several minutes to 24 hours.

Animals with brain diseases and metabolic or toxic disorders often have other clinical signs, such as abnormal behavior or gait, blindness, loss of appetite, vomiting, diarrhea, excessive thirst, frequent urination, weight loss, weakness, and general debilitation. Young animals may fail to grow normally.

🩺 Diagnostic Tests

Evaluation of an animal with seizures includes physical and neurologic examinations, routine laboratory tests, and sometimes x-rays. Additional tests may be recommended based on the results of these tests or if a metabolic or toxic cause is suspected.

Identification of specific brain disorders requires imaging of the brain, such as magnetic resonance imaging (MRI). Collection and examination of cerebrospinal fluid, which surrounds the brain, is often helpful in the diagnosis of certain inflammations or infections of the brain.

TREATMENT AND FOLLOW-UP

℞ Treatment Options

If an underlying cause is identified, specific treatment is started for that disorder. Depending on their frequency, duration, and severity, treatment may be recommended to control the seizures. In general, treatment is usually started if seizures occur more frequently than every 6-8 weeks, if multiple seizures occur within a 24-hour period, or if the underlying disease cannot be resolved. (For a detailed description of seizure treatments, see the handouts on **Seizures: Treatment** and **Seizures: Treatment of Resistant Cases**.)

🐾 Follow-up Care

If an underlying disease is identified, initial follow-up is defined by that disease. Rechecks are usually needed frequently at the beginning of seizure therapy and may be decreased to twice yearly once seizure control is achieved. It is helpful to keep a diary of the timing and frequency, duration, and severity of the seizures in order to establish patterns that can play a role in adjusting treatments.

Prognosis

Prognosis depends on the underlying cause. Prognosis is good if the underlying disease can be resolved and guarded if it cannot be treated. Prognosis for animals with idiopathic epilepsy is usually good, because many of these seizures can be controlled.

SPECIAL INSTRUCTIONS:

Seizures: Idiopathic Epilepsy

A. Courtenay Freeman, DVM
Marc Kent, DVM, DACVIM (Small Animal and Neurology)
Simon R. Platt, BVM&S, MRCVS, DACVIM (Neurology), DECVN

BASIC INFORMATION

Description

Idiopathic epilepsy is a disorder of recurring seizures of unknown cause. In dogs, a genetic or inherited influence has been proven for some breeds. All diagnostic tests used to search for the causes of seizures are normal in animals with idiopathic epilepsy. Idiopathic epilepsy is a common cause of seizures in dogs, but it is uncommon in cats.

Cause

It is theorized that an imbalance in brain chemistry causes an excess of excitatory nerve impulses and a deficiency of inhibitory nerve impulses. Consequently, the brain is predisposed to excessive stimulation, which results in seizures. Idiopathic epilepsy is diagnosed more commonly in purebred dogs such as the German shepherd dog, border collie, golden retriever, and Labrador retriever but can occur in any dog. Idiopathic epilepsy typically affects dogs from 1 to 5 years of age but may develop at any age.

Clinical Signs

Animals with idiopathic epilepsy have recurring seizures. Most seizures last 1 to 3 minutes, and they can occur at any time of the day. Time between seizures can be as short as minutes or as long as months. The time between seizures is called the *interictal* period. The Latin term *ictus* refers to a seizure. Affected animals are normal between seizures and do not have any neurologic abnormalities on physical examination.

Seizures can take many different forms. The most common form is a generalized seizure (grand mal seizure) in which the animal is unconscious and unresponsive. It may fall or lie down. The legs are often rigidly stretched out or drawn up toward the body. The limbs may jerk or paddle as if running. Chewing motions, excessive salivation, urination, or defecation may occur. For a Description of other manifestations of seizures, see the handout on **Seizures: Causes and Diagnosis**.

Diagnostic Tests

The diagnosis of idiopathic epilepsy requires eliminating all other diseases that can cause seizures. Evaluation of an animal with seizures includes physical and neurologic examinations, routine laboratory tests, and sometimes x-rays. Additional tests may be recommended based on results of these tests or if metabolic or toxic causes must be ruled out. Imaging of the brain using magnetic resonance imaging (MRI) or computed tomography (CT scan) and analysis of cerebrospinal fluid may also be recommended to evaluate for an underlying brain disease. Animals with idiopathic epilepsy have normal test results.

TREATMENT AND FOLLOW-UP

Treatment Options

Treatment is unlikely to prevent all future seizures in most animals. Instead, treatment is aimed at reducing the duration, severity, and frequency of seizures. Several antiepileptic drugs are available to control seizures. (For specific information regarding treatment, see the handouts **Seizures: Treatment** and **Seizures: Treatment of Resistant Cases**.)

Several factors require consideration prior to therapy, because treatment is lifelong and costly and has potential side effects. It is helpful to keep a diary of the seizures, to establish any patterns of frequency, duration, severity, and other characteristics. This information can affect the decision on when to begin antiepileptic therapy and can aid in determining the need to adjust therapy.

Treatment is generally recommended in the following situations:
- The seizures occur more frequently than once every 6-8 weeks.
- More than one seizure occurs during the first episode. More than one seizure in a 24-hour period is referred to as a *cluster seizure*.
- The first seizure lasted more than 20 minutes or multiple seizures occurred over a short period of time without the animal regaining normal consciousness and behavior in between. Continuous seizure activity is called *status epilepticus*.
- The animal's quality of life is impaired by the seizure activity.

Not every animal with idiopathic epilepsy requires treatment. For instance, an animal that has experienced only a single, isolated seizure is not usually started on medication. Instead, the affected animal may be monitored, and the frequency of any future seizures helps determine when to start therapy. Additionally, animals with infrequent seizures may require no treatment.

It is important to see a veterinarian immediately if more than one seizure occurs in a 24-hour period, if seizure activity continues beyond 5 minutes, or if recovery of consciousness and behavior is not complete between seizures.

Follow-up Care

Patient follow-up is described in the handouts on **Seizures: Treatment** and **Seizures: Treatment of Resistant Cases**.

Prognosis

Prognosis for animals with idiopathic epilepsy is usually good, because many of these seizures can be controlled. Animals that are well controlled on anticonvulsant medications can live normal, healthy lives with idiopathic epilepsy. The prognosis is guarded for animals with poorly controlled seizures.

SPECIAL INSTRUCTIONS:

Seizures: Treatment

A. Courtenay Freeman, DVM
Marc Kent, DVM, DACVIM (Small Animal and Neurology)
Simon R. Platt, BVM&S, MRCVS, DACVIM (Neurology), DECVN

Several drugs are available for controlling seizures. The goal of therapy is to decrease the frequency, duration, and severity of seizures. Despite appropriate treatment, most animals continue to have seizures. The following description of medications pertains to animals with idiopathic epilepsy, but these medications can also be used to control seizures from other underlying causes.

PHENOBARBITAL

Description

Phenobarbital is an effective antiepileptic drug and is often the first drug chosen to treat animals with epilepsy. Adequate seizure control may take up to 2 weeks, because it takes some time to build up the concentration of phenobarbital in the blood. For severe seizures, a high dose may be given initially and may result in excessive side effects, such as sedation. Phenobarbital comes in injectable, tablet, and liquid formulations, but the liquid form may not be palatable to cats and some dogs. Phenobarbital is eliminated from the body by the liver, so it is avoided in animals with liver disease.

Side Effects

The most common side effects are increased thirst, urination, and appetite. Some animals may become sedated and have an uncoordinated gait, but this effect typically wears off after several weeks. Rarely, animals may become hyperactive and restless.

More serious side effects include liver damage, blood disorders, and allergic skin reactions. Liver damage is most likely in dogs that receive high doses or take the medication for a long time. Blood disorders caused by phenobarbital include decreased levels of red blood cells, white blood cells, and platelets, which can result in lethargy, decreased appetite, increased susceptibility to infections, and spontaneous bleeding. In rare cases, phenobarbital can cause skin ulcerations.

Animals receiving phenobarbital should be examined at least every 6 months, with evaluation of routine laboratory tests to monitor for side effects. Specialized tests may be recommended to evaluate liver function in animals with suspected liver damage. For animals experiencing severe side effects, phenobarbital treatment may be slowly tapered and discontinued under the guidance of a veterinarian. Stopping phenobarbital abruptly can result in seizures and should not be done without consulting your veterinarian.

Monitoring

Repeated measurement of phenobarbital blood levels is used initially to adjust dosages, then every 6 months to make sure blood levels do not become too high. Excessive blood concentrations are often associated with side effects. Although there is a desired range for phenobarbital levels in the blood, some animals' seizures can be controlled even with low blood concentrations.

POTASSIUM BROMIDE

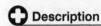 Description

Potassium bromide is another effective antiepileptic drug. It can be used alone or in combination with phenobarbital to control seizures. Combinations of potassium bromide and phenobarbital may control seizures that are not controlled by either drug alone. Potassium bromide is available through compounding pharmacies in capsule or liquid form.

Side Effects

The most common side effects are increased thirst, urination, and appetite. Animals may also become sedated and have an uncoordinated gait. Sedation typically wears off after several weeks. Vomiting may occur but can be reduced by administering the drug with food. Pancreatitis has been associated with potassium bromide, so animals that develop severe vomiting, lethargy, and lack of appetite should be evaluated by your veterinarian. Potassium bromide is not recommended in cats because it can cause severe respiratory problems.

Potassium bromide takes several (3-5) months to reach effective blood concentrations but may control seizures even before reaching these levels. With severe seizures, a high initial dose may be administered in an effort to achieve immediate therapeutic drug concentrations, but these loading doses are associated with severe side effects such as profound sedation. Dogs receiving a loading dose may require hospitalization.

Monitoring

Repeated measurement of potassium bromide blood levels is used initially to adjust dosages, then usually every 3-4 months for awhile. Eventually, blood levels may be checked only every 6 months to make sure they do not become too high. Excessive blood levels are more commonly associated with side effects. In some animals, seizures can be controlled despite a low concentration in the blood.

Blood levels are affected by the salt content of the diet. Animals should be fed a consistent diet, and any changes in diet should be made in consultation with your veterinarian. Specialized diets used in the management of other diseases can lead to excessive blood concentrations and side effects, so discuss these diets with your veterinarian.

Potassium bromide is eliminated from the body by the kidneys, so the drug is usually avoided or is given only in low doses to animals with kidney disease. Animals with liver disease may be treated safely with potassium bromide.

SPECIAL INSTRUCTIONS:

Seizures: Treatment of Resistant Cases

A. Courtenay Freeman, DVM
Marc Kent, DVM, DACVIM (Small Animal and Neurology)
Simon R. Platt, BVM&S, MRCVS, DACVIM (Neurology), DECVN

ANTIEPILEPTIC DRUGS FOR RESISTANT CASES

Treatment Options

Several newer drugs are available for treating seizures. They can be used in combination with phenobarbital and potassium bromide to improve seizure control in severely affected animals. These medications may also be tried as the sole treatment for seizures in some cases, but their effectiveness as a sole therapy is unknown at present. Most of these newer drugs are also expensive. Once seizure control has been achieved with any of these drugs, the dosage of phenobarbital or potassium bromide can often be decreased.

Levetiracetam

Levetiracetam (*Keppra*) is an antiepileptic drug that has few side effects and may offer good seizure control in dogs. It is effective in many cases refractory to other drugs. Levetiracetam is not eliminated from the body by the liver, so it can be used in animals with liver disease. Levetiracetam comes as a tablet and is usually given three times daily.

Gabapentin

Gabapentin (*Neurotin*) is also effective in many animals with seizures refractory to other drugs. The most common side effect is sedation. Gabapentin is eliminated from the body by the liver and kidneys but has not yet been shown to cause liver disease. Gabapentin comes as a capsule and is administered three times daily.

Zonisamide

Zonisamide (*Zonegran*) may be as effective as levetiracetam or gabapentin. It is well tolerated by dogs. Side effects include decreased appetite, sedation, and incoordination. Allergic reactions, decreased tearing (dry eye), and blood disorders are potential side effects. Zonisamide is eliminated from the body by the liver, so is avoided in animals with liver disease. It comes as a tablet and is administered twice daily.

EMERGENCY DRUGS

Diazepam

Diazepam (*Valium*) is not a new drug and is widely used in the emergency treatment of seizures. Diazepam is often used in hospitalized animals, because it is given intravenously during a seizure. Diazepam can also be administered into the nose or the rectum. Dogs with severe seizures can be given diazepam rectally at home to reduce seizure severity and to try and prevent repeated seizures. In dogs, the effect of diazepam is short lived, so the drug is not used for long-term management of seizures. On rare occasions, cats on oral diazepam can develop severe, often fatal, liver damage, so oral administration of diazepam is done with caution in cats.

Follow-up Care

Once antiepileptic therapy is started, treatment commonly continues for life. Many antiepileptic drugs have side effects, so follow-up evaluations and close monitoring are required. At the beginning of treatment, follow-up evaluations and telephone consultations are used to ensure the successful control of seizures via appropriate dosing. Once the seizures are controlled, the animal is evaluated at least every 6 months. In addition to drug blood levels, other routine laboratory tests are used to monitor for side effects and to evaluate the animal's general health. Always discuss any changes in medications with your veterinarian; it is dangerous to make dosage adjustments on your own. Even if side effects occur, antiepileptic drugs should not be abruptly discontinued without consultation with a veterinarian. Discontinuation of these drugs is usually done gradually, under the direction of your veterinarian.

SPECIAL INSTRUCTIONS:

Spinal Cord Trauma

A. Courtenay Freeman, DVM
Marc Kent, DVM, DACVIM (Small Animal and Neurology)
Simon R. Platt, BVM&S, MRCVS, DACVIM (Neurology), DECVN

BASIC INFORMATION

Description
The spinal cord is protected within the spinal column, which is composed of small bones called *vertebrae*. The spinal cord transmits neurologic information between the brain and the rest of the body. Spinal cord trauma can cause neurologic abnormalities and pain.

Causes
The most common causes are automobile accidents. Other causes include falling from a height or being struck by an object. Trauma to the spinal column may cause fractures or luxations (dislocations of the spine) that result in bruising, bleeding into, or compression of the spinal cord.

Clinical Signs
Signs are dependent on the area of spinal cord affected and the severity of the trauma. Often, other areas of the body are also injured, with loss of blood (hemorrhage), internal organ damage, broken bones, and/or trauma to the heart and lungs.

Neurologic abnormalities vary with the degree of spinal cord injury:
- Mild injury may result in only pain at the injured site.
- Moderate injury causes an uncoordinated gait, crossing over of the legs while walking, scuffing of the nails, and weakness.
- When the injury is more severe, animals lose the ability to move their legs and may have difficulty urinating on their own.
- With the most severe damage, animals cannot feel a painful stimulus applied to their toes and are paralyzed.

All four legs may be affected if the spinal cord in the neck is injured. Only the hind legs are affected if the damage occurs in the upper or lower back region.

Diagnostic Tests
Routine laboratory tests may be recommended to evaluate for blood loss and organ damage associated with the trauma. X-rays are used to evaluate injury to the chest, abdomen, and other bones.

X-rays of the spine may show a fracture, luxation, or malalignment of the spine. Additional imaging with computed tomography (CT scan) or magnetic resonance imaging (MRI) may be recommended to further evaluate the vertebrae and spinal cord. CT scans show more detailed images of bone that may be used for planning surgery in cases of fracture or dislocation. MRI allows detailed evaluation of the spinal cord for damage or compression.

TREATMENT AND FOLLOW-UP

Treatment Options
Animals with spinal cord trauma may be treated conservatively or surgically, depending on the severity of the signs and the stability of the spine. Conservative therapy is typically recommended when neurologic signs are mild and the spine appears on imaging studies to be stable and properly aligned.

Animals with mild injuries may be treated with exercise restriction and medication. Occasionally splints (back braces) are used to help support the spine. Exercise restriction involves strict confinement to a crate and leash walking only to allow the animal to urinate and defecate. Cats are confined in a small area with a litter box. Animals cannot be allowed to run, jump, or play during their confinement. Exercise restriction usually lasts 4-6 weeks, with gradual return to normal activity at the end of the confinement period.

Anti-inflammatory medications, such as nonsteroidal anti-inflammatory drugs or steroids, can be used, but these two classes of drugs are not used together because of their combined side effects. Pain medications may be needed to keep the animal comfortable.

Some animals require surgery to stabilize spinal fractures or luxations, realign the spinal column, and decompress (relieve pressure on) the spinal cord. Surgery involves the placement of orthopedic implants to fuse the spinal column and prevent additional movement. In some cases, the spinal canal may be opened and any bone fragments or blood clots removed to relieve compression on the spinal cord.

Depending on the overall condition of the affected animal, spinal surgery is sometimes delayed until the animal can be safely anesthetized. Animals also require strict cage rest for several weeks after surgery to allow their injuries to heal.

Follow-up Care
While the animal is hospitalized, neurologic functions are monitored on a daily basis. After discharge, periodic rechecks are often used to monitor for improvement. X-rays of the spine are usually performed to evaluate healing at 4-6 weeks after surgery.

Prognosis
Prognosis depends on the severity of spinal cord injury and other systemic abnormalities. Animals with the ability to feel a painful stimulus in their affected legs often walk again after surgery, but recovery can take several weeks to months. If the animal is unable to feel a painful stimulus in the affected legs, the prognosis for regaining the ability to walk is grave. Residual problems, such as incoordination and incontinence, are possible. Maximal improvement is usually seen within 3-4 months.

SPECIAL INSTRUCTIONS:

Spinal Tumors

A. Courtenay Freeman, DVM
Marc Kent, DVM, DACVIM (Small Animal and Neurology)
Simon R. Platt, BVM&S, MRCVS, DACVIM (Neurology), DECVN

BASIC INFORMATION

Description

The spine is a complex structure that is composed of vertebrae (bones), intervertebral discs (cartilaginous structures situated between vertebrae), and the spinal cord. Spinal tumors can arise from any of these anatomic structures (called *primary tumors*), or they can spread to the spine from nearby structures or from tumors elsewhere in the body (metastasis). These latter two types of tumors are referred to as *secondary tumors*. Although any animal can be affected, large-breed dogs are predisposed. These tumors occur more often in older dogs and cats.

Causes

Common vertebral tumors include osteosarcoma, fibrosarcoma, and hemangiosarcoma. These tumors usually affect only one vertebra and are the most common types of spinal tumors in dogs.

The brain and spinal cord are covered by layers of tissue called *meninges*. A meningioma is a tumor that arises from the meninges; it is a common spinal tumor in dogs.

Spinal tumors can also develop from the spinal cord itself, and these cancers are collectively known as *gliomas*. Tumors can also arise from the nerves exiting the spinal cord. (See handout on **Peripheral Nerve Sheath Tumors**.)

Some cancers arising from white blood cells can affect multiple vertebrae, including multiple myeloma, plasmacytoma, and lymphoma. Lymphoma may also develop within the spinal canal without affecting the vertebrae, and it is a common spinal tumor in cats.

Clinical Signs

Signs typically develop slowly; however, an acute onset is observed in some animals. All types of spinal tumors tend to produce similar signs. The most common, and sometimes the only, clinical sign is neck or back pain.

Clinical signs depend on the location of the tumor and the degree of associated spinal cord damage. Tumors of the neck can affect the function of all four legs, whereas those of the spine in the chest and back areas affect only hind leg function. As the tumor grows, it compresses (squeezes) the spinal cord, which results in weakness and incoordination. Inability to walk, paralysis, and inability to feel a painful stimulus (such as pinching a toe) can occur with severe compression.

Diagnostic Tests

A spinal problem may be suspected based on the history, signs, and results of neurologic examination. X-rays of the spine may reveal loss of vertebral bone suggestive of a tumor. Special imaging techniques are often required to make a diagnosis. Magnetic resonance imaging (MRI) allows detailed evaluation of the spinal cord and surrounding structures. Computed tomography (CT scan) or myelography may also be recommended. Myelography is an x-ray study of the spine that is done after a dye is injected around the spinal cord. Definitive diagnosis of a spinal tumor may require a biopsy, which often involves surgery.

Routine laboratory tests and x-rays of the chest and abdomen may be recommended to search for metastasis. A spinal tap and cerebrospinal fluid analysis may be helpful in eliminating other diseases that cause similar signs.

TREATMENT AND FOLLOW-UP

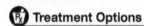

Treatment Options

Treatments options include medical, surgical, and/or radiation therapy, depending on the type and location of the tumor. Treatment that is solely designed to provide pain relief and temporarily improve clinical signs (palliative therapy) may be considered in some cases. Steroids are often used to reduce inflammation associated with a spinal tumor and thereby improve clinical signs. Steroids may also provide pain relief. Other medications, such as tramadol, can be used in conjunction with steroids to relieve pain.

Chemotherapy may be used for some spinal tumors, such as lymphoma and multiple myeloma. Depending on the location of the tumor, surgery may be performed to remove as much of it as possible. Although some tumors appear to be completely removed at the time of surgery, microscopic cells often remain. Despite this, surgery may provide temporary relief of pain and clinical signs. Spinal tumors that are not operable may be treated with radiation therapy. Radiation therapy can also be performed after surgery to treat any remaining cancerous tissue.

Follow-up Care

Follow-up examinations are needed to monitor for improvement or progression of the neurologic abnormalities. Animals receiving chemotherapy must also be rechecked frequently and laboratory tests repeated to monitor for side effects. Radiation therapy typically requires several weeks of treatment.

Prognosis

Overall, the prognosis for animals with spinal tumors is variable, depending on the type of tumor and the degree of spinal cord damage prior to treatment. Some types of spinal cancers can be treated successfully for long periods, but some types do not respond even to aggressive therapy.

SPECIAL INSTRUCTIONS:

Spondylosis Deformans

A. Courtenay Freeman, DVM
Marc Kent, DVM, DACVIM (Small Animal and Neurology)
Simon R. Platt, BVM&S, MRCVS, DACVIM (Neurology), DECVN

BASIC INFORMATION

Description

The spinal column is composed of small bones called *vertebrae*. The spinal cord runs through the center of these bones, within the spinal canal. Between adjacent vertebrae are discs (intervertebral discs) that act as cushions and provide strength and stability to the spine. These cushions allow the vertebrae some flexibility and movement with respect to each other.

Spondylosis deformans is the presence of bony growth beneath and around the spinal column that forms solid bridges between adjacent vertebrae. The bone growth can cover the entire space between vertebrae, surrounding the intervertebral disc.

Causes

Spondylosis deformans is a common degenerative or age-related change of older dogs. The cause is unknown, but it may result from slight instability of the spinal column. The presence of spondylosis deformans may also indicate underlying intervertebral disc disease. (See the handout on **Intervertebral Disc Disease**.)

Clinical Signs

Spondylosis deformans alone does not usually cause neurologic signs or pain. Rarely, the bony growth can extend into the spinal canal and compress the nerves and spinal cord. If spinal cord compression occurs, pain, an uncoordinated gait, and weakness may occur.

Diagnostic Tests

Spondylosis deformans can be seen on x-rays of the spine. A magnetic resonance imaging (MRI) procedure is necessary if neurologic signs are present.

TREATMENT AND FOLLOW-UP

Treatment Options

Treatment is typically not necessary. Rarely, if spinal cord compression occurs, surgery is needed to remove the compressive bone.

Follow-up Care

Spondylosis deformans is usually an incidental finding and does not require long term follow-up.

Prognosis

Prognosis is good, because spondylosis deformans does not typically cause neurologic abnormalities or clinical signs.

SPECIAL INSTRUCTIONS:

Steroid-Responsive Meningeal Arteritis

A. Courtenay Freeman, DVM
Marc Kent, DVM, DACVIM (Small Animal and Neurology)
Scott J. Schatzberg, DVM, PhD, DACVIM (Neurology)

BASIC INFORMATION

Description

Steroid-responsive meningeal arteritis (SRMA) is a disease in which the layers of tissue covering the brain and spinal cord (*meninges*) become inflamed (*meningitis*) due to an immune reaction. Animals with meningitis often exhibit pain and neurologic abnormalities. The disease is seen most commonly in young, large-breed dogs less than 2 years old. Breeds that are predisposed to the condition include the boxer, Bernese Mountain dog, and beagle.

Causes

The cause of this inflammation has yet to be determined. The inflammation arises when the animal's immune system becomes activated and attacks the meninges.

Clinical Signs

The most common clinical sign of SRMA is an acute (sudden) onset of pain. The pain typically is isolated to the neck but may be present along the entire spine. Affected dogs may be reluctant to walk, lift their head, or move their neck.

Other clinical signs include fever, lethargy, depression, and decreased appetite. Affected dogs occasionally have signs of inflammation in the joints of the legs (immune-mediated polyarthritis). Polyarthritis, which is an inflammation of multiple joints, may cause additional discomfort, lameness, reluctance to walk, and a short-strided gait.

Diagnostic Tests

SRMA may be suspected initially, based on the history and neurologic examination findings. Routine blood tests may indicate generalized inflammation. X-rays or other advanced imaging studies, such as magnetic resonance imaging (MRI), myelography, or computed tomography (CT scan) of the neck may be recommended to exclude other potential causes of neck pain and similar signs.

Cerebrospinal fluid (CSF) analysis is a key component in the diagnostic work-up for SRMA. A spinal tap is performed to collect the CSF, which typically shows increased numbers of a type of white blood cell called the *neutrophil* and elevated total protein levels. Measurement of a specific antibody, immunoglobulin A (IgA), in CSF may also be performed by specialized laboratories. Increased IgA levels in CSF are highly suggestive of SMRA.

Bacterial cultures and other tests are often needed to exclude infectious diseases from consideration, because many of the clinical signs and results of the CSF analysis are not specific for SRMA and may also occur in cases of infection. Consequently, the diagnosis of SRMA is made by a combination of history, examination findings, advanced imaging and CSF analysis, additional laboratory tests, exclusion of infectious agents, and response to therapy.

TREATMENT AND FOLLOW-UP

Treatment Options

Treatment of SRMA involves suppression of the immune reaction, most commonly through the administration of steroids. Dogs usually respond to treatment within a few days; however, treatment is continued for several months. As the clinical signs resolve, the dose of steroids is slowly decreased until the dog is weaned off the therapy, if possible, or until the lowest dose that controls the clinical signs is found. Occasionally, affected dogs require additional medications for pain and other clinical signs.

Follow-up Care

Affected dogs are re-evaluated frequently at first, to monitor response to treatment and to make decisions about tapering the steroids. Rechecks and monitoring are also needed to monitor for recurrence of the disease. Notify your veterinarian if any signs worsen or recur as the drugs are decreased. Occasionally, a spinal tap and CSF analysis may be repeated to evaluate for resolution of the inflammation.

Prognosis

Prognosis is good if affected dogs are treated early with immunosuppressive therapy; however, some dogs experience relapses. Occasionally, long-term medication is necessary to control clinical signs.

SPECIAL INSTRUCTIONS:

Tick Paralysis

A. Courtenay Freeman, DVM
Marc Kent, DVM, DACVIM (Small Animal and Neurology)
Scott J. Schatzberg, DVM, PhD, DACVIM (Neurology)

BASIC INFORMATION

Description

Tick paralysis is a form of generalized muscle paralysis of dogs that is caused by a neurologic toxin generated by certain species of ticks. The neurotoxin responsible for tick paralysis prevents the nerves from activating muscles by blocking a chemical called *acetylcholine*.

Causes

The two ticks most commonly associated with this condition are the *Ixodes* and *Dermacentor* ticks, both of which are natural parasites of dogs. Not every tick is capable of producing the disease. In order to cause tick paralysis, the tick must bite and feed on the animal. As the tick feeds, the neurotoxin is released into the blood of the animal. Signs typically appear after the tick has been attached for 3-5 days.

Clinical Signs

The most obvious clinical sign is generalized weakness involving all four legs. Signs appear suddenly (acutely) and steadily worsen over 1-3 days. Initially, the hind legs become weak, followed rapidly by weakness in the front legs. Decreased muscle tone is observed in all four legs, which makes the legs appear very limp. The dog often has difficulty standing, stands in a crouched position, and has a short-strided gait. Affected animals easily become tired when walking and often can walk only a few steps before having to rest. Severely affected animals become paralyzed.

If the tick is not removed, the muscles involved with breathing can become paralyzed, which can be life-threatening. Affected dogs are not in pain. Occasionally, jaw weakness and an inability to blink the eyelids are observed.

Diagnostic Tests

A presumptive diagnosis of tick paralysis can be made from a combination of clinical signs, neurologic examination findings, and finding a tick feeding on the affected animal. If a tick is not found but the animal improves after application of a product that kills ticks, tick paralysis may also be suspected. Specialized neurologic testing can be done to support the diagnosis but usually requires referral to a veterinary neurologist. Other tests are often recommended to rule out other diseases that cause similar clinical signs.

TREATMENT AND FOLLOW-UP

Treatment Options

Clinical signs rapidly resolve over 24-48 hours after removal of the tick. Severely affected dogs usually require hospitalization and intensive supportive care during the recovery period. Animals with difficulty breathing may be placed on a mechanical ventilator. Insecticide products that are safe for dogs are applied to kill any remaining ticks and prevent re-exposure.

Follow-up Care

Removal of the tick usually cures the disease. Long-term follow-up is not necessary in dogs that recover, but continuous, year-round tick prevention should be instituted.

Prognosis

Prognosis for recovery is excellent once the tick has been killed or removed. Prognosis is worse if muscles involved with breathing are affected or if pneumonia is present. Recurrence can occur if the dog is bitten by another tick capable of inducing the disease.

SPECIAL INSTRUCTIONS:

Tremor Syndrome

A. Courtenay Freeman, DVM
Marc Kent, DVM, DACVIM (Small Animal and Neurology)
Scott J. Schatzberg, DVM, PhD, DACVIM (Neurology)

BASIC INFORMATION

Description

Tremor syndrome is a disorder caused by mild inflammation of the covering of the brain and spinal cord (*meninges*) that produces fine tremors of the head and whole body. Tremor syndrome tends to affect young (1-5 years of age), small-breed dogs. Typical breeds affected include the Maltese, poodles, and West Highland white terrier. Tremor syndrome has been called "little white shaker disease" because it seems to be most common in small breed dogs with white hair coats; however, any dog can be affected, regardless of size and coat color.

Causes

The tremors are caused by inflammation of the covering of the brain and spinal cord, but an underlying cause has not been found. The inflammation may be caused by an immune-mediated process in which the animal's own immune system attacks the meninges, leading to inflammation (*meningitis*).

Clinical Signs

Head and body tremors are the predominant clinical signs. The tremors appear as fine shaking movements similar to shivering. They typically increase in severity during excitement and lessen with rest. Tremors are absent during sleep. Some dogs also have a high-stepping, uncoordinated gait, abnormal eye movements, and (rarely) seizures. Dogs with severe generalized tremors may have difficulty walking.

Diagnostic Tests

History and neurologic examination findings are important in the initial diagnosis of tremor syndrome. Routine blood tests (such as a complete blood count and biochemistry profile) and a urinalysis are usually normal or may suggest inflammation.

Advanced imaging of the brain may be performed using magnetic resonance imaging (MRI) or computed tomography (CT scan). Although the MRI is usually normal in dogs with tremor syndrome, imaging of the brain rules out other neurologic diseases that can produce similar clinical signs.

Cerebrospinal fluid (CSF) evaluation is important in the diagnostic work-up, and the fluid is obtained via a spinal tap. Animals with tremor syndrome have evidence of inflammation in their CSF, with increased numbers of white blood cells called *lymphocytes* and elevated protein levels.

TREATMENT AND FOLLOW-UP

Treatment Options

Tremor syndrome is treated with steroids. Initially, steroids are given at a high dose to suppress the immune system and decrease inflammation. The tremors usually decrease or stop within a few days to weeks after therapy is started, but medication is continued for several months to prevent a relapse. Over time, the steroid dose is tapered slowly in an attempt to wean the animal off the therapy or to find the lowest dose necessary to control the clinical signs.

Follow-up Care

Patients typically are re-evaluated every few weeks initially, to monitor for resolution of the tremors. Additionally, recheck appointments may be scheduled every few weeks while steroids are tapered to monitor for recurrence of clinical signs.

Prognosis

Prognosis for recovery is good. Tremors stop in most animals shortly (1-3 days) after initiating therapy. However, some dogs relapse when the medications are tapered or discontinued and require lifelong treatment to control the tremors.

SPECIAL INSTRUCTIONS:

SECTION 5

Digestive System

Section Editor: Craig G. Ruaux, BVSc, PhD, DACVIM (Small Animal)

Anal Sac Diseases
Cholangiohepatitis in Cats
Cleft Palate
Colitis, Acute
Colitis, Chronic
Copper Storage Hepatopathy in Dogs
Epulis in Dogs
Esophageal Foreign Body
Esophagitis and Esophageal Stricture
Exocrine Pancreatic Insufficiency
Fecal Incontinence
Gall Bladder Disease in Dogs
Gastric Dilatation-Volvulus
Gastric Foreign Body
Gastric Neoplasia
Gastritis, Acute
Gastritis, Chronic
Gastrointestinal Ulceration
Gingivitis
Hemorrhagic Gastroenteritis in Dogs
Hepatic Encephalopathy

Hepatic Lipidosis in Cats
Hepatitis in Dogs, Chronic
Inflammatory Bowel Disease in Cats
Inflammatory Bowel Disease in Dogs
Intestinal Neoplasia
Intestinal Obstruction
Intestinal Parasites
Lymphoplasmacytic Stomatitis in Cats
Megacolon in Cats
Megaesophagus
Oral Melanoma in Dogs
Oral Squamous Cell Carcinoma in Cats
Pancreatitis in Cats
Pancreatitis in Dogs
Perianal Fistula in Dogs
Perianal Tumors
Perineal Hernia in Dogs
Portosystemic Vascular Anomalies
Protein-Losing Enteropathy
Salivary Mucocele in Dogs

Anal Sac Diseases

Craig G. Ruaux, BVSc, PhD, DACVIM (Small Animal)

BASIC INFORMATION
Description
The anal sacs are two small pouches under the skin near the anus at the 4 and 8 o'clock positions. These sacs hold a thick, fatty liquid that is strongly scented and produced by the anal glands. This liquid is used by wolves and wild cat species to mark their territories. In the domestic dog and cat, the use of anal gland secretions for territorial marking is much reduced or completely absent; however, the glands and their associated sacs are still present. Occasionally the anal sacs become blocked (impacted) or infected. Anal sac disease occurs more commonly in dogs than in cats.

Normal emptying of the anal sacs occurs with defecation. When the anal sphincter muscle opens, it compresses the sac, causing it to empty through the small opening of the anal sac duct. Dogs and cats can also empty their anal sacs voluntarily, but they usually only do so if they are frightened.

Causes
Failure of the anal sacs to empty during defecation can occur when animals eat low-fiber diets that produce feces that are soft and do not stretch the anus. Hard, gritty material may accumulate within the sac, leading to swelling and possible obstruction. Infection of the anal sac duct, possibly from bacteria or fungal organisms living around the anus, can cause swelling of the duct and prevent the sacs from emptying. Sometimes the infection travels along the duct into the anal sac, and an abscess may form.

Clinical Signs

Any impaction or swelling of the anal sacs can cause anal discomfort in both dogs and cats. The most common clinical sign is scooting or dragging of the animal's rear end on the floor while it is seated. Other signs include excessive licking of the anal area, a foul odor, and sometimes the presence of a small hole under the tail that drains pus or gritty mucous material. The area around the anus is commonly swollen, red, and painful.

Diagnostic Tests

Your veterinarian may perform a rectal examination (using a gloved finger) to assess the size of the anal sacs and to look for masses or problems that can be confused with anal sac disease, such as an anal tumor or perineal hernia. Often the diagnosis of anal sac disease is obvious from clinical and rectal examinations.

Additional diagnostic tests are sometimes necessary in more complicated cases. A bacterial culture may be done if the anal sacs are infected. If any mass or lump is found near the anus, it may be aspirated with a needle. The material collected is then examined under the microscope. Laboratory tests may also be recommended, especially measurement of blood calcium, which can be elevated with certain anal sac tumors. X-rays may be considered prior to biopsy and removal of any masses.

TREATMENT AND FOLLOW-UP
Treatment Options
Uncomplicated impaction of the anal sacs can often be treated by manually expressing the sacs. After the sac is emptied, clinical signs usually disappear rapidly. Prevention of further impactions can be attempted by increasing fiber in the diet and ensuring that your pet has frequent opportunities to defecate.

Animals with infected anal sacs often need broad-spectrum antibiotics and manual expression of the sacs. In severe cases, surgical drainage of the abscessed gland may be needed. Surgical removal of the sacs may be recommended in animals with recurring impactions or infections. Cancer of the anal glands is treated by surgical removal of the tumor. Anal gland cancer can be very aggressive and can invade the lymph nodes of the abdomen, so referral to a veterinary oncologist may be recommended.

Follow-up Care

Most cases of impactions resolve with therapy and do not require frequent follow-up visits. Notify your veterinarian if any signs recur. Dogs with infected or abscessed anal glands are often re-examined after 1 week of antibiotic therapy. If any clinical signs worsen, if the animal's appetite decreases, or if new signs appear (such as a foul odor or pus near the anus), seek further veterinary care for your pet.

Prognosis
Prognosis for most dogs and cats with anal sac impaction is good, because most cases are easily managed with manual expression and dietary change. Dogs with infected or abscessed anal glands have a less certain prognosis, depending on the severity and depth of the infection. Dogs with anal gland tumors have a poor or grave prognosis, because these tumors often have spread to other parts of the body by the time they are detected.

SPECIAL INSTRUCTIONS:

Cholangiohepatitis in Cats

Craig G. Ruaux, BVSc, PhD, DACVIM (Small Animal)

BASIC INFORMATION

Description

One of the most important functions of the liver is the synthesis and release of a substance called *bile*, which is released into the small intestine to help digest fats. The importance of bile flow has been known for so long that our names for the parts of the liver that secrete and release bile are based on the medieval word for bile, *choler*. Cholangiohepatitis is inflammation of the vessels (cholangio) that carry bile through the liver, called the *biliary tree,* and of the liver itself (hepatitis). Cholangiohepatitis begins with inflammation of the biliary tree, and the liver becomes inflamed later in the disease.

Causes

Two major forms of cholangiohepatitis exist in cats. These two forms differ in the type of inflammation present and in their cause. In younger cats, the major form is *suppurative cholangiohepatitis*, which usually involves a bacterial infection of the bile system or liver. In older cats (usually older than 8 years of age), *lymphocytic cholangiohepatitis* is more commonly diagnosed. The cause of lymphocytic cholangiohepatitis is not well known, but it may arise from an abnormal reaction by the cat's own immune system (immune-mediated inflammation) to the liver and bile ducts.

Cholangiohepatitis is often diagnosed in association with inflammatory bowel disease (IBD) and pancreatitis. When all three problems are present together, the condition is called *feline triaditis*.

Clinical Signs

Clinical signs are often vague and variable. Probably the most common clinical sign is a decreased or absent appetite. Vomiting, jaundice (yellow color to the gums, whites of the eyes, or skin), weight loss, and fever may also be noted. In some cats loss of appetite is the only sign, and the diagnosis is not suspected until diagnostic tests have been run. Signs of IBD and pancreatitis may also be present. (See also the handouts on **Inflammatory Bowel Disease in Cats** and **Pancreatitis in Cats**.)

Diagnostic Tests

Diagnosis of cholangiohepatitis usually requires several different diagnostic tests. Blood tests typically show increased liver enzyme activities and often an elevated bilirubin, which is the chemical that causes the yellow color of jaundice. An abdominal ultrasound is often recommended to examine the liver, biliary tree, and gall bladder, which may be thickened or distorted. Samples of bile may be obtained for bacterial culture, and in some situations parts of the liver may be biopsied and cultured.

Because the treatment for suppurative cholangiohepatitis is different from that for lymphocytic cholangiohepatitis, biopsy of the liver can be extremely important in determining appropriate treatment. Other laboratory tests and x-rays may be recommended to rule out diseases that cause similar clinical signs.

TREATMENT AND FOLLOW-UP

Treatment Options

The main treatment for suppurative cholangiohepatitis is long-term (2-6 months) antibiotic therapy. Ideally, the antibiotic is chosen based on results of a bile or liver culture. If lymphocytic cholangitis is diagnosed, the main treatment is anti-inflammatory or immune suppressive doses of glucocorticoid drugs, such as prednisone.

Additional treatments may be recommended to help improve liver function and protect against further damage. These treatments may include antioxidant medications (such as SAMe or vitamin E), multiple vitamin supplements, appetite stimulants (such as mirtazapine or cyproheptadine), and drugs (such as ursodiol) that make the bile more watery so that it can be secreted more easily. All of these supportive treatments may make the cat feel better sooner, but they do not fix the underlying problem on their own.

Some extremely sick cats require hospitalization for fluids, intravenous antibiotics, and assisted feeding. Cats with cholangiohepatitis are at risk for developing hepatic lipidosis (fatty liver syndrome), particularly if they are overweight and stop eating completely. (See also the handout on **Hepatic Lipidosis in Cats**.)

Follow-up Care

Cat with cholangiohepatitis need regular follow-up visits to check their progress. Initially, progress checks may be recommended every 7-14 days; later, they may be decreased to once monthly, depending on the cat's response to the therapy. At the follow-up visits, blood samples are often drawn to recheck the liver tests, bilirubin levels, and other abnormalities.

Prognosis

Prognosis for cats with cholangiohepatitis is variable, depending on the type (suppurative or lymphocytic), the presence of other diseases (IBD, pancreatitis), and the willingness of the cat to take medications. Most cats with cholangiohepatitis can be successfully treated, but some cats die of this condition, particularly if they develop hepatic lipidosis.

SPECIAL INSTRUCTIONS:

Cleft Palate

Craig G. Ruaux, BVSc, PhD, DACVIM (Small Animal)

BASIC INFORMATION
Description

A cleft palate is a gap or hole in the roof of the mouth. The palate originally forms as two halves, on the left and right sides of the mouth. These two halves normally fuse during the development of the fetus. A cleft palate results when the two sides of the palate do not fuse properly prior to birth. The palate has a hard, bony part (hard palate) and a soft, membranous part (soft palate). A cleft may involve either or both of these parts. Clefts of the front part of the hard palate may also involve the upper lip. Cleft palates are more common in dogs than in cats.

Causes

A cleft sometimes forms in the palate after trauma to the head and mouth, such as being hit by a car. More commonly, a cleft palate is a congenital birth defect. Some drugs (steroids, hydroxyurea) are known to increase the risk of cleft palate in puppies if they are given to the mother early in pregnancy. Some dog breeds, particularly the brachycephalic breeds (breeds with flat faces, such as the Boston terrier, English bulldog, and pug) are at increased risk, probably because of a genetic anomaly within these breeds. However, affected puppies can be of any breed or a mixed breed.

Clinical Signs

Usually, the first clinical sign noticed is milk bubbling from the nose while the puppy is nursing or a defect in the upper lip. Puppies may cough or sneeze, and repeated nasal infections are common. Affected animals often fail to grow as fast as their littermates because they have problems swallowing milk and solid food. Aspiration pneumonia may occur when milk or food is inhaled into the lungs. Pneumonia can cause fever, lethargy, shortness of breath, and bad-smelling breath.

Diagnostic Tests

The diagnosis of a cleft palate is usually made by observing a space in the palate while examining the mouth. Sedation may be needed for a thorough examination and to assess how much tissue is absent, if surgery is to be attempted. Chest x-rays may be recommended if pneumonia is suspected.

TREATMENT AND FOLLOW-UP

Treatment Options

The best treatment option is to repair the cleft surgically. Surgical repair of cleft palate can be complex and may require several procedures. Depending on the severity of the lesion and the involvement of hard palate, soft palate, or both, your veterinarian may recommend referral to a veterinary surgeon. It is not unusual for the surgical site to heal slowly, and partial breakdown of the surgical site may occur, with one or more follow-up surgeries needed. Antibiotics are usually started in animals with pneumonia.

Follow-up Care

Patients require close monitoring after surgery. Chest x-rays are repeated in animals with aspiration pneumonia at 1- to 2-week intervals to assess response to therapy.

Prognosis

Prognosis depends on the complexity of the defect and how well it can be corrected with surgery. In many cases, the prognosis is guarded (uncertain) to poor, because surgical site breakdown and reopening of the cleft can occur. Neonates with a very severe cleft are often euthanized because their food intake is inadequate. If surgical repair of the cleft is successful, the prognosis is better, particularly if the animal is able to eat and drink successfully.

SPECIAL INSTRUCTIONS:

Colitis, Acute

Craig G. Ruaux, BVSc, PhD, DACVIM (Small Animal)

BASIC INFORMATION

Description

Colitis is an inflammation of the colon. Acute colitis typically develops rapidly, with clinical signs that appear and disappear within a very short period.

Causes

The most common causes of acute colitis in dogs and cats are dietary indiscretion (eating something that does not agree with them) and bacterial infection (possibly from spoiled food). Some parasites of the gastrointestinal tract and certain drugs (such as aspirin) also cause colitis. Stress, such as being put into a kennel or hospital, can sometimes lead to acute colitis in a dog or cat.

Clinical Signs

Because the colon is the last part of the intestinal tract before the rectum and anus, the major clinical sign is diarrhea.

- Increased urgency to defecate is common; the animal may be anxious, ask to go outside frequently, or have accidents in the house.
- When the animal attempts to pass a bowel movement a period of unproductive straining may occur, which can be confused with constipation.
- When a bowel movement is passed, it is usually very soft to watery and small in volume. Occasionally fresh, red blood and mucus (a slimy material) are seen in the stool.

Some animals with acute colitis develop a mild fever or lose their appetite. If there is excessive loss of body fluids from diarrhea, signs of dehydration (sunken eyes, lethargy, skin that does not slide easily) can be seen.

Diagnostic Tests

A fecal sample is usually tested for parasites. If your pet has a fever or signs of dehydration, blood tests to assess the degree of dehydration and its effects on other organs, such as the kidneys and liver, are often recommended. If your pet has a high fever or has possibly been exposed to raw poultry meat or dead birds, culture of the feces for *Salmonella* bacteria may be recommended. X-rays, an ultrasound of the abdomen, or both are sometimes needed to look for other problems (such as constipation) that can cause similar clinical signs. There is no specific laboratory test for colitis; instead, the diagnosis is usually made from the clinical signs and history. Although the disease can be confirmed with colonoscopy and biopsy, they are rarely done, because the colitis usually resolves quickly.

TREATMENT AND FOLLOW-UP

Treatment Options

Most cases of acute colitis are self-limited, meaning that the signs usually resolve without the need for specific therapy. As the cause of the problem resolves or is passed from the gastrointestinal tract, the clinical signs disappear. Antibiotics are not usually helpful and may make matters worse, because they interfere with the normal bacteria in the gastrointestinal tract. Maintenance of adequate fluid intake and feeding of a relatively bland, easily digested diet are usually sufficient, and clinical signs often subside within 2-4 days.

If fecal analysis shows evidence of a parasite infestation, then routine, broad-spectrum anti-parasite medications will be prescribed.

If a patient is showing evidence of severe dehydration, either on physical examination or on results of blood tests, hospitalization for intravenous fluid therapy may be necessary. Patients with a high fever may be treated with antibiotic drugs. If a *Salmonella* bacterial infection is detected, people must be very careful to wash their hand after handling the animal, because *Salmonella* can infect people as well as animals.

Follow-up Care

In most cases, the clinical signs resolve rapidly, and there is no need for follow-up visits. If clinical signs do not resolve within 2-3 days, notify your veterinarian If *Salmonella* infection has been detected and treated with antibiotics, follow-up fecal cultures are needed to be certain that the infection has been eliminated. To prevent a recurrence, avoid feeding the animal any suspect foods, and keep the animal away from substances or situations that caused the colitis.

Prognosis

The prognosis for recovery in most cases of acute colitis is good. Most animals recover with only maintenance of adequate fluid intake and a bland, easily digested diet. Clinical signs should resolve within 2-3 days.

SPECIAL INSTRUCTIONS:

Colitis, Chronic

Craig G. Ruaux, BVSc, PhD, DACVIM (Small Animal)

BASIC INFORMATION

Description

Colitis is inflammation of the colon or large intestine, the last part of the intestinal tract. Chronic colitis is suspected if clinical signs of colitis persist for longer than 7-10 days or recur frequently (sometimes up to 3-4 days per week).

Causes

The cause of chronic colitis is often hard to determine. Dietary allergies, food intolerance, and parasite infestations can cause similar signs and must be ruled out. In many cases, an underlying cause is never conclusively identified, so the condition is called *idiopathic chronic colitis*. The boxer breed may develop a specific form of chronic colitis called *histiocytic ulcerative colitis*, which is thought to arise from an infection in the large intestine. In other dog breeds, it is very unusual for infections to be the underlying cause.

Clinical Signs

The major clinical sign of chronic colitis is diarrhea:

- Increased urgency to defecate is common; the animal may be anxious, ask to go out frequently, or have accidents in the house. Cats may pass feces outside the litter box.
- When the animal has a bowel movement, a period of unproductive straining may occur, which can be confused with constipation.
- When a bowel movement is passed, it is usually very soft to watery and small in volume. Occasionally, blood and mucus (a slimy material) are seen in the stool.

Most animals with chronic colitis do not lose their appetite and maintain a normal body weight, unless they become systemically ill with the disease.

Diagnostic Tests

Initially, a fecal sample is checked for parasites. If your pet has a fever or signs of dehydration, blood tests are usually recommended to assess the degree of dehydration and the effects on other organs such as the kidney and liver. X-rays of the abdomen or an abdominal ultrasound are sometimes needed to look for other problems, such as constipation, that can cause similar clinical signs.

The most effective method of diagnosing chronic colitis is through colonoscopy. This procedure allows your veterinarian to view the lining of the colon and look for ulcers, tumors, and inflamed areas. Animals need to be fully anesthetized for this procedure. Biopsy samples can be obtained during the colonoscopy. Many animals with chronic colitis also have inflammatory bowel disease in the stomach and small intestine, so colonoscopy may be combined with upper gastrointestinal tract endoscopy during the same anesthetic procedure. Your veterinarian may recommend referral to an internal medicine specialist to have these tests performed.

TREATMENT AND FOLLOW-UP

Treatment Options

Often the treatment for chronic colitis is as simple as changing the diet, because in many cases a dietary intolerance or food allergy is the underlying cause. The new diet is either specifically manufactured to be hypoallergenic or composed of a completely new source of protein (for instance, lamb instead of chicken). The decision to use a hypoallergenic diet or a new protein source depends on the number of different diet types your pet has consumed in the past.

Usually, if the new diet is going to be beneficial, an improvement in clinical signs is seen within 14 days. If no improvement occurs with diet changes alone, anti-inflammatory drugs, such as steroids, may be given. If steroid medications are started, all other nonsteroidal anti-inflammatory drugs (such as those used for arthritis) must be stopped, or side effects are likely to occur.

For boxers with histiocytic ulcerative colitis, 3-4 weeks of antibiotic therapy is usually beneficial, although signs may recur in some dogs. Antibiotics are used less often in other dogs, but they may be of benefit in some individual cases. Certain sulfa drugs and oral administration of probiotic bacteria may also benefit some dogs.

Follow-up Care

Many patients show improvement in approximately 2 weeks following a diet change or treatment with anti-inflammatory drugs. Failure to improve often indicates a need for further testing and evaluation or the addition of other medications. After the signs resolve, drug therapy is slowly tapered and may eventually be stopped. Notify your veterinarian if any signs recur as the medications are decreased.

Prognosis

Prognosis for most animals with chronic colitis is good, because clinical signs resolve in many patients, and all medications can be stopped. Occasionally, medications and periodic monitoring are needed for life.

SPECIAL INSTRUCTIONS:

Copper Storage Hepatopathy in Dogs

Craig G. Ruaux, BVSc, PhD, DACVIM (Small Animal)

BASIC INFORMATION

Description

An important function of the liver is to remove toxic substances, such as copper, from the bloodstream. In some dogs, abnormalities can occur in the proteins that bind copper in liver cells. The liver of these dogs can still remove copper from the bloodstream, but it gradually accumulates to toxic amounts inside the liver cells. The affected cells die, which reduces the overall function of the liver. Breeds at high risk for copper storage hepatopathy include the Bedlington terrier, Doberman pinscher, Labrador retriever, cocker spaniels, West Highland white terrier, and Skye terrier. Abnormal copper accumulation can also occur with long-standing diseases of the bile system; however, the amount of copper that accumulates is significantly less than with primary copper storage hepatopathy.

Causes

In the Bedlington terrier, this disease arises from a mutation in the gene *COMMD1,* which contains the instructions for making a protein that is necessary for the excretion of copper from liver cells. In the other mentioned breeds, there is evidence that a genetic component may be involved, but the actual gene is not known at this time. Regardless of cause, clinical signs in affected dogs develop following the death of liver cells from excess copper.

Clinical Signs

Clinical signs of copper hepatopathy are the same as for most other liver diseases, and they can be vague and variable in the early phases of the disease. Dogs are often lethargic, may appear depressed, have decreased or complete loss of appetite, and have reduced exercise tolerance. In severely affected animals with diminished liver function, stupor or coma may develop, dogs may become extremely sleepy after eating, and excess fluid accumulation (ascites) may develop in the abdomen or under the skin.

Diagnostic Tests

Typically, the diagnosis is suspected when a dog of a breed known to be prone to this condition shows clinical signs of liver disease and routine laboratory tests indicate abnormal liver function. Additional laboratory tests, abdominal x-rays, and an ultrasound may be needed to confirm the presence of liver disease and to rule out diseases that can cause similar clinical signs.

Definitive diagnosis of copper storage hepatopathy requires a liver biopsy to measure the amount of copper that is present. Several methods are available for obtaining the liver biopsy, including needle biopsy under ultrasound guidance, laparoscopy surgery through a tiny keyhole incision, and a more routine surgical approach through an abdominal incision. The method chosen depends on the equipment available and the surgical experience and preference of your veterinarian. In some cases, your dog may be referred to a veterinary specialist for the procedure.

TREATMENT AND FOLLOW-UP

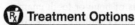 Treatment Options

The most important treatment for this hepatopathy is removal of the copper from the liver, which is done through a process called *chelation.* Chelation drug therapy with D-penicillamine binds the copper and releases it into the urine and feces. Once the amount of copper in the liver is decreased, steps are taken to reduce the accumulation of new copper by feeding a special diet that is extremely low in copper.

Additional drugs and supplements are commonly given, such as large amounts of vitamin C and zinc. Together, the vitamin C and the zinc make it more difficult for copper to be absorbed from the gut into the body. To work effectively, the zinc *must* be given at least 2 hours before the dog is fed. Some dogs have nausea and vomiting when zinc therapy is started, but these usually resolve within a week.

Follow-up Care

Regular follow-up visits and monitoring tests are needed during the initial phase of the therapy. A follow-up liver biopsy is often recommended after 2-3 months to measure the amount of copper present and determine whether drug therapy has been adequate. Once the low-copper diet has been started, liver tests may be rechecked every 3-6 months. Treatment and periodic monitoring are usually needed for the rest of the dog's life.

Prognosis

If the disease is caught early and treated appropriately, many affected dogs can lead normal lives. Prognosis is more guarded (uncertain) for dogs that have severe clinical signs, because they may not be able to regenerate enough liver tissue to function normally.

SPECIAL INSTRUCTIONS:

Epulis in Dogs

Craig G. Ruaux, BVSc, PhD, DACVIM (Small Animal)

BASIC INFORMATION

Description

An epulis is a small, rounded tumor found in the mouth of dogs at the edge of the gum line (the gingiva). These tumors arise from the tissues that hold the teeth in place. In some cases, the epulis can cause the teeth to change position, making it more difficult for the dog to eat. Most epulides are slow growing and may be present for several months before detection.

There are three main types of epulis, based on their manner of growth and the tissues involved:

- The most common types are the *fibromatous* and *ossifying* epulides. The ossifying epulis has areas of bone or tooth enamel within it. The fibromatous type contains bundles of connective tissue collagen.
- The rarest form, and the most worrisome, is the *acanthomatous* or squamous epulis. This type is able to invade the bone of the jaw and can lead to significant damage of the bones of the face or lower jaw if not treated appropriately and early.

Although an epulis is a type of tumor, it is usually benign. The acanthomatous type of epulis very rarely metastasizes (spreads to other parts of the body). Most commonly, this epulis invades the nearby bone.

Causes

There is no known cause of epulis in dogs. Some breeds, particularly the brachycephalic breeds (those with very short snouts, such as the pug, boxer, and English bulldog), seem to develop epulides more commonly, but the reason for this is unknown.

Clinical Signs

A very large epulis can affect eating. You may notice that the dog has trouble picking up food, drops food while chewing, or has trouble swallowing. Some dogs drool or have halitosis (bad-smelling breath) if the epulis becomes damaged and infected, or food particles become stuck in the epulis. A large epulis can also lead to distortion of the face and abnormal deviation of the teeth. If the epulis is damaged during chewing, blood may be seen on the lips or in food or water bowls.

Often, an epulis is only detected during a physical examination when your veterinarian checks the condition of the teeth and gums.

Diagnostic Tests

Diagnosis of an epulis is often made from the physical examination, based on observing a characteristic small tumor. Other forms of cancer in the mouth (such as oral melanoma and squamous cell carcinoma) are more worrisome than most forms of epulis, and tests may be needed to differentiate them from acanthomatous epulis. Your veterinarian may recommend x-rays or computed tomography (CT scan) of the jaw and skull, collecting cells from the tumor for examination under the microscope, or biopsy of the mass (which usually requires general anesthesia and surgery).

TREATMENT AND FOLLOW-UP

Treatment Options

Surgical removal of the epulis is the treatment most commonly recommended. It may involve the extraction of affected teeth as well. Failure to remove all of the affected tissue can allow the tumor to grow back. If the epulis is very large, especially if it is an acanthomatous epulis, large sections of jaw bone and multiple teeth may be extracted to improve the chance of a cure. In cases with invasion of the bone requiring extensive reconstructive surgery, your veterinarian may recommend referral to a surgery or oncology specialist.

Epulides are not usually responsive to chemotherapy. Radiation therapy is sometimes recommended for large acanthomatous epulides.

Follow-up Care

Most dogs recover from surgery for removal of an epulis rapidly and are soon back to normal. Sutures placed in the mouth may dissolve on their own over several weeks to months. After surgery, your dog's mouth may be tender, and its appetite may be reduced for 2-3 days. Dogs having major surgery for removal of a very large epulis or acanthomatous epulis may need to be hospitalized for several days, given medications for pain, and fed through a tube to allow the surgical wounds to heal.

Prognosis

The prognosis for a cure following removal of a fibromatous or ossifying epulis is good, as long as an adequate amount of tissue is removed. The prognosis for an acanthomatous epulis is more guarded (uncertain), because the chance of a surgical cure depends on the size of the tumor, amount of bony invasion, location within the mouth, and the skill of the surgeon carrying out the procedure.

SPECIAL INSTRUCTIONS:

Esophageal Foreign Body

Craig G. Ruaux, BVSc, PhD, DACVIM (Small Animal)

BASIC INFORMATION

Description

The esophagus is a muscular tube that carries swallowed food and water from the mouth to the stomach. Other than during swallowing, the esophagus should be empty. An esophageal foreign body is any item, either food or some other material, that has gotten caught somewhere in the esophagus.

The esophagus has several points where it becomes narrow and where material is most likely to get stuck. The narrow spots are at the beginning of the esophagus (upper esophageal sphincter), in the middle of the chest where the esophagus passes the heart, and at the very end where it enters the stomach (lower esophageal sphincter).

Causes

Esophageal foreign bodies occur when the animal attempts to swallow an object that is too large or sharp to pass smoothly through the esophagus. Swallowed fish hooks can lodge in the esophagus, but these do not usually cause complete obstruction.

Clinical Signs

Because the esophagus cannot work properly when a foreign body is present, food, water, and saliva are not swallowed properly. Regurgitation (similar to vomiting, but the food is not digested), drooling of saliva, and bad breath may occur. Regurgitation of blood-tinged fluid can be seen and is a worrisome sign. A fever may be detected.

Animals with an esophageal rupture or tear often have a high fever, are very depressed, are in pain, and may have shortness of breath.

Diagnostic Tests

If an esophageal foreign body is suspected, x-rays are taken of the chest and neck region. Some foreign materials, such as bones or metal, are readily seen on x-rays. Other foreign bodies are difficult to see with plain x-rays, and additional studies may be done after the animal is given an oral contrast agent (which shows up white on x-rays). This contrast procedure (esophagram) is often necessary with fabric foreign bodies (for instance, a swallowed sock), because they are difficult to see on plain x-rays.

Routine laboratory and other tests may be recommended to rule out diseases that cause similar signs, to assess any effects on other organs, and as a preoperative measure prior to surgery.

TREATMENT AND FOLLOW-UP

Treatment Options

Esophageal foreign bodies can be extremely serious problems. Animals with complete esophageal obstruction from a large foreign body need immediate therapy. Delaying therapy increases the risks of both short-term and long-term complications.

The best method of treatment is to remove the foreign body as soon as possible. Depending on the size of the animal and the foreign body, it may be possible to retrieve the foreign material through an endoscope that is passed through the mouth into the esophagus. Either a rigid or a flexible endoscope with grasping forceps may be used to view the foreign body and the lining of esophagus and to remove the material.

Surgery (via an incision into the esophagus) to remove the foreign body is very difficult, because the esophagus does not heal well. If a patient has a foreign body in the esophagus that requires surgical removal, your veterinarian may recommend referral to a veterinary surgery specialist for this procedure.

After the foreign body is removed, antibiotics, medications for pain, antacids, and medications to protect the lining of the esophagus are usually begun. Supportive care with intravenous fluids may also be started. Animals with severe esophageal damage may have a feeding tube placed into the stomach that allows the animal to receive food and water without passing them through the esophagus. The feeding tube usually stays in place for at least 2 weeks.

Follow-up Care

Intensive monitoring may be required following rupture of the esophagus. Postoperative visits are usually scheduled 1-2 weeks after removal. Notify your veterinarian if any signs of regurgitation, loss of appetite, or fever occur.

Prognosis

Prognosis for complete recovery is good if there is no damage to the lining of the esophagus. The amount of damage to the lining increases with the amount of time that the foreign body is left in place, so the prognosis becomes poorer with long durations.

Some animals that have severe damage to the esophagus will form a stricture at some time after removal of the obstruction. The stricture arises from scarring and reduces the diameter of the esophagus. If this happens, clinical signs of regurgitation will return.

Severe damage and rupture of the esophagus have a poor prognosis, because these cases are often complicated by infection that develops within the chest. In these cases, the condition can be life-threatening.

SPECIAL INSTRUCTIONS:

Esophagitis and Esophageal Stricture

Craig G. Ruaux, BVSc, PhD, DACVIM (Small Animal)

BASIC INFORMATION

Description

The esophagus is a muscular tube that carries swallowed food and water from the mouth to the stomach. The esophagus is very sensitive to damage from stomach acid, so any medical problem leading to excess stomach acid in the esophagus can cause inflammation, which is called *esophagitis*. In people, the same condition is called *heartburn* or *acid reflux disease*.

Some animals with severe esophagitis will later form an esophageal stricture—scarring that reduces the esophageal diameter. When the diameter of the esophagus is reduced by a stricture, the animal is less able to swallow food and water.

Causes

The esophagus can be exposed to stomach acid during profuse vomiting or gastric reflux, from eating high-fat foods, or during or after an anesthetic procedure. Esophagitis can also occur with some forms of food allergy, certain infections, and after trauma from ingestion of foreign bodies. Structural abnormalities of the esophagus, such as a hernia, may predispose the animal to esophagitis. Certain oral medications and the ingestion of irritating materials can also cause esophagitis.

Clinical Signs

Esophagitis can be painful, causing affected dogs and cats to lose their appetite. If the animal has difficulty swallowing, drooling of salvia and regurgitation of food or water may be seen.

When an esophageal stricture is present, food and water are less able to travel to the stomach, and the animal may act very hungry. Water and very soft food may be able to pass through the stricture, but harder foods, such as kibble or biscuits, may be regurgitated.

A possible complication of both esophagitis and esophageal stricture is aspiration pneumonia, which develops when food or liquids are inhaled into the lungs. If aspiration pneumonia is present, coughing, fever, lethargy, and halitosis (bad breath) may occur.

Diagnostic Tests

Initially plain x-rays of the neck and chest are often done to assess the esophagus. It is common for more specialized x-rays to be taken after the patient has been given an oral contrast material that shows up white on an x-ray. This procedure is called an *esophagram,* and it is particularly useful if an esophageal stricture is suspected.

In some animals, esophagoscopy, which is examination of the interior of the esophagus with a rigid or flexible endoscope, is needed. Esophagoscopy is done with the animal anesthetized.

The endoscope allows the veterinarian to see foreign bodies, strictures, or ulcers in the esophagus and also allows biopsy samples to be obtained. Examination of the stomach and upper small intestines may be done at the same time.

Other tests may be recommended to rule out diseases that cause similar signs and to determine the underlying causes of any acid reflux present.

TREATMENT AND FOLLOW-UP

Treatment Options

The esophagus is very susceptible to damage from stomach acid, so strong antacid medications are commonly prescribed. Other medications that help protect the esophagus from damage may also be started. Antibiotics and antifungal agents may be given for certain infections and for aspiration pneumonia. If regurgitation or vomiting is occurring, other drugs are administered to decrease these signs. Food is given in small meals, and usually softer foods are more readily accepted.

Animals with an esophageal stricture may require breakdown of the stricture. Strictures are usually treated by passing special water-filled balloon catheters into the esophagus while the animal is anesthetized. The catheter is passed into the area of the stricture and slowly expanded. Several such treatments may be necessary. Your veterinarian may recommend referral to a specialist who can perform this procedure.

Animals with severe esophageal damage may have a feeding tube placed into the stomach that allows the animal to receive food and water without passing them through the esophagus. The feeding tube usually stays in place for at least 2 weeks. Other therapies may be indicated, depending on the presence of any underlying cause of the esophagitis.

Follow-up Care

Uncomplicated cases of esophagitis are usually rechecked 7-10 days after starting therapy and then periodically for several months. More intensive monitoring is needed in cases with severe esophagitis or strictures and after insertion of a feeding tube.

Prognosis

Prognosis for recovery from uncomplicated esophagitis is usually good. Prolonged treatment may be required in some cases. Severe cases have a more guarded (uncertain) prognosis, particularly if aspiration pneumonia is present or a feeding tube is needed. Many animals with esophageal strictures return to more normal eating and esophageal function with treatment.

SPECIAL INSTRUCTIONS:

Exocrine Pancreatic Insufficiency

Craig G. Ruaux, BVSc, PhD, DACVIM (Small Animal)

BASIC INFORMATION
Description
The pancreas is a flat, glandular organ that is found in the upper part of the abdomen, near the stomach and liver. The pancreas has three major functions. One part of the pancreas, called the *endocrine pancreas*, produces the hormone insulin, which regulates blood glucose. The bulk of the pancreas, called the *exocrine pancreas,* produces the enzymes necessary to digest food. The last major function of the pancreas is to produce fluid and bicarbonate for mixing of food in the intestines. Exocrine pancreatic insufficiency (EPI) occurs when there is a loss of exocrine pancreas tissue and the animal cannot make enough enzymes for normal digestion. EPI can occur in both dogs and cats, but the disease is very rare in the cat.

Causes
The most common cause of EPI in the dog is a condition called *pancreatic acinar atrophy*. Dogs with this condition gradually lose the exocrine cells in the pancreas, for reasons that are unclear. Pancreatic acinar atrophy is most common in the German shepherd dog and the rough-coated collie. In these breeds, it is thought to be an inherited disease. Although EPI arises most often in these breeds, dogs of any breed can be affected. Cats and some smaller dog breeds may develop EPI if they have chronic pancreatitis for an extended period of time. Pancreatic acinar atrophy tends to occur in young adult dogs (often less than 2 years of age), whereas EPI associated with chronic pancreatitis tends to occur in middle-aged to older animals.

Clinical Signs
Because the animal is unable to digest food properly, signs of maldigestion are present. The most common sign is diarrhea. The animal usually passes feces that are very soft and pulpy, and the total volume of feces produced in a day is often dramatically increased. Since food is not being absorbed properly, the animal is unable to take in enough energy and usually loses weight or does not grow appropriately. Dogs often have a dramatically increased appetite and may eat their own feces (coprophagia). Cats are less likely to have an increased appetite and very rarely develop coprophagia. Vomiting may occur occasionally, and the hair coat may be of poor quality. (Also see the handouts on **Pancreatitis in Dogs** and **Pancreatitis in Cats**.)

Diagnostic Tests
Because the major clinical sign of exocrine insufficiency is diarrhea, other diseases that can cause diarrhea must be ruled out. Routine laboratory tests, fecal examinations, and x-rays may all be recommended.

To test the amount of pancreas tissue that is present, a specialized blood test is used. This test measures the amount of a digestive enzyme, called *trypsin*, in the bloodstream. Low levels of trypsin indicate that the pancreas is not producing enough enzymes. Other specialized tests for diseases of the small intestine are often run at the same time.

TREATMENT AND FOLLOW-UP
Treatment Options
The best treatment for EPI is to provide an oral supplement of digestive enzymes. These enzymes come in tablet and powder forms and are extracted from the pancreases of cows and pigs. Dietary supplements using plant enzymes do not work as well as enzymes from animal sources. The digestive enzymes are given with every meal and are usually required for the rest of the animal's life.

Feeding a lower-fat diet often helps to reduce the severity of the diarrhea. Vitamin supplements are often recommended, such as vitamins A, K, and B12. Some animals are also given antacid medications or antibiotics because of the presence of excessive numbers of bacteria in the small intestines.

Follow-up Care
Typically, a significant improvement in diarrhea and weight gain is seen within 14 days after starting the enzyme supplements. Body weight, consistency of the feces, appetite, and coprophagia are all monitored. High doses of enzymes may cause bleeding of the gums, which requires lowering the dose. Notify your veterinarian if initial signs do not improve or recur, or if new signs develop.

Prognosis
The prognosis for most dogs with EPI is good, assuming that the enzyme treatment is given properly. A poor response occurs in about 20% of affected dogs. Therapy is usually lifelong and can be expensive in large dogs. For cats, the prognosis is more guarded (uncertain). Cats are often harder to treat with the digestive enzymes because they avoid their food when the enzymes are added. Affected cats also tend to develop diabetes mellitus (sugar diabetes), which can be difficult to manage.

SPECIAL INSTRUCTIONS:

Fecal Incontinence

Craig G. Ruaux, BVSc, PhD, DACVIM (Small Animal)

BASIC INFORMATION
Description
Fecal incontinence occurs when a loss of control of the lower bowel and rectum allows feces to be passed at inappropriate times or places. Fecal incontinence may be neurogenic in origin (*neurogenic incontinence*) and associated with a failure of nervous sensation. In these cases, the animal does not realize that it is defecating (involuntary defecation) and does not assume the normal posture for defecation. In contrast, *urge incontinence* may occur with uncontrolled or strong urges to defecate. In these cases, the animal acutely needs to defecate and is aware of that need.

Causes
Diseases of the nerves in the lower spine, of the rectum and anus, and of the large intestine can all result in fecal incontinence. Diseases of the nerves in the lower spine include intervertebral disc disease and chronic arthritic changes. Masses or tumors in the wall of the rectum or in the pelvic canal can lead to excessive straining. Urge incontinence can result from inflammation of the lower colon or rectum. (See also the handout on **Acute Colitis**.) Some older animals develop incontinence from of a decline in their mental status (cognitive dysfunction, senility), which leads them to become less attentive to many aspects of daily life.

Clinical Signs
The major sign is the passing of feces at inappropriate times or places. Frequent, repeated requests to go outside to defecate, as well as repeated or unproductive straining are signs of colitis. Passing feces while walking; leaving bowel movements on the floor or bedding after rising; and continued dribbling of feces while being unaware of the defecation are typical of neurogenic fecal incontinence. In aged animals, loss of awareness of whether they are inside or outside, with indiscriminant defecation in a variety of locations, is often indicative of senile cognitive dysfunction.

Diagnostic Tests
Examination of the rectum and anus with a gloved finger is usually done to check the strength of the rectal sphincter and the presence of masses or other diseases. Routine laboratory tests, x-rays, and an abdominal ultrasound may be recommended to screen for pelvic, spinal, or other diseases. In some cases, computed tomography (CT scan) or magnetic resonance imaging (MRI) of the lower spine may be needed to assess the spinal cord and nerve roots in the lower back.

TREATMENT AND FOLLOW-UP
Treatment Options
If a primary cause of the incontinence can be identified, such as a slipped disc in the spine or severe degenerative joint disease in the lower back and pelvis, your veterinarian may recommend surgery. These types of surgery can be complex and difficult, so your pet may be referred to a veterinary specialist for further evaluation and care.

Animals with fecal incontinence from colitis generally respond well to changes in diet and/or anti-inflammatory drugs. Animals with fecal incontinence from cognitive dysfunction may be treated with drugs that stimulate mental activity, although these treatments do not produce a reliable positive response in all animals. No effective treatment is available for some forms of neurogenic incontinence.

Follow-up Care
Regular follow-up visits are recommended, especially during the initial phase of treatment of colitis or spinal disease. Once clinical signs are controlled, repeated follow-up visits may not be needed. Incontinence associated with more chronic conditions often requires long-term monitoring and follow-up.

Prognosis
Prognosis varies widely, depending on the cause of the fecal incontinence. Animals with urge incontinence from lower-bowel disease have a good prognosis once their condition is controlled. Prognosis for incontinence resulting from cognitive decline or neurologic disease is more variable and generally poorer, because these conditions are much more difficult to control.

SPECIAL INSTRUCTIONS:

Gall Bladder Disease in Dogs

Craig G. Ruaux, BVSc, PhD, DACVIM (Small Animal)

BASIC INFORMATION

Description

The gall bladder is a small pouch or sac that contains bile produced by the liver. The gall bladder stores bile until it is released into the small intestine, where it helps in the digestion of fat. In people, the most common disease of the gall bladder is gall stones. In dogs, inflammation of the gall bladder can occur, but the formation of hard stones is uncommon. The gall bladder can also become infected by bacteria, and some cancers can develop in the gall bladder, but these disorders are less common than the condition called *biliary mucocele*. A mucocele develops when bile becomes thickened and is retained in the gall bladder, causing it to become enlarged.

Causes

The cause of most gall bladder disease, particularly biliary mucocele, is not well defined in the dog. Many dogs with gall bladder disease have some sort of underlying metabolic or hormonal problem. Both hypothyroidism (low thyroid hormone levels) and hyperadrenocorticism (excessive steroid hormone levels) are associated with an increased risk of developing a biliary mucocele.

Clinical Signs

Common signs of gall bladder disease include a poor appetite, weight loss, vomiting, and diarrhea. In some dogs with severe obstruction of the gall bladder, the feces become a light tan to gray color due to lack of bile, which contains pigments that eventually turn the feces brown. The dog may also have jaundice (yellow discoloration of the gums, whites of the eyes, and skin). If the gall bladder is ruptured, bile peritonitis often develops, and the dog becomes severely ill. The dog may collapse, go into shock (with weak pulses), develop a high fever, have a painful abdomen, and be severely dehydrated.

Diagnostic Tests

Routine laboratory tests are used to assess the state of the liver, the presence of severe inflammation, and the degree of dehydration. X-rays of the abdomen may be recommended. The best method of assessing the gall bladder is an abdominal ultrasound. The gall bladder is usually easy to see on ultrasound. If a mucocele is present, marked thickening of the gall bladder wall is commonly present, and the gall bladder is filled with thick, dehydrated, sludge-like bile. The abnormal bile and thickened wall give the gall bladder an appearance similar to a cross-sectioned kiwi fruit. If a gall bladder mucocele is not identified on ultrasound, a biopsy of the liver and a bile sample may be submitted for microscopic examination and bacterial culture. Other tests may be recommended to rule out other diseases that cause similar signs.

TREATMENT AND FOLLOW-UP

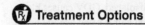

Treatment Options

A sick dog with a biliary mucocele is usually a surgical emergency, because the obstructed gall bladder must be removed before it ruptures. Rupture of the mucocele, particularly if it is infected by bacteria, leads to bile peritonitis, which can be life-threatening. If a mucocele is detected before the dog becomes ill, surgery to remove the gall bladder is still recommended. Gall bladder surgery can be technically challenging and carries significant risks, so your dog may be referred to a veterinary surgery specialist for the procedure.

If formation of the mucocele is incomplete, drugs may be tried that make the bile more watery and allow it to flow more easily. Dogs treated medically require close monitoring, because their condition can rapidly deteriorate if the mucocele worsens.

Follow-up Care

Frequent follow-up visits are usually needed when a mucocele is treated medically. At least monthly abdominal ultrasounds and laboratory testing are often recommended.

Following surgery, the dog is hospitalized and closely monitored for several days. Postoperative follow-up visits are often continued until all laboratory tests have returned to normal.

Prognosis

Surgery to remove a gall bladder mucocele is relatively risky. Even in the hands of experienced surgeons and with good intensive postoperative care, about 1 in 10 dogs die during surgery or immediately (24-36 hours) afterward. If the gall bladder has ruptured and bile peritonitis is present, the mortality rate increases to 1 in 4 dogs. If the gall bladder was infected when it ruptured, the dog may die during the surgery or within 24 hours of surgery.

If an underlying medical condition can be identified and drugs can dissolve the bile, the prognosis may be better but it is still guarded (uncertain), because these dogs can worsen rapidly even with appropriate treatment.

SPECIAL INSTRUCTIONS:

Gastric Dilatation-Volvulus

Rhea V. Morgan, DVM, DACVIM (Small Animal), DACVO

BASIC INFORMATION

Description

Gastric dilatation-volvulus (GDV) is an acute, life-threatening emergency. Gastric dilatation involves the sudden accumulation of gas and fluid in the stomach and is sometimes called *bloat*. Volvulus is the twisting of a bloated stomach so that the openings into and out of the stomach are blocked. As the stomach rotates, it may also cause the spleen to become displaced. GDV causes blood flow to the stomach to be compromised and is often accompanied by shock.

Causes

The exact reason for stomach bloating is unknown. Middle-aged or older, large- and giant-breed dogs are at the highest risk, but GDV can occur in small-breed dogs and cats (rare). The following are considered risk factors for bloat:

- Large- or giant-breed dogs with deep chests and lean body condition
- Dogs with close relatives that have experienced GDV
- Behaviors that promote the swallowing of air
- Stress and nervous temperament
- Feeding large volumes of food at each meal
- Feeding dry foods that contain high quantities of fat or oil
- Conditions that decrease outflow of material from the stomach

Clinical Signs

Restlessness and agitation may be the first signs noted. Affected dogs often pace, are reluctant to lie down, and retch or try to regurgitate; they may have excessive drooling. The abdomen may be noticeably distended and painful. As the duration of GDV increases, the animal may become weak, collapse, and have pale and/or dry gums. Rate and effort of breathing may also be increased.

Diagnostic Tests

A tentative diagnosis may be made by observing a distended, rigid abdomen in a dog of the appropriate age and breed. Certain changes on physical examination may allow your veterinarian to suspect the presence of GDV and shock. X-rays of the abdomen are used to assess the position of the stomach and to confirm the presence of dilatation and/or volvulus. However, x-rays are sometimes delayed until the dog has been stabilized with emergency procedures. Laboratory tests are commonly recommended to evaluate the effect of the GDV on other organs and body chemistries. An electrocardiogram may be indicated if an irregular heartbeat (arrhythmia) is detected.

TREATMENT AND FOLLOW-UP

Treatment Options

GDV is an emergency situation, and therapy is directed at both relieving the distention of the stomach and treating shock. Treatment for shock involves the administration of intravenous fluids and medications. The stomach is decompressed by passing a tube from the mouth into the stomach and evacuating all stomach contents. Decompression may not be possible if the stomach is twisted and the tube cannot be passed. In this instance, needles may be inserted into the stomach through the abdominal wall to release air, or a temporary opening may be made into the stomach through the side of the abdomen. Monitoring of the heart and administration of heart medications may also be started.

Once the animal is stable, surgery is usually performed to assess the health of the stomach; correct any volvulus and return the stomach and spleen to a normal position; remove any irreversibly damaged parts of the stomach and spleen; and permanently attach the stomach to the abdominal wall (gastropexy), so that the stomach cannot twist again in the future. Although some dogs with simple, short-lived bloat may not require surgery, most patients with GDV undergo surgery as soon as shock, heart arrhythmias, and other abnormalities are corrected.

Several surgical gastropexy techniques are available, including the incisional, belt-loop, and tube gastropexies, as well as others. Most of these techniques anchor the stomach wall to the right side of the abdomen.

Follow-up Care

Dogs with GDV require immediate intensive therapy, monitoring, and supportive care; without such care, the condition usually rapidly deteriorates and results in death. GDV can cause biochemical abnormalities, blood pressure problems, heart arrhythmias, secondary infections, damage to the lining and wall of the stomach, alterations in the spleen, and a life-threatening blood-clotting disorder, so laboratory tests and other monitoring procedures are commonly needed.

Postoperatively, intensive therapy is continued for several days. Food and water are usually withheld for 12-24 hours. Exercise is restricted until sutures are removed and the gastropexy site has healed. Your veterinarian may recommend changing the type, amount, and frequency of feedings.

Prognosis

Many dogs recover well, provided the GDV is diagnosed and treated quickly. Prognosis is poorest for animals with severe damage and perforation of the stomach and those with serious secondary infections (sepsis, peritonitis) or heart arrhythmias.

SPECIAL INSTRUCTIONS:

Gastric Foreign Body

Craig G. Ruaux, BVSc, PhD, DACVIM (Small Animal)

BASIC INFORMATION

Description

A gastric foreign body is any item, either food or nonfood material, that is present in the stomach and does not pass into the small intestine or is vomited. Some gastric foreign bodies can cause severe vomiting or intestinal obstruction, and others (such as coins or metal toys) can poison the animal.

Causes

Gastric foreign bodies occur when something is swallowed but cannot leave the stomach. They may include large pieces of bone, an item that the animal was playing with, accumulations of hair (hair balls), and abnormal material eaten (such as dirt, rocks, or kitty litter).

Some animals eat unusual items if they have nausea, such as can occur with gastritis. Some animals eat unusual items as part of a behavioral problem or as the result of a medical condition (such as anemia or Cushing's disease). The consumption of unusual items is called *pica*.

Clinical Signs

The most common clinical sign of a gastric foreign body is vomiting. Some animals also lose their appetite. If the foreign body is made of zinc, the animal may develop anemia (pale gums, lethargy, and weakness). If the foreign body is made of a heavy metal such as lead, signs of poisoning may occur. (See also the handouts on **Zinc Toxicosis** and **Lead Poisoning**.) Often, gastric foreign bodies are found when x-rays are performed on an animal with vomiting problems.

Diagnostic Tests

If a gastric foreign body is suspected, abdominal x-rays are commonly recommended. Routine laboratory tests and an abdominal ultrasound may also be recommended to rule out other conditions, such as liver, pancreatic, or kidney diseases that can cause vomiting.

A contrast study (gastrogram) of the stomach may be performed if a foreign body is suspected but not found on plain x-rays. In a gastrogram, barium or some other agent is administered orally to help highlight any foreign material. In some cases, foreign bodies are found during examination of the stomach with an endoscope (gastroscopy) or during exploratory surgery.

TREATMENT AND FOLLOW-UP

Treatment Options

The best treatment for a gastric foreign body is to remove it. Some foreign bodies can be removed with the use of an endoscope, but if the foreign body is large, abdominal surgery may be recommended. Surgical removal of gastric foreign bodies involves a procedure in which the stomach is opened, called a gastrotomy. Patients with gastric foreign bodies made of metals often require additional drug therapy to help bind and remove the metal from the rest of the body. Supportive care for anemia and other signs of toxicity may also be needed. Additional therapies may be started to address any underlying causes of pica.

Follow-up Care

Following a gastrotomy, food and water are often withheld for a period of time to allow the stomach to recover. Water is then initiated and is followed later by a bland diet if no vomiting occurs. The animal is also kept quiet until the sutures are removed, usually at 10-14 days after the surgery. Patients that have had a gastric foreign body removed with an endoscope have no sutures and tend to recover more quickly, with less follow-up care.

Prognosis

Prognosis for patients with gastric foreign bodies is usually good, assuming that the foreign body is removed with no complications and any underlying contributing disease is successfully treated. If the foreign body is not removed, obstruction of the small intestine may occur and can lead to severe vomiting and life-threatening illness.

SPECIAL INSTRUCTIONS:

Gastric Neoplasia

Craig G. Ruaux, BVSc, PhD, DACVIM (Small Animal)

BASIC INFORMATION

Description

Neoplasia is the term for tumor formation, and *gastric* pertains to the stomach. Gastric neoplasms can arise directly from tissues within the stomach, or they may develop when a tumor spreads to the stomach from other parts of the body (metastasis). Both benign and malignant tumors are found in the stomach, but most tumors in dogs and cats are malignant.

Cancer types that arise from components of the stomach include carcinoma (from the lining of the stomach), adenocarcinoma (from cells of stomach glands), fibrosarcoma (from connective tissue), lymphoma (from lymphocytes), plasmacytoma (from plasma cells), and leiomyosarcoma (from smooth muscles).

Leiomyoma is a benign tumor of the smooth muscles of the stomach wall. This tumor is most commonly diagnosed in older female dogs. Adenocarcinomas are the most common gastric tumors of dogs, and lymphoma is the most common tumor of cats. Malignant tumors are usually diagnosed in middle-aged or older dogs and cats, but lymphoma can also occur in younger cats.

Causes

There is no known cause for gastric cancers in the dog and cat.

Clinical Signs

The most common signs are vomiting and loss of appetite. Vomiting of blood or partly digested blood (that looks like coffee grounds) may occur. In some animals, the vomiting can be very severe and difficult to control. Vomiting causes the animal to lose fluids, so evidence of dehydration (dry and tacky skin and gums, sunken eyes) may be present.

Many animals have a poor appetite for a long time, and weight loss can be pronounced. Occasionally, your veterinarian may be able to feel a mass in the front part of the abdomen, but the stomach is located so deep in the abdomen that this is unusual.

Diagnostic Tests

Because the main signs of gastric tumors are vomiting and weight loss and many diseases can cause these signs, extensive laboratory tests and x-rays are usually recommended. An upper gastrointestinal contrast study (a series of x-rays taken after the animal has swallowed barium) can be particularly useful for showing masses inside the stomach. An abdominal ultrasound may be recommended, especially to look for spread of cancer to other organs in the abdomen. A mass in the stomach may not be seen on ultrasound because gas in the stomach usually gets in the way. If cancer is suspected based on these tests, chest x-rays may also be done to look for metastasis.

Gastric endoscopy, using a flexible fiberoptic tube, can be useful to identify a tumor or abnormalities in the stomach. Endoscopy also provides a means for obtaining biopsy samples and assessing the size of the lesion for planning additional surgery.

TREATMENT AND FOLLOW-UP

Treatment Options

Treatment options depend on the type of tumor present. Lymphomas and plasmacytomas are best treated with chemotherapy, sometimes involving several different drugs. Carcinomas, adenocarcinomas, and smooth muscle tumors are best treated by attempted surgical removal. Surgery may then be followed by chemotherapy for some of these tumors. Removal of gastric tumors can be challenging, especially if they are large and infiltrate much of the stomach, so your pet may be referred to a veterinary surgery specialist for the procedure, and a consultation may be requested from a veterinary oncologist (who specializes in cancer medicine).

Potent anti-vomiting and antinausea medications can be used to provide symptomatic relief for some animals, but many animals develop vomiting from these tumors that is almost impossible to stop. For some animals, euthanasia may be recommended, especially if the cancer has spread to or from other sites and there is little chance of providing a good quality of life.

Follow-up Care

Periodic follow-up visits are required after surgery and during chemotherapy for cancerous tumors, for the rest of the life of the animal. Laboratory tests, x-rays, and ultrasounds are often needed to monitor response to treatment, to detect evidence of spread of the tumor, and to check for side effects of the medications.

Prognosis

Older dogs with leiomyoma have a fair to good prognosis if the mass can be completely removed with surgery. The surgery is a major one, and recovery can be prolonged, particularly in old, frail dogs. Some animals with lymphoma and plasmacytoma have a good response to chemotherapy and survive for significant periods of time. (See also the handouts on **Lymphoma in Dogs** and **Lymphoma in Cats**.) Most animals with other gastric cancers die of their disease within 3-6 months after the diagnosis is made.

SPECIAL INSTRUCTIONS:

Gastritis, Acute

Craig G. Ruaux, BVSc, PhD, DACVIM (Small Animal)

BASIC INFORMATION

Description

Acute gastritis occurs when the stomach becomes inflamed. Inflammation of the stomach makes the stomach less able to handle food and water. The stomach produces acid and digestive enzymes that begin the breakdown of proteins and fats; when the stomach is inflamed, these processes are disturbed.

Causes

The most common cause of acute gastritis in dogs and cats is dietary indiscretion (eating something that does not agree with them or is foreign to the stomach). Some parasites of the gastrointestinal tract and drug reactions can also cause acute gastritis. Bacterial infections are extremely uncommon causes. Some drugs used to treat cancer can lead to acute gastritis and nausea; your veterinarian will warn you of this if those drugs are being used.

Clinical Signs

The most important clinical sign is vomiting. Acute gastritis develops rapidly. Your pet may appear normal in the morning yet have frequent vomiting in the afternoon. Loss of appetite is common, and some animals develop a mild fever. If there is excessive loss of body fluids from repeated vomiting, signs of dehydration (sunken eyes, lethargy, skin that does not slide around easily) can be seen. Affected animals sometimes seem to be in pain when you feel their abdomen.

Diagnostic Tests

Acute gastritis is not the only cause of vomiting. Many other diseases, particularly of the liver, kidneys, and pancreas, can lead to sudden onset of vomiting. For this reason, your veterinarian is likely to recommend blood tests to make certain these other diseases are not present. Blood tests are also useful for gauging the degree of dehydration that may be present. Some of these tests can be done quickly; others must be sent to specialized laboratories, and it may take several days for the results to become available.

The presence of a foreign body, such as a toy, bone, rocks, coins, or pieces of string, within the gastrointestinal tract can also lead to vomiting. Typically, routine abdominal x-rays are recommended to look for foreign bodies. In some cases, an abdominal ultrasound or other imaging techniques may be recommended to look at sections of the gastrointestinal tract that may be obstructed or moving abnormally.

TREATMENT AND FOLLOW-UP

Treatment Options

As long as other diseases have been ruled out, the treatment of acute gastritis is usually uncomplicated. The disease is typically self-limited; that is, the clinical signs usually resolve quickly, and supportive treatment is all that is necessary.

The stomach usually needs a period of rest to allow the inflammation to settle down. Withholding solid food for a period of 24 hours allows the stomach to rest. Medications (given either by injection or by mouth) are often prescribed for 2-3 days to stop vomiting and control nausea. While off solid food, most animals still tolerate liquids. It is important that adequate hydration be maintained, and if your pet can not tolerate liquids your veterinarian may recommend giving subcutaneous (injected under the skin) fluids.

After a period of stomach rest, food is gradually reintroduced. It is best to start with a low-fat, relatively bland diet. Commercial diets specifically made for gastrointestinal diseases may be recommended, or your veterinarian may suggest recipes for homemade diets. Small meals are given over the first few days, followed by a gradual return to the pet's normal diet over several days.

Animals with more severe dehydration or loss of electrolytes such as sodium or potassium may need to be hospitalized to allow administration of intravenous (IV) fluids. Insertion of an IV line also allows antivomiting and antinausea drugs to be given by injection, which helps if the patient cannot keep oral medications down.

Follow-up Care

If all signs resolve within 24-48 hours (most cases of acute gastritis), there may be no need for specific follow-up. If vomiting has not stopped completely within 3-4 days, if your pet becomes increasingly lethargic and has no appetite, if vomiting becomes more frequent and no liquids are kept down, or if blood is seen in the vomited material, contact your veterinarian for further assistance.

Prognosis

The prognosis for recovery from acute gastritis is good, with most patients showing compete recovery and return to normal within 3-4 days.

SPECIAL INSTRUCTIONS:

Gastritis, Chronic

Craig G. Ruaux, BVSc, PhD, DACVIM (Small Animal)

BASIC INFORMATION

Description

Gastritis is inflammation of the stomach. Gastritis makes the stomach less able to handle food and water the animal takes in. The stomach produces acid and digestive enzymes that begin the breakdown of proteins and fats; when the stomach is inflamed, these processes are disturbed. Chronic gastritis is suspected if clinical signs of gastritis have persisted for longer than 7-10 days or recur frequently (sometimes 3-4 days per week).

Causes

The cause of chronic gastritis is often hard to determine. In many cases, an underlying cause is never identified, and the condition is called *idiopathic chronic gastritis*. Dietary allergies, food intolerance, and parasite infestations can cause similar signs, so these conditions must be ruled out. The stomach may also become inflamed from several other diseases, such as kidney failure and liver disease.

Clinical Signs

The major clinical sign is vomiting, particularly after eating. Vomiting may also occur independent of eating. The vomitus may contain undigested food, bile (yellowish green material), fresh blood, or digested blood (looks like coffee grounds). If your animal vomits blood or coffee grounds–type material, seek veterinary care immediately.

Many animals with chronic gastritis have a steady or intermittently poor appetite. Signs can wax and wane, with some animals having days or weeks free of vomiting. Body temperature is usually normal, but weight loss can occur.

Diagnostic Tests

Although vomiting is the major clinical sign of chronic gastritis, this disease is not the only cause of vomiting. Many other diseases, particularly of the liver, kidneys, and pancreas, can result in vomiting. For this reason, your veterinarian is likely to recommend blood tests to make certain these other diseases are not present. Blood tests are also useful for gauging the degree of dehydration that may be present. Some of these tests can be done quickly; others must be sent to specialized laboratories, and it may take several days for the results to become available.

The presence of a foreign body, such as a toy, bone, rocks, coins, or pieces of string, within the gastrointestinal tract can lead to chronic vomiting. Typically, routine abdominal x-rays are recommended to look for foreign bodies. An abdominal ultrasound may also be recommended.

The most effective method of diagnosing chronic gastritis is through gastroscopy, which allows your veterinarian to view the lining of the stomach and look for ulcers, tumors, and inflamed areas. Any foreign bodies present can usually be removed during gastroscopy, and biopsies can be obtained. Animals must be fully anesthetized for this procedure.

Many animals with chronic gastritis also have inflammatory bowel disease, so gastroscopy is often combined with endoscopy of the small intestine. Your veterinarian may recommend referral to an internal medicine specialist for these tests to be performed.

TREATMENT AND FOLLOW-UP

Treatment Options

Often the treatment for chronic colitis is as simple as changing the diet, because many animals have a dietary intolerance or food allergy as the underlying cause. The new diet is either specifically manufactured to be hypoallergenic or is composed of a completely new source of protein (for instance, lamb instead of chicken). The decision whether to use a hypoallergenic diet or a new protein source depends on the number of different diets your pet has consumed in the past.

Usually, if the new diet is going to be beneficial, improvement is seen in 14 days. Antacids are also commonly administered as the diet is changed, because stomach acid aggravates any irritation to the stomach wall.

If no improvement occurs with diet changes alone, anti-inflammatory drugs, such as steroids, may be given. If steroid medications are started, all other nonsteroidal anti-inflammatory drugs (such as those used for arthritis) must be stopped, or side effects (such as stomach ulcers) are likely to occur. Additional medications may be recommended based on biopsy and laboratory test results.

Follow-up Care

Many patients show improvement in approximately 2 weeks following a diet change or treatment with antacids and anti-inflammatory drugs. If improvement does not occur, if any vomiting of blood or coffee grounds–looking material is seen, or if your pet becomes lethargic or pale, notify your veterinarian immediately or seek emergency veterinary care. In animals whose signs resolve, drug therapy is slowly tapered and may eventually be stopped. Periodic rechecks, and sometimes repeated gastroscopies, are used to assess response to treatment.

Prognosis

Prognosis for most animals is good, because many show substantial improvement with diet change, antacids, and anti-inflammatory drugs. Occasionally, medications and periodic monitoring are needed for life.

SPECIAL INSTRUCTIONS:

Gastrointestinal Ulceration

Craig G. Ruaux, BVSc, PhD, DACVIM (Small Animal)

BASIC INFORMATION

Description

Gastrointestinal (GI) ulceration occurs when the surface layer of the lining of the gut is damaged. The stomach, the lower part of the esophagus, and the first part of the small intestine are common places for ulcerations to develop, because they are exposed to stomach acid. Ulceration can occur at any location in the gut, particularly if severe inflammation is present, such as with inflammatory bowel disease.

Causes

Common causes of ulceration in the upper GI tract are nonsteroidal anti-inflammatory drugs (NSAIDs), such as aspirin, and steroid drugs, such as prednisone or dexamethasone. Animals given both NSAIDs and glucocorticoid steroids are at high risk for developing ulcers, so the combination is usually avoided.

Ulceration can also occur with gastric foreign bodies and ingestion of caustic materials; gastric dilatation (bloat); some types of cancer of the stomach and small intestine; mast cell tumors (see the handouts on **Mast Cell Tumors** and **Mastocytosis**); severe stress; or other illnesses, such as shock, kidney failure, or liver failure.

Clinical Signs

Bleeding into the esophagus and stomach usually causes vomiting. The material may look like coffee grounds (partially digested blood) or fresh red blood mixed with food or saliva. Ulceration in the small intestine often causes melena, which is the presence of dark, tarry, sticky feces. Melena represents digested blood in the stool.

Because blood loss can be substantial with a bleeding ulcer, anemia (pale gums, skin, vulva) is common. Vomiting and/or diarrhea can cause large amounts of body fluids to be lost, with secondary dehydration (dry, tacky gums, stiff skin, sunken eyes). Loss of appetite, weight loss, and fever are other common signs.

Diagnostic Tests

Because the main signs of GI ulceration (vomiting and loss of appetite) can be caused by many diseases, extensive testing is usually necessary to reach a diagnosis. Laboratory tests and x-rays of the abdomen are often recommended. X-rays taken after the animal has swallowed barium can be useful for showing GI ulcers. An abdominal ultrasound, fecal tests, and blood clotting assays may be recommended to rule out other diseases that cause similar clinical signs. Gastric endoscopy, using a long fiberoptic tube, allows identification and assessment of the size of any ulcer lesions and also provides a means for obtaining biopsy samples. Further testing may be needed to search for an underlying cause.

TREATMENT AND FOLLOW-UP

Treatment Options

Treatment involves several separate therapies, usually started together:

- Gastric acid is often a major contributor to ulceration, so powerful antacid medications, such as cimetidine, ranitidine, famotidine, or omeprazole, are given.
- The drug sucralfate is administered because it coats the lining of the gut and acts as a "bandage" by binding directly to the exposed tissue. This drug must be given at very specific times, depending on when the antacid medications are given. Your veterinarian will outline a treatment schedule for your pet.
- If the ulceration was caused by NSAID or steroid medications, special drugs, such as misoprostol, may be tried that work to counteract the effects of these drugs on the gut.

Many animals require hospitalization so that injectable medications and intravenous fluids may be given. GI ulceration can be quite painful, so strong pain medications may be started. Transfusions may be administered for shock and significant blood loss. Other supportive care may include antivomiting medications, antibiotics, motility agents to get the gut moving again, and drugs specifically directed at any underlying cause.

A perforating ulcer occurs when the ulcer has formed a hole through the gut into the abdomen. If a perforating ulcer is present, emergency surgery is commonly done to repair the damage.

Follow-up Care

Depending on the severity of the ulceration, the need for follow-up visits and repeated testing varies. Animals with mild disease are often rechecked 7-10 days after starting medical treatment, or sooner if clinical signs worsen. Animals with severe disease that require hospitalization or surgery may need intensive monitoring and laboratory testing while they are hospitalized. Follow-up visits and monitoring are also more intense during the first week after the animal is discharged from the hospital. Be sure to notify your veterinarian if any signs recur or if new signs develop after therapy is started.

Prognosis

Prognosis is variable for animals with GI ulceration, depending on the cause and severity of the ulceration. Some animals recover rapidly with simple medical therapy. Other animals may have serious underlying disease, develop life-threatening blood loss, or require emergency surgery.

SPECIAL INSTRUCTIONS:

Gingivitis

Craig G. Ruaux, BVSc, PhD, DACVIM (Small Animal)

BASIC INFORMATION

Description

The gingiva is the part of the gums that surrounds the teeth where they arise from the jaw. Gingivitis is inflammation of this area. Gingivitis is a component of *periodontal disease*, which is the most common dental disease of dogs and cats.

Because the gingiva lies in close proximity to the teeth and helps maintain the health of the tooth sockets, long-standing and severe gingivitis can increase the risk that teeth will be lost. When the gingiva is inflamed, it often recedes from the tooth, revealing the tooth roots.

Causes

The major cause of gingivitis in animals is accumulation of scale (plaque) and tartar on the base of the teeth. In cats, some viral infections (herpesvirus, calicivirus, feline immunodeficiency virus) are associated with gingivitis. Other medical conditions, particularly kidney disease or kidney failure, can lead to the formation of ulcers on the gum line and secondary gingivitis. Chemical irritants (such as cleaning products or caustic compounds) can also cause inflammation of the gums and gingiva.

Clinical Signs

In many animals, there are no obvious signs of gingivitis, and the condition may be noticed only when your veterinarian is doing an oral examination on your pet. Some cats with severe gingivitis have a loss of appetite, show pain on opening of the mouth, or have bleeding from the gums. (See the handout on **Lymphoplasmacytic Stomatitis in Cats**.) The gingiva are usually bright red and swollen. Gingivitis is often associated with heavy scale and tartar accumulation (brown to gray material caked on and around the teeth). Occasionally, a foul odor may be noticed in the mouth.

Diagnostic Tests

Gingivitis is usually diagnosed simply by observing redness and swelling of the gum margin, particularly when scale and tartar are present. Some animals develop a proliferative gingivitis, and the gingiva becomes dramatically swollen. This proliferation can look like a tumor or epulis (see the handout on **Epulis in Dogs**) and may require biopsy of the tissue to determine the nature of the condition. In affected cats, assays for the common viral diseases may be recommended. If serious periodontal disease is suspected, dental x-rays may be recommended.

TREATMENT AND FOLLOW-UP

Treatment Options

The main treatment for gingivitis that is associated with scale and tartar is to clean and polish the teeth with the animal under general anesthesia. Once the tartar and scale are removed, gingivitis can be reduced or prevented through a program of routine teeth cleaning. Your veterinarian will discuss teeth cleaning options and preventive care with you.

Cats with severe gingivitis associated with viral infections often need extractions of affected teeth to control the inflammation. Antibiotics may be started in some cases to decrease the bacteria present in the mouth, often prior to dental cleaning.

Follow-up Care

Most animals recover fully following dental cleaning or extraction procedures. Antibiotics may be continued postoperatively. Your veterinarian will outline a follow-up program to help monitor dental health and ensure that gingivitis does not recur.

Prognosis

Gingivitis is usually reversible. Prognosis for animals with gingivitis is good to excellent, assuming that an effective maintenance program of teeth cleaning is continued that prevents accumulation of scale and tartar.

SPECIAL INSTRUCTIONS:

Hemorrhagic Gastroenteritis in Dogs

Craig G. Ruaux, BVSc, PhD, DACVIM (Small Animal)

BASIC INFORMATION

Description

Hemorrhagic gastroenteritis (HGE) is an acute, severe form of diarrhea that occurs in dogs. The diarrhea causes large amounts of water to be lost from the body, resulting in severe dehydration. Substantial amounts of blood may also be lost into the gastrointestinal tract (gut), which can be a severe and life-threatening condition if left untreated.

Causes

The cause of HGE in dogs is not well defined. Some viral diseases (canine parvovirus, canine coronavirus) and parasites (whipworms) can cause similar signs, but HGE is thought to arise independent of these conditions. Some studies have suggested the involvement of certain bacterial toxins (moldy food), but in most cases no cause is found. Small breeds of dogs are affected more commonly than large dogs.

Clinical Signs

The most common clinical sign is a severe diarrhea that is notably bloody, which is why the disease is called *hemorrhagic gastroenteritis*. Clinical signs develop rapidly. Affected dogs may have a subnormal body temperature and shivering. The skin may feel dry and somewhat thick because of dehydration. The gums are often dry and tacky to the touch, and they may be a dark, red "brick" color.

Diagnostic Tests

Your veterinarian will recommend laboratory tests to gauge the degree of dehydration, to look for other diseases that cause similar signs, and to look for complicating conditions, such as kidney failure (caused by the dehydration). Tests may be done on a sample of the diarrhea to look for canine parvovirus and intestinal parasites. Other laboratory tests and x-rays may also be recommended.

Quick screening tests include measurement of the packed cell volume (PCV) and total protein (TP). Dogs with HGE usually have a high PCV with a normal TP, whereas dogs with dehydration from other causes usually have a high PCV and high TP. This distinction is very important in making the diagnosis of HGE.

TREATMENT AND FOLLOW-UP

Treatment Options

Dogs with HGE need intensive therapy, because they are often severely dehydrated, with sludging of the blood that can lead to failure of the kidneys, liver, and heart. Most patients require hospitalization for intravenous fluid therapy to replace lost fluids and to keep up with ongoing fluid losses from diarrhea. Dogs with HGE can deteriorate very rapidly and may die within hours after the onset of clinical signs if not treated appropriately.

Food is often withheld until vomiting resolves. Hospitalization may be continued for at least 1-2 days until the dog starts eating. Supportive care with antibiotics, electrolyte solutions, and anti-vomiting or antacid medications is also commonly provided during this time. If body protein levels decline from severe blood loss, special intravenous colloid solutions or plasma transfusions may be recommended.

Follow-up Care

Intensive monitoring of vital signs (such as heart rate, urine output, body temperature, and body weight) and laboratory tests may be required for severely ill dogs while they are hospitalized. Serial PCV, TP, and electrolyte testing is recommended for most dogs. Dogs that survive the initial crisis and respond to fluid therapy usually recover quickly and may need no further follow-up visits after discharge. If complications such as reduced kidney function occur, follow-up visits and repeat monitoring or testing are often needed.

Prognosis

HGE is an extremely serious disease in small dogs, and without treatment their prognosis is poor. With appropriate treatment, the prognosis is still uncertain in some dogs, depending on how badly dehydrated the dog was at the beginning of treatment. Even with the best intensive care, some dogs die of this disease. Dogs that survive the first 24 hours of treatment have a good prognosis. Recurrences are possible in some dogs at a later date.

SPECIAL INSTRUCTIONS:

Hepatic Encephalopathy

Craig G. Ruaux, BVSc, PhD, DACVIM (Small Animal)

BASIC INFORMATION
Description
Encephalopathy is altered brain function caused by some underlying disease. Hepatic encephalopathy arises when the liver is unable to work effectively and does not clear compounds that are toxic to the brain. In hepatic encephalopathy, much of the problem develops from substances that are produced when intestinal bacteria break down dietary proteins that are then absorbed into the body. Normally the liver removes these substances, but if blood is shunted away from the liver or the liver is too diseased to process them, these toxic substances build up in the bloodstream and eventually affect the brain.

Causes
A major cause in young animals is the presence of abnormal blood vessels that bypass the liver and shunt blood from the intestines around the liver and into the rest of the circulation. These vessels are called *portosystemic vascular anomalies* or *liver shunts.* (See the handout on **Portosystemic Vascular Anomalies**.)

In older animals, liver failure is the most common cause. Liver failure can occur rapidly with diseases such as acute hepatitis or toxin ingestion, or it may develop after many years of chronic inflammatory disease of the liver. (See the handouts on **Chronic Hepatitis in Dogs** and **Hepatic Lipidosis in Cats**.)

Clinical Signs
The most prominent signs are changes in behavior, mental dullness, depression or stupor, and seizures. Some animals act blind or wobbly; walk in circles or wander aimlessly; pant excessively; or walk into and press their heads (head pressing) against corners or walls. Often these signs are at their worst after a meal, especially one that is high in protein. Signs may also be precipitated by bleeding into the gut, transfusions, infections, and other conditions.

Additional signs of chronic liver disease include weight loss and fluid in the abdomen (ascites). Young animals with portosystemic vascular anomalies often grow slowly and are undersized; cats may show excessive drooling.

Diagnostic Tests
Routine laboratory tests and abdominal x-rays are often recommended initially if hepatic encephalopathy is suspected. Specialized tests, such as bile acid assays, are then needed to establish that liver function is reduced. An abdominal ultrasound may be used to gauge the size of the liver, to look for evidence of scarring and shrinkage (cirrhosis), and to search for abnormal, shunting blood vessels.

Detecting abnormal blood vessels requires a high level of skill, particularly in very small animals, and sometimes additional tests, such as a nuclear scan or a contrast x-ray procedure (portography) may be needed. In these cases, your veterinarian may recommend referral to a veterinary specialist for further testing. Other tests may be recommended to rule out other diseases that can cause encephalopathy.

TREATMENT AND FOLLOW-UP
Treatment Options
If a portosystemic vascular anomaly is detected, surgical closure of the abnormal vessel is usually recommended, if possible. If the encephalopathy is caused by chronic liver disease or a portosystemic vascular anomaly that cannot be repaired surgically, medical management is started.

Medical therapy involves measures to decrease the production and absorption of toxic substances in the gut. Decreasing the amount of protein in the diet lowers the production of these substances and is an important part of therapy. Absorption of toxins can be reduced by making the environment in the gut more acidic with a medication called *lactulose*. Lactulose is also a laxative, so the amount of time that proteins or feces remain in the gut is decreased. This may cause soft stools, mild diarrhea, and excessive gas (flatulence), especially in the first 7-10 days. Because bacteria are also involved in the production of toxic compounds, broad-spectrum antibiotics are commonly given along with the lactulose and low-protein diet. Other therapies may be recommended, depending on the type of underlying liver disease and the presence of complicating conditions.

Follow-up Care
Patients with vascular anomalies that undergo surgery require regular follow-up visits and testing for several months. Animals on medical therapy usually show an improvement in their signs within 1 week. Follow-up visits may be needed at weekly intervals for several weeks until the animal is stable, then every 2-3 months thereafter.

Prognosis
Prognosis is good for young animals with portosystemic vascular anomalies that can be successfully treated with surgery. Assuming there are no complications and recovery is uneventful, these animals often go on to lead entirely normal lives. Animals with inoperable vascular anomalies or end-stage liver disease have a guarded (uncertain) to poor prognosis. They usually require lifelong treatment, and their clinical signs typically worsen over time. Eventually these animals may die or be euthanized.

SPECIAL INSTRUCTIONS:

Hepatic Lipidosis in Cats

Craig G. Ruaux, BVSc, PhD, DACVIM (Small Animal)

BASIC INFORMATION

Description

Hepatic lipidosis is infiltration of the liver with fat (lipid). This condition tends to arise when a cat suddenly stops eating or reduces its food intake for some reason. When the cat stops eating, fat reserves in the body are mobilized and move to the liver to generate energy. The fat cannot be processed properly if protein intake is also inadequate, so it remains in the liver cells. When the liver cells become filled with fat, they no longer work properly, which further makes the cat feel sick and less willing to eat. Because unwillingness to eat is at the root of this problem, the lipidosis gets dramatically worse.

Causes

Cats that are overweight are more likely to develop lipidosis if they stop eating, but any cat can develop this problem. The main cause of the lipidosis is the cessation of eating, which may be secondary to many conditions, such as trauma to the jaw, dental disease, and various conditions of other organs (such as the kidney, pancreas, or liver). A large part of dealing with hepatic lipidosis is identifying the cause of the loss of appetite.

Clinical Signs

The main sign is a loss of appetite. Vomiting, lethargy, depression, and dehydration are also common. The signs present may be associated with the lipidosis or with the underlying disease that led to the lipidosis. In some cats with severe lipidosis, jaundice (yellow color of the gums, whites of the eyes, and skin) develops from liver failure.

Diagnostic Tests

Diagnosis of hepatic lipidosis usually requires several different diagnostic tests. Blood tests typically show increased liver enzyme activities, and an elevated bilirubin (the chemical that causes the yellow color) if the cat is jaundiced. An abdominal ultrasound is often recommended to examine the liver. Hepatic lipidosis is diagnosed by examination of a sample of liver tissue obtained by needle aspiration or biopsy. Needle aspiration provides a smear of individual cells that are examined under the microscope (cytology), whereas a biopsy provides a larger section of tissue.

Additional tests, including specialized tests for diseases of the small intestine and pancreas, are often recommended in an effort to identify the underlying cause. In many cases, treatment is started prior to obtaining all the test results, because delaying food intake further aggravates the situation.

TREATMENT AND FOLLOW-UP

Treatment Options

The most important aspect of treatment is to make certain food intake is adequate. Because most cats with hepatic lipidosis are not eating voluntarily, placing a feeding tube is often the easiest and best way to provide nutrients. Feeding tubes may be inserted into the back of the cat's throat (pharyngostomy tube), into the cat's esophagus further down the neck (esophagostomy tube), or into the stomach (percutaneous endoscopic gastrotomy or PEG tube). These procedures are usually performed under general anesthesia.

Most cats must take in more food than what they are willing to eat for a period of several weeks, so providing adequate food intake via feeding tubes is easier to accomplish for both the cat and the owner. Forced feeding with a syringe is difficult to do in cats, usually makes them less willing to eat on their own, and is often avoided.

The most important component of the diet that helps return liver function to normal is an amino acid called *arginine*. Arginine is usually added as a supplement to the diet of cats with hepatic lipidosis. Other vitamins and antioxidant supplements are also commonly given during the recovery process.

For very severely affected cats, hospitalization may be recommended for fluid therapy, possible blood transfusions, and other supportive care. Antivomiting agents and antacids may be given as food is gradually introduced. Specific therapy for underlying diseases is also begun.

Follow-up Care

Regular follow-up visits and monitoring are needed after discharge from the hospital. Tube feeding is continued until the cat is eating on its own. PEG feeding tubes are left in place for at least 10 days to allow proper healing around the entry site into the abdomen. Recovery from hepatic lipidosis can take longer than 4-6 weeks in some cats.

Prognosis

Prognosis for cats with hepatic lipidosis is guarded (uncertain) and varies with the underlying cause of the loss of appetite. Many cats recover adequately with assisted feeding. Some cats die from their lipidosis, as a result of severe liver failure, difficulty in re-establishing normal blood electrolytes during tube feeding, or progression of the underlying disease.

SPECIAL INSTRUCTIONS:

Hepatitis in Dogs, Chronic

Craig G. Ruaux, BVSc, PhD, DACVIM (Small Animal)

BASIC INFORMATION

Description

Hepatitis is inflammation of the liver, a very large organ found in the front part of the abdomen. Hepatitis comes in two forms, acute and chronic. Inflammation leads to a loss of function and, over time, loss of liver tissue from necrosis (death of liver cells) and fibrosis/cirrhosis (scarring and shrinkage). Several potential causes of chronic hepatitis exist in the dog, but often no specific cause is found. Some dog breeds, particularly the Doberman pinscher, Labrador retriever, American and English cocker spaniels, and German shepherd dog, are at higher risk, but this disease can be diagnosed in any breed. It is most common in middle-aged to older dogs.

Causes

Canine adenovirus infection, some bacterial diseases (such as leptospirosis), and long-term treatment with certain drugs (such as anticonvulsants or antifungal medications) can lead to chronic hepatitis. Some forms of chronic hepatitis are immune mediated; that is, the dog's immune system attacks liver tissue for reasons that are unclear. In most cases, the disease has been present for so long and so much damage has been done to the liver that it is no longer possible to identify a cause.

Clinical Signs

Lethargy, loss of appetite, and vomiting are common. With marked reduction in liver function, jaundice (yellowing of the skin, gums, and whites of the eyes), ascites (fluid in the abdomen), and behavioral changes can occur. Many of the clinical signs are vague, and the disease may not be suspected until routine blood tests are done.

Diagnostic Tests

Initial diagnostic tests include laboratory tests specific for the liver (abbreviated as ALT, AST, and GGT) and the bile duct system (abbreviated as ALP). Blood albumin (a protein), cholesterol, and glucose are often abnormal; blood urea may also be low. X-rays and an abdominal ultrasound often show a small liver. Bile acid tests may be recommended to assess liver function. Further testing may be needed to look for an underlying cause or to rule out other diseases that cause similar clinical signs.

Ultrasound examination is particularly useful, because it allows biopsy samples of the liver to be obtained. In some cases, surgery may be needed to biopsy the liver. Before liver biopsy is done, blood clotting tests are usually performed. Although other tests can suggest the presence of chronic hepatitis, the only definitive test is a biopsy. Results of biopsies can also be extremely valuable in guiding the type of therapy used.

TREATMENT AND FOLLOW-UP

Treatment Options

If a cause of the hepatitis is identified, treatment is directed toward the cause. If no specific cause is identified, the goals of therapy are to reduce inflammation, decrease fibrosis in the remaining liver, and reduce clinical signs such as nausea, vomiting, decreased appetite, behavioral changes, and ascites.

If significant active inflammation is present in the biopsy sample, it is common for anti-inflammatory steroid drugs to be used. In some dogs, the use of steroids is associated with side effects such as increased water consumption, increased appetite, panting, and anxiety. If these side effects are severe, additional anti-inflammatory drugs, such as azathioprine, may be used so that the steroids can be decreased.

A large number of nutraceutical and vitamin supplements are available for dogs with liver disease, any of which may potentially be beneficial in certain cases. Antinausea and antacid medications are commonly prescribed. Dogs with very severe hepatitis may be started on a special low-protein diet; however, in most cases it is more important that the dog eats sufficient calories and protein to maintain weight and to help potentially regenerate liver tissue.

Follow-up Care

Periodic laboratory tests are needed initially to assess response to treatment and to watch for side effects of the medications. Retesting is usually needed long term, both at set intervals and any time an apparent change in the dog's condition is noted. Notify your veterinarian if any signs worsen or recur.

Prognosis

Canine chronic hepatitis is typically irreversible and worsens over time. Some dogs with this condition eventually die or are euthanized because of loss of liver function, complications arising during treatment, or severe behavioral changes (potentially seizures or coma) associated with liver failure. Some dogs live out their lives and die of other unrelated conditions, particularly if the rate of deterioration of chronic hepatitis can be slowed with drug therapy. The development of ascites (fluid in the abdomen) is a poor prognostic sign; most dogs with chronic hepatitis and ascites die within 1 year of diagnosis.

SPECIAL INSTRUCTIONS:

Inflammatory Bowel Disease in Cats

Craig G. Ruaux, BVSc, PhD, DACVIM (Small Animal)

BASIC INFORMATION

Description

Inflammatory bowel disease (IBD) is the name given to several common conditions in which the walls of the gastrointestinal tract (gut) become inflamed. Clinical signs vary depending on the part of the gut that is inflamed. IBD in cats is not the same as irritable bowel syndrome in people, and treatments designed for the control of human irritable bowel syndrome do not help IBD in cats.

Causes

The cause of IBD in most cats is never completely determined. Dietary intolerances or allergies seem to play an important part in triggering IBD in many cats. The cat may be allergic to a particular part of the diet (usually the protein source) or may develop intolerance to one of the many different types of bacteria that live in the gut.

Clinical Signs

Clinical signs of this disease are highly very variable. The most common signs are poor appetite, vomiting, diarrhea, and/or weight loss. Some cats develop dry, scaly skin and matting of the fur, particularly if they have secondary vitamin deficiencies. Signs can vary in type and severity from day to day. In some cats, excessive gas, bloating and flatulence, or even constipation can occur. Clinical examination sometimes reveals a thickened intestinal tract on palpation of the abdomen, but this is not a reliable finding.

Diagnostic Tests

Because the clinical signs of inflammatory bowel disease are very vague and can arise with many other diseases, a large number of tests may be necessary to reach a diagnosis:

- Initially, routine laboratory tests and fecal examination for parasites may be done. If another disease is found, it should be treated, but its presence does not mean that IBD is not also present.
- More specialized tests of intestinal function are commonly recommended when small intestinal disease is suspected. These tests measure the amounts of certain vitamins and digestive enzymes in the bloodstream and are run by specialized laboratories, so results may not be available for several days.
- Abdominal x-rays and/or an ultrasound are useful in searching for other diseases, but they cannot rule out a diagnosis of IBD.
- The most definitive way to diagnose IBD is through biopsy of the intestinal tract. Depending on the part of the gut that is affected, biopsy samples may be obtained with the use of an endoscope (a flexible tube passed into the intestines through the animal's mouth) or abdominal exploratory surgery.
- Typically, all or most of the laboratory tests are performed before endoscopy or surgery is recommended.

TREATMENT AND FOLLOW-UP

Treatment Options

Often the treatment for IBD is as simple as changing the diet, because many cats have a dietary intolerance or allergy as the underlying condition. The new diet is either specifically manufactured to be hypoallergenic or is composed of a completely new source of protein (for instance, lamb instead of chicken). The decision whether to use a hypoallergenic diet or a new protein source depends on the number of different diets your pet has consumed in the past.

Usually, if the new diet is going to be beneficial, an improvement in clinical signs is seen within 14 days.

If no improvement occurs with diet changes alone, anti-inflammatory drugs, such as steroids, may be given. If your cat is placed on steroid medications, it is very important to consult with your veterinarian prior to giving other anti-inflammatory medications, such as aspirin or meloxicam.

Some cats with IBD develop severe vitamin deficiencies that must be treated with injectable vitamin supplements.

Follow-up Care

Follow-up examinations and repeated laboratory testing are often used to assess response to treatment and make adjustments in medications. If no or little improvement occurs within 2-3 weeks following a diet change or treatment with steroids, the dose of steroids may be increased, or other immune suppressive drugs may be added. After all signs have disappeared, it may be possible to slowly taper the medications, based on the recommendations of your veterinarian. If drugs are tapered, notify your veterinarian if any signs recur.

Prognosis

Prognosis for most cats is good, because many show substantial improvement with diet changes and anti-inflammatory drugs. Some cats have more severe disease that is difficult to control, and in these cases the prognosis is poor to guarded (uncertain). Occasionally, cats with IBD develop intestinal lymphoma and require more aggressive therapy.

SPECIAL INSTRUCTIONS:

Inflammatory Bowel Disease in Dogs

Craig G. Ruaux, BVSc, PhD, DACVIM (Small Animal)

BASIC INFORMATION

Description

Inflammatory bowel disease (IBD) is the name given to several common conditions in which the walls of the gastrointestinal tract (gut) become inflamed. Clinical signs vary depending on the part of the gut that is inflamed. IBD in dogs is not the same as irritable bowel syndrome in people, and treatments designed for the control of human irritable bowel syndrome do not help IBD in dogs.

Causes

The cause of IBD in most dogs is never completely determined. Dietary intolerances or allergies seem to play an important part in triggering IBD in many dogs. The dog may be allergic to a particular part of the diet (usually the protein source) or may develop intolerance to one of the many different types of bacteria that live in the gut.

Clinical Signs

Clinical signs of this disease are highly very variable. The most common signs are poor appetite, vomiting, diarrhea, and/or weight loss. Signs can vary in type and severity from day to day. In some dogs, excessive gas, bloating and flatulence, or even constipation can occur. Clinical examination sometimes reveals a thickened intestinal tract on palpation of the abdomen, but this is not a reliable finding.

Diagnostic Tests

Because the clinical signs of inflammatory bowel disease are very vague and can arise with many other diseases, a large number of diagnostic tests may be necessary:

- Initially, routine laboratory tests and fecal examination for parasites may be done. If another disease is found, it should be treated, but its presence does not mean that IBD is not also present.
- More specialized tests of intestinal function are commonly recommended when small intestinal disease is suspected. These tests measure the amounts of certain vitamins and digestive enzymes in the bloodstream and are run by specialized laboratories, so results may not be available for several days.
- Abdominal x-rays and/or ultrasound studies are useful in searching for other diseases, but they cannot rule out a diagnosis of IBD.
- The most definitive way to diagnose IBD is through biopsy of the intestinal tract. Depending on the part of the gut that is affected, biopsy samples may be obtained with the use of an endoscope (a flexible tube passed into the intestines through the animal's mouth) or abdominal exploratory surgery.
- Typically, all or most of the laboratory tests are performed before endoscopy or surgery is recommended.

TREATMENT AND FOLLOW-UP

Treatment Options

Often the treatment for IBD is as simple as changing the diet, because many dogs have a dietary intolerance or allergy as the underlying the condition. The new diet is either specifically manufactured to be hypoallergenic or is composed of a completely new source of protein (for instance, duck or rabbit instead of chicken). The decision whether to use a hypoallergenic diet or a new protein source depends on the number of different diets your pet has consumed in the past.

Usually, if the new diet is going to be beneficial, an improvement in clinical signs is seen within 14 days.

If no improvement occurs with diet changes alone, anti-inflammatory drugs, such as steroids, may be given. If your pet is placed on steroids, it is very important not to give other pain or anti-inflammatory medications without consulting your veterinarian first.

Some dogs with IBD develop severe vitamin deficiencies that must be treated with injectable vitamin supplements. Antibiotics may be recommended if secondary overgrowth of bacteria in the gut is suspected.

Follow-up Care

Follow-up examinations and repeated laboratory tests are often used to assess response to treatment and make adjustments in medications. If no or little improvement occurs within 2-3 weeks following a diet change or treatment with steroids, the dose of steroids may be increased, or other immune suppressive drugs may be added. After all signs have disappeared, it may be possible to slowly taper the medications, based on the recommendations of your veterinarian. If drugs are tapered, notify your veterinarian if any signs recur.

Prognosis

Prognosis for most dogs with IBD is good, because many show substantial improvement with diet changes and anti-inflammatory drugs. Some dogs have more severe disease that is difficult to control, and in these cases the prognosis is guarded (uncertain).

SPECIAL INSTRUCTIONS:

Intestinal Neoplasia

Craig G. Ruaux, BVSc, PhD, DACVIM (Small Animal)

BASIC INFORMATION
Description

Several types of neoplasms (tumors) can arise in the intestines. They may be benign or malignant (cancer). Intestinal tumors can develop from cells that line the inside of the intestinal tract (carcinoma, adenocarcinoma), from inflammatory and white blood cells in the wall of the intestine (lymphoma, mast cell tumor, plasmacytoma, others), or from the muscles of the gut (leiomyoma, leiomyosarcoma). Benign polyps, fibromas, lipomas, and adenomas may also occur.

The most common tumors in dogs are adenocarcinomas and lymphomas, both of which are malignant. Lymphoma is the most common tumor in cats and may be either B-cell or T-cell in origin. In general, B-cell tumors are the more aggressive type. Other, less common types of tumors may also arise in the intestine or invade it from nearby structures.

Causes

No cause has been identified for most intestinal tumors in dogs. Some breeds are prone to certain forms of intestinal tumors. The golden retriever, boxer, Chinese shar-pei, English springer spaniel, Doberman pinscher, Labrador retriever, and German shepherd dog have a higher risk for lymphoma. The Bernese Mountain dog and the flat-coated retriever develop histiocytic sarcomas more often than other breeds. Leiomyosarcoma occurs most often in the German shepherd dog. Cats with inflammatory bowel disease or previous exposure to or infection with feline leukemia virus are more prone to intestinal lymphoma.

Clinical Signs

Clinical signs often depend on the location, type, and aggressiveness of the tumor. Common signs include weight loss, poor appetite, vomiting, and diarrhea. The latter two signs are more likely if the intestinal mass is obstructing the movement of food. Diarrhea (sometimes with mucus and straining) is common with tumors of the large intestine.

Some tumors bleed into the intestines, which can cause signs of anemia (pale gums, weakness) and either fresh, red blood or dark, tarry material (melena or digested blood) in the stools. If the intestine is affected as part of a widespread cancer (some forms of lymphoma, plasmacytoma, histiocytic sarcoma, others), then other signs may be present, lymph nodes (glands) and other organs may be enlarged, and other masses may be detected.

Diagnostic Tests

Because the main signs of intestinal tumors are vomiting, poor appetite, and weight loss and many diseases cause these signs, extensive laboratory tests and x-rays are usually recommended. An abdominal ultrasound may be used to detect masses, assess nearby lymph nodes, and search for cancer in other abdominal organs. In some cases, fine-needle aspiration (extracting cells with a needle), done under ultrasound guidance, may reveal the type of tumor present. A gastrointestinal contrast study (a series of x-rays taken after the animal has swallowed barium) can be particularly useful for showing masses in the small intestines. Endoscopy, using a flexible fiberoptic tube, is useful to identify tumors in the upper small intestine or in the colon and also provides a means for obtaining biopsy samples and assessing the size of the lesion for planning additional surgery.

Obtaining a biopsy specimen is critical to making an accurate diagnosis of the type of neoplasia present, so that appropriate treatment can be planned and a prognosis can be given. If the tumor is not at the beginning or the end of the intestinal tract, the best method to obtain a biopsy is through abdominal exploratory surgery. If cancer is suspected, then chest x-rays may be recommended. Other testing may also be needed to rule out diseases that cause similar signs.

TREATMENT AND FOLLOW-UP

Treatment Options

Intestinal lymphoma is usually treated with chemotherapy. (See handouts on **Lymphoma in Dogs** and **Lymphoma in Cats**.) Surgical removal is usually recommended for other tumors. Some tumors can be completely cured by surgery, especially the benign tumors. For many malignant tumors, some form of additional chemotherapy or radiation therapy may be recommended.

Follow-up Care

Periodic follow-up visits are required after surgery and during chemotherapy for cancerous tumors, for the rest of the life of the animal. Laboratory tests, x-rays, and ultrasounds are often needed to monitor response to treatment, to detect evidence of spread of the tumor, and to check for side effects of the medications.

Prognosis

Prognosis is good for benign tumors that can be removed completely with surgery. Surgery and follow-up chemotherapy can extend the life of many animals with intestinal cancer, often by 6-12 months, but the long-term prognosis is poor, because many of these tumors recur. Prognosis is grave for animals with tumors that cannot be entirely removed or have already metastasized.

SPECIAL INSTRUCTIONS:

Intestinal Obstruction

Craig G. Ruaux, BVSc, PhD, DACVIM (Small Animal)

BASIC INFORMATION

Description

For the intestinal tract to work properly, fluid and food material must be able to pass through its entire length. When the passage of material is obstructed, nutrients cannot be absorbed, fluids are lost from the body, and the animal can rapidly become severely ill. Obstructions may be partial or complete, with the latter being more serious.

Causes

The most common cause is a foreign body (such as a toy, piece of string, or fabric) or an indigestible food item (bone, large piece of cartilage) that has been swallowed by the animal. This type of obstruction tends to be more common in younger animals. Other diseases of the intestines or nearby organs can lead to intestinal obstruction, including intestinal tumors, abscesses, strictures, adhesions, intussusception (telescoping of the bowel onto itself), and enlargement of other organs.

Clinical Signs

The main signs are vomiting and loss of appetite. Because the intestinal tract constantly produces fluids, vomiting may continue even if the animal is not drinking. Loss of fluids from vomiting causes dehydration, which is manifested as stiffening of the skin, sunken eyes, and dry, tacky gums. Along with the water that is lost, essential electrolytes such as sodium and potassium are usually lost, leading to muscular weakness, lethargy, and depression.

Fever is also common, possibly from complicating bacterial infections. Diarrhea and abdominal pain may also occur. In some animals, the obstruction can be felt when the veterinarian palpates the abdomen, but some abdomens feel normal even when severe obstructions are present.

Diagnostic Tests

Typically, when an obstruction is suspected, x-rays of the abdomen are recommended. Bone or metallic foreign material is visible on x-rays, but other foreign bodies may not be. Other tests, such as a barium study (series of x-rays taken after the animal has swallowed barium) or an abdominal ultrasound may be done. An ultrasound is also useful for assessing other organs, such as the liver, spleen, or nearby lymph nodes (glands).

Animals with an intestinal obstruction are usually dehydrated and have lost significant amounts of essential electrolytes. Routine laboratory tests are used to measure electrolytes and look for evidence of complications, such as kidney problems and infections. Other tests may be recommended to rule out diseases that cause similar signs and to search for metastasis if cancer is suspected.

Occasionally, the presence of an intestinal obstruction is not detected until an abdominal exploratory surgery is performed.

TREATMENT AND FOLLOW-UP

Treatment Options

The best treatment for intestinal obstruction is to remove the cause and relieve the obstruction. In most instances, intestinal surgery is required. In rare cases, obstructing objects can be removed from the first part of the small intestine with the use of an endoscope (a flexible fiberoptic tube that is introduced through the animal's mouth).

Dehydrated and severely ill animals must be stabilized with intravenous fluids and electrolytes prior to surgery. Other medications that may be administered include antibiotics, antivomiting drugs, and pain medications. With complete obstructions, surgery is performed as soon as the animal is stable.

A variety of surgical techniques are available for relieving obstructions. They include simple incisions into the intestines to remove foreign bodies, removal of segments and reconnection of the intestines, re-rotation of twisted sections of the intestine, repair of herniated or telescoped bowel, and other procedures.

Follow-up Care

Following surgery, most animals are hospitalized for 1-4 days for continued fluid therapy and administration of injectable drugs. All liquids and foods are commonly withheld for a period of time to allow the intestines to recover. Liquids are started initially, and then food is introduced if no vomiting occurs. Close monitoring of severely ill animals is required postoperatively.

Most animals are discharged with skin sutures (stitches) or staples that need to be removed 10-14 days after surgery. Dietary and exercise restrictions may be imposed during the recovery period.

Prognosis

Most animals recover fully if a foreign body was the source of the obstruction. In these cases, the main factors that influence the likelihood of survival are the severity of dehydration and electrolyte abnormalities present prior to surgery, the time that elapsed between the onset of complete obstruction and surgery, and the presence of other complications. Prognosis for intestinal obstructions from causes other than foreign bodies is highly variable. Animals with intestinal obstruction that do not have surgery usually die of other organ failure.

SPECIAL INSTRUCTIONS:

Intestinal Parasites

Craig G. Ruaux, BVSc, PhD, DACVIM (Small Animal)

BASIC INFORMATION
Description
Numerous parasitic organisms can live inside the gastrointestinal (GI) tract (gut) of dogs and cats. Some of these parasites (roundworms, hookworms, whipworms) cause clinical signs, whereas others have little impact on the health of the animal. Some intestinal parasites of dogs and cats can potentially infect humans, which is of particular concern when young children are handling or playing with animals that are infested or in areas (such as sandboxes) where infected animals have defecated.

Causes
Most GI parasites of dogs and cats are obtained from their environment. The methods by which animals are infected vary depending on the particular parasite involved. Some parasites have a direct life cycle, in which infective larvae (young worms) develop from eggs in the feces and are able to immediately infect a new host when eaten. Other parasites have complicated life cycles that require them to infect other (intermediate) hosts before infecting the dog or cat. Roundworms (*Toxocara canis*) can be transmitted from the mother before birth or through the mother's milk.

📋 Clinical Signs
Parasites that have little impact on the health of their host, such as most forms of tapeworm, may cause no clinical signs. Tapeworm eggs are passed in packages called *proglottids* that are sometimes seen in the feces or crawling on the skin around the anus. The most common type of tapeworm proglottid looks like a moving grain of white rice. Tapeworm segments can cause irritation to the skin around the anus and may lead to tail-dragging or scooting behaviors.

Many roundworms can cause to diarrhea, weight loss, failure to grow, and a poor hair coat. Hookworms and whipworms eat blood that they suck from the walls of the intestines. This can cause intestinal bleeding, with dark, tarry diarrhea and anemia (pale gums and tongue, weakness). Severely affected animals, particularly puppies and kittens, may develop pot bellies because of muscle weakness and malnutrition.

A protozoan (single-celled organism) called *Giardia* is a common cause of chronic diarrhea in some areas of the country. Giardiasis can affect animals of any age. Human beings can also become infected with *Giardia*, but the strain of the *Giardia* organism that affects people is different than that infecting dogs and cats.

🔬 Diagnostic Tests
Because of the wide variety of parasites that can infect the gut, several different diagnostic tests may be recommended. For some parasites, such as tapeworms, simply identifying tapeworm segments by sight is all that is necessary to make the diagnosis.

Most intestinal parasites are diagnosed by finding their eggs in a fecal sample. Direct smears and floatation or concentration procedures may be performed, with samples examined under a microscope. Some fecal flotation methods for certain parasites require 12-24 hours before results are available. Certain intestinal parasites are diagnosed by more complicated tests that are sent to an outside laboratory, and in these cases results usually are not available for a few days.

Fecal examinations are a common component of wellness examinations in animals. Because animals are exposed to parasites in their environment throughout their life, routine fecal examinations allow many parasites to be treated before they can cause any clinical signs or be spread to other animals and humans. However, a negative fecal sample does not rule out the presence of an intestinal parasite, because not all samples will contain parasites or their eggs.

TREATMENT AND FOLLOW-UP
℞ Treatment Options
The specific drug recommended depends on the type of parasite diagnosed. Some antiparasitic drugs contain one ingredient that kills one type of parasite, whereas others are combination products that kill a wider group of parasites. Decreasing parasite numbers in the environment through good kennel hygiene, washing of bedding, bathing the animal during treatment, and killing intermediary hosts (such as fleas) is important for preventing infection and reinfection.

🐾 Follow-up Care
Repeated fecal testing may be recommended to determine whether the parasite infestation has been eradicated. Repeat treatments may be needed at specific intervals to completely control the infestation.

Prognosis
Prognosis for most animals with intestinal parasites is good, providing effective antiparasitic medications are given correctly. Because many parasites exist in large numbers in the animal's environment, it is very common for animals to become reinfected and require repeated treatment. Recommendations for regular treatment to eliminate and control parasite infections vary depending on the climate in which you live. Your veterinarian will design a comprehensive testing and prevention program for your pet.

SPECIAL INSTRUCTIONS:

Lymphoplasmacytic Stomatitis in Cats

Craig G. Ruaux, BVSc, PhD, DACVIM (Small Animal)

BASIC INFORMATION

Description

Stomatitis is inflammation of the mouth, particularly the area in the back of the mouth just behind the tongue. Lymphoplasmacytic stomatitis is a specific form of stomatitis that can result in severe inflammation, often in association with inflammation of the gum line (gingivitis) and the tissues around the teeth (periodontitis). The condition receives its name from the type of cells that are present in the inflammation, a mixture of lymphocytes and plasma cells. Both of these cells are white blood cells, and plasma cells produce antibodies.

Causes

Although the exact cause of lymphoplasmacytic stomatitis is not well defined, it may be an immune-mediated disease in which the cat's immune system attacks its own tissues. Viral infections, such as feline calicivirus and feline immunodeficiency virus (FIV), may contribute to the disease. These infections may occur alone or together. The body's immune reaction against cells infected with these viruses may cause or aggravate the inflammation.

Clinical Signs

The most common clinical sign is reduced appetite. The cat often appears to be hungry but is unwilling to eat. Swallowing can be painful or difficult, particularly when the back of the mouth is severely inflamed. Halitosis (bad breath) and drooling of saliva may be present in some cats.

On oral examination, the back of the mouth, gum margins, and base of the teeth are usually very red and inflamed. Bleeding of the gums, tooth loss, exposed teeth, growth of the gums over the teeth, or raised proliferative lesions in the back of the mouth may be seen.

Diagnostic Tests

Lymphoplasmacytic stomatitis can look similar to other diseases in the mouth, such as eosinophilic granuloma and squamous cell carcinoma (a form of cancer). To definitively diagnose lymphoplasmacytic stomatitis, samples are collected for microscopic examination. Scrapings of the affected tissues may be examined under the microscope (cytology), or surgical biopsies may be submitted for histopathologic examination. Most sample collection techniques require a short period of general anesthesia. Other routine laboratory tests may be recommended to look for effects on other organs. Tests for the related viruses may also be recommended.

TREATMENT AND FOLLOW-UP

Treatment Options

In some cats, aggressive cleaning of the teeth (descaling and polishing) and scrupulous maintenance of dental hygiene are effective treatments. In some cats, multiple teeth must be extracted. Antibiotics are often helpful to control secondary bacterial infections.

In many cases, anti-inflammatory or immune-suppressive drugs are required to control the inflammation. High doses of oral or injectable glucocorticoid steroid drugs (prednisone, methylprednisolone, triamcinolone, or others) are commonly used. If the disease does not respond adequately to steroids, then other immune-suppressive drugs, such as chlorambucil and aurothioglucose, may be added to the therapy.

Follow-up Care

Cats receiving anti-inflammatory or immune-suppressive therapy require regular recheck visits, typically at 14-day intervals, during the initial period of therapy. Once the inflammation is under control, recheck visits become less frequent. Substantial clinical improvement may take several weeks.

Side effects such as increased water consumption, weight gain, and occasional restlessness or irritability may occur with high-dose steroids and other immune-suppressive drugs, so notify your veterinarian if any new signs appear. Laboratory tests may be repeated to determine the response to therapy and to monitor for side effects of the medications.

Prognosis

Prognosis for cats with lymphoplasmacytic stomatitis is fair to guarded (uncertain). If the cat responds to dental hygiene measures, tooth extraction, and immune-suppressive therapy with return of a good appetite, prognosis is favorable. Even when the signs resolve, treatment may only control the disease; it is hard to cure.

Clinical signs in some cats are difficult to control, and increasingly powerful immune-suppressive therapy carries a greater chance of side effects. Some cats are euthanized because of a poor response to therapy and persistent oral discomfort.

SPECIAL INSTRUCTIONS:

Megacolon in Cats

Craig G. Ruaux, BVSc, PhD, DACVIM (Small Animal)

BASIC INFORMATION

Description

The colon or large intestine contains the remains of digested material and dehydrates it to form feces. The colon ends at the rectum and anus. If the passage of feces is altered or delayed and feces remain in the colon for prolonged periods, the colon continues to extract water from the feces. As a result, the feces becomes very dry and hard, which makes it harder for them to move. Subsequently, more and more feces accumulate, which stretches the colon and greatly increases its size. A chronically enlarged colon that is often filled with dried feces is called a *megacolon*.

Causes

Of the two main causes of megacolon in cats, the more common one is unrelieved or recurrent constipation. Constipation may arise from narrowing of the pelvis due to an old fracture, paralysis of the anal region from neurologic damage or disease, chronic intestinal diseases, or other diseases that cause persistent dehydration (such as kidney disease). If constipation is not relieved, the distended colon loses normal muscle strength, which further aggravates the constipation.

A second form of megacolon develops from loss of normal nerve function within the wall of the colon. The nerve problem decreases muscle strength, which leads to constipation. Constipation is an effect, not a cause. The cause of the nerve dysfunction is not often identified. Regardless of the underlying cause, the end result is a colon that is dramatically larger than normal.

Clinical Signs

The most common sign is severe constipation. Cats may strain for long periods in the litter box, passing only small amounts of feces. Some cats vomit and lose their appetite. Occasionally, a liquid part of the feces is passed (paradoxical diarrhea), while solids are left behind. On clinical examination, an enlarged colon often can be felt within the abdomen. The cat may have signs of dehydration (tacky mucous membranes, stiff skin that tents up when pulled).

Diagnostic Tests

X-rays of the abdomen and spine are often recommended to look for problems in the skeleton (such as old pelvic fractures), to assess the degree of constipation, and to search for other problems that may be contributing to constipation. Routine laboratory tests and an abdominal ultrasound are sometimes recommended to look for contributing diseases and evidence of dehydration.

TREATMENT AND FOLLOW-UP

Treatment Options

In most cases, it is important to correct any dehydration with subcutaneous (under the skin) or intravenous fluids prior to treating the constipation. This is particularly important if the cat has kidney disease. Treatment of the constipation and megacolon involves several options. The approach taken depends on the cause of the disease. Treatment options include the following:

- Relief of severe constipation often requires general anesthesia and administration of multiple enemas to soften the fecal material, combined with manual kneading and extraction of the stool. Multiple rounds of anesthesia and administration of enemas over several days may be needed to relieve the constipation.
- In cats with less severe constipation (particularly if they can still pass some feces), warm-water enemas, drugs (such as cisapride, nizatidine, ranitidine) to increase muscular contraction of the colon, laxatives (such as lactulose, docusate sodium), and dietary changes (increased fiber) may be tried.
- If constipation arises from a mechanical problem, such as an old pelvic fracture that is impeding passage of feces, surgery may be needed to enlarge the pelvic canal.
- For colons that have lost all muscle strength and ability to move feces, partial removal of the colon (subtotal colectomy) may be considered. Your veterinarian may refer your cat to a veterinary surgery specialist for this procedure.

Follow-up Care

Cats that are treated with medications and laxatives are usually monitored closely with follow-up visits until the constipation has resolved. Long-term preventive medical therapy and periodic rechecks are often advisable, because constipation can recur. After subtotal colectomy, the initial postoperative period can be challenging, because bowel movements may be soft for a period of time. Eventually their consistency often returns to normal. Medical therapy is not often needed after surgery, but periodic rechecks may be recommended.

Prognosis

Prognosis for cats with megacolon that are treated medically is usually guarded (uncertain). If muscle function returns and constipation resolves with therapy, the prognosis is reasonable; however, recurrence is common in many cats. Cats can suffer severe, life-threatening illness as a result of long-term constipation. The prognosis for recovery from surgery is good if no complications occur.

SPECIAL INSTRUCTIONS:

Megaesophagus

Craig G. Ruaux, BVSc, PhD, DACVIM (Small Animal)

BASIC INFORMATION

Description

The esophagus is the muscular tube that carries swallowed food and water from the mouth to the stomach. Diseases that affect the muscles of the esophagus interfere with the passage of food and water through the esophagus. Under normal circumstances the esophagus is collapsed, but loss of muscle tone causes it to become relaxed and distended. A distended, enlarged esophagus that lacks good muscle tone is called a *megaesophagus*. Megaesophagus is more common in dogs than in cats.

Causes

In some dogs, myasthenia gravis causes megaesophagus. In this disease, antibodies are produced that interfere with muscle function, causing the esophagus to become paralyzed. Some hormonal problems (hypoadrenocorticism, possibly hypothyroidism) can potentially lead to megaesophagus in dogs. In puppies, a birth defect involving the blood vessels leaving the heart can cause narrowing of the esophagus, with formation of a dilated section in front of the heart. (See the handout on **Persistent Right Aortic Arch.**)

Congenital megaesophagus is an inherited trait in the wirehaired fox terrier, miniature schnauzer, and possibly the Chinese shar-pei. Megaesophagus may arise with certain infections (canine distemper, tetanus) and poisonings (botulism, lead, organophosphates).

In both dogs and cats, megaesophagus may develop in front of an esophageal stricture and with dysautonomia, a rare neurologic disease. In many animals, no specific cause is ever identified, and the disease is referred to as *idiopathic megaesophagus*.

Clinical Signs

The main clinical sign is regurgitation of undigested food, water, saliva, or mucus. Some animals have problems swallowing, which can be worse with certain types of food (dry kibble versus canned).

The presence of megaesophagus increases the risk of aspiration pneumonia from inhalation of food or fluid into the lungs. Coughing, fever, depression, lethargy, and loss of appetite are common with pneumonia. Occasionally the enlarged esophagus can be felt at the opening of the chest. Other signs may be present, depending on the underlying cause.

Diagnostic Tests

Chest x-rays are commonly recommended in animals with regurgitation or suspected pneumonia. Additional x-rays or a video x-ray (fluoroscopy) may be done after food containing barium is swallowed (esophagram). The barium highlights the walls of the esophagus.

Laboratory tests are often done to look for evidence of infection and inflammation from pneumonia. Hormonal assays, tests for myasthenia gravis, and tests for toxins may also be submitted. Many of these are submitted to outside laboratories, and results may take some time. Further tests may also be recommended to rule out other diseases that cause similar signs.

TREATMENT AND FOLLOW-UP

Treatment Options

Animals with aspiration pneumonia usually require hospitalization for intravenous fluids, antibiotics, and intensive nursing care. If a specific underlying disease or cause of the megaesophagus, such as hypothyroidism or myasthenia gravis, is identified, treatment is directed at that disease. Most underlying diseases are treated medically, but surgery is required for a persistent right aortic arch.

Animals with idiopathic and other types of megaesophagus require special feeding techniques so that they can take in adequate amounts of food and the risk of aspiration pneumonia is decreased.

- The most common technique is to feed the animal from an elevated position. Very small dogs and most cats can be held upright by one person while another feeds the animal. Large dogs are best fed and watered by placing their bowls on a tall platform.
- After feeding, the animal is held upright for at least 15 minutes so that the food gently falls into the stomach.
- Feeding several, small meals is often better than feeding large meals.
- The best consistency of the food to feed varies among animals. Some do better with gruels, whereas others do better with solid, meatball-shaped materials.

In some patients, adequate intake of food and water cannot be accomplished with these techniques, and placement of a feeding tube into the stomach may be necessary.

Follow-up Care

Animals with megaesophagus require regular and consistent follow-up, often at weekly intervals initially. Close monitoring is done until the underlying disease and the megaesophagus are under control or successfully managed. If at any time your animal develops trouble breathing or sudden onset of a cough or fever, seek immediate veterinary care.

Prognosis

Prognosis for most animals is guarded (poor to uncertain) unless a treatable underlying cause is found. Even with successful treatment of the cause, megaesophagus often persists. Dogs with idiopathic megaesophagus may develop aspiration pneumonia at any time, and any particular episode of pneumonia can be life-threatening.

SPECIAL INSTRUCTIONS:

Oral Melanoma in Dogs

Craig G. Ruaux, BVSc, PhD, DACVIM (Small Animal)

BASIC INFORMATION

Description

Melanoma is a tumor that arises from cells (melanocytes) that produce a dark brown pigment known as *melanin*. Melanomas in the mouth of dogs are often malignant and require early, aggressive treatment for the best outcome. Oral melanoma is one of the more common malignant cancers of dogs but it is rare in cats.

Causes

No direct cause of oral melanoma has been identified in dogs. Dogs with darkly colored gums and black hair coats (such as the Scottish terrier) may be at higher risk. The tumor can occur in any breed, but it is more common in certain breeds, such as the cocker spaniel, German shepherd dog, poodles, dachshund, and golden retriever. Middle-aged or older dogs (average age, 10-12 years) are affected most often.

Clinical Signs

The main finding is a mass inside the mouth. The mass may be black or pink in color. It may arise from the gum near the teeth (gingival), from the inside of the cheek, high on the gums above the teeth, from the palate (roof of the mouth), or even on the tongue. Halitosis (bad breath), bleeding from the mouth and gums, loss of appetite, face rubbing, and trouble chewing or swallowing may occur. In some cases, the mass is only found during a regular physical examination.

Metastasis (spread) of the cancer to the lymph nodes (glands) under the jaw is possible. Melanomas may invade nearby bone, which causes the teeth to become loose and malaligned.

Diagnostic Tests

Diagnosis and management of oral melanoma can be challenging. It is very important to differentiate these lesions from an epulis (see handout on **Epulis in Dogs**), because treatment and outcome are often very different. Definitive diagnosis is obtained by histopathology, which requires surgical removal or biopsy of the tumor. These tumors can invade deeper tissues and can be aggressive, so surgery to obtain a biopsy specimen must be carefully planned to avoid problems that might complicate future surgical treatment. Some oral melanomas can be diagnosed by fine-needle aspiration (extracting cells with a needle) and examination of the cells under the microscope (cytology). However, cytology is not 100% reliable for identifying whether the tumor is a melanoma.

Laboratory tests, x-rays of the chest, and an abdominal ultrasound are often recommended to search for spread (metastasis) of the tumor. The process of assessing the amount of cancerous tissue present in the body is called *staging the cancer*. In some cases, x-rays, computed tomography (CT scan), or magnetic resonance imaging (MRI) of the jaw is done to establish the extent of tumor growth within the mouth. Your veterinarian may recommend referral to a veterinary oncologist (cancer specialist) for staging and treatment planning.

TREATMENT AND FOLLOW-UP

Treatment Options

The main treatment is surgical removal of the tumor. Wide margins (at least 1 inch or 2 cm) of apparently normal tissue must be removed in addition to the tumor, and this can be difficult to achieve in the mouth. Obtaining wide margins may require removal of teeth, a portion of the jaw (mandibulectomy), or a section of cheek bone (maxillectomy). Because radical surgery is often needed, your dog may be referred to a veterinary surgery specialist for the procedure. Following surgical removal, radiation therapy is sometimes recommended to kill any cells that may have been left behind.

A recently introduced therapy for oral melanoma involves administration of a vaccine that causes the dog's own immune system to kill melanoma cells. This treatment is usually administered after surgery has been done, and the vaccine is available only from a veterinary oncologist. The vaccine is most effective in cases in which the original mass was 1 cm (½ inch) or less in diameter, successful surgery was performed, and there is no evidence of metastasis to the lymph nodes or lungs.

Follow-up Care

The schedule for follow-up visits varies, depending on the treatment method used. Following oral surgery, soft foods are fed until healing of the site is complete. Antibiotics may be given for any secondary infections, and an Elizabethan collar may be applied to prevent self-trauma. Laboratory tests and chest x-rays may be repeated periodically to monitor for spread of the disease.

Prognosis

Oral melanoma has a poor prognosis in dogs. Even with aggressive surgery, radiation, and vaccine therapy, many dogs die within 6-12 months of the diagnosis.

SPECIAL INSTRUCTIONS:

Oral Squamous Cell Carcinoma in Cats

Craig G. Ruaux, BVSc, PhD, DACVIM (Small Animal)

BASIC INFORMATION

Description

Squamous cell carcinoma (SCC) is a form of malignant cancer that arises from cells in the outer layer of the skin and gums. An oral SCC is diagnosed when this cancer is found in the mouth. Oral SCC is the most common form of oral cancer in cats and is a very serious disease. Early, aggressive treatment is necessary to provide the best chance for good control of clinical signs and good quality of life.

Causes

No direct cause of oral SCC has been identified in cats. Exposure to cigarette smoke, canned fish, and flea collars are suspected to increase the risk of oral SCC in cats, but none of these is a proven cause. Exposure to sunlight, particularly in cats that lack protective pigment in white skin or pink areas on the gums and lips, increases the risk of development of oral SCC in these light-colored tissues. Although the ears are more commonly affected by exposure to sunlight, lesions that arise on the lips can extend into the mouth. Chronic inflammation from periodontal disease and eosinophilic ulcers may contribute in some cases.

Clinical Signs

Oral SCCs are aggressive, rapidly growing lesions that tend to form ulcers. The most common clinical signs are bleeding from the mouth, drooling, apparent pain when chewing or swallowing, and loss of appetite. The cancer is usually easy to see when it develops on the gum line or adjacent to the teeth. In some cats, SCC affects the tongue or the deeper tissues in the back of the mouth. In these cases, deep sedation or general anesthesia may be needed to allow adequate examination of the whole mouth.

Diagnostic Tests

It is very important to distinguish oral SCC from other, similar looking lesions in the mouth, such as severe inflammation and other forms of cancer that have different treatments and outcomes. Depending on the location and size of the lesion in the mouth, your veterinarian may recommend fine-needle aspiration (extracting cells with a needle), impression smears, or surface scrapings to obtain cells for examination under the microscope (cytology) or removal of a portion of the mass (biopsy) for histopathology. These tumors can invade deeper tissues and can be aggressive, so surgery to obtain a biopsy specimen must be carefully planned to avoid problems that might complicate future surgical treatment.

Laboratory tests, x-rays of the chest, and an abdominal ultrasound are often recommended to search for spread (metastasis) of the tumor. The process of assessing the amount of cancerous tissue present in the body is called *staging the cancer*. In some cases, x-ray studies, computed tomography (CT scan), or magnetic resonance imaging (MRI) of the jaw is done to establish the extent of tumor growth within the mouth. Your veterinarian may recommend referral to a veterinary oncologist (cancer specialist) for staging and treatment planning.

TREATMENT AND FOLLOW-UP

Treatment Options

Treatment options for oral SCC in cats are limited. The best option for prolonging a good quality life is well-planned, aggressive surgery to remove the cancer. Surgery may require removal of teeth, a portion of the jaw (mandibulectomy), or a section of cheek bone (maxillectomy). Because radical surgery is often needed, your cat may be referred to a veterinary surgery specialist for the procedure.

Removal of just the mass itself may have little effect on survival time, because these cancers recur very rapidly if any cells are left behind. Following surgery, local radiation therapy, chemotherapy, or other treatments may be recommended. In some cats, palliative therapy (treatment aimed at keeping the cat comfortable) may be tried, with medications for pain and insertion of a feeding tube.

Follow-up Care

The schedule for follow-up visits varies depending on the treatment method used. Following oral surgery, soft foods are fed until healing of the site is complete. A feeding tube may also be inserted in to the stomach, to allow the mouth time to heal. Antibiotics may be given for any secondary infections, and an Elizabethan collar may be applied to prevent self-trauma. Laboratory tests and chest x-rays may be repeated periodically to monitor for spread of the disease (metastasis) and for side effects from chemotherapy.

Prognosis

Oral SCC is an aggressive disease that severely impacts the cat's health and quality of life. Very few cats survive longer than 1 year after diagnosis, regardless of the treatment they receive. Cats that receive no therapy usually die or are euthanized within 6 weeks of the diagnosis.

SPECIAL INSTRUCTIONS:

Pancreatitis in Cats

Craig G. Ruaux, BVSc, PhD, DACVIM (Small Animal)

BASIC INFORMATION

Description

The pancreas is a flat, thin organ located in the front of the abdomen, near the stomach, that contains two major types of cells. One group of cells (*endocrine pancreas*) produces hormones (insulin, glucagon) that regulate blood sugar, and the other group (*exocrine pancreas*) produces digestive enzymes that are released into the intestine to break down food.

Pancreatitis is inflammation of the exocrine part of the pancreas. When the pancreas becomes inflamed, it becomes painful and swollen and may affect the stomach, small intestine, and parts of the liver. Swelling and irritation of the stomach, small intestine, pancreas, and parts of the liver are responsible for most of the clinical signs seen.

Causes

In most cats, the cause of pancreatitis is unknown. Many cats with pancreatitis also have inflammatory small bowel disease (IBD) and/or inflammation of the liver and gall bladder (cholangiohepatitis). An underlying problem may lead to any or all of these diseases in a particular cat. Many cats with IBD or cholangiohepatitis are sensitive to the types of protein in their diet, and the inflammation may represent a dietary allergy in some cats.

Two forms of pancreatitis exist: acute and chronic pancreatitis. In the cat, chronic pancreatitis is far more common that acute pancreatitis. Most cats with pancreatitis have a long history of clinical signs that are often vague or misleading.

Clinical Signs

The most common sign in the cat is lethargy, followed by a poor appetite. Vomiting, dehydration, and a painful abdomen on palpation are seen occasionally, particularly during flare-ups. It is very common for signs of chronic pancreatitis to come and go in the cat; even when the cat seems to feel better, the pancreas can still be inflamed. Some cats with chronic pancreatitis develop diabetes mellitus if the insulin-producing cells are damaged. Bouts of chronic pancreatitis make the diabetes more difficult to regulate.

Diagnostic Tests

Reaching a diagnosis of pancreatitis in the cat can be quite complicated. Your veterinarian may recommend several types of blood tests and x-rays:

- Routine blood tests are used to look for other diseases that cause similar signs.
- A specialized test measures a form of digestive enzyme in the bloodstream that is increased with inflammation of the pancreas. Your veterinarian may combine this test, called the *feline specific pancreatic lipase test* (SpecfPL), with other function tests of the small intestine.

An abdominal ultrasound is commonly done to look for an enlarged, swollen pancreas. The pancreas of the cat can be difficult to see on ultrasound, so your veterinarian may refer your cat to a veterinary specialist for this examination.

TREATMENT AND FOLLOW-UP

Treatment Options

Cats with acute pancreatitis often require hospitalization for fluid therapy and medications to treat pain and to stop vomiting. Some may need insertion of a feeding tube to provide necessary nutrition. Severe acute pancreatitis is rare in the cat, but it can be life-threatening and can deteriorate rapidly if not treated promptly.

Many cats with chronic pancreatitis do not need to be hospitalized. In many of these cats the underlying problem is a dietary intolerance or allergy, so a diet change may be necessary. Your veterinarian can suggest a novel diet, based on the history of diet types that your cat has previously eaten.

If the cat does not respond to the new diet, anti-inflammatory medications may be tried. These drugs must be used with care, because they can have significant side effects. Steroid medications are particularly problematic for cats with diabetes mellitus.

Chronic pancreatitis can be a frustrating disease to control, and several different treatment approaches and fine-tuning of the therapies may be required.

Follow-up Care

Frequency and number of follow-up visits vary depending on the severity and frequency of the clinical signs. Remember that many cats show little or no signs of their chronic pancreatitis except during flare-ups. Repeating the SpecfPL blood test is often the only way to know whether the treatments are truly helping. Cats that require glucocorticoid steroid drugs must be monitored closely for the development of complications, particularly diabetes mellitus.

Prognosis

Prognosis for cats with pancreatitis requiring hospitalization is difficult to predict. Some cats die of this disease, even with the best possible care. Prognosis for cats with chronic pancreatitis is generally good, particularly if a change of diet is all that is needed to control the inflammation. Your pet must be monitored closely for the development of complications, particularly diabetes mellitus.

SPECIAL INSTRUCTIONS:

Pancreatitis in Dogs

Craig G. Ruaux, BVSc, PhD, DACVIM (Small Animal)

BASIC INFORMATION

Description

The pancreas is a flat, thin organ located in the front of the abdomen, near the stomach, that contains two major types of cells. One group of cells (*endocrine pancreas*) produces hormones (insulin, glucagon) that regulate blood sugar, and the other group (*exocrine pancreas*) produces digestive enzymes that are released into the intestines to break down food.

Pancreatitis is inflammation of the exocrine part of the pancreas. When the pancreas becomes inflamed, it becomes painful and swollen and may affect the stomach, small intestine, and liver. Swelling and irritation of the pancreas and these other organs are responsible for most of the clinical signs seen.

Causes

Two forms of pancreatitis exist: acute and chronic. Dogs most commonly develop acute pancreatitis, but chronic pancreatitis can occur and is more common in some breeds than in others. In many cases, the cause of pancreatitis is unknown, but eating foods that are unusual (such as human food or garbage) or high in fat is known to increase the risk for acute pancreatitis. Other risk factors include obesity and the presence of diseases of the liver, small intestine, or adrenal glands (hyperadrenocorticism). Occasionally pancreatitis develops following abdominal trauma or surgery, or from tumors near the pancreas or certain infections.

Clinical Signs

The most common signs of acute pancreatitis are vomiting, dehydration, a painful abdomen, lethargy, and fever. These signs are vague and may arise with diseases of many other organs, which must be ruled out.

Dogs with chronic pancreatitis usually have a poor appetite and lethargy. Vomiting, dehydration, and a painful abdomen occur occasionally, particularly during flare-ups. It is very common for signs of chronic pancreatitis to come and go in the dog; even when the dog seems to feel better, the pancreas can still be inflamed.

Over time, persistent inflammation can cause loss of exocrine pancreas tissue, which leads to diarrhea from poor digestion of food. Some dogs with chronic pancreatitis develop diabetes mellitus if the insulin-producing cells are damaged. Bouts of chronic pancreatitis also make diabetes more difficult to regulate in dogs.

Diagnostic Tests

Reaching a diagnosis of pancreatitis can be quite complicated. Your veterinarian may recommend several types of blood tests and x-rays:

- Routine blood tests are used to look for other diseases with similar signs.
- A specialized test measures a form of digestive enzyme in the bloodstream that is increased with pancreatitis. Your veterinarian may combine this test, called the *specific pancreatic lipase immunoreactivity test* (SpecPL), with other tests that assess the function of the small intestine.

An abdominal ultrasound is commonly used to look for an enlarged, swollen pancreas. The pancreas can be difficult to see on ultrasound, so your veterinarian may refer your dog to a veterinary specialist for this examination.

TREATMENT AND FOLLOW-UP

Treatment Options

Dogs with acute pancreatitis often require hospitalization for fluid therapy, medications for pain and vomiting, and other supportive care. Food and water are initially withheld to allow the pancreas to heal. A feeding tube may be recommended in some dogs. Severe acute pancreatitis can be life-threatening and can rapidly deteriorate if not treated promptly.

Many dogs with chronic pancreatitis do not require hospitalization; however, those with severe bouts may be hospitalized for intravenous fluid therapy. For dogs with chronic pancreatitis, every effort is made to identify any other abdominal diseases, such as inflammatory bowel disease (IBD) or cholangiohepatitis, because the presence of these diseases can make recovery more complicated and prolonged.

With diagnosis of pancreatitis, the diet is changed to one with a lower fat content. If the dog does not respond to the new diet within 2-3 weeks, anti-inflammatory medications may be tried. These drugs must be used with care, because they can have significant side effects. Steroid medications are particularly problematic for dogs with diabetes mellitus.

Chronic pancreatitis can be a frustrating disease to control, and several different treatment approaches and fine-tuning of the therapies may be required.

Follow-up Care

Follow-up visits are usually done periodically based on the severity of the disease. The SpecPL test is often repeated after 2-3 weeks to gauge whether the inflammation is improving.

Prognosis

Prognosis for dogs with severe, acute pancreatitis requiring hospitalization and fluid therapy is often difficult to predict. Some dogs die of this disease, even with the best possible care. Prognosis for dogs with chronic pancreatitis is generally good, particularly if a change to a lower-fat diet is all that is necessary to control the inflammation and the clinical signs.

SPECIAL INSTRUCTIONS:

Perianal Fistula in Dogs

Craig G. Ruaux, BVSc, PhD, DACVIM (Small Animal)

BASIC INFORMATION

Description

A perianal fistula is a track or tunnel between the anus and the adjacent skin. The term *perianal* means around or near the anus. Perianal fistulas are often associated with severe skin infections, especially if they allow material from the anus to be pushed under the skin.

Causes

The underlying cause of perianal fistulas in dogs is not known with certainty, but they are most commonly diagnosed in the German shepherd dog, which suggests that there is a heritable, genetic component to the disease. Since many cases respond to immune-suppressive therapy, the condition may be an immune-mediated disease in some dogs. It is speculated that excessive immune responses to bacteria in the dog's colon, to some component of the diet, or to an external allergen may be involved. Serious skin infections and the moist environment under a broad tail (common in many German shepherd dogs) probably contribute to the severity of the disease but are not essential to its development.

Clinical Signs

Some dogs have no clinical signs, and the disease is only found during a routine physical examination. Dogs with clinical signs commonly show excessive licking at the anus and perianal region. Examination of the anal region in most dogs shows draining sores and matting of the hair, along with a foul odor and moist inflammation of the skin. The extent and depth of each fistula can be much greater than initially suspected, and clipping of the hair from around the anus is necessary to fully gauge the amount of tissue involved.

Excessive straining or discomfort while passing stools often occurs. Fresh blood may be seen in the feces. Affected dogs may show pain when the tail is lifted or the area around the anus is touched.

Diagnostic Tests

The appearance of the lesions, particularly in a predisposed breed, is strongly suggestive of the diagnosis. Other conditions that can look like perianal fistulas include abscesses of the anal sacs (see handout on **Anal Sac Diseases**) and tumors of the tissue surrounding the anus (see handout on **Perianal Tumors**). Differentiation of perianal fistulas from these other conditions may require a rectal examination, insertion of a cannula into the fistula to determine its origin, or surgical removal of a tissue sample for biopsy and histopathology. If anesthesia is anticipated for the biopsy, then preoperative laboratory tests may be recommended.

TREATMENT AND FOLLOW-UP

Treatment Options

Initially, most dogs with perianal fistulas are given immune-suppressive medications. Examples of oral medications include steroids (such as prednisone), cyclosporine, and azathioprine. Tacrolimus in a topical ointment form is sometimes used for mild lesions or in addition to oral medications. Your veterinarian will discuss these various options and their potential side effects with you.

If medical management does not work adequately, surgical removal of the affected tissue may be recommended. Surgery may include removal of the anal sacs, because they often become involved secondarily. Tail amputation may also be recommended in cases that recur despite prior medical or surgical therapy. Surgery alone, without medical therapy, has had mixed results.

Follow-up Care

Frequent follow-up is recommended during the first 4-6 weeks of medical therapy, because recovery times can be prolonged. Dogs on medical therapy also require periodic laboratory testing to monitor for side effects of the medications. Fecal incontinence is a potential complication of surgery, especially with severe or extensive lesions.

Prognosis

If the dog responds well to medical therapy, the prognosis is fair to good, but the disease may require lifelong therapy. The prognosis for dogs with more severe disease or disease that requires both surgery and medical therapy is more guarded (uncertain). Fistulas may heal, only to return at a later date.

SPECIAL INSTRUCTIONS:

Perianal Tumors

Craig G. Ruaux, BVSc, PhD, DACVIM (Small Animal)

BASIC INFORMATION

Description

Perianal tumors are tumors that develop on or close to the anus. Dogs and cats have several types of glands around the anus. Some of the material they produce is stored in the anal sacs, which are two small pouches located beside and slightly below the anus. (See handout on **Anal Sac Diseases**.) Perianal tumors most commonly arise from the glands or from the anal sacs; however, certain skin tumors can develop in the perianal region. Perianal tumors include benign (adenoma) and malignant (adenocarcinoma, carcinoma) masses of the perianal glands, the anal sacs, and the anus itself. Perianal tumors are most commonly diagnosed in dogs but are occasionally found in cats.

Causes

There is no known cause for tumors that arise from the anal sacs. Benign perianal adenomas occur most commonly in older male dogs that have not been castrated. In these dogs, the tumors seem to develop because of long-term exposure to the male hormone testosterone.

Clinical Signs

Perianal tumors may cause no signs and be found only on physical examination, or they may rupture and bleed, which can cause excessive licking at the anal area. In dogs with short tails, a mass may be visible. If the mass involves the anus, straining to defecate and blood on the feces may be noted. Perianal adenomas may arise as single or multiple masses, or they may produce a thickened ring of tissue that surrounds the anus (hepatoid circumanal adenoma).

Perianal adenocarcinoma may cause other clinical signs, such as increased water consumption and urine production if blood calcium is increased, as well as decreased appetite, lethargy, and reduced exercise tolerance. In many animals, an anal sac adenocarcinoma is first suspected when high blood calcium level is detected on screening laboratory tests.

Diagnostic Tests

If a perianal adenoma is found on physical examination, laboratory testing may be recommended prior to surgery. Animals with suspected perianal adenocarcinoma require more extensive diagnostic evaluation, because these tumors have the potential to spread to other parts of the body (metastasize) and to cause changes in body chemistry (elevated blood calcium concentrations) that can lead to kidney failure. Besides laboratory tests, chest and abdominal x-rays and an abdominal ultrasound are commonly recommended. Examination of cells taken by fine-needle aspiration (cytology) allows differentiation between benign and malignant tumors in some cases, but in others, confirmation of the type of tumor requires a surgical biopsy.

TREATMENT AND FOLLOW-UP

Treatment Options

Castration is often recommended for benign perianal tumors. Bleeding or fast-growing tumors are often surgically removed at the same time. Small tumors may regress following castration. In dogs with slow-growing hepatoid circumanal adenomas, no specific therapy may be recommended, but if the skin of the anus becomes irritated or ulcerated, soothing creams may be prescribed.

Wide surgical removal is usually recommended for perianal and anal sac adenocarcinomas (along with the affected anal sac), as well as for anal carcinomas. Medical therapy to lower blood calcium and improve kidney function may be needed prior to surgery. Surgery to remove these tumors can be challenging, so your pet may be referred to a veterinary surgery specialist for the procedure. If the tumor has spread to other organs, effective treatment is difficult. Since surgical removal of all tumor cells is impossible in these cases, additional radiation and chemotherapy may be recommended.

In dogs with inoperable malignant tumors, only palliative treatment may be possible. This therapy aims at improving the quality of life but has no effect on the dog's survival time. Palliative measures may include administration of drugs that reduce blood calcium, pain, and nausea.

Follow-up Care

Dogs with hepatoid circumanal adenoma may be monitored periodically. Notify your veterinarian if any changes occur in the ring of tissue. Dogs treated only with castration are often monitored for 1-3 months to ensure that the tumor is shrinking. Animals with malignant tumors require frequent follow-up visits, particularly if they are receiving radiation or chemotherapy.

Prognosis

Prognosis for dogs with benign tumors is very good. Complications (fecal incontinence, anal strictures, infections) may arise after surgery but are uncommon unless the tumor is large or deep. In most cases of malignant tumors, the dog dies from the tumor and its side effects or is euthanized because of recurrence of the disease. Surgery, chemotherapy, and palliative therapy may extend the dog's life and provide better quality of life, but most dogs die within 1 year after diagnosis of a malignant tumor.

SPECIAL INSTRUCTIONS:

Perineal Hernia in Dogs

Craig G. Ruaux, BVSc, PhD, DACVIM (Small Animal)

BASIC INFORMATION

Description

A perineal hernia forms when the muscles surrounding the posterior part of the pelvis, rectum, and anus become weakened. The rectum bulges into the weakened muscles of the pelvic canal, forming a diverticulum (outpouching). This causes the dog to strain, and the straining causes the muscles of the pelvic canal to break down even more. Parts of the rectum, bladder, or prostate can move through the gap in the pelvic muscles and become entrapped in the hernia.

Causes

Perineal hernias are most common in older, male dogs that have not been castrated. Changes in hormone concentrations (decreasing testosterone, possibly increasing estrogen) are thought to cause muscle weakening, which can eventually lead to hernia formation. Constipation or enlargement of the prostate gland may also be important factors in some dogs, but these conditions do not need to be present for a perineal hernia to form. Perineal hernias are very rare in cats.

Clinical Signs

The hernia may be visible as a large, soft swelling over the rear end, near the anus. A hernia may develop on one or both sides. Dogs often strain repeatedly as if attempting to pass stool, giving the impression they are constipated. If the bladder or prostate gland is caught in the hernia, the dog may have severe abdominal pain or may strain repeatedly as if trying to urinate. If the bladder is trapped in the hernia for a long period, a form of kidney failure occurs from the urinary obstruction, which causes the dog to become very ill rapidly. Signs of prostatitis may be present in some dogs.

Diagnostic Tests

The presence of a hernia can usually be confirmed by your veterinarian through a rectal examination using a gloved finger. Rectal examination is also necessary to define the size of the defect in the wall of the pelvic canal. If trapping of the bladder or prostate gland in the hernia is a possibility, abdominal x-rays may be recommended. Laboratory tests and chest x-rays are often performed prior to surgery.

TREATMENT AND FOLLOW-UP

Treatment Options

Treatment of perineal hernia requires surgery to reduce the hernia (push the contents back into their normal locations) and repair the muscular wall of the pelvic canal. If the dog has not previously been castrated, castration at the time of the surgery may decrease the chance of a recurrence.

If the dog is seriously ill from a urinary obstruction and the bladder is entrapped in the hernia, then emergency measures may be necessary prior to surgery. Urine can be withdrawn from the bladder by insertion of a catheter in some dogs or by the use of a needle and syringe in other dogs. Urine is removed until the bladder is small enough to be manually pushed into the abdomen, or a urinary catheter can be inserted. Intravenous fluids and other therapy for kidney failure are instituted, and surgery to repair the hernia is delayed until the dog is stable. If the bladder cannot be repositioned, then emergency surgery may be needed.

After surgery, most dogs are started on laxatives and low-residue, high-moisture food. These measures soften the stool and decrease straining during defecation, helping to ensure a good postoperative result. Usually, conservative therapy with laxatives, low-residue diets, and manual removal of feces without surgery are not sufficient to manage the problem, because the underlying muscle weakness and herniation are not corrected. These measures may be tried, however, in dogs that are unable to withstand surgery because they are high anesthetic risks.

Because the muscles of the pelvic canal are weakened, the surgical repair may not be strong enough to resist forces that are exerted when the dog strains to defecate, and the repair may break down. If the hernia is large and affects both sides, or if the hernia has recurred after surgery, your pet may be referred to a veterinary surgery specialist for more advanced surgery that could involve moving muscles from the upper leg and inner thigh to reinforce the repair, insertion of synthetic meshes, or other procedures.

Follow-up Care

Following surgery, the dog should be kept quiet until the sutures are removed in 10-14 days. Notify your veterinarian if any straining or signs recur after the surgery.

Prognosis

Prognosis for a perineal hernia is uncertain because of the possibility of recurrence following surgery. Fecal incontinence may occur after surgery if hernias were repaired on both sides. Some dogs die from complications such as kidney failure.

SPECIAL INSTRUCTIONS:

Portosystemic Vascular Anomalies

Craig G. Ruaux, BVSc, PhD, DACVIM (Small Animal)

BASIC INFORMATION
Description
Blood leaving the gut passes to the liver through a special system of blood vessels, called the *portal circulation*. In the liver, nutrients and toxic substances are absorbed and processed before they reach the rest of the body. A portosystemic vascular anomaly (shunt) is an abnormal blood vessel that allows blood from the gut to bypass the liver.

There are two major types of portosystemic vascular anomalies, congenital and acquired. A congenital anomaly is one that is present at birth, whereas acquired anomalies develop later in life, usually from liver disease. Congenital anomalies may be intrahepatic (within the liver) or extrahepatic (outside the liver) in location.

Causes
The cause of congenital portosystemic vascular anomalies is unknown. A genetic component may be involved in certain breeds, such as the Irish wolfhound, pug, Havanese, Maltese, Dandie Dinmont terrier, miniature schnauzer, Cairn terrier, and Yorkshire terrier, because they have a higher risk for developing these anomalies.

Acquired anomalies develop from scarring and cirrhosis of the liver (see the handout on **Chronic Hepatitis in Dogs**), which cause pressure to increase in the portal blood vessels. New, abnormal vessels form that alleviate this pressure as the vessels bypass the liver.

Clinical Signs
Most animals with acquired shunts have very advanced liver disease, with signs such as poor appetite, weight loss, lethargy, depression, increased water consumption, and fluid accumulation in the abdomen or under the skin (ascites or edema). Young animals with congenital anomalies usually fail to grow properly and are small in comparison to their littermates.

Affected animals become mentally depressed or behave oddly after they have eaten, because of a sudden influx of toxic compounds into the circulation as food is digested. These behavioral changes are a form of hepatic encephalopathy. (See handout on **Hepatic Encephalopathy**.)

Diagnostic Tests
Routine laboratory tests and abdominal x-rays are often recommended initially. X-rays may show a small liver and kidneys that are larger than normal. Bile acid assays are often run, because with portosystemic anomalies, bile acid levels are typically extremely elevated after a meal, which indicates that blood from the gut is bypassing the liver. An abdominal ultrasound may be used to gauge the size of the liver, to look for evidence of scarring and

shrinkage of the liver, and to search for abnormal blood vessels. Detecting abnormal vessels requires a high level of skill, particularly in very small animals, and sometimes additional tests, such as a nuclear scan or a contrast x-ray procedure (portography) may be needed. In these cases, your veterinarian may recommend referral to a veterinary specialist for further testing. Other tests may also be recommended to rule out other diseases that can cause similar signs.

TREATMENT AND FOLLOW-UP
Treatment Options
If a portosystemic vascular anomaly is detected, surgical closure of the vessel is usually recommended, if possible. Depending on the size, complexity, and position of the shunt in the abdomen, surgery may or may not be feasible. Your pet may be referred to a veterinary surgery specialist for the procedure.

If an anomaly is present that cannot be repaired surgically, medical management is started. Medical therapy involves measures to decrease the production and absorption of toxic substances in the gut. Decreasing the amount of protein in the diet lowers the production of these substances and is an important part of therapy. Absorption of toxins can be reduced by making the environment in the gut more acidic with a medication called *lactulose*. Lactulose is also a laxative, so the amount of time that proteins or feces remain in the gut is decreased. It may cause soft stools, mild diarrhea, and excessive gas (flatulence), especially in the first 7-10 days.

Since bacteria are also involved in the production toxic compounds, broad-spectrum antibiotics are commonly given along with the lactulose and a low-protein diet.

Follow-up Care
Patients with vascular anomalies that undergo surgery require regular follow-up visits and testing for several months. Animals on medical therapy usually show an improvement in their signs within 1 week. Follow-up visits may be needed at weekly intervals for several weeks until the animal is stable, and then every 2-3 months.

Prognosis
Prognosis is good for young animals with anomalies that can be successfully treated with surgery. Assuming there are no complications and recovery is uneventful, these animals often go on to lead normal lives. Animals with inoperable anomalies or end-stage liver disease have a more guarded to poor prognosis. They require lifelong treatment, and their clinical signs typically worsen over time.

SPECIAL INSTRUCTIONS:

Protein-Losing Enteropathy

Craig G. Ruaux, BVSc, PhD, DACVIM (Small Animal)

BASIC INFORMATION

Description

Protein-losing enteropathy (PLE) is a term used to describe conditions of the gastrointestinal tract (gut) that cause protein to be lost in the feces. When excessive amounts of protein are lost from the gut, nutrient and caloric intake is inadequate and weight loss occurs. Loss of protein from the body can develop with a wide variety of diseases, many of which must be ruled out before reaching a diagnosis of PLE.

Causes

Protein loss can occur with inflammation in the gut, such as with inflammatory bowel disease (IBD) and certain infections (viral, fungal, bacterial). Protein may also be lost with bleeding into the gut from ulcers or tumors or from intestinal parasites (especially hookworms, whipworms, and giardiasis in dogs).

More significant and severe protein loss can occur with abnormalities in the vessels that remove lymph (fluid containing white blood cells) from the intestines (a condition called *lymphangiectasia*), with partial obstructions of the small intestines, and with some forms of cancer. Certain dog breeds are at higher risk for the development of PLE from lymphangiectasia, which implies that PLE may be a genetic disorder in some dogs. Examples include the Yorkshire terrier, Maltese, and Norwegian lundehund.

Clinical Signs

Signs are of PLE are often vague and can wax and wane, so an initial suspicion may not arise until preliminary diagnostic tests have been run. Usually dogs with PLE have signs of gastrointestinal disease, such as diarrhea, vomiting and lack of appetite. Animals with severe PLE may develop edema (swelling) of the limbs and skin, difficulty breathing from fluid in the chest, and enlargement of the abdomen from fluid accumulation (ascites). Weight loss is common.

Diagnostic Tests

PLE is often first suspected when total protein and/or albumin protein content of the blood is found to be low. In more severe cases, globulin protein is also low, and other laboratory abnormalities may be detected. When low proteins are discovered, several fecal tests may be recommended to look for parasites or bleeding in the gastrointestinal tract. In dog breeds that are known to be at risk for PLE, such as the soft-coated wheaten terrier, silky terrier, and Rottweiler, a specialized fecal test can be used to look for protein loss.

Protein loss from other sites must also be ruled out through tests such as a urinalysis and urine protein/creatinine ratio to look for protein loss from the kidneys; x-rays of the chest; x-rays and an ultrasound of the abdomen; and specialized tests of liver function, such as a bile acid test. If the liver is working properly, no protein is being lost in the urine, and no abnormalities are detected in the chest, then the most likely cause of the low protein is PLE.

With more severe disease, particularly if surgery is planned, your veterinarian may recommend tests to assess the blood's ability to clot, because the proteins that control blood clotting tend to be lost along with albumin. Any fluid retrieved from the abdomen and chest may be sent for analysis. Some forms of PLE, particularly lymphangiectasia, are best diagnosed with intestinal biopsies.

TREATMENT AND FOLLOW-UP

Treatment Options

The main treatment for PLE from lymphangiectasia is to feed an extremely low-fat diet. Fat in the diet is absorbed through the lymph vessels in the gut, so feeding a low-fat diet decreases the amount of lymph that is made. If other causes of PLE, such as IBD, intestinal tumors, intestinal obstructions, or parasites, are found, treatment is directed toward the primary disease.

If fluid is present in the abdomen or chest, diuretics are often given to help remove the fluid. Large volumes of fluid are sometimes drained from the chest or abdomen with a needle or catheter. Dogs with abnormal blood clotting may be given medications to help reduce the risk of blood clots in large veins or arteries (thrombosis). Plasma transfusions may be used in some cases to replace blood-clotting proteins.

Follow-up Care

Follow-up visits and repeated testing are usually needed, with their frequency depending on the severity of the protein loss and the presence of complications, such as ascites or blood clotting problems.

Prognosis

Prognosis for dogs with PLE is variable. If a condition can be identified that is treatable and potentially curable, the prognosis is good. Examples include intestinal parasites, certain infections, and IBD. Dogs with intestinal cancer or lymphangiectasia have a poor or guarded (uncertain) prognosis. Many dogs with persistent PLE eventually die from complications such as thrombosis or severe ascites.

SPECIAL INSTRUCTIONS:

Salivary Mucocele in Dogs

Craig G. Ruaux, BVSc, PhD, DACVIM (Small Animal)

BASIC INFORMATION

Description

A salivary mucocele or sialocele is an accumulation of saliva under the skin in a sac-like swelling. Several sets of salivary glands are present on both sides of the mouth and head. Mucocele swellings are usually located under or behind the lower jaw, alongside the face, or occasionally under the tongue. When a salivary mucocele develops under the tongue, it is called a *ranula*. Salivary mucoceles arise more commonly in dogs than in cats, and the most common mucocele of the cat is the ranula.

Causes

Salivary mucoceles usually develop when saliva leaks from a salivary duct or a portion of a salivary gland. The specific cause of a salivary mucocele is often unclear. Blunt trauma (blows, automobile accidents) or penetrating trauma (bite wounds, foreign bodies) to the jaw or side of the head and face can lead to rupture of a salivary duct and leakage of saliva into the surrounding soft tissues. Rarely, gritty deposits or stones composed of saliva and minerals, called *sialoliths*, obstruct a salivary duct and cause it to rupture.

When saliva leaks into the soft tissues, it stimulates a strong inflammatory reaction. This reaction can lead to scar tissue formation, which further obstructs the salivary duct and worsens leakage of saliva. Eventually, a sac-like structure forms that keeps the saliva collected in one area.

Clinical Signs

Salivary mucoceles vary in their appearance, size, and texture. They may be soft, flabby, and nonpainful or large, firm, and painful. In dogs, the most common locations are under the lower jaw or on the side of the head, behind the jaw. When a ranula forms, a reddish fluid-filled swelling can be seen, usually on one side, under the base of the tongue. Ranulas can interfere with eating, and the animal may drool excessively or have foul breath. If the salivary gland under the eye is affected, the eye may protrude on that side and/or a soft swelling may be seen below the eye.

Diagnostic Tests

The diagnosis of a salivary mucocele or ranula is often suspected based on the appearance and location of the swelling. Aspiration of the swelling using a small needle and syringe reveals fluid that contains saliva and mucoid material. Evacuation of fluid and collapse of the swelling helps to rule out tumors of the salivary glands, which may occur in the same locations but are usually solid.

In many cases, the salivary gland that is affected is obvious from the location of the swelling, but with some large mucoceles (except for ranulas) it can be hard to tell which gland is involved. A number of techniques can be used to identify the gland, including the following:

- Plain x-rays may be taken to search for sialoliths.
- A special x-ray procedure called *sialography* may be performed. A liquid that shows up white on x-rays is injected into the salivary duct that is believed to be involved, in order to determine if the duct is leaking or obstructed.
- Advanced imaging, such as computed tomography (CT scan) or magnetic resonance imaging (MRI), often identifies the gland involved.
- The mucocele can be surgically explored and the leakage traced back to its origin.

Your veterinarian may be able to perform some of these procedures and may recommend referral to a veterinary specialty practice or institution for the others.

TREATMENT AND FOLLOW-UP

Treatment Options

In some cases, surgery to drain the saliva and mucus is all that is necessary. Some mucoceles recur after drainage, and surgical removal of the entire affected salivary gland, with the mucocele, must be performed. Depending on the gland in question, referral to a veterinary surgery specialist may be recommended, because some of the salivary glands are very close to important blood vessels and nerves, and the surgery can be very intricate.

Follow-up Care

Postoperative follow-up is usually scheduled 7-14 days after surgery for removal of sutures. If simple drainage was the only procedure performed, further recheck visits may be needed to monitor for recurrence. In these instances, notify your veterinarian if the swelling recurs.

Prognosis

Prognosis for most salivary mucoceles is good, although recurrence is possible if the gland is not removed with the mucocele. Surgical removal of the entire affected salivary gland, while invasive, has an extremely good chance of a complete cure. Salivary mucoceles are not immediately life-threatening, but they may become painful and disfiguring if not treated appropriately.

SPECIAL INSTRUCTIONS:

SECTION 6

Endocrine System

Section Editor: Rhea V. Morgan, DVM, DACVIM (Small Animal), DACVO

Diabetes Insipidus
Diabetes Mellitus in Cats
Diabetes Mellitus in Dogs
Hyperadrenocorticism (Cushing's Disease) in Dogs
Hypercalcemia

Hyperlipidemia
Hyperthyroidism in Cats
Hypoadrenocorticism (Addison's Disease)
Hypoglycemia
Hypothyroidism in Dogs

Diabetes Insipidus

Rhea V. Morgan, DVM, DACVIM (Small Animal), DACVO

BASIC INFORMATION

Description

Diabetes insipidus (DI) is also called *water diabetes,* because it is characterized by excessive drinking and urination. It is a separate disease from sugar diabetes. There are two major forms of diabetes insipidus, and both conditions are uncommon:

- Central DI arises from decreased output of vasopressin (antidiuretic hormone) in the brain. Vasopressin acts on the kidneys to increase the concentration of the urine (that is, to decrease its water content).
- Nephrogenic DI arises when the kidneys do not respond to vasopressin hormone.

Causes

Central DI may occur as a congenital defect (rare and present at birth) or may arise following infections, inflammation, trauma, or tumors of the brain.

Nephrogenic DI may also rarely occur as a congenital defect. More often, the nephrogenic form develops after an infection of the kidneys or uterus or as a consequence of chronic renal failure. It may also develop with certain metabolic problems, such as high calcium and low potassium levels, hyperadrenocorticism (too much circulating cortisone hormone in the body), and hyperthyroidism (high thyroid hormone levels). Certain drugs may also cause nephrogenic DI.

Clinical Signs

The main signs of DI are dramatic thirst and the passage of very dilute (watery, light-colored) urine. Thirst can be so severe that the animal may seek out water from unusual places, such as toilets or ponds. Increased frequency of urination is usually noted. Urinary accidents in the house are common in dogs that do not have ready access to the out-of-doors. Weight loss, decreased appetite, and neurologic signs are sometimes seen.

Diagnostic Tests

- Urine is very dilute or watery and almost clear in color.
- Other routine laboratory tests are often normal in cases of central DI. Kidney tests, urine cultures, and other tests may be abnormal

in cases of nephrogenic DI. It is often necessary for a number of laboratory tests to be run to search for the cause of DI and to rule out other causes of increased thirst and urination.

- Specific tests that may be used to diagnose (confirm the presence of) the disease include a water deprivation test and administration of manufactured vasopressin.
- The water deprivation test involves careful withdrawal of water to determine whether the urine becomes concentrated. There are several techniques for performing this test; some require hospitalization, and all must be done with careful monitoring for dehydration and kidney problems.
- The vasopressin test involves giving the hormone and then monitoring the kidneys' response to it. There are also several ways to perform this test.

TREATMENT AND FOLLOW-UP

Treatment Options

Treatment of central DI involves giving vasopressin hormone. The hormone is currently available as eye drops and in pill form; nasal drops have been available in the past. The hormone is expensive and often must be given twice daily.

Nephrogenic DI is difficult to treat because there are no direct remedies available. Certain diuretics sometime help the symptoms of nephrogenic DI.

With both conditions, the animal must be allowed unlimited access to water, or severe dehydration and kidney failure may occur.

Follow-up Care

Close monitoring of water consumption and urine concentration are required while medication dosages are being adjusted.

Prognosis

The prognosis is variable, depending on the underlying cause and form of the disease. If the response to vasopressin is good, then it can be used long term. The disease is usually irreversible.

SPECIAL INSTRUCTIONS:

Diabetes Mellitus in Cats

Rhea V. Morgan, DVM, DACVIM (Small Animal), DACVO

BASIC INFORMATION

Description

Diabetes mellitus (DM) is also known as sugar diabetes. The word *mellitus* means "sweet" and refers to the increased blood and urine sugar levels that occur with this disease. DM arises when the pancreas gland does not produce enough insulin. Insulin is the hormone that allows many tissues of the body to utilize blood sugar (glucose). As insulin levels falls, blood sugar becomes elevated, producing many adverse side effects in the body.

Causes

The most common cause of DM in the cat is the destruction of beta cells in the pancreas. Beta cells are responsible for insulin production. This destruction often arises from chronic inflammation of the pancreas gland. This type of diabetes is known as type I DM.

Type II DM, which arises either from the development of resistance to insulin or from a decreased action of insulin within the body, is uncommon in cats.

Clinical Signs

- DM affects many different breeds and types of cats. The disease is most often seen in neutered male cats, 10 years of age or older.
- Common clinical signs include increased thirst and urination, increased appetite, and weight loss. Because glucose cannot be utilized by the body, it is almost as if the cat is starving in the midst of plenty.
- Some cats are also lethargic and weak and may walk with the hocks (ankles) of their hindlegs dropped to the floor.

Diagnostic Tests

DM is diagnosed when the fasting blood sugar concentration is significantly elevated. Cats that are stressed have the ability to temporarily raise their blood sugar to levels above normal, so repeated blood glucose tests and the testing of urine for the presence of glucose may be needed to confirm the disease.

Additional tests are often indicated to look for other diseases (such as urinary tract infection or fatty infiltration of the liver) that may accompany DM. Such tests include a complete blood count, biochemistry profile, urinalysis, urine culture, abdominal x-rays, etc.

Because older cats are also prone to hyperthyroidism (elevated production of thyroid hormone), thyroid tests may also be submitted.

TREATMENT AND FOLLOW-UP

Treatment Options

Cats with type II DM or very mild type I DM may respond to an oral medication (glipizide) that lowers blood sugar.

Most cats, however, require injections of insulin to control their disease. Several forms of insulin are available, and each has a different duration of action:

- Protamine zinc insulin (PZI) is preferred in many cats because it can often be given just once daily. It is not always readily available, however. Other types of insulin that may be tried in the cat are Ultralente and NPH insulin.
- Glargine (*Lantus*) is a new sustained-release insulin that has been tried in small numbers of cats, using a once- or twice-daily dosing schedule. Until more cats are treated with this insulin, initial dosing can be tricky.
- Vanadium, an oral supplement, is occasionally given to cats that require large doses of insulin, in an attempt to lower the amount of insulin they need each day.

In addition to insulin, the diet may be changed to a low-fat, high-fiber type of diet that contains complex carbohydrates. Several such foods are available by prescription through your veterinarian. Although it is difficult to train cats to eat meals, it is best if they eat around the time the insulin injection is given.

Follow-up Care

Diabetic cats can be difficult to monitor at home because collection of their urine can be tricky, they often eat throughout the day rather than eating their meals all at one time, and they become stressed and may not eat when hospitalized.

Most monitoring is done by checking the level of glucose in small blood samples. Samples may be taken by your veterinarian at specific times during the day or throughout the day, over a prolonged period.

Monitoring may also be done at home in some instances, through pinprick sampling and testing of those samples on glucometers designed for use in diabetic people.

It is important to work closely with your veterinarian to establish a method for monitoring blood sugar and/or urine sugar while the cat is on insulin therapy.

Prognosis

The prognosis for many cats with DM is good, as long as the disease can be regulated and other ancillary problems can be controlled or resolved.

Successful treatment of this disease requires that the owner learn to give injections, become familiar with the signs of insulin overdosage and underdosage, and learn how to adjust insulin dosages.

With dedication on the part of the owner, many diabetic cats live active, normal lives for many years.

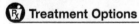

SPECIAL INSTRUCTIONS:

Diabetes Mellitus in Dogs

Rhea V. Morgan, DVM, DACVIM (Small Animal), DACVO

BASIC INFORMATION

Description

Diabetes mellitus (DM) is also known as sugar diabetes because of the increased blood and urine sugar levels that occur with this disease. DM arises when the pancreas gland does not produce enough insulin. Insulin is the hormone that allows many tissues of the body to utilize blood sugar (glucose). As insulin levels falls, blood sugar becomes elevated, producing many adverse side effects in the body.

Causes

The most common cause of DM in the dog is the destruction of beta cells in the pancreas. Beta cells are responsible for insulin production. This destruction often arises from chronic inflammation of the pancreas gland. This type of diabetes is known as type I DM.

In the keeshond breed, type I DM is an autosomal recessive trait in which one abnormal gene is inherited from each parent.

Type II DM, which arises either from the development of resistance to insulin or from a decreased action of insulin within the body, is rare in dogs.

Clinical Signs

- The miniature schnauzer, miniature poodle, toy poodle, Samoyed, and pug are at increased risk. The usual age at onset is 7-9 years. Females develop DM more often than males.
- Common clinical signs include increased thirst and urination, increased appetite, and weight loss. Because glucose cannot be utilized by the body, weight loss occurs even with more food intake.
- Some dogs may develop cataracts very suddenly and go blind.
- A severe form of complicated DM called *diabetic ketoacidosis* may cause the animal to become terribly ill, with vomiting, depression, weakness, dehydration, and rapid breathing.

Diagnostic Tests

DM is diagnosed when the fasting blood sugar concentration is significantly elevated. A urinalysis may also show sugar (glucose) and ketones in the urine.

Additional tests are often indicated to look for other diseases (such as urinary tract infection or inflammation of the pancreas) that may accompany DM. Such tests include a complete blood count, biochemistry profile, urinalysis, urine culture, abdominal x-rays, etc. If Cushing's disease (overactivity of the adrenal glands) is also suspected, hormonal tests may be performed.

TREATMENT AND FOLLOW-UP

Treatment Options

Most dogs with DM require injectable insulin to control their disease. Insulin comes in three forms: short-acting (regular insulin—*Humulin R, Novolin R*), intermediate-acting (NPH or PZI—*Humulin N, Novolin N, Vetsulin, Caninsulin, PZI Vet*), and long-acting (glargine—*Lantus*). Regular insulin is used most often for diabetic ketoacidosis. Twice-daily injections are needed by most dogs, even when the longer-acting insulins are given.

In addition to insulin, the diet may be changed to a low-fat, high-fiber type of food that contains complex carbohydrates. Several such foods are available by prescription through your veterinarian. Exercise and activity levels are often regulated so that they do not fluctuate widely from day to day.

Dogs with diabetes ketoacidosis usually require hospitalization with administration of intravenous fluids, multiple injections of regular insulin, and frequent monitoring of blood sugar.

Because other hormones effect DM, intact female dogs should be spayed, and other hormonal abnormalities (Cushing's disease, hypothyroidism) should be corrected. Dogs with cataracts must have their DM well regulated prior to surgery.

Follow-up Care

Monitoring is extremely important to keep the blood sugar within the desired range. Too much insulin or too little food intake (poor appetite, vomiting) may result in hypoglycemia (low blood sugar). Too little insulin results in persistently high blood sugar that may lead to ketoacidosis.

Home monitoring often involves keeping track of water intake and the frequency of urinations, checking urine for sugar and ketones, using a glucometer and pricking the skin or the ear to measure blood sugar, and monitoring appetite and food intake.

In-clinic monitoring involves checking blood sugar, possibly as a glucose curve. A glucose curve is produced by measuring blood sugar several times over the course of the day, after insulin is administered and the dog is fed as usual. Other laboratory tests may be repeated to ensure that the complications of DM are resolving.

Sometimes glucose curves can be obtained at home with the use of a glucometer or a continuous, subcutaneous device.

Based on test results, the dose of insulin is adjusted. It is increased when blood sugar is high and decreased when blood sugar is low.

Prognosis

DM can be challenging to regulate and may require patience and persistence, but it can be successfully managed in most dogs. It is necessary for owners to educate themselves about the disease and to remain in close contact with their veterinarian. Most dogs readily accept the injections and the necessary monitoring.

SPECIAL INSTRUCTIONS:

Hyperadrenocorticism (Cushing's Disease) in Dogs

Rhea V. Morgan, DVM, DACVIM (Small Animal), DACVO

BASIC INFORMATION
Description

Hyperadrenocorticism arises from overproduction of glucocorticoid hormones by one or both adrenal glands (Cushing's disease) or from chronic or excessive administration of steroid medications (Cushing's syndrome). In atypical cases, other adrenal hormones, such as sex hormones, may also be elevated.

Causes

Pituitary-dependent hyperadrenocorticism (PDH) develops when a tumor of the pituitary gland produces high levels of adrenocorticotropic hormone (ACTH), which subsequently causes the adrenal glands to become overactive. PDH is the most common cause (85%) of Cushing's disease in the dog. Most pituitary tumors are small (microadenoma) and do not cause neurologic signs, but large tumors (macroadenoma) occur in about 30% of affected dogs. Since ACTH influences both adrenal glands, both glands are usually enlarged with this form of the disease.

Adrenal tumors occur in 15% of affected dogs, and about half of these tumors are malignant. Often, only one adrenal gland is affected and enlarged.

Iatrogenic hyperadrenocorticism arises from prolonged or excessive administration of glucocorticoid medications (such as prednisone, dexamethasone, hydrocortisone, triamcinolone, or methylprednisone). Since the pituitary gland constantly detects high levels of steroids in the blood, it decreases the production of ACTH, which causes both adrenal glands to shrink.

📋 Clinical Signs

Most affected dogs are middle-aged or older. The miniature poodle, dachshund, boxer, Boston terrier, and beagle are predisposed to the disease. Adrenal tumors occur more often in female, large-breed dogs. Common clinical signs include the following:

- Increased thirst, urination, appetite
- Obesity ("pot belly" appearance), lethargy, muscle weakness
- Symmetrical thinning or loss of hair coat, especially on the trunk
- Thinning or darkening of the skin, skin that bruises easily
- Panting, heat intolerance
- Urinary tract and skin infections

Less common clinical signs include hypertension and hemorrhages within the eyes, infertility, congestive heart failure, acute breathing problems from blood clots in the lungs, and ruptured ligaments in the knees.

🔬 Diagnostic Tests

Cushing's syndrome is usually suspected based on a history of prolonged exposure to steroid medications and can be confirmed through laboratory evidence of low adrenal gland function (low cortisol levels and poor response to an ACTH stimulation test).

The diagnosis of Cushing's disease requires laboratory and other testing, because no clinical sign is specific for the disease. Routine tests may show elevations in liver enzymes, cholesterol, blood sugar, and white blood cells. Urinalysis and urine culture may indicate infection.

Several *screening tests* are available that involve measurement of cortisol hormone levels in the blood. They include the low-dose dexamethasone test, ACTH response test, urine cortisol/creatinine ratio, and the modified high-dose dexamethasone test. Most of these tests require blood samples to be taken at timed intervals.

Once the diagnosis of Cushing's disease is tentatively made, it is necessary to determine what type (PDH or adrenal tumor) is present. Tests that help differentiate these two conditions are the high-dose dexamethasone test, measurement of blood ACTH, abdominal x-rays, ultrasound of the adrenal glands, and advanced imaging of the pituitary gland.

Cushing's disease can be difficult to diagnose, because test results may not be clear-cut. Multiple tests or repeated testing may be needed to achieve a diagnosis.

TREATMENT AND FOLLOW-UP

℞ Treatment Options

Cushing's syndrome is treated by slow, tapered withdrawal of steroid medications. Rapid withdrawal of drugs should not be done, because it takes some time for the adrenal glands to start producing hormones again. Acute hypoadrenocorticism can occur if steroids are withdrawn suddenly.

PDH is most often treated with medications, namely mitotane (*Lysodren*) or trilostane. Ketoconazole and L-deprenyl may be used in certain circumstances but are often less effective. Radiation therapy of some pituitary tumors may also be considered.

Adrenal tumors may be treated by surgical removal, or medical therapy with mitotane or trilostane may be tried. Surgery is most successful when only one adrenal gland is involved and the tumor has not invaded the surrounding aorta or renal blood vessels. Postoperative care is challenging because the other adrenal gland is often not capable of secreting normal levels of hormone for some time. Malignant tumors may also metastasize to other locations in the body.

🐾 Follow-up Care

Treatment of this disorder is complicated and requires frequent adjustment of drug dosages and repeated laboratory testing, which can be expensive. In addition, the drugs are potentially toxic, and the effects of mitotane persist for several days even after it is terminated. A thorough understanding of the effects and side effects of these drugs is crucial.

Prognosis

Although most animals with PDH improve with therapy, not all clinical abnormalities are reversible, and the disease may shorten the dog's overall life span.

SPECIAL INSTRUCTIONS:

Hypercalcemia

Rhea V. Morgan, DVM, DACVIM (Small Animal), DACVO

BASIC INFORMATION

Description

Hypercalcemia is higher-than-normal blood calcium levels.

Causes

The most common cause in animals is cancer:

- *Hyperparathyroidism* is overproduction of parathormone (PTH) by the parathyroid gland. PTH increases calcium in the blood. A common cause is a benign tumor (adenoma) of the parathyroid gland. Older animals are usually affected, with an average age of 11 years in dogs and 13 years in cats. The keeshond and Siamese breeds are prone to this disease.
- *Lymphoma,* a malignancy of white blood cells, may cause hypercalcemia by production of PTH-like substances.
- *Other tumors,* especially in dogs, can also cause hypercalcemia. Examples in dogs include tumors of the anal sac, thymus, pancreas, stomach, bone, mammary glands, nose, and multiple myeloma, among others. Examples in cats include squamous cell carcinoma and certain leukemias.

Hypercalcemia can be a complication of *hypoadrenocorticism* (low levels of cortisol hormone).

Other causes include *vitamin D overdosage* through accidental ingestion of synthetic vitamin D3 drugs, such as calcipotriene (Dovonex), calcitriol (Rocaltrol), or calcipotriol (Calcijex), or ingestion of cholecalciferol rodenticides such as Quintox, Rampage, Ceva True Grit, or Orthos Mouse-B-Gone.

Occasionally, *kidney disease* and *certain inflammatory conditions* are also causes.

Clinical Signs

Signs are often vague and may pertain to the underlying cause. Increased thirst and urination, decreased appetite, vomiting, constipation, lethargy, weakness, and weight loss may occur. Because a high circulating calcium concentration is toxic to the kidneys, renal failure may occur. Kidney and bladder stones develop in one third of animals with hyperparathyroidism. Severe hypercalcemia may cause neurologic signs, such as muscle twitching, seizures, and coma, as well as alterations in heart rhythm.

Diagnostic Tests

Accidental vitamin D overdosage may be suspected based on the history of ingestion of certain drugs or mice or rat poisons.

In all other cases, a thorough search for the underlying cause is needed. First, the calcium test is often repeated to make sure the result is reliable, or a different (ionized) calcium test is performed. Subsequent tests may include routine blood tests, urinalysis and urine culture, measurement of PTH and adrenal hormones (cortisol), specialized serum protein tests if myeloma is suspected, chest and abdominal x-rays, abdominal ultrasound, aspiration or biopsy of any masses or of the bone marrow, and, occasionally, measurement of serum vitamin D levels. Surgery of the neck to assess the parathyroid glands may be required in some cases of suspected hyperparathyroidism.

The cause of hypercalcemia can be very difficult to determine in certain cases of cancer, because the tumor can be quite small and still cause serious hypercalcemia.

TREATMENT AND FOLLOW-UP

Treatment Options

Immediate lowering of blood calcium is important to minimize kidney damage.

- Encouraging removal of calcium through the urine is done by administration of intravenous (IV) saline and diuretic medications (such as furosemide or thiazides). In emergency situations, IV biphosphonate and calcitonin medications may be tried in dogs but may not be readily available. Oral phosphate binders (*Amphojel*) may lower the blood phosphorus concentration, which helps prevent calcification of soft tissues in the body.
- Once the diagnosis is achieved, prednisone (a steroid medication) may help lower blood calcium. It is initially avoided in cases of suspected tumors, because it can make some tumors (such as lymphoma, leukemia, or myeloma) more difficult to find.

Once the underlying cause is determined, specific treatment is undertaken:

- Surgery is needed to remove most parathyroid tumors.
- Chemotherapy is the treatment of choice for lymphoma, multiple myeloma, and leukemia.
- Surgery, chemotherapy, and/or radiation therapy may be needed for other tumors.
- See the handout on **Hypoadrenocorticism (Addison's Disease)** for treatment options.
- Cases of vitamin D and cholecalciferol rodenticide toxicosis are treated with calcium-lowering therapies and supportive care.

Supportive care involves use of agents to decrease nausea and protect the stomach, such as sucralfate, famotidine, or other antacids. Treatment for kidney failure may also be needed.

Follow-up Care

Blood calcium and kidney assays are repeated frequently until there is evidence of improvement and then periodically. Other monitoring and recheck visits depend on the underlying cause and its treatment, as well as the degree of damage done to the kidneys. Postoperative monitoring of the blood calcium concentration is important for several days after parathyroid surgery.

Prognosis

Prognosis for animals with cancer depends on whether the tumor can be effectively treated and whether the hypercalcemia has caused kidney damage. Prognosis is very poor in animals with renal failure, regardless of the underlying cause. Prognosis is good for animals with benign parathyroid tumors if the kidneys are healthy.

SPECIAL INSTRUCTIONS:

Hyperlipidemia

Rhea V. Morgan, DVM, DACVIM (Small Animal), DACVO

BASIC INFORMATION
Description
Hyperlipidemia refers to increased circulating fat (lipids) in the blood. It may involve high levels of triglyceride, cholesterol, or lipoproteins. *Lipemia* is a white discoloration of the blood serum caused by circulating lipids.

Causes
Hyperlipidemia is common after eating but should diminish within 12 hours. This form of lipemia is considered normal. Mild elevations in cholesterol may occur in animals on high-fat diets. Persistent hyperlipidemia is abnormal and may be primary or secondary.
* Primary hyperlipidemia is usually an inherited disorder of triglyceride and lipoproteins (miniature schnauzers), cholesterol (briard, rough collie) or chylomicrons (domestic cats). The exact genetic defect that causes abnormal lipid levels in these animals has not been defined in most breeds.
* Secondary hyperlipidemia develops as a complication of some other disease, such as hypothyroidism, diabetes mellitus (sugar diabetes), pancreatitis, hyperadrenocorticism, liver disease, and certain forms of kidney disease (nephrotic syndrome). It may also arise with use of glucocorticoid (steroid) or progestogen (especially megestrol acetate in cats) medications.

Clinical Signs
Signs of primary hyperlipidemia are quite variable:
* Miniature schnauzers may be normal or have abdominal discomfort, gastrointestinal signs, and increased thirst. Pancreatitis may develop more easily in these dogs.
* Most briards and collies act normal and have few clinical changes.
* Animals with inherited hyperchylomicronemia develop lipid deposits in abnormal locations, such as the skin, eye, and other soft tissues, or they may develop fatty tumors (xanthomas).

Signs of secondary hyperlipidemia are often vague but can include abdominal pain, vomiting and diarrhea, decreased appetite, and deposition of lipid in abnormal locations or organs. Occasionally, seizures may occur. Elevated cholesterol may lead to atherosclerosis (hardening of the arteries), which can affect the heart and blood pressure.

Diagnostic Tests
Blood samples taken after an animal has eaten are often lipemic and may have elevations in triglyceride and cholesterol. These changes should diminish or disappear in samples taken after a 12-hour fast. Persistent elevations warrant close scrutiny of the dietary fat content or testing for the causes of secondary hyperlipidemia. Tests for secondary hyperlipidemia may include routine blood tests, urinalysis, tests for pancreas function, hormonal assays, specialized kidney and liver function tests, abdominal x-rays, and ultrasound studies.

Primary hyperlipidemia is diagnosed when all of the causes of secondary hyperlipidemia have been ruled out. Other blood tests may be run to identify which specific lipids are elevated.

TREATMENT AND FOLLOW-UP
Treatment Options
For secondary hyperlipidemia, treatment is directed at the underlying cause, and a low-fat food is started. Treatment of primary hyperlipidemia is indicated when it is associated with clinical signs and mainly involves feeding a low-fat diet. Several commercial diets are available for both dogs and cats that are low in fat. Some of these are prescription diets and available only through veterinarians.

Drugs that lower cholesterol and triglyceride have not been studied much in dogs and cats and are not recommended at this time because of their potential side effects. Fish oil supplements are considered safe, but their benefit in treating hyperlipidemia remains to be determined.

Follow-up Care
Fasting blood lipid tests are usually repeated 4-6 weeks after changing the diet or starting therapy for an underlying disease and then repeated periodically. Other monitoring is based on the underlying condition.

Prognosis
Secondary hyperlipidemia often resolves with successful treatment or correction of the original problem. Primary hyperlipidemia is more difficult to treat but does not usually become a serious, life-threatening problem.

SPECIAL INSTRUCTIONS:

Hyperthyroidism in Cats

Rhea V. Morgan, DVM, DACVIM (Small Animal), DACVO

BASIC INFORMATION

Description

Hyperthyroidism is an excess of circulating thyroid hormones. It results in a high metabolic state, which causes changes in many different body organs.

Causes

In most cats, the cause of this disorder is unknown. It may be related to environmental, nutritional, or other factors.

There are two thyroid glands, one on either side of the larynx (voice box). In about 70% of affected cats, both glands become overactive and enlarged. In about 10%, one or both thyroid glands may form a benign tumor (adenoma). In 1-2%, a malignant tumor (carcinoma) develops.

Clinical Signs

Most cats are middle-aged (average age at onset, 12-13 years). Signs are often gradual in onset, become more severe over time, and include:

* Weight loss, muscle wasting, decreased ability to jump onto objects
* Increased appetite
* Vomiting
* Increased thirst and urination
* Nervousness, hyperactivity, increased vocalization

Less commonly, diarrhea, weakness, lethargy, intolerance to heat or stress, panting, loss of appetite, and sudden blindness from hypertension-induced retinal detachments may occur.

Physical examination may reveal a palpably enlarged thyroid gland or glands, thin body condition, heart murmur or irregular heartbeat or both, high heart rate, excessive shedding and matting, or poor quality hair coat. Muscle weakness, abnormal gait, retinal hemorrhages or detached retinas, apathy, and dehydration may also be noted.

Diagnostic Tests

Hyperthyroidism is diagnosed by measurement of a thyroid hormone (T4) in the blood.

* Circulating T4 is increased in 95% of affected cats.
* T4 may be falsely low or normal in cats with other illnesses, so the diagnosis can be difficult to make. Repeat measurement of T4, measurement of other thyroid hormones, or other tests on the thyroid glands may be needed to reach a diagnosis.

Routine laboratory tests may reveal alterations in white blood cell count, elevated liver tests, and low potassium concentration. Laboratory tests may also show the presence of kidney disease, which is common in older cats. Chest x-rays, an electrocardiogram (ECG), and an echocardiogram (heart ultrasound) may be needed to evaluate heart function. Blood pressure measurement may be done to check for hypertension (elevated blood pressure).

TREATMENT AND FOLLOW-UP

Treatment Options

Several options exist, including medical therapy, surgery, radiation therapy with radioactive iodine, and injection of the thyroid gland with ethanol.

* The most common medication used is methimazole, which comes in pill form or can be compounded into a paste to apply to the ear. It is given once or twice daily and can be given in the presence of kidney disease. Periodic monitoring is needed to adjust the dosage and to detect side effects. Side effects are most common in the first several months of treatment and include loss of appetite, vomiting, facial sores, low white blood cell or platelet counts, and liver problems.
* Surgery involves removal of one or both thyroid glands. Thyroid glands that have migrated to other areas of the neck or are in the chest can be difficult to find. Because the parathyroid glands lie on the surface of the thyroid glands, they may also be removed, which can cause some problems in the days following surgery. Poor kidney function may also show up after surgery with a return to normal fluid circulation.
* Radioactive iodine (I-131) can be used if kidney function is normal. The iodine is given once by injection, and the cat is hospitalized until it has been cleared in the urine. It is generally easy on the cat but is less available and more expensive than other treatments.
* Destruction of the thyroid gland by injection of ethanol is done under ultrasound guidance by a radiologist experienced in the technique. Potential side effects include damage to the nerves near the thyroid gland.

Follow-up Care

Routine laboratory and T4 assays are done after many of the treatments and are repeated periodically for cats on medical therapy. Post-treatment problems, such as low calcium after surgery or hypothyroidism (very low T4) and secondary heart changes, may also require medication.

Prognosis

Most clinical signs improve with treatment, but some heart and eye changes can be permanent. Cats with kidney disease and hyperthyroidism tend to be more difficult to manage.

SPECIAL INSTRUCTIONS:

Hypoadrenocorticism (Addison's Disease)

Rhea V. Morgan, DVM, DACVIM (Small Animal), DACVO

BASIC INFORMATION

Description

Hypoadrenocorticism (Addison's disease) arises from decreased secretion of hormones by the adrenal gland. The adrenal gland makes several types of hormones, and usually mineralocorticoid and glucocorticoid hormones are both decreased. In atypical Addison's disease, only glucocorticoids are diminished.

Causes

Primary hypoadrenocorticism may develop when the adrenal glands are attacked by the immune system. The triggering event for this problem is unknown. Lymphoma may cause hypoadrenocorticism in the cat. Prolonged administration of steroid medications, brain tumors and trauma, and congenital defects of the pituitary gland may cause *secondary hypoadrenocorticism*. The pituitary gland is responsible for secreting the hormone that activates the adrenal gland (adrenocorticotropic hormone [ACTH]), and ACTH falls in all of these latter conditions.

Clinical Signs

Hypoadrenocorticism occurs most often in young, female dogs of many different breeds. Certain families of Leonbergers and standard poodles may be affected. The disease can occur in young cats of any breed or gender.

Clinical signs include intermittent vomiting, diarrhea, decreased appetite, weight loss, and sometimes dark, bloody diarrhea. Lethargy, depression, and weakness are also common. Sometimes hair loss and increased thirst and urination occur.

In some animals, signs wax and wane; in others, an acute crisis develops, with the animal showing signs of collapse, dehydration, and shock. Although pulses can be weak, the heart rate may remain slow because of high blood levels of potassium.

Diagnostic Tests

The diagnosis often requires laboratory testing, because no clinical sign is specific for Addison's disease:

• A blood count may reveal anemia and elevated white blood cells.
• Classic findings on a chemistry profile of the blood include low sodium, high potassium, low chloride, and sometimes high calcium levels. Animals with atypical Addison's disease do not have these blood abnormalities, because they are caused by a mineralocorticoid deficit. Low blood sugar can also occur during shock.
• An ACTH response test shows abnormally low blood cortisol levels and confirms the diagnosis.

• With primary hypoadrenocorticism, the circulating ACTH level in the blood is high; with secondary hypoadrenocorticism, it is low.

Other tests that may be run, depending on the presenting clinical signs, include chest and abdominal x-rays, an electrocardiogram (ECG), a urinalysis, abdominal ultrasound, and fecal examination.

TREATMENT AND FOLLOW-UP

Treatment Options

Animals in an acute crisis require hospitalization for intravenous fluids, injectable steroids, and medications to lower blood potassium levels. Shock must be treated aggressively, and blood or plasma transfusions may be required if the animal is hemorrhaging into the gut. The acute crisis can be life-threatening and reversed only through intensive care.

For most dogs with hypoadrenocorticism, lifelong supplementation with mineralocorticoids is needed. This may involve administration of oral fludrocortisone (usually once daily) or injections of desoxycorticosterone pivalate (DOCP) every 25-40 days. Oral glucocorticoids (steroids such as prednisone or dexamethasone) are also given for life. For dogs with atypical Addison's disease, only glucocorticoids may be required.

Cats with hypoadrenocorticism are often treated with DOCP every 3-4 weeks and with either oral or injectable steroid medications.

Follow-up Care

During an acute crisis, intensive monitoring with repeated blood tests is often needed to ensure that all laboratory abnormalities are resolving. Frequent rechecks and blood tests are needed in newly diagnosed patients until correct dosages of medications are determined. Once regulated, periodic rechecks are performed usually for the rest of the animal's life. Blood potassium levels may remain a little elevated, even with adequate treatment.

Prognosis

If the animal survives an acute crisis, then the disease is often very manageable. Treatment of the disease can be rewarding, because most animals respond well to the medications. Because adrenal gland hormones help to combat stress, however, affected animals often do not handle physical stresses very well. During periods of stress (such as surgery or other illnesses), extra steroid supplementation may be needed, and close monitoring for signs of relapse is important.

SPECIAL INSTRUCTIONS:

Hypoglycemia

Rhea V. Morgan, DVM, DACVIM (Small Animal), DACVO

BASIC INFORMATION
Description
Hypoglycemia refers to a low concentration of glucose (sugar) in the blood or serum.
Causes
Hypoglycemia has many different causes.
- Neonatal and juvenile hypoglycemia. Puppies and kittens, as well as toy-breed dogs, have inadequate stores of glycogen (which can be converted to glucose) in the liver. They also may have physical problems that make it hard for them to maintain normal blood sugar, such as poor nutrition, diarrhea, intestinal parasites, or hypothermia.
- Overdosage of insulin in diabetic animals
- Ingestion of hypoglycemic drugs or agents. In cats, this may involve overdosage with glipizide or glyburide. In dogs, ingestion of xylitol in sugar-free gum can cause hypoglycemia.
- Hypoadrenocorticism (low levels of cortisol hormone)
- Insulinoma (a tumor of the cells of the pancreas that secrete insulin)
- Other malignant tumors. Some tumors have the ability to secrete substances that act like insulin. Examples include malignant tumors of the liver, kidneys, and fat cells.
- Liver failure
- Overwhelming infection (sepsis)
- Exertional hypoglycemia. Hypoglycemia may develop in hunting, sled-dog, and other breeds under extreme working conditions. It arises from depletion of stored glycogen in the liver and increased demand for blood sugar.
- Inherited glycogen storage diseases, which are congenital defects that affect normal liver function. They have been documented in the Norwegian forest cat, Akita, English springer spaniel, German shepherd dog, Lapland (Swedish Lapphund), and others.

Clinical Signs

Signs are often neurologic in nature, with the severity proportional to how fast, how long, and how low the blood sugar drops. Mild signs include weakness, tremors, increased appetite, mental dullness, and bizarre behavior. Serious signs include collapse, seizures, stupor or coma (unconscious), and blindness.

Diagnostic Tests

Because glucose assays can be affected by the storage of samples and other factors, the test is often repeated if it is initially low. Repeated evidence of low blood sugar confirms the presence of hypoglycemia.

In some cases, the origin of the low blood sugar is suspected based on the animal's age, size, and circumstances (such as a puppy that became hypothermic during shipping, a hunting dog that collapsed at the end of the day, a dog seen swallowing a pack of sugar-free gum, or a diabetic cat that did not eat breakfast after insulin was given).

In other cases, the cause is not obvious, and an exhaustive search must be undertaken to find the origin. Such tests include a blood count, biochemistry profile, insulin assays, chest and abdominal x-rays, abdominal ultrasound, specialized tests for liver and adrenal function, aspiration or biopsy of any masses found, and surgical exploration of the abdomen (especially for a suspected insulinoma).

TREATMENT AND FOLLOW-UP

Treatment Options

Symptomatic treatment of low blood sugar is important. If the animal is conscious, it can be offered food. If the animal is unconscious, intravenous glucose is given. Intravenous fluids and antiseizure drugs may be needed for animals that do not respond to glucose alone. Maintenance of body temperature and supportive care are given until the animal recovers.

Specific treatment is started once the underlying cause is determined:
- Frequent feedings may prevent neonatal, juvenile, and exertional hypoglycemia.
- Continuous or intermittent oral or injectable glucose is given for ingestion of hypoglycemic agents, insulin overdosage, sepsis, or liver failure.
- Treatment of insulinoma and other tumors may involve surgical removal. Oral diazoxide is used in some cases of insulinoma, because it helps maintain blood sugar levels.
- Steroids such as prednisone may be helpful in cases of hypoadrenocorticism, insulinoma, or other tumors.
- No effective therapy has been developed for glycogen storage diseases.

Follow-up Care

Blood glucose assays are repeated until the animal and glucose blood levels have returned to normal. Other vital signs are monitored frequently in animals with seizures. Following insulinoma surgery, blood sugar may rise dramatically and may require transient insulin injections.

Prognosis

Animals with neonatal, juvenile, or exertional hypoglycemia and animals that have ingested hypoglycemic agents or received too much insulin frequently respond well to supplemental glucose. Animals with severe seizures, however, carry a poorer prognosis. Animals with insulinoma may do well following complete surgical resection, but metastasis is common within 1 year after surgery.

Prognosis for animals with other tumors depends on whether the tumor can be effectively treated. Sepsis and liver failure are both difficult to treat, and recovery from these diseases is variable. No treatment is available for inherited glycogen storage diseases, and most animals deteriorate over months. For more information on hypoadrenocorticism, see the client handout on **Hypoadrenocorticism (Addison's Disease)**.

SPECIAL INSTRUCTIONS:

Hypothyroidism in Dogs

Rhea V. Morgan, DVM, DACVIM (Small Animal), DACVO

BASIC INFORMATION
Description
Hypothyroidism develops from a decrease in circulating thyroid hormone levels in the blood. It is one of the more common hormonal problems in the dog. Because thyroid hormone is needed to maintain normal metabolism, hair growth, activity levels, reproduction, heart function, and other bodily functions, the manifestations of hypothyroidism may involve many organs.

The thyroid gland produces two hormones, T3 and T4, and both are usually low in hypothyroidism.

Causes
Primary hypothyroidism develops from inflammation of the thyroid gland, which may be caused when the body's immune system attacks the gland. Destruction and scarring of the gland may also arise from infections, tumors, or trauma.

Secondary hypothyroidism develops when the brain does not produce thyroid-releasing hormone (TRH) or thyroid-stimulating hormone (TSH, the hormone that tells the thyroid gland to make thyroid hormone).

* Congenital hypothyroidism (called *cretinism*) is very rare in the dog. Inherited goiter is also rare but can occur in toy fox terriers.
* TRH or TSH deficiency has been seen in giant schnauzers and boxers.

Hypothyroidism can also develop with use of the trimethoprim-sulfa drugs and following surgery or radiation therapy of the thyroid gland or neck region.

True hypothyroidism must be differentiated from the significant and temporary effects that other diseases and certain drugs can have on thyroid hormone levels. In this instance, hormone levels fall during the illness or while the drug is being given, and they usually return to normal after the illness has subsided and the drugs are withdrawn.

Clinical Signs
Most dogs are middle-aged, and spayed females and castrated males may be affected more often than others. The disease is common in golden retrievers, Doberman pinschers, and certain other breeds. Signs are often gradual in onset and can be quite variable and include the following:

* Dermatologic signs: symmetrical hair loss, dull and poor-quality coat, seborrhea
* Metabolic signs: lethargy, seeks warm areas, weight gain and obesity, inability to exercise
* Cardiovascular signs: low heart rate, atherosclerosis (hardening of the arteries)
* Neurologic signs: muscle weakness, shrinkage of muscles, paralysis of the larynx (vocal cords) resulting in breathing problems, paralysis of some nerves around the head
* Reproductive signs: infertility, abnormal or failure of heat cycles
* Cretinism: growth and mental retardation, retention of puppy coat, overly large head, skeletal dwarfism

Diagnostic Tests
Hypothyroidism is diagnosed by measuring thyroid hormone levels in the blood.

* Blood tests can be done for T3, T4, freeT4 (separation of T4 from its carrier proteins), and TSH.
* T4 testing alone is often used as a screening test and to monitor the effects of therapy. Full assays of all four hormones are needed in some animals to reach a diagnosis.

Routine laboratory tests may reveal other abnormalities, such as anemia, high cholesterol and triglyceride levels, and altered liver function. Laboratory tests are also necessary to rule out other causes of the clinical signs seen. Other tests that can be run in certain cases include thyroid antibody assays, and thyroid scans, and ultrasounds. Sometimes the diagnosis of hypothyroidism can require repeated testing, because initial results may be unclear or nondiagnostic.

TREATMENT AND FOLLOW-UP

Treatment Options
Hypothyroidism is treated by supplementation with oral L-thyroxine, the commercially available form of T4. Dosages require adjustment in each individual animal, with some dogs requiring once-daily and some twice-daily administration.

Follow-up Care
Thyroxine pills are usually given for 2-6 weeks, after which thyroid assays are repeated to determine whether the hypothyroidism has improved. T4 levels are measured at a specific time after the thyroid pill is given; your veterinarian will instruct you as to when the test should be run. Depending on the results, the dosage may be raised, lowered, or left the same. Continued, periodic monitoring of T4 is needed throughout the course of the dog's life to ensure that thyroid values remain in the normal range. Most dogs require lifelong therapy, because most thyroid glands do not recover normal function.

Prognosis
Most clinical signs begin to improve within 3-4 weeks, except for neurologic signs, which can take several months. Exercise and activity levels often improve dramatically, and appetite usually returns to normal. Many hair coat problems also resolve with time. Dogs usually do well on the thyroid supplement and go on to live normal lives.

SPECIAL INSTRUCTIONS:

SECTION 7

Urinary System

Section Editor: Cathy E. Langston, DVM, DACVIM (Small Animal)

Acute Kidney Failure
Anemia of Chronic Kidney Disease
Benign Prostatic Hypertrophy in Dogs
Bladder Cancer
Bladder Stones in Cats
Bladder Stones in Dogs
Bladder Trauma
Chronic Kidney Disease in Cats
Chronic Kidney Disease in Dogs
Cystitis in Cats
Cystitis in Dogs
Ectopic Ureter in Dogs
Fanconi Syndrome in Dogs
Kidney Dysplasia in Dogs
Kidney Stones in Cats

Kidney Toxins (Nephrotoxicosis)
Perinephric Pseudocysts in Cats
Polycystic Kidney Disease in Cats
Prostate Cancer in Dogs
Prostatic and Paraprostatic Cysts in Dogs
Prostatitis and Prostatic Abscessation in Dogs
Protein-Losing Nephropathy in Dogs
Pyelonephritis (Kidney Infection)
Renal Neoplasia
Ureteral Obstruction in Cats
Urethral Obstruction in Cats
Urethral Prolapse in Dogs
Urethritis
Urinary Incontinence in Dogs

Acute Kidney Failure

Cathy E. Langston, DVM, DACVIM (Small Animal)

BASIC INFORMATION

Description

Acute kidney or renal failure (ARF) is not a common problem in dogs and cats, but it can be devastating when it occurs. ARF ranges from a mild disease that is readily responsive to treatment to complete shutdown of the kidneys. When the kidneys fail, urea and other waste products are retained in the body (uremia) and cause the animal to become very ill.

Causes

ARF can be caused by toxins, infections, or poor blood flow to the kidneys. Common toxins include antifreeze (ethylene glycol), drugs (nonsteroidal anti-inflammatory drugs, certain antibiotics), grapes and raisins in dogs, and lily plants in cats. Bacterial infections can be a cause. Leptospirosis is a common kidney infection that affects dogs but not cats. Anything that decreases blood flow to the kidney can cause ARF, such as dehydration, low blood pressure, shock, heat prostration, and anesthesia. ARF is sometimes associated with other severe diseases in the body, such as elevated blood calcium levels, pancreatitis, and other abdominal disorders. In cats, obstruction of urinary outflow by kidney stones or scar tissue is becoming a common cause of ARF.

Clinical Signs

An abrupt increase in water intake may be one of the first signs of ARF; it is frequently associated with a poor appetite and vomiting. Diarrhea, lethargy, and depression may also occur. Signs may rapidly worsen. In severe cases, the kidneys completely shut down and stop making urine. High blood potassium levels that develop with ARF can cause the heart to slow down and stop. In other cases, the heart and respiratory rates may be high. Ulcerations may develop in the mouth, and halitosis (foul breath odor) may occur from the uremia.

Diagnostic Tests

Laboratory tests (biochemistry panel and complete blood count), urinalysis, and a urine culture are used to diagnose ARF. Evaluation of blood electrolytes is also important, because severe electrolyte problems, such as dangerously high potassium levels (hyperkalemia), can occur.

Further testing is often needed to determine the underlying cause. For example, in cats, an abdominal x-ray or ultrasound, or both, are generally helpful in determining whether a urinary obstruction is present. In dogs, a blood test for leptospirosis is usually warranted. If there is a suspicion of antifreeze ingestion, a special ethylene glycol test performed on the first day may be helpful.

Occasionally a kidney biopsy is recommended, along with tests to rule out other diseases that cause similar clinical signs.

TREATMENT AND FOLLOW-UP

Treatment Options

ARF is a serious disease that requires hospitalization in most cases. The mainstay of treatment is intravenous (IV) fluids. Careful monitoring of the patient is necessary, because the volume of urine produced can change dramatically and rapidly, leading to either dehydration or fluid retention. Diuretics, which increase the volume of urine produced, may be tried but are not always effective.

Drugs to control nausea and vomiting are usually needed. Medications may be given IV to correct severe electrolyte imbalances, such as high potassium levels and acidosis of the blood. Some patients with persistent vomiting and lack of appetite may be helped by insertion of a temporary feeding tube. Specific treatments for the underlying cause are also started. (See the handouts on **Antifreeze Poisoning**, **Leptospirosis**, and **Ureteral Obstruction in Cats**.)

If standard medical therapy is ineffective, advanced treatment options may be considered. These include hemodialysis (removal of uremic toxins by passage of the blood through a kidney dialysis machine), continuous renal replacement therapy (CRRT, a form of dialysis), or peritoneal dialysis (administration of fluids into the abdomen that absorb some of the uremic toxins, followed by removal of as much of the fluid as possible). These therapies are generally offered only by specialized hospitals, so your pet may be referred to a veterinary specialist for these treatments.

Follow-up Care

Intensive monitoring is required during hospitalization and often includes measurements of blood pressure, heart and respiratory rates, body temperature and weight, blood electrolytes, kidney function tests, and urine output. After discharge from the hospital, follow-up visits generally involve examinations and laboratory tests. If the ARF completely reverses, long-term monitoring may not be necessary, although yearly blood and urine tests are prudent.

Prognosis

ARF is a serious disease, and only about half of affected animals survive it. Patients with infections, urinary obstruction, or low blood flow as the cause tend to do better than those that developed ARF from a toxin. Of the animals that survive, about half have residual kidney damage.

SPECIAL INSTRUCTIONS:

Anemia of Chronic Kidney Disease

Cathy E. Langston, DVM, DACVIM (Small Animal)

BASIC INFORMATION

Description

Anemia is a low red blood cell (RBC) count. RBCs carry oxygen to the tissues of the body. If RBC numbers are low, body tissues may be deprived of adequate oxygen.

Causes

As RBCs age, they are taken out of circulation and replaced with new, younger RBCs. The kidneys make a hormone, erythropoietin, which stimulates the bone marrow to make these new RBCs. As the kidneys fail, they make less erythropoietin, and fewer RBCs are produced to replace the cells that are removed. This failure to replenish RBC numbers creates a slowly worsening anemia. Another cause of anemia in patients with kidney disease is a bleeding ulcer in the stomach.

Clinical Signs

Anemia often produces signs of tiredness (lethargy), weakness, fast heart rate, rapid breathing, and poor appetite. On physical examination, pale gums, a heart murmur, and weak pulses may be detected.

Diagnostic Tests

Hematocrit and packed cell volume (PCV) are very similar blood tests that measure the percentage of blood composed of RBCs. These values are low with anemia. The reticulocyte count determines the number of new RBCs being produced. This value is also typically low with anemia from chronic kidney disease. In some cases, bone marrow aspiration is recommended to rule out other causes of anemia.

TREATMENT AND FOLLOW-UP

Treatment Options

If stomach ulcers are known or suspected to be causing anemia, treatment is usually recommended with antacids, such as famotidine (*Pepcid*), and the gastric protectant, sucralfate. B vitamin supplements may help the anemia a little.

Blood transfusions immediately increase the PCV and improve signs associated with anemia. In emergency situations, transfusions are the best choice; however, transfused RBCs generally only last few weeks. To sustain an anemic animal long term would require repeated transfusions, and with each transfusion the risk of

a transfusion reaction increases, even if blood cross-match tests are performed prior to each transfusion to check for compatibility.

Commercial erythropoietin can be used to replace the natural hormone the kidneys are failing to make. Two forms are available; both are given by injection under the skin (subcutaneous). Erythropoietin (*Epogen, Procrit*) is initially given three times per week until the PCV is normal, then usually once weekly to maintain the PCV. Darbepoetin (*Aranesp*) is initially given weekly and can often be decreased to every other week.

Unfortunately, both of these hormones are made for people. Although they work in animals, the immune system of some animals can recognize them as foreign substances and form antibodies against the drugs. If this happens, the immune system inactivates the hormone that has been injected, as well as any natural hormone the kidneys may still be making. This inactivation makes the anemia worse than it was before hormone shots were started. About 20% of patients on erythropoietin and 10% on darbepoetin develop this immune reaction. Some patients can partially recover from it, but many will be dependent on blood transfusions afterward.

Because of this potential reaction, treatment with hormone shots is usually delayed until the signs of anemia are moderate to severe. Other side effects of hormone shots include high blood pressure (hypertension) and seizures. Despite the possibility of adverse effects, most patients feel much better, are more interactive, and eat more while receiving these injections.

Because RBCs contain iron, iron supplements are needed when the animal is receiving hormone shots. Oral iron pills are available, or monthly iron shots may be administered.

Follow-up Care

With hormone treatment, weekly rechecks are often scheduled that include a PCV, blood pressure measurement (if available), and reticulocyte count (ideally) until the anemia has improved. The frequency of rechecks can be gradually decreased if the anemia improves.

Prognosis

Anemia decreases the quality of life of dogs and cats with chronic kidney disease. The combined signs of chronic kidney disease and anemia may cause the animal to feel so poorly that euthanasia is considered. Successful treatment of the anemia often prolongs and improves the quality of the animal's life.

SPECIAL INSTRUCTIONS:

Benign Prostatic Hypertrophy in Dogs

Cathy E. Langston, DVM, DACVIM (Small Animal)

BASIC INFORMATION

Description

The prostate is a small gland that surrounds the beginning of the urethra. The urethra is the tube that carries urine from the bladder to the outside. The normal prostate has two lobes, one on each side of the urethra, with a small indentation between the lobes. The prostate makes fluid that is secreted into the urethra during ejaculation of semen.

Benign prostatic hypertrophy or hyperplasia (BPH) is a symmetrical enlargement of the prostate that occurs in intact (unneutered), older, male dogs. It is the most common prostatic disease of dogs.

Causes

Testosterone causes certain types of cells in the prostate to grow in number (hyperplasia) and to enlarge in size (hypertrophy). Over time, this effect causes the prostate to become enlarged (prostatomegaly). A large prostate is normal in intact male Scottish terriers and should not be confused with BPH.

Clinical Signs

Most dogs with BPH do not have any clinical signs. Some dogs may strain to defecate, because the enlarged prostate presses on the colon. Rarely, the prostatic enlargement may partially obstruct the urethra, which leads to straining during urination. Other potential signs include a yellow or bloody penile discharge that is not associated with urination and blood in the urine.

In most dog, BPH is discovered during a physical examination. An enlarged prostate can be felt by rectal palpation, but the gland is not painful or irregular.

Diagnostic Tests

An enlarged prostate can be seen on plain x-rays. An abdominal ultrasound may be recommended, because it can confirm that the internal architecture of the prostate is preserved, even though the gland is enlarged. A urinalysis and urine culture may be performed to rule out a urinary tract infection. Rarely, biopsy is needed to distinguish BPH from other causes of prostatic disease, such as prostatic infection or cancer.

TREATMENT AND FOLLOW-UP

Treatment Options

Castration is an effective treatment for BPH and is the recommended procedure. After termination of testosterone production (by removal of the testicles), the prostate typically shrinks to a normal size within 3-6 weeks. If castration is not performed, the effects of testosterone on the prostate can be blocked with the medication, finasteride (*Proscar, Propecia*). After finasteride is started, the prostate usually decreases in size by 70% within 10 weeks. If the drug is stopped, the BPH will return within 8 weeks. Finasteride can cause birth defects and should not be handled by pregnant women.

Monitoring alone may be chosen for some dogs with mild BPH and no symptoms. Despite anecdotal reports, Saw palmetto extract is not effective for treating prostate disease in dogs.

Follow-up Care

After castration surgery, the prostate is usually palpated again in 3-4 weeks to ensure that it is shrinking as expected. If the gland is not shrinking, then other diseases (such as prostatic cancer or infection) may be involved, and further testing for those diseases is often recommended. In asymptomatic dogs on no treatment, periodic examinations with rectal palpation are used to assess the prostate.

Prognosis

BPH is a benign disease, but it predisposes the dog to prostatic infections if left untreated. Prognosis is excellent with castration, because the surgery usually cures the condition.

SPECIAL INSTRUCTIONS:

Bladder Cancer

Cathy E. Langston, DVM, DACVIM (Small Animal)

BASIC INFORMATION

Description

Bladder cancer includes all malignant tumors of the bladder and accounts for fewer than 1% of all cancers in dogs and cats. Most tumors of the bladder are malignant. Inflammatory polyps are the most common benign tumors of the bladder.

Causes

The most common type of bladder cancer is transitional cell carcinoma. Breeds predisposed to this tumor include the Scottish terrier, Shetland sheepdog, collie, Airedale terrier, and beagle. Other types of bladder tumors include squamous cell carcinoma, lymphoma, adenocarcinoma, and rhabdomyosarcoma. Although most bladder cancers occur in older pets, rhabdomyosarcoma occurs in young, large-breed dogs. Bladder cancer may be more common in female than in male dogs, and it is rare in cats.

Clinical Signs

The most common signs are blood in the urine, straining to urinate, and urinating small volumes of urine frequently. If the tumor is large, it can sometimes be felt by your veterinarian when palpating the animal's abdomen. Because these tumors can grow into the urethra (the tube that carries urine from the bladder to the outside), they can sometimes be felt during rectal palpation.

If the tumor blocks the urethra, dogs may strain to urinate without producing any urine. The bladder can become very large because of the retained urine, even if the blockage is not complete. If the tumor blocks one ureter (the tube that carries urine from the kidney to the bladder) as it enters the bladder, clinical signs may not be apparent. If both ureters become blocked, kidney failure occurs.

Diagnostic Tests

Initially, blood and urine tests (urinalysis, culture) are often recommended to investigate the clinical signs. Standard urinalysis is not likely to show cancer cells. A special urine test, called a *bladder tumor antigen test*, can be used to screen for bladder cancer. Any disease of the bladder, including a simple bladder infection, can cause the test to be positive (false-positive result), but a negative test means that the chance that cancer is present is extremely low. This test can be used to screen older dogs at risk for bladder cancer (especially Scottish terriers) before they develop any signs of bladder disease.

X-rays cannot usually detect bladder tumors, so other tests are needed. An abdominal ultrasound can detect bladder masses but cannot determine whether the mass is benign or malignant.

A contrast study may be performed by infusing either carbon dioxide gas (negative contrast) or a liquid dye (positive contrast) into the bladder via a urinary catheter and then taking a series of x-rays. Cystoscopy, which involves passing a small fiberoptic viewing scope into the bladder through the urethra, can be used to identify and biopsy a bladder mass.

The type of cancer present can only be determined with a biopsy. In some cases, the biopsy is obtained at the time of surgery. If cancer is suspected, chest x-rays may be recommended to look for metastasis (spread of tumor).

TREATMENT AND FOLLOW-UP

Treatment Options

Most bladder cancers arise in the region of the bladder where the openings of the ureters and urethra enter the bladder, which makes complete surgical removal difficult. Transplantation of the ureters into other areas of the bladder and diversion of the urethra to the outside of the abdomen may be required.

An experimental technique using laser therapy (with cystoscopy and ultrasound) is being developed to remove portions of bladder tumors. When the tumor regrows, this procedure can be repeated. If the tumor blocks the urethra, a metal tube (stent) can be placed in the urethra to hold it open so that patient can empty the bladder; alternatively, a tube can be placed directly from the bladder to the outside to allow urine drainage. If the tumor blocks the ureters, a stent may also be attempted.

Transitional cell carcinoma does not readily respond to chemotherapy. Piroxicam, a nonsteroidal anti-inflammatory drug, may have some benefit in dogs. Secondary infections are treated with antibiotics.

Follow-up Care

Monthly ultrasounds may be done to monitor tumor progression. Cystocentesis, a method of obtaining urine by inserting a needle into the bladder, should be avoided in dogs with bladder cancer, because it could spread cancer cells along the needle track. Urine cultures (of samples obtained by a catheter or collected at home) are often performed every 2 to 3 months.

Prognosis

Prognosis for transitional cell carcinoma is poor, with average survival times of several months. Causes of euthanasia include obstruction of the urethra, kidney failure, metastasis, and poor quality of life.

SPECIAL INSTRUCTIONS:

Bladder Stones in Cats

Cathy E. Langston, DVM, DACVIM (Small Animal)

BASIC INFORMATION

Description

Bladder stones (cystoliths, cystic calculi) are physical aggregations of minerals and other substances in the bladder. They may rub and irritate the lining of the bladder, increase the risk of bladder infections, or lodge in the urethra (the tube that carries urine from the bladder to outside the body), causing an obstruction.

Causes

The two most common types of bladder stones in cats are calcium oxalate stones and struvite stones. They occur with about equal frequency. Calcium oxalate stones are more likely to develop in acidic urine, whereas struvite stones are more likely to form in alkaline urine. Complex interactions between the animal's diet and stone formation affect the development of both of these types of stones.

Urate stones are uncommonly encountered in cats and are usually associated with liver disease or vascular shunts. Other types of stones are rare in cats.

🖐 Clinical Signs

Signs of bladder irritation include frequent trips to the litter box, voiding of small volumes of urine, blood in the urine, pain on urination, and urinating outside the litter box. Bladder stones may lodge in the urethra, causing a complete urinary obstruction. Urinary obstruction is more common in male cats. Signs of obstruction include straining to urinate without producing any urine and abdominal pain. Urinary obstruction is an emergency situation. (See the handout on **Urethral Obstruction in Cats**.)

🔬 Diagnostic Tests

Diagnostic steps that are often recommended include routine blood and urine tests (urinalysis, culture) and abdominal x-rays. Urinalysis may show microscopic calcium oxalate or struvite crystals. It is important to note that cats can have crystals in their urine without having stones, and they can have stones without having crystals.

Both calcium oxalate stones and struvite stones show up on plain x-rays, making x-rays an excellent test for detecting stones. Some stones are too small to be seen on x-rays, but an abdominal ultrasound can usually detect them.

Analysis of stones is necessary to be sure of their composition, so stones that are physically removed from the bladder are submitted for analysis.

TREATMENT AND FOLLOW-UP

℞ Treatment Options

Struvite stones can often be dissolved by feeding a special, prescription diet (Hill's S/D). The cat must eat this diet exclusively; no supplemental treats or other foods are allowed. On average, it takes 3-4 weeks to dissolve struvite stones.

Calcium oxalate stones cannot be dissolved with dietary changes or medications. The only effective therapy is physical removal of the stones, which generally means bladder surgery (cystotomy) done through an abdominal incision. In certain cases, particularly in a large female cat with a solitary stone, the stone can be fragmented with a laser during cystoscopy (passage of a small fiberoptic viewing scope into the bladder) and the fragments flushed out. However, few veterinary hospitals have the equipment needed for cystoscopy and laser therapy. Surgery is generally a faster procedure. If the cat is a large female and the stones are small, it may be possible to flush them out with the animal under anesthesia.

With other types of stones, medications may be useful for dissolving them or preventing recurrence. After the stones are removed, preventive measures may include feeding a moist food and certain prescription diets. Prescription diets that are designed to simultaneously prevent struvite and calcium oxalate stones include Hill's Multicare C/D and Royal Canin's SO.

🐾 Follow-up Care

Following surgery, a recheck visit is usually scheduled at 10-14 days for suture removal. When medical therapy is used to dissolve the stones and also after surgery, urine pH (a measure of acidity) and x-rays are usually repeated at 1, 3, and 6 months to monitor for improvement or recurrence of stones. Longer-term monitoring may also be recommended.

Prognosis

Prognosis for resolution of bladder stones is excellent. For calcium oxalate and struvite stones, dietary management can decrease the risk of recurrence, although some cats develop more stones within 3-5 years.

SPECIAL INSTRUCTIONS:

Bladder Stones in Dogs

Cathy E. Langston, DVM, DACVIM (Small Animal)

BASIC INFORMATION

Description
Bladder stones (cystoliths, cystic calculi) are physical aggregations of minerals and other substances in the bladder. They may rub and irritate the lining of the bladder, increase the risk of bladder infection, or lodge in the urethra (the tube that carries urine from the bladder to outside the body), causing an obstruction.

Causes
Several types of bladder stones occur in dogs. Struvite stones (triple magnesium phosphate), occur in the presence of bladder infections. Female dogs are predisposed to struvite stones. Calcium oxalate stones occur with higher frequency in certain breeds of dogs, such as the miniature schnauzer, shih tzu, bichon frise, Lhasa apso, Yorkshire terrier, and miniature poodle. They may also develop secondary to other diseases, such as hyperadrenocorticism (Cushing's disease) or hypercalcemia (high blood calcium). Urate stones occur with liver problems, such as portosystemic vascular shunts and other inherited defects of the liver. The Dalmatian and English bulldog breeds are predisposed to urate stones. Other types of stones, such as cystine, calcium phosphate, xanthine, and silica stones, are rarely encountered.

Clinical Signs
Signs of bladder stones include frequent urination and urgency, voiding of only small volumes of urine, and pain on urination. Blood may occur throughout the urine stream or may be worse at the end of urination. Bladder stones may lodge in the urethra, causing blockage. Urinary obstruction from stones is more common in male dogs. Signs include straining to urinate without producing any urine and abdominal pain. Urinary obstruction is an emergency situation.

Diagnostic Tests
Diagnostic steps that are often recommended include routine blood and urine tests (urinalysis, culture) and abdominal x-rays. Urinalysis may show microscopic crystals. It is important to note that dogs can have crystals in their urine without having stones, and they can have stones without having crystals. Urine culture is important, because urinary infections may cause stones, and stones may cause infection.

Struvite and calcium oxalate stones show up on plain x-rays, making x-rays an excellent screening test. Some very small stones and stones of other types may not be apparent on x-rays, but an abdominal ultrasound can usually detect them.

Analysis of stones is necessary to be sure of their composition, so stones that are physically removed from the bladder are submitted for analysis.

TREATMENT AND FOLLOW-UP

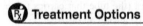 Treatment Options
Struvite stones can often be dissolved with a special diet (Hill's S/D) and control of any underlying infection with antibiotics. The dog must eat this diet exclusively; no supplemental treats or other foods are allowed. On average, it takes 1-3 months to dissolve struvite stones.

Calcium oxalate stones cannot be dissolved with dietary changes or medications. The only effective therapy is physical removal of the stones, which generally means bladder surgery (cystotomy) done through an abdominal incision. In certain cases, particularly in female dogs with a solitary stone, the stone can be fragmented with a laser during cystoscopy (passage of a small fiberoptic viewing scope into the bladder) and the fragments flushed out. However, few veterinary hospitals have the equipment needed for cystoscopy and laser therapy. Surgery is generally a faster procedure. If the dog is a female and the stones are small, it may be possible to flush them out with the animal under anesthesia. After removal, the urine is kept dilute (watery) by feeding moist food, and urine pH is maintained in the alkaline range to help prevent recurrence.

With other types of stones, medications may be useful for dissolving them or preventing recurrence. For urate stones in Dalmatians, a special diet (Hill's U/D) and the oral drug, allopurinol, may help dissolve stones and prevent recurrences.

Follow-up Care
After removal or dissolution of struvite stones, monitoring for infection with urine cultures is recommended on a monthly basis until three negative cultures in a row are obtained. Because urate stones do not show up on plain x-rays, ultrasounds are needed to monitor for recurrence.

Following surgery to remove calcium oxalate stones, a recheck visit is usually scheduled at 10-14 days for suture removal. Future rechecks consist of urinalyses and x-rays at 1, 3, and 6 months, then every 6 months thereafter. The goal is to detect recurrence of stones while they are small enough to flush out, without the need for surgery.

Prognosis
Bladder stones can be removed surgically, leading to full recovery. Certain types of stones may recur, but appropriate preventive measures may work for years.

SPECIAL INSTRUCTIONS:

Bladder Trauma

Cathy E. Langston, DVM, DACVIM (Small Animal)

BASIC INFORMATION
Description
Traumatic injury to the bladder may cause bruising, bleeding, or rupture of the bladder. The most serious damage is rupture of the bladder, which results in urine leakage into the belly (abdomen).
Causes
Trauma to the bladder may occur from blunt forces (automobile accidents, falls from heights) or penetrating injuries (gunshot, knife, or stick wounds). It can also occur with surgery of the bladder. Occasionally, catheterization, cystocentesis (obtaining urine by needle aspiration of the bladder), or palpation of the bladder results in mild trauma in a diseased bladder. Sometimes the bladder ruptures with no or minimal trauma, especially if it is diseased (such as with cancer) or blocked (obstructed) for a prolonged period.

Clinical Signs
Bloody urine is a very common sign of bladder trauma. Other external signs of trauma may be present, such as bruising, wounds of the abdominal wall, and difficulty walking (fractured pelvis or hips). Inability to urinate may occur if the bladder ruptures, but the ability to pass urine does not exclude bladder rupture. Progressive distension of the belly may indicate urine leakage into the abdomen. The abdomen is also typically very painful, because urine is irritating. Over time, toxins in the urine are absorbed into the bloodstream from the abdomen, leading to signs of kidney failure and potentially widespread infection.

Diagnostic Tests
The history and physical evidence of trauma in the area of the abdomen, along with urinary symptoms, allows a tentative diagnosis of urinary tract trauma. X-rays may show fluid in the belly, but they cannot determine whether the fluid is urine. An abdominal ultrasound helps identify rupture of the bladder or other parts of the urinary tract. A partially filled bladder may be seen on ultrasound (or even felt on palpation of the belly) despite the presence of a partial tear in the bladder. Instillation of contrast material (a liquid dye that shows up white on x-rays) into the bladder through a urinary catheter may reveal leakage into the abdomen, thereby confirming a rupture.

Urine leakage can also be confirmed by testing fluid obtained from the belly by simple needle aspiration (paracentesis). If the creatinine level in belly fluid is higher than the creatinine level in the blood, urine is leaking into the abdomen. Measurement of creatinine is the best test, because substances such as urea may be partially reabsorbed into the bloodstream, making confirmation difficult.

TREATMENT AND FOLLOW-UP
Treatment Options
If the bladder is bruised, no specific treatment is necessary, because the bruising resolves with time. If large blood clots are present in the bladder, they also usually dissolve over time. If the blood clots are causing an obstruction, a urinary catheter may be inserted for a few days to allow urine to drain.

If the bladder has ruptured, a urinary catheter is placed in the bladder to allow urine to drain out of the body instead of into the belly. If the hole in the bladder is small, the hole may seal on its own if the bladder is kept empty with the urinary catheter. It generally takes several days for small holes to seal.

If the hole in the bladder is large or continues to leak, surgery is necessary to repair the tear. If the patient is too unstable for general anesthesia, either because of trauma elsewhere in the body (such as severe lung bruising from an automobile accident) or because of kidney failure caused by the bladder rupture, drainage of urine from the belly may be necessary for several days. A peritoneal catheter can be placed directly into the abdomen to provide drainage. In some cases, peritoneal dialysis (instilling fluid and then draining it to remove toxins) may also be helpful. Surgery is then performed once the patient is stable.

Follow-up Care
After a urinary catheter is removed, urinations are monitored closely. A contrast procedure may also be performed when the catheter is removed to make sure no urine is still leaking. Blood tests for kidney function and electrolytes are often repeated for several days.
Prognosis
With appropriate treatment in the hospital, simple bladder ruptures are likely to heal. Surgical repair of a traumatic bladder rupture is also usually successful. If the bladder ruptured because of severe underlying bladder disease, such as cancer or prolonged blockage, the remaining bladder wall is often unhealthy and there is a substantial risk of urine leakage from the surgery site. Prognosis is poorer in these latter cases.

SPECIAL INSTRUCTIONS:

Chronic Kidney Disease in Cats

Cathy E. Langston, DVM, DACVIM (Small Animal)

BASIC INFORMATION

Description

Chronic kidney disease (CKD), also called *chronic renal failure*, is long-standing (greater than 3 months) kidney dysfunction that is manifested by dilute urine (urine that is not as concentrated as it should be) and retention of urea (uremia) and other waste products in the body. CKD is a common problem in older cats but can also occur in young and middle-aged cats.

Causes

In many cases, the underlying cause of CKD is never discovered. Identifiable causes include kidney infections and stones, obstruction of the ureter (the tube that carries urine from the kidney to the bladder), incomplete recovery from previous damage to the kidney (such as acute renal failure), polycystic kidney disease (an inherited condition common in long-haired cats), and certain tumors (such as lymphoma). In young cats, congenital kidney disease (such as kidney dysplasia) may be the cause. Kidney stones are common in middle-aged cats.

Clinical Signs

CKD may be detected on routine screening of blood and urine prior to the onset of signs. Diagnosis at this stage allows treatments to be started that may slow the progression of CKD. Early clinical signs may include increased water intake and urine production, decreased appetite, and nausea. In later stages, vomiting, lethargy, and dehydration may be apparent. Physical examination findings may include dehydration, weight loss or muscle loss, poor hair coat, small or irregular kidneys, and a uremic odor to the breath.

Diagnostic Tests

Initially, a biochemistry panel, complete blood test, and urinalysis are usually recommended. With CKD, kidney function tests, such as blood urea nitrogen (BUN) and creatinine, are elevated. Levels of blood electrolytes (potassium) and certain chemicals (phosphorus, calcium) may also be abnormal. Urinalysis is crucial to determine the ability of the kidneys to concentrate the urine and to look for protein in the urine.

Additional diagnostic tests may include a urine culture to screen for infection, blood pressure measurement (especially if there is protein in the urine) to check for high blood pressure (hypertension), and a complete blood count to look for anemia. Abdominal x-rays and an ultrasound are often done to look for kidney stones, evidence of infection, or other changes. In some cases, a kidney biopsy may be recommended, along with laboratory tests to rule out other diseases that can cause similar signs.

TREATMENT AND FOLLOW-UP

Treatment Options

Currently, no treatments are available that will reverse CKD. The goals of treatment are to slow progression of CKD and treat the clinical signs. Feeding a special kidney diet, which contains less protein and phosphorus, is the most effective method of slowing progression of CKD. Cats eating a kidney diet can live twice as long as those eating a regular maintenance diet. These diets can be started even before signs occur. Control of blood phosphorus levels is also necessary. If dietary changes alone do not accomplish this, drugs to bind the phosphorus in the food can be given with each meal.

If chronic dehydration is present, injections of fluid under the skin (subcutaneous fluids) may be helpful. The frequency varies from daily to twice weekly, and the injections can be given at home. If hypertension is present, a variety of drugs can be used to control it. Hypertension is more common in early stages of CKD in cats. Excess protein in the urine is rare in cats and can be treated with angiotensin-converting enzyme (ACE) inhibitor drugs.

Potassium supplements may be needed in some cats, as well as drugs to treat excess acid in the blood. Severe, advanced anemia can be treated with hormone injections to stimulate the production of red blood cells, but some cats develop side effects from the hormone the longer it is used. Antacids, such as famotidine, are frequently prescribed for vomiting, and appetite stimulants may be given.

Follow-up Care

Follow-up visits often involve examinations, laboratory tests, and blood pressure measurements (when available). Frequency of visits depends on the severity of CKD, with monthly visits recommended in advanced cases. Cats with early, stable disease may only need to be checked every 3-6 months.

Prognosis

CKD is a progressive disease that slowly worsens, but the rate of progression is highly variable. Cats diagnosed with early disease have an average survival time of 3 years. Those with moderate disease live an average of 2 years. Those with advanced disease generally succumb to CKD within months. Despite these general rates, the survival time of any individual cat is impossible to predict.

SPECIAL INSTRUCTIONS:

Chronic Kidney Disease in Dogs

Cathy E. Langston, DVM, DACVIM (Small Animal)

BASIC INFORMATION

Description

Chronic kidney disease (CKD), also called chronic renal failure, is long-standing (greater than 3 months) kidney dysfunction that is manifested by dilute urine (urine that is not as concentrated as it should be) and retention of urea (uremia) and other waste products in the body. CKD is a common problem in older dogs but can also occur in young and middle-aged dogs.

Causes

In many cases, the underlying cause of CKD is never discovered. Identifiable causes include kidney infections and stones, incomplete recovery from previous damage (such as acute kidney failure), and diseases of the glomerulus (filtering structure) in the kidney (such as protein-losing nephropathy or glomerulonephritis). In young dogs, congenital kidney disease (such as kidney dysplasia) may be the cause. CKD may also arise as the kidneys deteriorate with age in older dogs.

Clinical Signs

CKD may be detected on routine screening of blood and urine prior to the onset of signs. Diagnosis at this stage allows treatments to be started that may slow the progression of CKD. Early clinical signs may include increased water intake and urine production, decreased appetite, and nausea. In later stages, vomiting, lethargy, and dehydration may be apparent. Physical examination findings may include dehydration, weight loss or muscle loss, small or irregular kidneys, and a uremic odor to the breath.

Diagnostic Tests

Initially, a biochemistry panel, complete blood test, and urinalysis are usually recommended. With CKD, kidney function tests, such as blood urea nitrogen (BUN) and creatinine, are elevated. Levels of certain blood chemicals (especially phosphorus) may also be abnormal. Urinalysis is crucial to determine the ability of the kidneys to concentrate the urine and to look for protein in the urine.

Additional diagnostic tests may include a urine culture to screen for infection, blood pressure measurement (especially if there is protein in the urine) to check for high blood pressure (hypertension), and a complete blood count to look for anemia. Abdominal x-rays and an ultrasound are often done to look for kidney stones, evidence of infection, or other changes. In some cases, a kidney biopsy may be recommended, along with laboratory tests to rule out other diseases that can cause similar signs.

TREATMENT AND FOLLOW-UP

Treatment Options

Currently, no treatments are available that will reverse CKD. The goals of treatment are to slow progression of CKD and treat the clinical signs. Feeding a special kidney diet, which contains less protein and phosphorus, is the most effective method of slowing progression of CKD. Dogs eating a kidney diet can live twice as long as those eating a regular maintenance diet. These diets can be started even before signs occur.

Control of the blood phosphorus levels is also necessary. If diet alone does not accomplish this, drugs to bind the phosphorus in the food can be given with each meal. Administering a form of vitamin D (calcitriol) may also help delay an increase in phosphorus. If chronic dehydration is present, injections of fluid under the skin (subcutaneous fluids) may be helpful. The frequency varies from daily to twice weekly, and the injections can be given at home.

Excess protein in the urine can be treated with angiotensin-converting enzyme (ACE) inhibitor drugs. If hypertension is present, a variety of drugs can be used to control it. Dogs rarely develop low blood potassium levels from CKD, but potassium supplements may be needed in some cases. Severe, advanced anemia can be treated with hormone injections to stimulate production of red blood cells, but some dogs develop side effects from the hormone the longer it is used. If vomiting is present, antacids (such as famotidine or omeprazole) or antiemetics (such as metoclopramide, ondansetron, or dolasetron) may be prescribed.

Follow-up Care

Follow-up visits often involve examinations, laboratory tests, and blood pressure measurements (when available). Frequency of visits depends on the severity of CKD, with monthly visits recommended in advanced cases. Dogs with early, stable disease may only need to be rechecked every 3-6 months.

Prognosis

CKD is a progressive disease that slowly worsens, but the rate of progression is highly variable. Some dogs may worsen over months, and others over 2-3 years, before reaching a point where quality of life deteriorates to an unacceptable level.

SPECIAL INSTRUCTIONS:

Cystitis in Cats

Cathy E. Langston, DVM, DACVIM (Small Animal)

BASIC INFORMATION
Description
Bladder inflammation (cystitis) is common in young adult to middle-aged cats. The term *feline lower urinary tract disease* (FLUTD) refers to any condition that causes inflammation of the bladder of cats. It is not a specific disease. When cats show signs of bladder disease, testing is necessary to determine the underlying cause, so that specific therapy, if available, can be started.

Causes
Bladder stones account for about 15% of cystitis cases in cats. Bladder infections are not common in cats and account for fewer than 2% of cystitis cases. Structural abnormalities, such as bladder cancer, inflammatory polyps, and ectopic ureters, account for fewer than 10% of the cases. Behavioral problems also account for fewer than 10%.

In more than half of cats with signs of cystitis, no underlying cause can be found. If appropriate tests to exclude all other causes of cystitis are performed and are found to be negative, the term *feline idiopathic cystitis* (cystitis of unknown cause) is used.

Clinical Signs
Common signs of cystitis in cats include difficulty urinating or straining to urinate, pain on urination, urinating small volumes frequently, frequent trips to the litter box, urinating outside the litter box, and blood in the urine. Cystitis can progress to obstruction of urine outflow in male cats. (See also the handout on **Urethral Obstruction in Cats.**)

Diagnostic Tests
Urinalysis may show blood in the urine, white blood cells, or crystals. The presence of crystals may be normal in cats without signs of bladder disease. Crystals can been seen only under the microscope, and their presence does not mean that stones are present. Urine culture may be performed, although infections are rare.

Laboratory tests may also be recommended to rule out kidney disease and other medical conditions. X-rays of the abdomen are used to search for bladder stones. If the stones are too small or do not contain calcium, they will not be seen on x-rays. In these cases, an abdominal ultrasound may be needed.

Additional diagnostic tests may include contrast cystography to evaluate the thickness of the bladder and cystoscopy to look for any irregularities in the lining of the bladder. Positive contrast cystography involves taking x-rays after injecting a dye (that shows up white on x-rays) into the bladder through a urinary catheter.

With double-contrast cystography, air may be instilled first, followed by the dye. Cystoscopy involves passing a tiny, fiberoptic viewing scope into the bladder with the animal under anesthesia. This latter procedure is not widely available, however.

TREATMENT AND FOLLOW-UP
Treatment Options
If a cause is found, such as stones or infection, it is treated. Since infection is rarely the cause of cystitis in cats, antibiotics are not often needed. If an underlying reason is not apparent (the majority of cases), certain general treatments can be tried. Diluting the urine by feeding food with higher water content (canned or moist foods) can be tried. Access to fresh water is important, and water fountains may encourage cats to drink more.

Enriching the cat's environment also helps decrease the frequency and severity of signs. Providing toys and active playtime can help. Windows that allow outside viewing and increased time for interactions with owners may also be helpful. The litter box should be cleaned fastidiously (scooped daily and changed weekly). Provide one litter box for each cat in the household, plus one extra box. Avoid covered litter boxes and scented litter. Different cats have different preferences for the type of litter, so experimentation may be needed. More information and advice can be found at *www.indoorcatinitiative.com.*

Medications are often used as a last resort. Pain medications and certain sedatives or relaxants may be helpful. Amitriptyline (*Elavil*) is a tricyclic antidepressant that helps relax the bladder and may be useful for long-term treatment. It does not help in the short term. Feline pheromone spray (*Feliway*) may help some cats. Anti-inflammatory medications may be tried in some cats.

Follow-up Care
Because stress plays a role in idiopathic cystitis, frequent recheck visits to the veterinary hospital are sometimes counterproductive. Preventive measures, such as environmental enrichment, are important.

Prognosis
Most episodes of idiopathic cystitis resolve in 4-7 days, regardless of treatment. About half of affected cats have a recurrence of signs, which may be exacerbated by stress. The frequency, severity, and duration of signs seem to decrease as the cat gets older.

SPECIAL INSTRUCTIONS:

Cystitis in Dogs

Cathy E. Langston, DVM, DACVIM (Small Animal)

BASIC INFORMATION

Description

Cystitis is a general term for inflammation of the bladder. In dogs, the term is often used to describe infections of the bladder, but many other conditions can cause cystitis.

Causes

The most common cause of cystitis in dogs is urinary tract infection. Bladder infections are common in female dogs and can occur in male dogs. Conditions that increase the risk of bladder infection include bladder stones, anatomic abnormalities (such as congenital ectopic ureters), urinary incontinence, diseases that impair the immune system's ability to fight infection (such as Cushing's disease, diabetes mellitus, or chronic kidney disease), inability to completely empty the bladder (common with severe back problems), chronic skin infections around the vulva of female dogs, and prostate infections in male dogs. Bladder infections are not contagious.

Bladder stones, which irritate the lining of the bladder, can cause cystitis. Other causes include bladder cancer and benign, inflammatory polyps. Idiopathic (unknown cause) cystitis, which is common in cats, is very rare in dogs.

Clinical Signs

Common signs include frequent urination of a small volume of urine, straining and urgency to urinate, pain while urinating, and blood in the urine. Affected dogs may urinate in the house because they cannot hold the urine. They are aware they are urinating (for example, a female dog will squat). Urinary incontinence (unconscious release of urine) also can occur with cystitis, and it can be difficult to distinguish inappropriate, voluntary urination from incontinence if the dog is not observed.

Diagnostic Tests

Physical examination findings may include skin infections around the vulva or the presence of folds of skin that partially cover the vulva, thereby trapping moisture and increasing the risk of skin infection. Obesity makes those skin folds larger, and weight loss is necessary to control this problem. Assessment of nerve function in the back legs, tail, and anus may help identify problems that are also affecting the bladder.

Urinalysis and urine culture are usually done for dogs with signs of cystitis. The ideal way to obtain a urine sample for culture is to remove the urine directly from the bladder with a needle (cystocentesis). This is a simple procedure, similar to drawing a blood sample. The second best method to obtain urine for culture is to pass a urinary catheter into the bladder. Because a few bacteria are normally present at the opening of the urethra, it is possible to contaminate the urine when samples are collected in this fashion. Urine samples caught when the patient is voluntarily urinating (voiding) may also have normal bacteria in them, making interpretation of cultures difficult. If voided samples are used, they should be collected in the middle of urination, and the urine should not touch the fur as the dog is urinating.

Additional potential diagnostic tests include laboratory tests to rule out kidney disease and other medical conditions, abdominal x-rays to look for bladder stones, and an abdominal ultrasound to look for bladder stones, polyps, cancer, or other problems. In some cases, other specialized tests such as cystoscopy or contrast x-ray studies may be recommended.

TREATMENT AND FOLLOW-UP

Treatment Options

For bacterial infections, antibiotics are usually effective. The choice of antibiotic is ideally based on results of urine culture. Culturing identifies the specific bacteria involved and predicts the response to various antibiotics. A simple bladder infection can usually be cured in 5-7 days. With long-standing infections, recurrent infections, or infections complicated by untreatable causes, a longer course of antibiotics may be needed. In rare cases, the infection is never completely cured and long-term or intermittent antibiotics is required to control it.

For other causes of cystitis, correction of the underlying problem usually improves the signs. For example, removing bladder stones decreases irritation within the bladder. If benign bladder polyps are present, anti-inflammatory medications may be needed in addition to antibiotics.

Follow-up Care

For simple bladder infections, signs generally improve within a few days of starting antibiotics. Urine may be cultured 3-7 days after the antibiotics are completed, to ensure that the infection has been eradicated. For complicated cases, urine culture may be performed monthly for several months to make sure the infection does not return.

Prognosis

Simple bladder infections have an excellent prognosis. If the underlying cause of the cystitis cannot be cured, the cystitis may persist (continuously or intermittently). Long-term concerns include secondary infection of the kidney, which can cause kidney failure.

SPECIAL INSTRUCTIONS:

Ectopic Ureter in Dogs

Cathy E. Langston, DVM, DACVIM (Small Animal)

BASIC INFORMATION

Description

The ureter is the tube that carries urine from the kidney to the bladder. An ectopic ureter is a ureter that enters the bladder in an abnormal position. Normally, the ureter empties into the bladder in front of the bladder sphincter, the muscle that keeps the bladder closed so that urine does not leak out. When the opening of the ectopic ureter is beyond the bladder sphincter, urine constantly dribbles out as it is formed. This manifests as urinary incontinence.

Causes

Ectopic ureter is a congenital defect, meaning that it is present at birth. In some cases, it appears to be inherited. Breeds that are predisposed to ectopic ureters include the Siberian husky, Labrador retriever, golden retriever, Newfoundland, English bulldog, West Highland white terrier, fox terrier, Skye terrier, and miniature and toy poodles. The condition is rare in cats. Ectopic ureter can involve one or both ureters and is sometimes complicated by abnormalities of the bladder wall or sphincter.

Clinical Signs

The most common sign of ectopic ureters is urinary incontinence in a young dog. Affected dogs may constantly dribble urine or leak urine while sleeping. In female dogs, the fur under the tail and back legs may be wet or discolored from the constant urine leakage. Bladder infections may be present. In most cases, the problem is present from an early age, but occasionally signs do not occur until middle age. Normal urinations are also usually seen.

Diagnostic Tests

Initially, blood and urine tests (urinalysis, culture) are often recommended to assess kidney function, check for bladder infections, and search for other causes of increased urine production. Following these tests, some form of advanced imaging is needed to diagnose ectopic ureters.

- Cystoscopy is one of the best tests for diagnosing ectopic ureters, because the opening of the ureters can be seen by passing a tiny, fiberoptic viewing scope into the bladder with the animal under anesthesia. This procedure is not widely available, however.
- An excretory urogram can be performed at most hospitals. It involves giving an intravenous injection of a contrast agent (a dye that shows up white on x-rays) and then taking a series of x-rays that follow the dye as it goes through the kidneys and ureters to the bladder. In larger dogs, the accuracy of this test is increased by using computed tomography (CT scan) instead of plain x-rays.
- In some cases, the ectopic ureter can be identified on abdominal ultrasound.
- Retrograde urethrography may be tried but does not always identify the ectopic ureter. With this procedure, dye is injected into the bladder through a urinary catheter, and x-rays are taken. If the dye enters the ureter, then its location may be visible on the x-rays.

Measurement of the strength of the bladder sphincter can give additional information, but the equipment for this test is not commonly available.

TREATMENT AND FOLLOW-UP

Treatment Options

The best treatment is to surgically move the ureter to a normal location in the bladder, especially if the kidney on that side is functioning normally. Various surgical techniques are available to accomplish this and many require use of an operating microscope or some form of magnification to improve the outcome. Your pet may be referred to a veterinary surgery specialist for this procedure.

A newer treatment option that is not yet widely available involves use of a laser to redirect the opening of the ureter to further inside the bladder. This laser technique is done via cystoscopy and does not require open-abdominal surgery, but it can only be used for certain types of ectopic ureter.

If the ectopic ureter is not fixed, urinary incontinence continues. These dogs are at risk for bladder infections that can spread upstream to the kidneys (pyelonephritis), which can be life-threatening.

Follow-up Care

If surgery was performed, the animal is kept quiet postoperatively until suture removal (in 10-14 days). After correction, urine may be cultured at the first follow-up visit to check for persistent infections. If surgery is successful, long-term follow-up is not necessary, but further testing may be needed if incontinence persists.

Prognosis

Prognosis with surgery or laser treatment is good, in that the majority of dogs are not incontinent afterward, or any residual incontinence can be controlled with medications. In some cases, the incontinence persists after surgery, particularly in those animals with additional abnormalities of the bladder sphincter.

SPECIAL INSTRUCTIONS:

Fanconi Syndrome in Dogs

Cathy E. Langston, DVM, DACVIM (Small Animal)

BASIC INFORMATION

Description

Fanconi syndrome arises when function of the kidneys is altered, so that certain substances are lost in the urine. The urine contains excessive amounts of sugar, amino acids (the building blocks of proteins), protein, bicarbonate, potassium, and phosphorus. Kidney failure, associated with increased values of blood urea nitrogen and creatinine, is not always present initially but frequently develops over time.

Causes

Fanconi syndrome may be inherited or acquired from other causes. The most common form of Fanconi syndrome is an inherited disorder in the Basenji dog. A recent increase in the number of cases of acquired Fanconi syndrome in non-Basenji dogs is potentially linked to ingestion (eating) of chicken jerky treats, but this association is only speculative at this point. Rare causes of Fanconi syndrome include heavy metal intoxication (lead, copper, mercury, organomercurials, Lysol, maleic acid), drugs (gentamicin, cephalosporins, cisplatin, aspirin, outdated tetracycline), and some miscellaneous causes.

Clinical Signs

In Basenjis, Fanconi syndrome may be diagnosed with routine screening tests prior to the onset of signs. Early signs include excessive drinking and urination, weight loss, and a poor hair coat.

With acquired Fanconi syndrome, kidney failure may be a prominent feature, with additional signs of nausea, poor appetite, vomiting, and lethargy.

Diagnostic Tests

The presence of sugar in the urine when the blood sugar is normal is typical of Fanconi syndrome. A blood biochemistry panel may show elevated blood urea nitrogen or creatinine levels or low levels of potassium or bicarbonate. Special urine tests can be performed to confirm the amino acid loss, different from the ones commonly used to detect protein in the urine. The presence of Fanconi syndrome may also be confirmed by evaluating blood and urine samples collected at the same time and comparing the relative amounts of certain substances (especially potassium and phosphate) in both samples.

If heavy metal toxicity is suspected, tests may be submitted to measure the levels of certain heavy metals in the blood. Other tests may be recommended to rule out diseases that cause similar signs.

TREATMENT AND FOLLOW-UP

Treatment Options

When Fanconi syndrome is associated with kidney failure, standard treatments for kidney failure, such as fluid therapy, will be started. Fluids may be given intravenously in acute or severe situations or subcutaneously (under the skin) if the disease is chronic. In many cases of acquired Fanconi syndrome, a temporary feeding tube is recommended, because it may take a few weeks for appetite to return.

Replacement of the substances that are lost in the urine is an important part of treatment. Potassium can be supplemented by administration of potassium gluconate or potassium citrate. Potassium supplementation also improves the acid buildup in the blood (acidosis) that occurs with this disease. Sodium bicarbonate tablets may also be needed for the acidosis. Amino acid supplements and multiple vitamins are frequently given. A common treatment plan, referred to as the *Gonto protocol*, that utilizes many of these medications and supplements is popular with Basenji owners. For an explanation of this protocol, visit *www.zandebasenjis.com/protocol.htm*.

Follow-up Care

Frequent rechecks and monitoring are needed if renal failure is present. (See also the handouts on **Acute Kidney Failure** and **Chronic Kidney Disease in Dogs**.) For uncomplicated Fanconi syndrome, a biochemistry panel and venous blood gas analysis are usually rechecked 8-10 weeks after starting therapy, again in 6 months, and then annually if the dog is stable and no dosage adjustments are needed. Potassium levels are usually rechecked weekly after any dose adjustment. Urine cultures are commonly performed at least every 6 months, because these patients are at risk for urinary tract infections.

Prognosis

For Basenjis with Fanconi syndrome, lifespan may not be substantially reduced from normal. Kidney failure is the most common cause of death in dogs with the syndrome.

SPECIAL INSTRUCTIONS:

Kidney Dysplasia in Dogs

Cathy E. Langston, DVM, DACVIM (Small Animal)

BASIC INFORMATION

Description

Kidney dysplasia is abnormal development of the kidneys that is present at birth (congenital).

Causes

In some breeds of dogs, kidney dysplasia is an inherited condition that is passed to the puppy in the genes from one or both parents. Breeds that are predisposed include the shih tzu, Lhasa apso, soft-coated wheaten terrier, Samoyed, Alaskan malamute, Norwegian elkhound, cocker spaniels, standard poodle, and Doberman pinscher. Kidney dysplasia can also occur as a spontaneous problem, perhaps as a result of prenatal (prior to birth) infections.

Clinical Signs

Clinical signs associated with kidney dysplasia are the same as the signs of chronic kidney failure. Often, excessive water intake and production of large volumes of urine are present from the time of weaning. Some affected puppies are smaller than their healthy littermates. As the disease progresses, more signs are likely to develop, including poor appetite, weight loss, nausea, and vomiting. Seizures may occur when levels of toxins (retained waste products that are not cleared by the kidneys) are extremely high. Often, signs may be present at a very early age; however, in milder cases, they may not become apparent until the dog is several years old.

Diagnostic Tests

The initial diagnostic tests for kidney dysplasia are the same as for chronic kidney disease and include blood and urine tests, along with blood pressure measurement (when available). An abdominal ultrasound and abdominal x-rays typically show small, irregular, and scarred kidneys. Kidney biopsy is sometimes performed to confirm the diagnosis. The dysplasia in various breeds of dogs may have characteristic findings on the biopsy. Researchers are currently searching for a genetic test to detect the disease at an early age.

TREATMENT AND FOLLOW-UP

Treatment Options

Treatment for kidney dysplasia is the same as for chronic kidney disease and includes kidney diets, medications, and fluid therapy. (See the handout on **Chronic Kidney Disease in Dogs**.) There is no treatment specific for kidney dysplasia.

Follow-up Care

The frequency of follow-up visits depends on the severity of the disease. Follow-up visits often involve examinations, laboratory tests, and blood pressure measurements.

Prognosis

Chronic kidney failure from kidney dysplasia will worsen. The time frame for progression is highly variable and ranges from months to years.

SPECIAL INSTRUCTIONS:

Kidney Stones in Cats

Cathy E. Langston, DVM, DACVIM (Small Animal)

BASIC INFORMATION

Description

Kidney stones are formed in the kidney. They may remain in the kidney without causing obvious problems; they may lead to progressive kidney damage; or they may block the outflow of urine from the kidney, resulting in a nonfunctional kidney. Kidney stones can also pass into the ureter, the tube that carries urine from the kidney to the bladder. Once in the ureter, they may pass all the way to the bladder or become lodged in the ureter, leading to acute kidney failure.

Causes

Most kidney stones in cats are calcium oxalate or other calcium-containing stones. Although other types of stones are possible, they are rarely encountered in the kidney. Over the past 10-15 years, the incidence of kidney stones in cats has increased, for unknown reasons.

Clinical Signs

Kidney stones may be discovered incidentally when x-rays are taken for other reasons. About half of cats with chronic kidney disease have kidney stones. The stones are likely to be seen on x-rays or on an ultrasound that is performed to evaluate the kidneys. Whereas severe pain is a common feature of passing kidney stones in people, passage of stones does not seem to be a painful condition in most cats. If the stone blocks the ureter, however, swelling of the kidney can be quite painful, making the cat uncomfortable when it is picked up.

Signs of a sudden blockage to urine flow include a decrease in appetite, lethargy, and possibly vomiting. Even with a blockage, some cats continue to make urine from the other kidney. For kidney failure to occur, both kidneys must be affected. In some cats, one kidney is damaged and becomes nonfunctional, but this goes undetected because the other kidney is working well. Then, when the remaining functional kidney becomes blocked, the cat suddenly goes into kidney failure.

Diagnostic Tests

Incidental kidney stones are found on abdominal x-rays or an ultrasound. X-rays are better at showing stones in the ureters; an ultrasound is better at identifying evidence of blockage of urine flow. When kidney failure is present, laboratory tests often reveal elevations in blood urea nitrogen, creatinine, and potassium levels, as well as other abnormalities.

If it is suspected that kidney stones are blocking urine flow, a series of x-rays (excretory urography) may be taken after administration of a contrast material (a dye that shows up white on x-rays). In some cases, the contrast material is given intravenously (IV). If the kidney is thought to be completely blocked, the contrast material may be injected directly into the kidney under anesthesia. Occasionally, computed tomography (CT scan) is needed to see smaller stones or multiple stones.

TREATMENT AND FOLLOW-UP

Treatment Options

Not all kidney stones require removal. Sometimes, removing the stones can cause more damage to the kidney than leaving them in place. Stones are usually removed if they are blocking urine flow, causing infections, or enlarging in size (despite appropriate diets and medications). Surgical removal may also be performed if the stones are lodged in the ureter. Because cat ureters are very small, surgery is challenging, and magnification is necessary. Surgery may require referral to a veterinary surgery specialist.

Another treatment, lithotripsy, involves shattering the stones into fragments that are small enough to pass on their own. Few veterinary hospitals have the ability to perform lithotripsy on cats. There is also a chance of bruising the kidney with this treatment. If the stones cannot be removed, it may be possible to insert a tube from the kidney to the bladder that bypasses the stones and allows urine to flow freely.

Treatments to decrease formation of new stones include feeding a canned diet, increasing water intake, and, possibly, medications to make the urine alkaline.

Follow-up Care

For cats with asymptomatic kidney stones, abdominal x-rays or an ultrasound, blood tests, a urinalysis, and a urine culture are usually performed every 3-6 months. If the stone is obstructing urine flow or causing kidney failure, monitoring frequency depends on the severity of the problem.

Prognosis

The presence of nonobstructing kidney stones in cats with chronic kidney disease does not appear to affect their survival time. In cats with kidney stones that are causing blockage, removal of the stones improves survival compared to medical management. About 80% of cats with stones removed live for more than 2 years, whereas only 66% of cats treated with medical management live more than 2 years.

SPECIAL INSTRUCTIONS:

Kidney Toxins (Nephrotoxicosis)

Cathy E. Langston, DVM, DACVIM (Small Animal)

BASIC INFORMATION

Description

A variety of substances encountered by dogs and cats can injure the kidney, potentially leading to kidney failure.

Causes

The following substances are known to cause kidney failure and are the most commonly encountered poisonings. There are *many* other substances that are not included on this list.

- Household substances: antifreeze or other substances that contain ethylene glycol, such as paint thinner; rat poisons that cause calcium elevation; potentially, certain chicken jerky treats (unproven); solvents
- Plants: grapes and raisins (apparently dogs only), lily plants (apparently cats only), certain toxic mushrooms
- Drugs: nonsteroidal anti-inflammatory drugs, such as ibuprofen, carprofen, and others; certain antibiotics, such as aminoglycosides, sulfonamides, and outdated tetracycline or doxycycline; psoriasis creams; immunosuppressive drugs, such as cyclosporine and azathioprine; amphotericin B (antifungal agent); acyclovir (an antiviral drug); chemotherapeutic agents, such as cisplatin, carboplatin, methotrexate, and doxorubicin; high doses of diuretics; and others
- Heavy metals: mercury, arsenic, nickel, copper, lead, and others
- Venoms: certain snake and bee venoms

Clinical Signs

Many toxins that cause kidney failure also cause vomiting shortly after ingestion, but this is variable. Another common sign is a sudden increase in water consumption and urine production. In some cases, increased urine production is followed by a decrease in production to below normal. The onset of kidney failure varies, depending on the specific toxin. It can start within hours after ingestion of a toxin, or it can be delayed by several days.

Diagnostic Tests

In the case of known exposure to a kidney toxin, initial steps include tests to evaluate kidney function (blood urea nitrogen and creatinine concentrations) and a urinalysis to evaluate the ability of the kidney to concentrate the urine. A test for ethylene glycol (antifreeze) is available but must be performed within a few days after the ingestion. A delay in testing can cause the test to be negative despite exposure. On the other hand, certain commonly administered drugs may cause the test to be falsely positive. (See the handout on **Antifreeze Toxicity**.)

In some cases, kidney function tests are found to be elevated when vomiting or other signs are investigated. In these cases, extensive testing may be needed to determine the underlying cause and may include abdominal x-rays, an abdominal ultrasound, urine culture, serologic tests for infections that may affect the kidneys, and others.

TREATMENT AND FOLLOW-UP

Treatment Options

If ingestion of a kidney toxin is detected within several hours, vomiting maybe induced (by your veterinarian) to remove the toxin from the body before it has been absorbed. In some cases, oral activated charcoal may be given to bind any toxin that remains in the gut. Intravenous fluid therapy can help flush out some toxins and decrease kidney damage. If the kidneys completely shut down, medications that stimulate urine production (diuretics) may be helpful, or some type of dialysis may be required.

See the handouts on **Antifreeze Poisoning** and **Cholecalciferol Rodenticide Poisoning** for details on treatment of these conditions.

Follow-up Care

Intensive monitoring is needed for animals in kidney failure, as outline in the handout on **Acute Kidney Failure**. Frequent follow-up visits are often needed until kidney function recovers. Long-term monitoring may be necessary if kidney function does not recover completely.

Prognosis

Kidney damage from toxins can be quite severe. If complete kidney shutdown occurs and dialysis is necessary, about 20% of these animals survive. For less severe damage, prognosis is variable, with up to 50-60% survival. Permanent kidney damage is possible in some cases.

SPECIAL INSTRUCTIONS:

Perinephric Pseudocysts in Cats

Cathy E. Langston, DVM, DACVIM (Small Animal)

BASIC INFORMATION

Description

A perinephric pseudocyst is an accumulation of fluid around the kidney. The fluid accumulates inside the renal capsule, a fibrous tissue that normally surrounds the kidney. These cysts may occur on one or both kidneys.

Causes

The cause of perinephric pseudocysts is unknown.

Clinical Signs

Abdominal distention may occur from extremely large cysts and may be visible as a swelling in the abdomen behind the ribs. Sometimes pseudocysts are detected when an abdominal mass or enlarged kidney is found on a routine physical examination. In about half of the cases, chronic kidney failure is present at the time of diagnosis. Signs of chronic kidney failure include excessive thirst and urination, poor appetite, lethargy, weight loss, poor hair coat, and anemia. Rarely, pseudocysts may rupture and the fluid inside drains into the belly (causing abdominal distention) or into the chest (causing difficult or rapid breathing).

Diagnostic Tests

The most useful diagnostic test is an abdominal ultrasound (sonogram). On the ultrasound, the fluid around the kidney is easily seen and is clearly contained within the kidney capsule. The kidney may appear to be floating in the fluid. The kidney may look normal, or it may be small and scarred. Laboratory tests, a urinalysis, and urine culture are often performed to look for evidence of kidney failure and urinary infection. X-rays may be done to rule out other causes of abdominal masses.

An intravenous pyelogram (excretory urogram) may be recommended in some cases. It involves intravenous injection of a type of dye that is taken up by the kidneys, followed by a series of timed x-rays. Occasionally fluid is retrieved from the cyst and submitted for analysis. Other tests may be recommended to rule out other causes of chronic kidney disease.

TREATMENT AND FOLLOW-UP

Treatment Options

If the pseudocyst is an incidental finding (that is, it is not causing the cat any problems), treatment may not be necessary. Draining the fluid by inserting a needle through the skin into the pseudocyst is relatively simple but is not encouraged because the procedure may cause the cat to become dehydrated or may cause an infection to develop in the cyst.

If the pseudocyst is so large that it causes abdominal discomfort, drainage of fluid may be helpful. The pseudocyst usually refills with fluid after simple needle drainage, however. Surgical removal of the capsule around the kidney allows the fluid to drain into the belly, where other tissues can resorb it.

In general, diminished kidney function does not recover after removal of the capsule, although there have been rare reports of improvement in kidney function after this surgery. Treatment for chronic kidney disease is started as needed. (See the handout on **Chronic Kidney Disease in Cats**.)

Follow-up Care

If the pseudocyst was incidentally discovered and kidney function is normal, examination of the cat every 6 months is prudent. If kidney function is impaired, examinations and laboratory tests are performed based on the severity of the kidney dysfunction.

Prognosis

Prognosis for cats with perinephric pseudocysts depends primarily on the presence and severity of any kidney failure.

SPECIAL INSTRUCTIONS:

Polycystic Kidney Disease in Cats

Cathy E. Langston, DVM, DACVIM (Small Animal)

BASIC INFORMATION

Description

Polycystic kidney disease (PKD) is a disorder that causes multiple cysts to develop in the kidneys. As these cysts enlarge, they compress the surrounding kidney tissue. As more and more normal kidney tissue is crowded out by the cysts, kidney function declines.

Causes

PKD is an inherited condition that is transmitted by a dominant gene, the mutant *PKD1* gene. If either the mother or the father cat carries the gene, the kitten can inherit the gene and develop the disease. This disease occurs most commonly in the Persian, Himalayan, and other longhaired breeds of cats. It can also occur in the Scottish fold, British shorthair, and any other cats with an affected cat in their background.

Clinical Signs

The cysts usually cause no clinical signs themselves (that is, they are not painful) until they destroy enough kidney tissue for kidney (renal) failure to occur. Clinical signs usually develop around 3-10 years of age, with an average age at onset of 7 years. Signs are similar to those from other causes of chronic kidney disease and include excessive drinking and urinating, poor appetite, lethargy, vomiting, and weight loss. Sometimes enlarged kidneys can be felt by your veterinarian during a physical examination, even before kidney failure occurs.

Diagnostic Tests

Laboratory and urine tests will detect kidney failure if it is present. In these cases, blood urea nitrogen (BUN) and creatinine levels are elevated, and urine specific gravity (a measure of the kidney's ability to concentrate the urine) is relatively low. Abdominal x-rays may show enlarged, irregular kidneys. An abdominal ultrasound (sonogram) readily detects the cysts by the time kidney failure is present.

It is possible to screen cats for PKD prior to the onset of kidney failure. Abdominal ultrasounds can reliably detect cysts in affected cats older than 9 months of age and are fairly reliable in cats as young as 4 months of age. A genetic test is available for kittens over 8 weeks of age that detects the *PKD1* gene. The test involves submission of a simple swab of the cells in the mouth. The swab is sent to the Veterinary Genetics Laboratory at the University of California-Davis (*www.vgl.ucdavis.edu*).

TREATMENT AND FOLLOW-UP

Treatment Options

No specific treatment exists to slow the enlargement of the cysts or to reverse PKD. Once renal failure has developed, general treatments that slow the progression of chronic kidney disease are used, including kidney diets; phosphorus restriction; medications for protein in the urine (if present); and blood pressure medications for any hypertension. Fluid therapy, potassium supplements, and treatment of accompanying anemia are also administered as needed. (See also the handout on **Chronic Kidney Disease in Cats**.) Once kidney failure is nearing the point where the kidneys can no longer sustain a good quality of life (end-stage kidney failure), kidney transplantation can be considered.

Follow-up Care

In the early years of the cat's life, before kidney function tests become abnormal, annual blood monitoring is recommended. Once the blood tests are found to be abnormal, more frequent monitoring is needed. The specific frequency of recheck visits and laboratory testing depends on how sick the individual cat is, and generally ranges from every month to every 3 months.

Prognosis

Eventually, kidney failure worsens and death will occur or euthanasia will be considered. The rate of progression of PDK is variable. Cats may survive 2-3 years or longer from the time abnormal kidney blood values are found. Cats with PKD should not be used for breeding. Genetic screening is also advised for cats from breeds with a high incidence of this condition before they enter a breeding program.

SPECIAL INSTRUCTIONS:

Prostate Cancer in Dogs

Cathy E. Langston, DVM, DACVIM (Small Animal)

BASIC INFORMATION

Description

Prostate cancer is the development of a malignant tumor of the prostate. It occurs in both intact (unneutered) and neutered male dogs, in contrast to other prostatic diseases, which occur almost exclusively in intact male dogs. Although castration protects against other prostatic diseases, it does not always prevent prostate cancer. Castration does not increase the risk of prostate cancer, however.

Causes

The most common type of prostate cancer is prostatic adenocarcinoma. Transitional cell carcinoma can also occur in the prostate, but it generally spreads from the bladder or urethra. Other types of cancer can occasionally develop within the prostate or spread to the prostate from distant locations. It can be difficult to distinguish between the various types of prostate cancer.

Clinical Signs

Initially, clinical signs may be absent. As the tumor enlarges, bloody urine, bloody or yellow discharge from the penis, straining to urinate, painful or frequent urinations, or straining to defecate make occur. If the tumor grows into the urethra, it can obstruct urine flow. Pain or swelling of the prostate gland or lymph nodes (glands) near the prostate may cause an abnormal gait when the dog walks. Prostate cancer can spread (metastasize) to the backbone, leading to pain or difficulty walking. Prostate cancer can also metastasize to the lungs, which can lead to coughing (with or without blood). Fever, lethargy, and depression occur in some cases.

An enlarged, irregular prostate gland that is stuck (adhered) to nearby structures may be detected by rectal palpation when your veterinarian examines the dog. Enlargement of lymph nodes in the region may also be detectable by rectal palpation.

Diagnostic Tests

Initially, blood and urine tests (urinalysis, culture) are often recommended to investigate the clinical signs. Standard urinalysis is not likely to show cancer cells. On plain x-rays, the prostate and nearby lymph nodes may be enlarged, and areas of mineralization (calcification) may be visible in the prostate. An abdominal ultrasound often confirms the presence of a mass in the prostate. Chest x-rays may be recommended to search for metastasis.

Examination of tissue specimens is necessary to confirm the diagnosis. Cells may be collected by needle aspiration of the prostate through the skin, but there is some risk of spreading tumor cells along the needle track. Cells obtained in this fashion are examined under the microscope (cytology). Biopsy can be performed at the time of abdominal surgery.

TREATMENT AND FOLLOW-UP

Treatment Options

Surgical removal of the prostate (prostatectomy) may be attempted to treat the tumor. Prostatectomy has many complications, including urinary incontinence. A laser can be used to partially remove the prostate (called transurethral resection of the prostate, or TURP), but the equipment for this procedure is not readily available. If the cancer is obstructing the urethra, an expandable metal tube (stent) can be inserted to keep the urethra open and re-establish urine flow.

Prostatic cancer does not usually respond well to chemotherapy, but it may improve with oral piroxicam, a nonsteroidal anti-inflammatory drug. Side effects of piroxicam include stomach upset and kidney disease. External-beam radiation therapy tends to cause unacceptable side effects. Intraoperative radiation therapy (applying radiation directly to the tissue during surgery) may provide some benefit and has fewer side effects. Castration is usually recommended, because it may help lessen the clinical signs associated with the tumor.

Follow-up Care

Frequent monitoring of clinical signs and prostate size are needed. Repeated urinalyses, laboratory tests, and abdominal imaging may be recommended, as well as periodic chest x-rays.

Prognosis

Prognosis for prostate cancer is poor. Almost 40% of affected dogs have metastasis by the time the prostate cancer is diagnosed, even if metastasis is not seen on chest x-rays. When metastasis is present, average survival time is about 3 months. If metastasis is not present, some dogs may live for up to 9 months with treatment.

SPECIAL INSTRUCTIONS:

Prostatic and Paraprostatic Cysts in Dogs

Cathy E. Langston, DVM, DACVIM (Small Animal)

BASIC INFORMATION

Description

Prostatic cysts are fluid-filled pockets in the prostate. They range in size from small to large, and they may be single or numerous. Paraprostatic cysts are large cysts that lie next to the prostate gland and are usually connected to the prostate by a stalk. Paraprostatic cysts do not open into the urethra (as normal prostatic ducts do). All prostatic cysts are more likely to occur in intact (unneutered) male dogs. The cat has only a rudimentary prostate gland, so these cysts are very rare in the male cat.

Causes

Prostatic cysts are thought to arise from blockage of ducts in the prostate, with subsequent expansion of the cyst due to accumulation of prostatic secretions. Paraprostatic cysts were previously thought to be a remnant of a fetal structure, but they are now thought to arise in the same fashion as prostatic cysts.

Clinical Signs

Dogs with prostatic cysts may have no signs until the cysts are large enough to impinge on surrounding structures. At that point, straining to defecate or urinate and difficult urination may develop. The urine may be bloody or cloudy. If the cyst becomes quite large, the abdomen may be distended. Occasionally paraprostatic cysts become infected, and the dog may develop lethargy, decreased appetite, abdominal pain, and fever. When rectal palpation is performed by your veterinarian, the cysts or an enlarged prostate can sometimes be felt.

Diagnostic Tests

Initially, blood and urine tests (urinalysis, culture) and abdominal x-rays are often recommended to investigate the clinical signs. Urinalysis and urine culture may indicate a urinary tract infection. X-rays may show an enlarged, irregular prostate, or they may show two structures that look like two bladders in the abdomen (in the case of a paraprostatic cyst). Both prostatic and paraprostatic cysts are readily apparent on an abdominal ultrasound.

A contrast study may be recommended. This procedure involves taking a series of x-rays after infusion of contrast material (a dye that shows up white on x-rays) into the urethra via a urinary catheter. With a paraprostatic cyst, the contrast study may show a mass near the prostate that does not fill with the dye. The contrast medium usually enters the prostatic tissue surrounding the urethra when prostatic cysts are present.

It can be difficult to differentiate a prostatic cyst from a prostatic abscess unless a sample of the fluid is obtained by needle aspiration (for microscopic and bacteriologic analysis), either under sedation with ultrasound guidance or at surgery. In some cases, the diagnosis can be confirmed only by abdominal exploratory surgery and submission of biopsy samples.

TREATMENT AND FOLLOW-UP

Treatment Options

Small prostatic cysts may be managed with castration and antibiotic therapy (if the cysts are infected). After termination of testosterone production (by removal of the testicles), the prostate typically shrinks to a normal size within 3-6 weeks, and the cysts subside.

Larger cysts, particularly paraprostatic cysts, may require surgical removal or drainage in addition to castration. Drainage may involve the placement of indwelling tubes that allow the cyst fluid to exit the body, or it may involve temporary drainage of the cyst during surgery and placement of omentum (tissue that covers the abdominal organs) into the cyst cavity. Infected paraprostatic cysts are treated similarly to prostatic abscesses. (See the handout on **Prostatitis and Prostatic Abscessation in Dogs.**)

Follow-up Care

For uncomplicated prostatic cysts, the prostate is usually palpated at the time of suture removal, and again 3-4 weeks after castration, to ensure that the prostate is shrinking as expected. If the gland is not shrinking, then other diseases (such as prostatic cancer or persistent infection) may be involved, and further testing for those diseases is often recommended. If the cysts were originally infected, urine culture is usually recommended 7 days after finishing the antibiotics, to ensure that the infection has resolved. Periodic follow-up visits to check indwelling drains and to repeat laboratory tests and abdominal imaging are usually required following surgery for large paraprostatic cysts.

Prognosis

If present, clinical signs are not likely to resolve without surgery for these cysts. Prognosis for simple prostatic cysts is good following castration and antibiotic therapy (if needed). With surgical removal or drainage, the prognosis is good for noninfected paraprostatic cysts, although recurrence of the cyst is possible in rare cases.

SPECIAL INSTRUCTIONS:

Prostatitis and Prostatic Abscessation in Dogs

Cathy E. Langston, DVM, DACVIM (Small Animal)

BASIC INFORMATION

Description

Prostatitis is inflammation of the prostate caused by infection. Prostatitis can be acute (sudden onset) or chronic. If the infection produces a pocket of liquefied material, it is a *prostatic abscess*. Prostatic infections usually occur in intact (unneutered) male dogs. The male cat has only a rudimentary prostate gland, so these infections almost never occur.

Causes

Infection generally comes from the urinary tract, especially the bladder and urethra. In some cases, infection can come from the kidneys. The presence of benign prostatic hypertrophy, prostatic cysts, or tumors predisposes dogs to prostatic infections. Other medical problems or treatments that suppress the immune system can occasionally predispose to prostatitis, including diabetes mellitus, steroid drugs, and chemotherapy.

Bacterial infection is the most common cause of prostatitis. Common examples include *Escherichia coli* (most common), staphylococci (staph), *Klebsiella*, and *Pseudomonas*. Brucellosis may involve the prostate gland but more often infects the testicles. Fungal infections of the prostate are uncommon.

Clinical Signs

Signs of *chronic prostatitis* include penile discharge (yellow or bloody), constipation or straining to defecate, infertility, and recurrent bladder infections. The bladder infections may cause frequent urination, urgency to urinate, or straining and pain on urination.

Signs of *acute prostatitis* are similar to those of chronic prostatitis. In addition, affected dogs may be lethargic, and have a poor appetite and fever. Other potential signs of acute prostatitis are reluctance to rise, stiff gait, arched back, and a tense abdomen (indicators of prostatic pain).

Signs of a prostatic abscess can be similar to those of acute or chronic prostatitis. If the abscess ruptures and infection leaks into the belly, peritonitis develops that can become complicated by widespread, overwhelming infection (sepsis) and shock. When rectal examination is performed by your veterinarian, most infected prostates are found to be enlarged and painful.

Diagnostic Tests

Initially, blood and urine tests (urinalysis, culture) and abdominal x-rays are often recommended to investigate the clinical signs. Blood tests may show an elevated white blood cell count. Changes in kidney and liver values may be detected if an overwhelming infection is present.

Urinalysis may show white blood cells and bacteria. Although prostatitis and prostatic abscesses are infections, cultures of urine obtained from the bladder are sometimes negative, especially if the infection is confined within the prostate.

Abdominal x-rays may show an enlarged prostate and evidence of peritonitis if a prostatic abscess has ruptured. An abdominal ultrasound usually shows an enlarged prostate with prostatitis, or pockets of fluid if an abscess is present. Semen analysis may reveal bacteria, but because ejaculation is painful in animals with prostatic infection, it is difficult to collect prostatic fluid samples.

Definitive diagnosis requires a positive culture from the prostate and/or biopsy. In many cases of prostatitis, these tests are not performed, and diagnosis is confirmed by a positive response to appropriate therapy.

TREATMENT AND FOLLOW-UP

Treatment Options

Chronic prostatitis may be treated with long-term antibiotics (6-8 weeks) in conjunction with measures to control any underlying predisposing factors. For example, it is important to treat accompanying benign prostatic hypertrophy with castration or finasteride, and prostatic cysts with castration.

For seriously ill dogs with acute prostatitis, intravenous (IV) antibiotics and fluid therapy may be needed initially. After the acute phase of the disease subsides, long-term antibiotics (at least 4 weeks) are usually administered, and castration is performed to prevent recurrence.

Prostatic abscesses that rupture into the abdomen are surgical emergencies. Even an abscess that has not ruptured is usually managed with surgery, because prostatic tissue around the infection can become thickened (as the body attempts to wall off the infection), which makes it difficult for antibiotics to enter the abscess. With surgery, the abscess is opened and drained, and the cavity is often filled with omentum (tissue that covers the abdominal organs). Surgery removes the infection and helps make the infected area more accessible to the immune system. Treatment with antibiotics alone is unlikely to be successful when an abscess is present.

Follow-up Care

Intensive monitoring is required if peritonitis is present. Repeated ultrasounds may be recommended after surgery. For prostatitis, re-examination, urinalysis, and urine culture are often recommended 1 week after finishing antibiotics.

Prognosis

Ruptured prostatic abscesses that lead to sepsis can be life-threatening, but with current surgical techniques, fatalities are uncommon. Reinfection and recurrence of abscess are common. Reinfection within months of stopping antibiotics is common with chronic prostatitis. Castration may prevent recurrences in some cases.

SPECIAL INSTRUCTIONS:

Protein-Losing Nephropathy in Dogs

Cathy E. Langston, DVM, DACVIM (Small Animal)

BASIC INFORMATION

Description

Protein-losing nephropathy (PLN) refers to any kidney disease that results in excess protein loss in the urine. Such conditions include glomerulonephritis (an inflammation of the glomerulus in the kidney), inherited glomerulopathy (noninflammatory disease of the glomerulus), and amyloidosis (a deposition of abnormal protein in the kidneys).

Causes

Glomerulonephritis can be caused by many different diseases. Generally, the kidney damage is caused by the immune system's response to various infections, widespread inflammation, or cancer. Glomerulonephritis can be a component of other immune diseases, such as systemic lupus erythematosus (called lupus or SLE) or polyarthritis. In about half of the cases, no underlying cause or triggering event is ever found.

As part of the immune response, immune complexes are deposited in the glomerulus, which damages the filtering membranes and allows proteins to leak into the urine. Breeds of dogs predisposed to glomerular diseases include the beagle, Bernese Mountain dog, bullmastiff, bull terrier, English cocker spaniel, Rottweiler, Samoyed, and soft-coated wheaten terrier.

Amyloidosis is the buildup of an abnormal protein material (amyloid) in the kidney, which also leads to increased loss of protein in the urine. Dog breeds that are predisposed to this disease include the Chinese shar-pei, beagle, and English foxhound. Abyssinian, Oriental shorthair, and Siamese cats are predisposed to amyloidosis. Amyloidosis can also be caused by chronic inflammation in the body or be associated with cancer.

Clinical Signs

In the early stages, no clinical signs specifically associated with PLN may occur, although signs of the underlying disease condition may be apparent. By the time clinical signs appear, substantial damage has usually already occurred in the kidneys. Signs include increased water consumption and urine output, poor appetite, weight loss, and poor hair coat. With very substantial protein loss, edema of the legs and abdomen may develop. Signs of kidney failure, such as vomiting, depression, dehydration, and uremic odor to the breath, may also be noted.

Diagnostic Tests

With PLN, a urinalysis shows increased amounts of protein in the urine, which can be measured with a urine test called a *urine protein/creatinine ratio*. Routine urinalysis as part of wellness or recheck examinations (for other forms of kidney disease) can detect excess protein in the urine in the early stages of this disease.

Other tests are commonly performed to look for the underlying cause, such as routine laboratory tests, urine culture, heartworm test, tests for Lyme disease and other infectious diseases, blood pressure measurement, chest and abdominal x-rays, and an abdominal ultrasound. Depending on the results of these tests, further testing may also be indicated. A kidney biopsy can provide much information about the type and severity of disease present.

TREATMENT AND FOLLOW-UP

Treatment Options

Specific therapy is started for the underlying cause of the PLN. Standard treatment for PLN itself includes feeding a special kidney diet that helps decrease the amount of protein lost in the urine. Drugs that decrease protein loss, such as angiotensin-converting enzyme (ACE) inhibitors (enalapril, benazepril, and others), may be recommended. Aspirin is usually given (after kidney biopsy), because PLN increases the risk of blood clots. If hypertension is present, it can be difficult to control and may require a combination of medications.

In some cases, drugs that suppress the immune system are used, but they often have variable results. Examples include steroids in cats and azathioprine, cyclophosphamide, and cyclosporine in dogs. Dogs with spontaneous amyloidosis may be treated with drugs such as colchicine, but these drugs are not very effective if kidney failure is present. Other treatments for chronic kidney disease are used as needed.

Follow-up Care

After starting an ACE inhibitor or other blood pressure medications, as well as when dosages are increased, laboratory tests (including creatinine and potassium), blood pressure measurement (when available), and urine protein/creatinine ratios are usually rechecked within 2 weeks. After all results and signs become stable, examinations and laboratory tests may be scheduled every 3 months (at least). Other monitoring may be recommended, depending on any underlying cause identified.

Prognosis

The use of ACE inhibitor drugs helps slow the progression of kidney damage, and dogs diagnosed early in the disease (prior to abnormal blood test results) can live for more than 1-2 years. Once the kidneys begin to fail and blood creatinine levels are moderately to severely elevated, the prognosis is poor and survival times are usually much shorter (months). In some cases, progression is very rapid, with the animal surviving only days.

SPECIAL INSTRUCTIONS:

Pyelonephritis (Kidney Infection)

Cathy E. Langston, DVM, DACVIM (Small Animal)

BASIC INFORMATION

Description

Bacterial infection of the kidney is termed *pyelonephritis*. Infection may occur within kidney tissue or in the renal pelvis, the area of the kidney where urine collects before being transported to the bladder.

Causes

In most cases, a urinary tract infection starts in the bladder and the bacteria travel upstream to the kidney. Anything that decreases the free flow of urine, such as obstruction of the urethra (tube that carries urine from the bladder to the outside), bladder, ureter (tube that carries urine from the kidney to the bladder), or kidney, increases the risk that the infection will spread to the kidney. The presence of stones and growths in the bladder and kidney also increases the risk. Other contributing factors include chronic kidney disease, diabetes mellitus, and conditions that impair the immune system or cause dilute (watery) urine.

The most common bacterial infection in the kidney is with *Escherichia coli*. Other bacteria may also be involved, and fungal infections occur rarely.

Clinical Signs

If only one kidney is infected, no clinical signs may be noted, and blood and urine tests may also be normal. If both kidneys are infected, signs may be those of kidney failure, such as increased volume of urine, increased thirst, poor appetite, vomiting, nausea, and lethargy. Signs of a bladder infection, such as frequent urination of small volumes of urine, pain on urination, and straining, may also be present. Blood in the urine can arise with infection in the kidneys or the bladder.

If the infection causes acute kidney failure, decreased or no urine production may occur, and the kidneys may become painful and swollen. Fever and a high white blood cell count may be present, but the absence of either of these does not exclude kidney infection. With chronic kidney infections, clinical signs may be minimal or absent. Chronic infection causes damage to the kidney; however, that results in scar tissue and shrinkage of the kidneys.

Diagnostic Tests

Initial diagnostic tests typically include blood tests to evaluate kidney function and urine tests to evaluate urine concentrating ability. A urine culture is performed, but it is not uncommon for culture of urine collected from the bladder to be negative despite infection in the kidney. Abdominal x-rays and an ultrasound may be recommended.

Although culture of a piece of kidney tissue obtained by biopsy increases the chance of finding the infection, the invasiveness of the procedure makes it too risky for general use (the biopsy would need to be taken from deeper within the kidney than the average kidney biopsy). Contrast x-ray studies, such as an excretory urogram (intravenous pyelogram), are sometimes helpful. An excretory urogram involves taking a series of x-rays after a dye (that shows up white on x-rays) is given intravenously. Other tests may be recommended to rule out diseases that cause similar clinical signs and other causes of kidney disease.

TREATMENT AND FOLLOW-UP

Treatment Options

Antibiotics are the mainstay of treatment of bacterial pyelonephritis and are often chosen based on a urine culture. If the urine culture is negative, a good antibiotic choice is one that is effective against *E. coli*. Kidney infections take much longer to cure than simple bladder infections, so antibiotics are usually continued for 4-6 weeks. If infection is related to a complete or partial blockage, removal of the obstruction may be necessary to achieve resolution of the infection.

Follow-up Care

With acute infections that cause complete kidney shutdown, improvement in kidney function may be seen within 4-7 days of starting antibiotics. With chronic kidney infections, no improvement in kidney function may occur, but decreasing the amount of ongoing damage in the kidney is still beneficial.

Repeating a urine culture 5-7 days after starting antibiotics is sometimes recommended to make sure the infection is resolving. Culture is often recommended about a week after completing the antibiotics, and again a month later. Blood tests for kidney function are usually performed at the same time. The need for repeated abdominal ultrasounds to monitor the course of the disease is variable.

Prognosis

Kidney infections can be serious, life-threatening conditions, but of all the causes of complete, acute kidney shutdown, they are one of the most treatable. About 75% of affected animals recover from an acute infection. The success rate for chronic infections is much lower. The rate of progression of kidney failure with chronic infections is variable; however, many animals can live for years after an infection.

SPECIAL INSTRUCTIONS:

Renal Neoplasia

Cathy E. Langston, DVM, DACVIM (Small Animal)

BASIC INFORMATION

Description

Renal neoplasia is the development of a tumor in the kidney. In most animals, the tumor is cancerous (malignant). Neoplasia is an uncommon cause of kidney disease in dogs and cats.

Causes

The most common tumor that involves the kidneys is lymphosarcoma, which is actually a cancer of a type of white blood cells (lymphocytes). It usually affects both kidneys but can involve only one. Lymphosarcoma (lymphoma) may also be present in other locations (liver, spleen, intestines, lymph nodes, central nervous system, other organs) when it is discovered in the kidneys, or the kidneys may be the first organs affected.

Other types of cancer in the kidney are relatively rare. Renal carcinoma can affect one or both kidneys. In 30% of carcinoma cases, the tumor has already metastasized (spread) by the time it is diagnosed. Renal carcinomas occur most often in older (average age, 7-9 years), male dogs. Renal adenoma is a benign tumor of the kidney.

German shepherd dogs are predisposed to renal cystadenoma. This tumor is inherited as a dominant trait and is often accompanied by uterine tumors and a certain skin disease. Young dogs (less than 1 year of age) very rarely develop a nephroblastoma. Metastasis has already occurred in about 65% of dogs with nephroblastoma at the time of diagnosis. Other types of kidney cancer include transitional cell carcinoma, hemangiosarcoma, and certain sarcomas. Cancer may also spread to the kidneys from other primary sites.

Clinical Signs

If lymphosarcoma is present in both kidneys, signs of kidney failure may be present, such as lethargy, poor appetite, increased water drinking, increased urination, weight loss, and vomiting. Blood may be seen in the urine with some kidney cancers. With lymphosarcoma, both kidneys may be swollen on physical examination; they may be smooth or lumpy. With other tumors, a mass may be present that involves the kidney and may be large enough to be felt (palpated) by your veterinarian. In other cases, no tumor or mass can be palpated. Rarely, the kidney tumor makes a hormone that increases the red blood cell count.

Diagnostic Tests

Abdominal x-rays may show an irregular kidney outline. Abdominal ultrasound may reveal a mass in one of the kidneys or swelling of both kidneys (lymphosarcoma). These findings increase the suspicion of cancer but do not prove its presence.

Laboratory tests (blood and urine) are usually recommended, and x-rays of the chest may be done to search for tumors in the lungs.

Additional potential diagnostic tests include needle aspiration or biopsy of the kidney. In some cases, particularly lymphosarcoma, inserting a needle into the kidney under sedation may provide enough cells for examination under a microscope (cytology) to determine whether cancer is present. In other cases, an actual biopsy is needed to confirm the presence of a tumor and identify the type of cancer. Kidney biopsies may be obtained through a keyhole incision or via surgical exploration of the abdomen, both of which require general anesthesia.

A contrast study, such as an excretory urogram (intravenous pyelogram), may be recommended in some cases to determine the extent of the cancer within the kidney and to provide a rough estimation of how well the other kidney is functioning. This contrast study involves taking a series of x-rays or computed tomography (CT) scans after intravenous injection of a dye that shows up white on x-rays. Renal scintigraphy scans can also be used to assess function of the other kidney.

TREATMENT AND FOLLOW-UP

Treatment Options

Lymphosarcoma is treated with chemotherapy, which in many patients can induce complete remission. (See also the handouts for **Lymphoma in Dogs** and **Lymphoma in Cats**.) For other malignant kidney tumors, removal of the affected kidney is usually considered, as long as the other kidney is normal. If the other kidney is diseased, removing the cancerous kidney could cause kidney failure.

Follow-up Care

Follow-up depends on the type of cancer and the treatment administered. Frequent recheck visits and laboratory testing are required for patients on chemotherapy. Postoperative monitoring may also involve periodic chest and abdominal x-rays and an abdominal ultrasound.

Prognosis

Cat with lymphosarcoma that receive chemotherapy have an average survival time of 3-6 months, although some live much longer. Dogs with renal carcinoma live on average another 8 months, if the tumor has not spread and the cancerous kidney is removed. Prognosis is very poor for the other malignant kidney tumors. Since renal adenomas are benign tumors, long-term survival is possible in these cases.

SPECIAL INSTRUCTIONS:

Ureteral Obstruction in Cats

Cathy E. Langston, DVM, DACVIM (Small Animal)

BASIC INFORMATION
Description
Ureters are the tubes that carry urine from the kidney to the bladder. If they become obstructed, urine flow stops and pressure builds up in the kidney, causing the kidney to cease functioning. Because one kidney can provide enough function to sustain the entire body, obstruction of one ureter may cause no visible signs. If both ureters are blocked or if the other kidney is not functioning well, serious kidney failure can develop rapidly. Ureteral obstruction from kidney stones can also occur in the dog but is less common than in the cat.

Causes
The most common cause of ureteral obstruction in the cat is a kidney stone that becomes lodged in the ureter. Some kidney stones are small enough to pass all the way to the bladder, but they may damage the ureter as they pass. Scarring that forms at the site of damage may eventually block urine flow.

Tumors of the ureter are very rare but they can obstruct urine flow. Abdominal masses and trauma may also affect the ureter. An occasional complication of ovariohysterectomy (spay surgery) is accidental ligation of the ureter near where the uterus is clamped and tied. All of these conditions usually affect only one ureter.

🗎 Clinical Signs
If only one ureter is affected, no clinical signs may be noted, and laboratory measurements of kidney function may remain normal. If the other kidney is impaired as well, either from previous damage or from simultaneous infection or blockage of both ureters, severe kidney failure may occur. Signs of kidney failure include poor appetite, lethargy, and vomiting. An increase in water consumption may occur. Urine volume may be increased, or no urine may be produced at all.

Although severe abdominal pain is common in people who are passing kidney stones, severe pain does not appear to be associated with ureteral stones in most cats. In some cats; however, abdominal pain may be detected on physical examination.

🔬 Diagnostic Tests
Initially laboratory and urine tests may be recommended to search for a cause of the clinical signs. Abdominal x-rays may sometimes show stones in the ureter, enlargement of the kidney, an abdominal mass, or some other abdominal problem. Abdominal ultrasound shows enlargement of the kidney when urine flow is blocked, and it may also show stones if they are near the kidney.

An excretory urogram may be needed to identify an obstruction. This procedure involves giving an intravenous injection of a contrast agent (a dye that shows up white on x-rays) and then taking a series of x-rays that follow the dye as it goes through the kidneys and ureters to the bladder. If kidney function is severely decreased by the obstruction, the kidney may not take up enough dye to provide a good study.

TREATMENT AND FOLLOW-UP

℞ Treatment Options
In some cases, kidney stones pass by themselves over hours to days. X-rays may be repeated to follow their course. If the stone does not move and the patient is in kidney failure or the obstruction is caused by scar tissue, surgery is needed to re-establish urine flow. Surgery to remove the stone requires some form of magnification, because cat ureters are extraordinarily small.

If the obstruction is very close to the bladder, the diseased portion of the ureter can be removed and the ureter reattached to the bladder. If scar tissue is present, a tube (stent) can be placed in the ureter that extends from the kidney to the bladder. The stent remains entirely inside the cat and can be left in place long term. Your pet may be referred to a veterinary surgery specialist for these procedures.

If the kidney is nonfunctional because of damage caused by an obstruction, it may be removed along with the ureter. If surgery is not performed, the resulting kidney failure may be managed similar to chronic kidney disease of other causes.

🐾 Follow-up Care
Follow-up care depends on the degree of kidney dysfunction and may involve laboratory tests for kidney function, urine culture, x-rays, and ultrasounds.

Prognosis
Prompt removal of an obstruction (within 4 days) increases the chance of recovery of normal kidney function. If removal is delayed by a week, recovery is still possible but will not be complete. After a month, minimal recovery is expected.

Following surgical removal of stones, 90% of cats are still alive after 2 years, compared to 66% of cats treated medically without stone removal.

SPECIAL INSTRUCTIONS:

Urethral Obstruction in Cats

Cathy E. Langston, DVM, DACVIM (Small Animal)

BASIC INFORMATION

Description

Urethral obstruction (UO) is a condition in which the urethra, which is the tube that carries urine from the bladder to outside the body, becomes blocked. This condition occurs primarily in male cats, because the urethra is extremely narrow as it passes through the penis. Female cats have a much wider and shorter urethra, which is unlikely to become blocked.

Causes

A variety of conditions can cause the urethra to become obstructed. Sometimes the obstruction is a physical blockage, such as a stone that does not completely pass. Gritty material that forms in the bladder may cause bladder inflammation that produces thick secretions. These secretions mix with the gritty material and form a substance that has the consistency of toothpaste. It is so thick that it may block the urethra. Excessive scar tissue from a stone that lodged previously or from prior urethral catheterization can cause a UO. In some situations, no physical obstruction is present but severe urethral spasms prevent urine from being passed.

Clinical Signs

The most common signs of UO are frequent trips to the litter box, generally associated with pain (crying) and straining to urinate, without producing any urine. As the problem progresses, kidney failure can develop and cause lethargy, vomiting, poor appetite, depression, and collapse. If the UO is not relieved in a timely manner, death can occur.

On physical examination, the bladder is usually distended, hard, and painful. The penis may be protruded and discolored (purple). If severe kidney failure is present, the heart rate may be slow due to high blood potassium levels. This is a critical problem that must be addressed immediately or the heart will stop.

Diagnostic Tests

The presence of a UO is usually diagnosed on physical examination. In about half of the cases, the exact underlying cause is not determined. Abdominal x-rays that include the urethra may reveal stones. An abdominal ultrasound may show sediment (sludge) in the bladder, although this does not prove that the sediment is causing the obstruction.

In some cases, particularly when obstruction recurs, a contrast study (urethrogram) may be helpful. With the animal under heavy sedation, liquid contrast material (a dye that appears white on x-rays) is injected into the urethra via a urinary catheter, and x-rays are taken. This technique can document the presence and location of a physical obstruction.

In addition to tests that look for a cause of the UO, blood tests to assess kidney function and electrolytes (potassium, sodium, and others) are usually performed.

TREATMENT AND FOLLOW-UP

Treatment Options

The first step is to stabilize any life-threatening conditions, such as a high blood potassium concentration. An intravenous (IV) catheter is placed so that fluids and emergency drugs can be given through the IV. The urinary bladder is often temporarily emptied by cystocentesis, which involves passing a needle through the abdominal wall into the bladder and aspirating the urine.

After the patient is stabilized, the blockage is relieved. A urinary catheter is inserted into the urethra and passed into the bladder. Injection of saline solution into the urethra as the catheter is passed sometimes flushes obstructing material back into the bladder. If the UO has developed from urethral spasms, a small amount of a numbing agent (lidocaine) may help relax the spasm enough to allow passage of the catheter.

IV fluids may be needed for a few days to treat any kidney damage. If an identifiable cause of the UO is detected, treatment of that condition is also necessary. For example, bladder surgery may be done to remove any stones.

Cats with frequent recurrence or persistent UOs may be treated with a surgical procedure called a *perineal urethrostomy* (PU). This procedure removes the penis (penile amputation) and the smallest part of the urethra, which is the area that becomes blocked most often. This procedure may increases the risk of bladder infections in some cats.

Prevention of UOs generally involves feeding a diet designed for urinary problems. Feeding moist food keeps the urine less concentrated and also decreases the risk of recurrence.

Follow-up Care

Intensive monitoring is needed for cats that are seriously ill, are in kidney failure, or require prolonged use of a urinary catheter. Urinalysis and urine culture are often repeated about 2 weeks after an episode.

Prognosis

Most cats with UOs survive and are discharged from the hospital. The risk of recurrence of signs is about 50%, and about 33% of these cats will experience obstruction again.

SPECIAL INSTRUCTIONS:

Urethral Prolapse in Dogs

Cathy E. Langston, DVM, DACVIM (Small Animal)

BASIC INFORMATION

Description

Urethral prolapse is a condition in which the tip of the urethra becomes everted through the opening of the penis.

Causes

The exact cause is unknown, but prolonged sexual excitement, the presence of urethral stones (calculi) or infection, and increased abdominal pressure (from coughing, straining to urinate, or straining to defecate) have all been implicated. English bulldogs are predisposed to this condition.

Clinical Signs

A prolapsed urethra looks like a small, red or purple mass at the tip of the penis. The mass may have a donut-shaped appearance. The tissue easily becomes inflamed. Blood may be seen in the urine, or a bloody discharge may be present. Affected dogs may strain to urinate or excessively lick the prepuce (the sheath around the penis).

Diagnostic Tests

Urethral prolapse is generally diagnosed by direct physical examination. A urinalysis, urine culture (to look for infection), and either abdominal x-rays or an ultrasound (to look for stones) are often recommended. Because English bulldogs are predisposed to urate and cystine stones in the bladder and these types of stones do not show up on x-rays, an ultrasound is generally preferred. If it is unclear whether the donut-shaped tissue is cancer or a urethral prolapse, cytology (evaluation of cells under a microscope) may be helpful. Other tests may be recommended to investigate the cause of any underlying coughing or straining.

TREATMENT AND FOLLOW-UP

Treatment Options

In some cases, the prolapsed tissue can gently be replaced using a urinary catheter. Then a temporary suture is placed at the opening of the penis to prevent the tissue from prolapsing again. Unfortunately, recurrence is common with this technique. The preferred treatment is to surgically remove the prolapsed tissue. Castration is often recommended to prevent recurrence from sexual excitement.

Follow-up Care

Bleeding is common and may persist for up to 2 weeks following surgery. The patient must be prevented from traumatizing the surgery site. Sedation and an Elizabethan collar help prevent licking of the site. During recovery, the dog must be kept from becoming excited. It should be isolated from other pets and kept away from all female dogs until recovery is complete.

Prognosis

Recurrence of the prolapse is likely if the exposed tissue is not surgically removed and castration is not performed. Prognosis is excellent with surgery. The condition is not life-threatening.

SPECIAL INSTRUCTIONS:

Urethritis

Cathy E. Langston, DVM, DACVIM (Small Animal)

BASIC INFORMATION
Description
Urethritis is inflammation of the urethra. The urethra is the tube that carries urine from the bladder to the outside. Because the bladder sphincter muscle (which keeps the bladder closed) lies at the beginning of the urethra, urethritis may cause urinary incontinence. Conversely, urethral disease may also obstruct urine flow. The urethra of females is relatively short and wide, so it is not prone to urethral diseases. The urethra of male cats is moderately long but also very narrow and is commonly affected. The urethra of male dogs is very long and travels through the prostate.

Causes
Urethritis may be caused by anything that irritates the urethra. Bladder stones may become lodged in the urethra or may cause damage as they pass. Infection in the bladder may also cause infection in the urethra. Bladder cancer may extend into the urethra. Prostate disease in male dogs may cause urethritis. In male cats, urethritis may be caused by obstruction (complete or partial) resulting from mucus debris, stones, blood clots, or muscle spasms.

Clinical Signs
Pets with urethritis typically have pain during urination. They make frequent attempts to urinate, strain while urinating, and have urgency to urinate. Blood in the urine may be more pronounced at the beginning of urination. The urethra may feel thickened or irregular when your veterinarian does a rectal examination (dogs).

Diagnostic Tests
Initially, blood and urine tests and abdominal x-rays are often recommended to investigate the clinical signs. Urinalysis and urine culture may show evidence of urinary infection. Abdominal x-rays that include the entire urethra may reveal stones in the bladder or urethra. An abdominal ultrasound may show stones or masses (tumors, polyps) in the bladder.

A contrast urethrogram may be recommended. This involves taking a series of plain x-rays or video x-rays (fluoroscopy) after injection of contrast material (a dye that shows up white on x-rays) into the urethra via a urinary catheter. This test evaluates whether any areas of the urethra are blocked by stones, tumors, or scar tissue.

Cystoscopy involves passing a fiberoptic viewing scope into the urethra with the animal under anesthesia. A rigid cystoscope can be used in female dogs and cats (those weighing more than 6 pounds), because the urethra is relatively straight in females.

A flexible cystoscope is necessary for evaluating the urethra of male dogs, because the urethra is long and curved. A specialized, tiny, flexible (to semirigid) cystoscope can be used for male cats. Cystoscopy allows the entire length of urethra to be examined, but the equipment is not widely available.

A urethral biopsy may be necessary to document cancer and to distinguish it from severe, benign inflammation. Biopsy may be performed via cystoscopy. If abnormal urethral tissue extends to the external tip of the penis, biopsies can be obtained without cystoscopy.

TREATMENT AND FOLLOW-UP
Treatment Options
Treatment is primarily directed at correction of the underlying disease. If a stone is obstructing the urethra, it may be flushed back into the bladder with the animal under anesthesia and retrieved surgically by bladder surgery (cystotomy). If the stone does not budge in male dogs, an incision can be made into the urethra to remove the stone. In male cats, it may be necessary to surgically remove the blocked part of the urethra in a procedure called a *perineal urethrostomy*.

If no physical obstruction is present, spasms of the urethra may be treated with muscle relaxants or antispasmodic drugs. A commonly used drug is phenoxybenzamine. In addition to relaxing urethral spasms, phenoxybenzamine may decrease blood pressure. A sign of excessively low blood pressure is profound sluggishness. Prazosin is a related drug that can also be tried. Oral diazepam (*Valium*) can relax urethral muscles. Side effects include sedation. Occasionally, severe liver damage can occur in cats from diazepam, so the drug is rarely used in cats. Anti-inflammatory drugs may be used in some cases.

Follow-up Care
The ability to urinate is closely monitored in animals with urethritis. If repeated straining occurs and no urine is produced, notify your veterinarian immediately. Frequency of follow-up examinations depends on the underlying cause as well as the severity and recurrence of signs.

Prognosis
Urethral spasm that contributes to urethral obstruction in cats can be a recurrent problem, and it leads to euthanasia in about 25% of affected cats. Like bladder tumors, urethral tumors do not usually respond well to treatment. Urethritis from a bladder infection often resolves completely when the infection is controlled.

SPECIAL INSTRUCTIONS:

Urinary Incontinence in Dogs

Cathy E. Langston, DVM, DACVIM (Small Animal)

BASIC INFORMATION

Description

Urinary incontinence is the involuntary release of urine from the bladder. Incontinence differs from urinary accidents where the dog is aware of the urination (for example, squats to urinate) but may be unable to wait for an appropriate time or place to urinate. Incontinence may arise when problems of the bladder sphincter (the muscle that keeps the bladder closed) or the beginning of the urethra allow urine to leak from the bladder. Urinary incontinence is uncommon in the cat.

Causes

Urinary incontinence can be caused by many different problems. A common cause in young, large-breed dogs is primary urethral sphincter incompetence (also known as *spay incontinence* or *estrogen-responsive incontinence*, although these names are inaccurate). In this condition, the urethral sphincter is weak.

Another common cause in young dogs is ectopic ureters. Secondary causes of incontinence that affect dogs of various ages include inflammation of the urethra or bladder, such as bladder infection, urethritis, stones, or cancer of the bladder or urethra. Spinal diseases can also cause loss of control of the bladder.

Clinical Signs

Urine may dribble constantly or only when the dog is relaxed (sleeping or lying down). In some cases, urine leaks only when the dog jumps or barks. With primary urethral sphincter incompetence, other signs of bladder disease, such as straining to urinate or painful urination, are usually absent. Dogs with this disease usually urinate normally when outside. If other bladder signs are present, such as urgency, pain, straining, or bloody urine, a secondary cause of incontinence is more likely.

Diagnostic Tests

Tests are usually recommended to evaluate the common causes of bladder disease; these may include a urinalysis, urine culture, abdominal x-rays, and an abdominal ultrasound. Cystoscopy (direct inspection of the urethra and bladder with a fiberoptic viewing scope) or a contrast study (injection of dye into a vein or into the bladder followed by a series of x-rays) may detect ectopic ureters or other anatomic abnormalities.

If all initial diagnostic tests are normal, special tests may be indicated to measure the strength of the bladder wall and the urethra. These tests are not commonly available in practice, so your pet may be referred to a veterinary specialty center for these procedures.

TREATMENT AND FOLLOW-UP

Treatment Options

Surgical or laser correction of ectopic ureters is indicated if that condition is present. (See the handout on **Ectopic Ureter in Dogs**.) With secondary urinary incontinence, treatment of the underlying problem usually cures the incontinence. Such treatment may include antibiotics for infection, removal of stones, and other measures.

Medication is helpful in controlling or decreasing the incontinence in cases of primary urethral sphincter incompetence. The drug, phenylpropanolamine, helps the sphincter contract more tightly. It is usually given two to three times daily. Side effects of this medication include high blood pressure (hypertension) and hyperactivity, but most dogs tolerate the medication well. An alternative medication, estrogen pills, can be given twice weekly. Phenylpropanolamine and estrogen can be used together if one drug fails to control the incontinence. Newer drugs are available for use in people, but experience with them in dogs is limited.

If medical management is unsuccessful, collagen injections may be beneficial in some dogs. With the animal under anesthesia, a cystoscope is used to inject a bulking agent (usually collagen, but other substances have been used) into the wall of the urethra. The bulking agent narrows the opening of the urethra, which may allow a weak sphincter to better control urine flow. Over time, the urethra will open again, and some patients require repeated injections every 3-12 months to remain continent. Hydraulic occluder devices have been placed in some dogs. Other surgical procedures have been described to treat severe cases of incontinence that have not responded to medications, but the success of surgery has been variable.

Follow-up Care

Dogs with primary urethral sphincter incompetence that is controlled with phenylpropanolamine and/or estrogen are often monitored with a urinalysis and urine culture every 6 months to ensure that no infection has developed.

Prognosis

In general, urinary incontinence is not a life-threatening disease. In most dogs, the incontinence can be controlled with medications, but in a small number of dogs it is resistant to all forms of therapy.

SPECIAL INSTRUCTIONS:

SECTION 8

Reproductive System
Section Editor: Ronald M. Bright, DVM, MS, DACVS

Agalactia
Cryptorchidism in Dogs and Cats
Dystocia in Dogs and Cats
Eclampsia in Dogs
Infertility in Bitches
Infertility in Male Dogs
Infertility in Queens
Infertility in Toms
Mammary Fibroadenomatous Hyperplasia
Mammary Tumors in Cats
Mammary Tumors in Dogs
Mastitis

Ovarian Remnant Syndrome
Paraphimosis in Dogs
Penile Tumors in Dogs
Phimosis
Pregnancy Loss in Bitches
Pseudocyesis
Pyometra Complex
Subinvolution of Placental Sites in Dogs
Testicular Tumors in Dogs
Uterine Prolapse
Vaginal Edema in Dogs
Vaginitis in Dogs

Agalactia

Ronald M. Bright, DVM, MS, DACVS

BASIC INFORMATION

Description

Agalactia is the absence of milk secretion in a female that has just given birth. It represents either a failure of milk production or failure of the release of milk into the teat canal. Normally, milk is not continuously released after it is produced. Instead, it is stored in the mammary gland (breast tissue) until the gland is stimulated to release the milk, which is called *milk let-down*. Lactation is the production of milk; it usually begins just before the mother gives birth.

Causes

A rare cause of agalactia is complete failure of the mammary glands to develop in the female. Why breast tissue does not develop is not well understood.

Milk let-down may fail to occur from either hormonal causes or psychological abnormalities. First-time pregnancies in young animals or the presence of anxiety or nervousness may prevent the mother from being relaxed enough to allow the litter to suckle. In highly stressed animals, adrenalin is secreted and interferes with the hormone, oxytocin, which enhances milk let-down.

Generalized debilitating conditions, such as infection of the uterus, mammary glands, or other systemic organs, can lead to agalactia. Nutritional deficiency of the dam can cause agalactia but is uncommon in most pets on well-balanced diets.

Clinical Signs

The mammary glands of the mother may or may not be well developed. The offspring attempt to suckle the mother but have no success in getting milk. Both the mother and offspring may become agitated, and the puppies or kittens may cry continuously.

Diagnostic Tests

The mammary glands often look normal on close examination, but no milk is visible on evaluation of the teat canal.

TREATMENT AND FOLLOW-UP

Treatment Options

It is not possible to treat congenital mammary abnormalities, and affected females should not be bred.

In nervous mothers, tranquilizers may be tried, not only to help them relax but because some tranquilizers also increase milk production indirectly. Drugs (such as metoclopramide) that increase the secretion of prolactin, a hormone that helps with milk production, may be given. Metoclopramide must be use cautiously, however, because it may cause hyperactivity or depression.

Suckling by the litter helps stimulate milk let-down. In some instances, when milk production by the mother is adequate, the administration of oxytocin stimulates milk let-down. If the cause of agalactia is poor nutrition or a systemic disease, correction of these conditions may reverse the agalactia.

Follow-up Care and Prognosis

In those mothers with no milk production at all, it often is not possible to reverse the agalactia. In these cases, the offspring must be hand reared. Your veterinarian may recommend that these females not be bred again, because the problem may recur with subsequent pregnancies.

The nervous dam can often be persuaded to allow the offspring to suckle, and milk production may then occur spontaneously. Some of these dogs also respond to oxytocin therapy. For a few days, the offspring may need supplemental feedings. Mothers that suffer from a milk let-down problem may not have the problem with subsequent litters.

SPECIAL INSTRUCTIONS:

Cryptorchidism in Dogs and Cats

Ronald M. Bright, DVM, MS, DACVS

BASIC INFORMATION
Description
Cryptorchidism is the failure of one or both testes to descend into the scrotum; descent usually occurs within 6-8 weeks after birth but may take as long as 6 months. The undescended testicle may be located within the inguinal canal (the groin), in the abdominal cavity, or alongside the penis and prepuce (sheath for the penis) at the base of the scrotum. Cryptorchidism usually involves only one testicle and is more likely to affect the right testis. A testicle that is not in the proper location is termed an *ectopic* testis.

Causes
This is a congenital anomaly that has a reported incidence of approximately 1-10% in dogs and up to 2% in cats. The anomaly is thought to be a trait that can be inherited.

Small-breed dogs are 2.7 times more likely to have this problem. Dog breeds thought to be more commonly affected include the Chihuahua, German shepherd dog, miniature schnauzer, Pomeranian, poodle, Shetland sheepdog, Siberian husky, and Yorkshire terrier. The Persian cat may also be affected.

Clinical Signs

There are usually no signs directly related to the retained testicle. Most signs are related to the development of one or more tumors within the retained testicle. Dogs with a retained testicle are about 14 times more likely to develop a testicular tumor.

Some tumors produce clinical signs associated with their production of estrogen. Dogs may take on female characteristics such as large nipples, hair loss, decreased size of the prepuce, and attraction of other males. The excess estrogen may also cause anemia, bleeding problems, and prostatic disease.

Testes that are not in the normal location are also more susceptible to testicular torsion (twisting of the testicle around its cord). Testicular torsion usually affects testes retained in the abdominal cavity, because of greater mobility compared with the usual location within the scrotum. Dogs with this condition often present with acute abdominal pain, vomiting, abdominal distention, fever, and lethargy.

Diagnostic Tests

Diagnosis of cryptorchidism, especially in the younger animal, can be difficult due to the location of the testis or its small size. Ectopic testes outside the abdomen can often be palpated (felt with

the finger tips), but they are usually smaller than normal, which makes palpation in some cases very difficult. Intra-abdominal testes are almost impossible to palpate unless they are enlarged because they are tumorous or a torsion is present. If a tumor or testicular torsion is suspected, abdominal x-rays or ultrasound help confirm the diagnosis.

TREATMENT AND FOLLOW-UP

Treatment Options

Some medical and surgical attempts (orchiopexy) to move ectopic testes into the scrotum have been largely unsuccessful and probably should not be done, because the condition may be inherited.

- Although a retained testicle should always be removed because of its potential for developing a tumor, both testicles (assuming one has descended correctly into the scrotum) are usually removed at the same time because of the likelihood this anomaly will be passed on to future generations.
- Removal of the ectopic testis may require a skin incision over the testicle or may require abdominal exploratory surgery.
- Testicles that have developed tumors can become very large, but removal may still be worthwhile, because many of these tumors are benign.
- The clinical signs related to increased estrogen that is secreted by some tumors usually subside—even the anemia, which in some cases can become severe.
- The overall health of the prostate gland may also improve from removal of the estrogen-secreting tumor.

Dogs with testicular torsion require stabilization prior to surgery, which is considered an emergency procedure. These dogs often have acute and unrelenting abdominal pain, and they may become seriously ill very quickly.

Follow-up Care

Most animals undergoing cryptorchid surgery do well postoperatively. However, if the surgery is done for a tumor or testicular torsion, the convalescent period is longer, and more intense monitoring and treatment are usually needed.

Prognosis
Prognosis is good if the testicle is removed before any problems develop. Long-term outlook in dogs castrated for testicular torsion or neoplasia is fair to good.

SPECIAL INSTRUCTIONS:

Dystocia in Dogs and Cats

Ronald M. Bright, DVM, MS, DACVS

BASIC INFORMATION

Description

Dystocia is the inability to initiate the act of labor or the delivery of pups or kittens at the end of a pregnancy. Dog breeds at increased risk for dystocia include the Yorkshire terrier, miniature poodle, Pomeranian, English bulldog, dachshund, Chihuahua, and Scottish terrier.

Causes

The causes of dystocia can generally be classified into those caused by the mother and those caused by the fetus.

Uterine inertia is a condition in which the uterine muscles either do not contract (primary uterine inertia) or become fatigued during labor (secondary uterine inertia) from persistent straining against an obstruction within the birth canal. Secondary uterine inertia is almost never the sole cause of dystocia.

A narrow birth canal caused by a previous fracture of the pelvis can prevent passage of the fetus. The head of the fetus may be too large to pass through the birth canal, or the fetus may be oversized or malformed. Sometimes an improper position of the fetus as it approaches the birth canal makes passage difficult.

Psychological stress can delay the onset of labor. A rare cause of dystocia is twisting of the uterus on itself (uterine torsion).

Clinical Signs

The following are signs of dystocia:

- Active straining has occurred for more than 30-60 minutes without the birth of a fetus.
- Straining for 2 or more hours has not resulted in delivery of a fetus.
- The resting stage between expulsion of fetuses is greater than 4 hours and there is no sign of straining even though it is known that more fetuses remain in the uterus.
- Signs of systemic illness, such as vomiting, weakness, or fever, are present.
- Abnormal vaginal discharge, such as frank blood or pus, is present.
- The pregnancy is known to be a high risk (predisposed breed); only one, large fetus is present; or narrowing of the birth canal has occurred from a prior pelvic fracture.
- Attempts to expel a fetus are painful.
- Obvious signs of distress are present.

Diagnostic Tests

The diagnosis of dystocia is often derived from the clinical signs and a thorough physical examination. Other tests that may be recommended include x-rays, an abdominal ultrasound, and laboratory tests, such as measurement of blood calcium levels. Low blood calcium may be associated with uterine inertia. Commercially available external whelping monitors can be used to detect diminished fetal viability (fetal stress) and abnormal patterns in the uterine contractions.

TREATMENT AND FOLLOW-UP

Treatment Options

The treatment of dystocia varies, depending on the underlying cause. If a fetus has passed part of the way through the birth canal but is now caught, it may be possible to dislodge the fetus through cautious use of fingers or instruments. Administering a tranquilizer to relieve stress in an apprehensive bitch or queen may be helpful.

If uterine inertia is diagnosed, medical therapy may be attempted, provided that the birth canal is a normal size, the cervix is open, the fetus is not too large to pass through the canal, and no other obstruction is identified. Medical therapy involves administration of the hormone, oxytocin, to stimulate uterine contractions. If calcium levels are low, supplementation of calcium is indicated, because it enhances uterine contractions and increases the effects of oxytocin.

If medical therapy fails, surgery to perform a cesarean section (C-section) is indicated. Your veterinarian may discuss the option of spaying the mother at the time of the cesarean section. If there are no further plans for breeding the mother or if a uterine rupture is present, ovariohysterectomy (spaying) may be recommended.

Follow-up Care and Prognosis

Following resolution of the current dystocia, emphasis must be placed on preventing dystocia during future pregnancies. Such measures include providing consistent and adequate amounts of exercise during the pregnancy and making sure the mother is fed a well-balanced diet.

To increase the chances of an optimal litter size, it is often recommended that bitches be bred 2 days after ovulation. All queens and bitches should be provided a quiet, dark, stress-free, and sanitary birthing environment.

SPECIAL INSTRUCTIONS:

Eclampsia in Dogs

Ronald M. Bright, DVM, MS, DACVS

BASIC INFORMATION
Description
Eclampsia is sudden onset of weakness, tremors, collapse, or seizures that is caused by low calcium levels in a nursing (lactating) bitch. The condition is also known as *puerperal tetany* or *postpartum hypocalcemia*. It is most often seen in small-breed dogs that are nursing large litters. It occurs only rarely in the cat.

Causes
Eclampsia develops when calcium stores in the mother's body are depleted due to calcium loss in the milk and calcium intake is inadequate. Heavy lactation (milk production and nursing) usually occurs for 2-3 weeks after delivery, and calcium loss can be quite high during this time.

Factors that promote the development of eclampsia include low calcium levels during pregnancy and poor nutrition after whelping. Supplementation of calcium during pregnancy may also precipitate this condition by suppressing the dog's normal regulation of calcium levels in times of greater need.

Clinical Signs
The onset of signs is very sudden (acute). Restlessness and panting may be seen early in the disease. Other typical signs include muscle twitching and spasms, pawing at the face, disorientation, weakness and wobbliness, and seizures. The dog may collapse and enter a coma that is followed by death. Muscles spasms and continuous seizures may result in extremely high body temperatures.

Diagnostic Tests
The diagnosis of eclampsia is suspected based on a history or physical evidence that the dog is lactating and the presence of typical clinical signs. Further evidence may include the timing of the onset of signs, the presence of a large litter, and the size of the dog. A blood test may be recommended to measure calcium levels. Low calcium levels or a positive response to the administration of calcium confirms the diagnosis.

TREATMENT AND FOLLOW-UP
Treatment Options
Restoring calcium levels to normal is the goal of therapy. Intravenous calcium is given to those bitches that have severe signs (seizures, continuous muscle spasms, coma). Severely affected dogs often require hospitalization with supportive fluid therapy and measures to lower their body temperature. On discharge from the hospital, the pups are removed from the bitch for 24 hours or longer. The dog may be sent home on oral calcium, vitamin D, and an improved diet.

For those bitches that are only mildly affected, oral calcium supplements and vitamin D may be tried. The puppies may continue to nurse mildly affected dogs, as long as signs do not worsen.

Follow-up Care
If signs were severe or if the signs return or worsen despite therapy, then it is necessary to hand rear the puppies after removing them from the bitch. Should this bitch be bred again, calcium supplementation started at the beginning of lactation may be helpful.

Prognosis
If treatment is started promptly, most bitches usually respond well to calcium treatment, and eclampsia is successfully controlled. Dogs that become comatose or have extremely high body temperatures for a long period have a worse prognosis.

SPECIAL INSTRUCTIONS:

Infertility in Bitches
Ronald M. Bright, DVM, MS, DACVS

BASIC INFORMATION
Description
An unspayed (intact) female dog is referred to as a *bitch*. Infertility in the bitch is present anytime there is a failure to conceive and become pregnant or when a pregnancy does not proceed to normal whelping (birth of live pups). A normal estrous (heat) cycle is necessary for a successful pregnancy.

Causes
Many different factors can affect the fertility of a bitch, including the following:
- Lack of a normal heat cycle can occur due to malnutrition, stress, generalized diseases, previous removal of the ovaries, ovarian cysts, or certain genetic problems. Sometimes the ovaries are normal and active but no obvious, external signs of heat occur (called a *silent heat*). Lack of exposure to other cycling bitches may also affect the heat cycle.
- The most common reason for many breeding problems in normally cycling bitches is improper breeding management, especially mistimed or an inadequate number of breeding episodes. Ovulation timing can help increase the chances of a successful breeding and is accomplished by running a series of blood tests measuring levels of progesterone or luteinizing hormone (LH).
- An infection of the uterus can create an unfavorable environment for survival of the sperm after breeding. Canine brucellosis is a specific uterine infection that can cause infertility.
- Some bitches have inadequate thyroid hormone levels or lack adequate amounts of LH or progesterone, which adversely affect their heat cycle.
- A number of congenital defects of the genital tract, especially of the vagina, can cause pain or prevent successful penetration by the male.
- Some animals have abnormal sexual organs that do not develop appropriately or enough to allow heat cycles. An example of this is the male pseudohermaphrodite, a dog that has the external appearance of a female but contains abdominal testicles and therefore will show no signs of heat (estrus).

Clinical Signs
An abnormal heat cycle may be noted. The bitch may refuse to breed. Abnormal vaginal discharge can indicate a possible infection of the vagina or uterus. Sometimes no clinical signs are detected, yet the female fails to become pregnant or the puppies are not carried to full term.

Diagnostic Tests
If the heat cycle is normal, the male dog may be the problem and should have its fertility assessed. (See handout on **Infertility in Male Dogs**.) A general health screening with a physical examination and laboratory tests is also indicated for the bitch. Testing is done for brucellosis. A sample may be collected from the vagina during early signs of heat to check for a bacterial infection. If infection is present, it is treated with appropriate antibiotics. Increasing the chance of a successful breeding by pinpointing the best time to breed can be done by measuring progesterone levels and doing vaginal cell analysis.

If a normal heat cycle is not occurring, then husbandry and nutritional factors must be evaluated. A thyroid function test is also performed when the heat cycle is absent.

TREATMENT AND FOLLOW-UP
Treatment Options
Management strategies may include providing optimal nutrition, parasite control, and adequate preventive medicine, as well as a sanitary environment. Correction of any congenital vaginal abnormalities may allow a natural breeding. Correction of problems detected with various diagnostic tests, such as low thyroid function, infection of the genital tract, or lack of heat cycles, may involve, respectively, thyroid supplementation, antibiotics, or the use of hormones to induce a heat cycle.

A bitch that is positive for brucellosis poses a health risk to all other dogs in the household or kennel, and if complete eradication of the disease is desired, then euthanasia of the infected bitch is necessary. Brucellosis can also be transmitted to humans, especially if they are young, old, or immune suppressed. Individual bitches with brucellosis that are not exposed to other dogs may be treated with spaying and long-term antibiotics.

Optimizing the time of breeding by employing proper breeding practices may correct the infertility problem. Artificial insemination using chilled semen may be needed to ensure a pregnancy. A chromosome test may help define a sexual developmental problem, and affected dogs should be removed from the breeding program.

Follow-up Care and Prognosis
Prognosis depends on the cause of the infertility. Approximately one half of infertility problems can be corrected by combining vaginal cell analysis with measurement of progesterone levels and initiation of better management strategies. Elimination of any genital bacterial infections also improves success. Brucellosis and genetic sexual developmental problems are usually irreversible.

SPECIAL INSTRUCTIONS:

Infertility in Male Dogs

Ronald M. Bright, DVM, MS, DACVS

BASIC INFORMATION

Description

A male dog is considered infertile when it is unable to breed a female or when breeding a female at an appropriate time (during ovulation) and multiple times does not result in pregnancy. If there is sporadic success in siring a litter of puppies, or if fewer puppies are produced in the litter than what is normal for the breed, the condition is called *subfertility* or *low fertility*.

Causes

One cause of infertility is inability to mate with the female, for either physical or behavioral reasons.

Behavioral problems may be related to inexperience or anxiety, attempting to breed a dominant female that does not allow the male to mount, or introduction of the male to a nonreceptive female. Males that have been reprimanded for mounting behavior (especially at times unassociated with breeding) are not likely to show normal mounting behavior when it is desired for breeding.

Failure of erection or an erection without ejaculation can occur in some males from physical or behavioral causes. In some dogs, ejaculation occurs but the semen travels backward into the bladder (retroejaculation). Even if the male is an experienced stud, ejaculation may not occur without the presence of a teaser bitch in heat. Physical conditions that prevent the male from assuming the proper position for mounting or locking with the female include spinal or hind leg pain and diseases of the prostate.

Poor semen quality can contribute to lack of conception. Bacterial infections of the genital tract (testicles, prostate), such as brucellosis, can result in poor semen quality. Other causes of low sperm counts include malnutrition, poor general body condition, recent illness, and hormonal problems. Decreased libido (desire to mate) may occur in some dogs.

Congenital causes of infertility include underdevelopment of the testes, abnormal sexual development of the female, and abnormalities or underdevelopment of the penis or sheath.

Clinical Signs

Many dogs have no outward clinical signs other than disinterest in the breeding process or inability to complete the act of mating. Decreased thyroid function is suspected in dogs with low energy, weight gain, or symmetrical hair loss. It is sometimes hard to tell whether the male or the female is the source of the infertility problem.

Diagnostic Tests

Often the diagnosis is based on historical evidence that the dog does not breed well or fails to produce a pregnancy. Close observation of attempts to mate and a thorough physical examination may reveal underlying physical problems. A urinalysis, semen analysis, and bacterial cultures may be recommended. Laboratory testing for brucellosis is commonly done. A thyroid hormone test may be performed. Rectal examination, x-rays, and an ultrasound may be recommended to rule out prostatic disease.

It may be helpful to biopsy the testicles or prostate, especially when other, more common causes of infertility are not found. If abnormal libido is present, measurement of testosterone levels in the blood may be helpful.

TREATMENT AND FOLLOW-UP

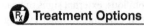 Treatment Options

Administering certain hormones can help correct poor or diminished libido, and some cases of retroejaculation into the bladder also respond to medications. Surgical correction may be attempted for congenital deformities of the penis and sheath. A chromosome test may help define a sexual developmental problem, and affected dogs should be removed from the breeding program.

Prostatic disease can sometimes be treated successfully, depending on the specific cause. Thyroid supplementation usually corrects hypothyroidism (low thyroid levels) and often reverses the male's infertility.

Brucellosis cannot be successfully treated and infertility is irreversible in most cases. Euthanasia is often recommended for brucellosis-positive dogs that live in a kennel environment, because they can transmit the disease to other dogs. Brucellosis can also be transmitted to people, especially if they are old, young, or immune suppressed.

Certain behavioral problems may be helped with hormonal supplementation, or natural mating can be substituted with artificial insemination.

Follow-up Care and Prognosis

The successful return to fertility in the male dog depends on the cause of the problem. Dogs with poor semen quality (decreased sperm count or poor sperm motility) are more likely to be successfully treated than those with complete absence of sperm. Dogs with testicles of a normal size and texture are more likely to become successful breeders than those with shrunken or scarred testicles. Sometimes a testicular biopsy helps predict the dog's ability to return to a fertile status after treatment.

SPECIAL INSTRUCTIONS:

Infertility in Queens

Ronald M. Bright, DVM, MS, DACVS

BASIC INFORMATION

Description

Infertility is suspected when an intact female cat (called a *queen*) either fails to have normal heat cycles or is unable to breed or conceive after mating with an intact, fertile male cat (called a *tom*).

Causes

Numerous causes of infertility exist, such as the following:

- Queens that remain indoors may not have predictable heat cycles as a result of not receiving enough duration or intensity of light. Normally, queens must be exposed to approximately 12-14 hours of daylight to initiate their heat cycle.
- A progesterone-secreting cyst or tumor of the ovary may prevent a heat cycle.
- Some queens do not have normal sexual development, which prevents them from coming into heat.
- Cats that have outward anatomic features of being a queen but have abdominal testes (*pseudohermaphrodites*) will never manifest a heat cycle.
- Some cats that have been surgically sterilized (spayed) but have remnants of ovarian tissue left behind will later come into heat, but they are unable to conceive because they lack a uterus. (See also the handout on **Ovarian Remnant Syndrome.**)
- Some cats may experience an abnormal heat cycle, with a prolonged period of being in heat, as a result of an estrogen-producing ovarian tumor or cyst.
- The queen may refuse to breed because of incompatibility with a particular sexual partner. Young and inexperienced queens may not want to breed with the tom.
- An anatomic abnormality of the vagina may prevent the tom from penetrating the female during mating.
- Queens rely on multiple copulations with a tom to induce ovulation. If multiple matings do not occur, the queen may not conceive.
- Bacterial or viral infections of the genital tract can prohibit a successful pregnancy.
- Infection of the uterus during a specific period of the heat cycle can also result in infertility.
- Congenital abnormalities of the uterus are rare but may render the queen infertile.

Clinical Signs

Signs vary depending on the cause of the fertility. Some cats lack of any obvious evidence of a normal heat cycle. Other cats remain in heat indefinitely or for prolonged periods. Signs of uterine infection include vaginal discharge, an unkempt hair coat, weight loss, lethargy, abdominal distention, fever, increased thirst, and increased urination.

Diagnostic Tests

Sometimes a diagnosis can be made based on a detailed history given by the owner, combined with physical examination by a veterinarian and a thorough evaluation of the reproductive organs. Laboratory tests, x-rays, and an abdominal ultrasound may be recommended to rule out certain illnesses, such as genital and urinary tract diseases and abnormalities. Testing for contagious diseases, such as feline leukemia virus, feline immunodeficiency virus, and feline infectious peritonitis (FIP) may be done.

Measurement of estrogen-related hormones may help identify infertility related to ovarian cysts or tumors. Measurement of progesterone levels can help identify the stage of the heat cycle the cat is experiencing and whether the cat has ovulated. Hormone levels commonly fluctuate, so tests are usually repeated at various intervals. Interpretation of hormonal assays can be difficult, and the results must be assessed in light of other clinical findings.

Chromosomal assays can be performed for certain genetic problems of sexual development. Certain anatomic abnormalities may only be detected via exploratory abdominal surgery.

TREATMENT AND FOLLOW-UP

Treatment Options

Treatment is directed at the primary source of the infertility and any underlying causes. Options include, but are not limited to, the following measures:

- Exposing the queen to 12-14 hours of daylight per day
- Housing the queen with other females that are cycling or with a known fertile male
- Surgical removal of any functional ovarian cysts or tumors
- Allowing the queen and tom to mate multiple times
- Intravaginal or surgical artificial insemination
- Administering drugs known to stimulate ovulation after natural or artificial insemination
- Treating any existing infections with appropriate drugs

Queens with uterine infections may require surgical sterilization, especially if they are systemically ill.

Prognosis

Prognosis varies depending upon the cause of the infertility. In cases where an underlying medical condition or anatomical cause of the infertility can be corrected, the problem may be reversible. Those queens with chromosomal defects, pseudohermaphroditism, and congenital abnormalities of the reproductive tract are permanently infertile. Serious infections of the uterus resulting in the need for surgical removal of the uterus and ovaries also render the queen infertile.

SPECIAL INSTRUCTIONS:

Infertility in Toms

Ronald M. Bright, DVM, MS, DACVS

BASIC INFORMATION

Description

Infertility may be suspected when a male cat (called a *tom*) does not engage in breeding activity with a female cat (called a *queen*) that is known to be in heat. Infertility may also be present if a tom has successfully mated with a known fertile queen but no subsequent pregnancy occurs.

Causes and Clinical Signs

Numerous causes of infertility exist, such as the following:

- Behavioral factors, such as a dominant or aggressive queen, may prevent the tom from mating, especially if the tom is inexperienced.
- A history of negative mating experiences may inhibit future acts of breeding (copulation).
- Sometimes living in a close, restricted environment may exaggerate negative behavioral factors.
- Faulty or abnormal sexual development can result in infertility.
- Decreased libido (disinterest in mating) may be present and is usually worse when the tom is immature. It may have a genetic basis in Persian cats.
- Physical limitations may play a role, such as the presence of a band of tissue preventing extrusion of the penis from its sheath, hair rings at the base of the penis, retrograde ejaculation, or underdeveloped testicles.
- Semen quality or quantity may be abnormal. Factors that affect semen include immaturity of the tom, testicular underdevelopment, and certain chromosomal defects (such as occurs in tortoiseshell-colored males). If the testicles are located in the abdomen (cryptorchidism) instead of in the scrotum, normal mating behavior may occur but the quantity of sperm may be low.
- A variety of chronic illnesses can affect either libido or the quality of the semen.
- Infections of the reproductive tract are uncommon causes of infertility in the tom. Rarely, feline infectious peritonitis (FIP) virus causes inflammation of the testes and infertility.

Diagnostic Tests

Sometimes a diagnosis can be made based on a detailed history given by the owner, combined with physical examination by a veterinarian and a thorough evaluation of the reproductive organs. Semen evaluation may uncover the source of the infertility. Motility of the sperm and the volume of the semen are the two most important parameters analyzed.

Laboratory tests may be recommended to rule out certain illnesses, such as urinary tract diseases. Testing for contagious diseases, such as feline leukemia virus, feline immunodeficiency virus, and FIP, may be done. Thyroid function testing may be recommended.

Measurements of the male hormone, testosterone, may be done in an effort to determine whether a tom has undescended testicles or is castrated. Chromosomal assays can be performed for certain genetic problems of sexual development.

TREATMENT AND FOLLOW-UP

Treatment Options

Treatment is directed at the primary source of the infertility and any underlying causes. Options include, but are not limited to, the following measures:

- Changes in housing and husbandry may be recommended.
- Keeping the tom and queen apart until the actual time of breeding may be helpful.
- Artificial insemination can be done in cats but is not as widespread as in the dog.

Your veterinarian may recommend referral to a reproductive specialist for further evaluation, as well as for help in developing corrective measures or accomplishing artificial insemination.

Prognosis

In many cases in which an underlying medical condition or anatomic cause of the infertility can be corrected, the problem is reversible. Confirmation of a chromosomal problem as the cause of abnormal sexual development carries a grave prognosis, because the affected tom will never be fertile.

SPECIAL INSTRUCTIONS:

Mammary Fibroadenomatous Hyperplasia

Ronald M. Bright, DVM, MS, DACVS

BASIC INFORMATION

Description

Mammary fibroadenomatous hyperplasia causes a significant increase in the size of one or more mammary glands (breasts). It usually develops in young cats that are either cycling in and out of heat or are pregnant.

Cats that have been spayed can develop this condition if they have been given the female hormone, progesterone, or progesterone-type drugs. Rarely, dogs can also develop the disorder when given progesterone-type drugs.

Causes

The cause of fibroadenomatous hyperplasia is not well understood. It may be related to increased levels of circulating progesterone in cats that are going through their heat cycle. The high level of progesterone may subsequently increase the amount of growth hormone secreted by the mammary tissue, which causes the tissue to enlarge. Prolonged administration of progestogen compounds for other conditions may cause the same changes.

Clinical Signs

Affected breasts become enlarged, and the enlargement is often smooth and rounded. Glands on both sides are usually affected in a similar fashion, so that the swelling is symmetrical. Because of the distribution of mammary tissue, more masses may arise than the actual normal number of mammary glands.

Affected glands are usually nonpainful and soft to the touch. The glands may become quite large, ranging from 1 to 5 inches (2-10 cm) in diameter. Sometimes the skin overlying the masses becomes stretched, red in color, and ulcerated (covered in raw, oozing sores). If the glands become inflamed, they may be painful.

The presence of active milk secretion is uncommon.

Diagnostic Tests

Making the diagnosis is helped by knowing the age, sexual status, and reproductive history of the animal (including administration of progesterone drugs). Obtaining a biopsy of the mass is the best way to diagnose this disease, and in many cases it may be done without removing the whole gland.

The most important conditions to differentiate from fibroadenomatous hyperplasia are mastitis (infection) and tumors of the mammary glands. Your veterinarian may recommend further tests to rule out these conditions.

TREATMENT AND FOLLOW-UP

Treatment Options

Removing the source of the progesterone is the primary goal of treatment, because the condition often regresses spontaneously once the hormone is withdrawn.

- The treatment of choice in the young cat that is going through heat cycles is to surgically remove the ovaries. Removal of the ovaries is usually combined with removal of the uterus (ovariohysterectomy or spaying of the cat). Regression often occurs within 3-4 weeks after the spay surgery, although it is occasionally delayed for up to 5-6 months.
- Antiprogesterone drugs can be tried and, if successful, will result in regression of the masses in 3-4 weeks. These drugs should not be given to pregnant cats, because they may cause abortion.
- If progesterone drugs have been used in the cat, discontinuation of the drug usually results in complete resolution of the lesions in 5-6 months.

Surgical removal of the affected glands can be done, but there is some controversy surrounding this option. It is generally recommended for those cats that do not respond to conventional therapy or when there is evidence of trauma or infection of the gland.

Follow-up Care

Follow-up visits are often needed to monitor the glands once a specific therapy has begun.

Prognosis

Prognosis is good when the source of progestogen is completely removed. Similarly, prognosis is also good after surgical removal in those rare instances where it is indicated.

SPECIAL INSTRUCTIONS:

Mammary Tumors in Cats

Ronald M. Bright, DVM, MS, DACVS

BASIC INFORMATION

Description

Mammary gland tumors are benign or malignant masses that develop in breast tissue. They are the third most common tumor in the cat and account for about 17% of all tumors in the female cat.

Older, intact (unspayed) cats are most often affected. Siamese cats are at twice the risk for developing mammary tumors and often develop them at an earlier age. Male cats may rarely develop mammary tumors but usually at an older age than the females.

Causes

Cats can develop mammary tumors secondary to the influence of estrogen or progesterone hormones. Intact cats have a seven-fold increased chance of developing a mammary tumor if they are not spayed before 6 months of age. Use of progesterone-like drugs also increases the chance that a cat will develop a mammary tumor.

Clinical Signs

The breasts toward the front of the chest are affected most commonly. Mammary tumors are usually in an advanced state when they are first noticed, because they have an aggressive nature. They are often attached to underlying structures, and approximately 25% of the masses are ulcerated on the surface (the skin over the mass has raw sores). The nipples are often swollen and red and may drain tan or yellow material. In more than 50% of affected cats, multiple glands are involved.

Breathing problems related to spread of the cancer to the lungs may be present, and some cats are thin and ungroomed.

Diagnostic Tests

The presence of a mass in a mammary gland in an older, intact female cat is highly suggestive of a mammary tumor. Fine-needle aspiration of the tumor and examination of the cells under the microscope usually confirms the presence of a malignant tumor and helps rule out other tumors not arising from mammary tissue.

If a malignant tumor is suspected or confirmed, it is important to determine whether the tumor has spread beyond the borders of the mammary tissue. Laboratory tests may be normal but are often recommended prior to biopsy or surgery. X-rays of the lungs and an ultrasound may be recommended to check for spread (metastasis) of the tumor. Aspiration of nearby lymph nodes (glands) with a fine needle may also help detect metastasis.

TREATMENT AND FOLLOW UP

Treatment Options

Surgery is the most common treatment for mammary tumors in the cat.

- In most cases, because of the aggressive nature of mammary tumors in cats, radical surgery is necessary. This may include removal of one or both mammary chains (complete mastectomy) depending on the location of the tumors.
- Because these tumors often invade into deeper structures such as the muscle, additional tissues must often be removed.
- Sometimes removal of nearby lymph nodes is also recommended at the time of surgery.

Removal of the ovaries and uterus is considered part of the treatment of these tumors, since ovarian and uterine disease often coexists with mammary tumors. Spaying of the cat is often delayed until the mastectomy surgery has healed and the cat has fully recovered. Radiation therapy and chemotherapy have not been very helpful (so far) in killing these tumors.

Follow-up Care

When a radical mastectomy is done, especially if both sides of the mammary chain are removed, the wound is often inflamed and has some degree of swelling along the suture line. A soft, padded bandage is often placed over the surgical site for several days to make the cat more comfortable and to protect the wound. Certain postoperative medications may be recommended in these cases.

Recheck visits are usually needed after surgery to monitor healing. Periodic laboratory tests and x-rays may be done to monitor for metastasis if the tumor was malignant.

Prognosis

In cats, the size of the malignant tumor is an important prognostic factor. The average survival time after surgery can vary from 4 months to more than 3 years, depending on the size of the tumor. It is important to realize that early diagnosis, combined with aggressive treatment, provides the best chance for prolonged survival in cats with malignant mammary tumors. In most cats, the more radical the surgery (mastectomy involving all mammary tissue compared to regional mastectomy), the better the survival times. The success of surgery is often compromised in the cat, however, because of the invasive nature of these tumors.

SPECIAL INSTRUCTIONS:

Mammary Tumors in Dogs

Ronald M. Bright, DVM, MS, DACVS

BASIC INFORMATION

Description

Mammary gland tumors are benign or malignant masses that develop in breast tissue. They usually affect older, female dogs. They are the most common tumors found in the female. These tumors usually occur in intact (unspayed) females or in dogs that were spayed later in life.

Causes

Since half of all mammary tumors contain hormone receptors, their development may be linked to estrogen or progesterone hormones. Dogs given progesterone to prevent heat cycles are at a greater risk of developing mammary tumors.

The risk of developing mammary tumors is directly related to the number of heat cycles the dog has experienced. If the dog is spayed before the first heat cycle, the risk is as low as 0.05%. Relative risk increases to 8% after one heat cycle and to 26% after a second heat cycle.

Clinical Signs

A swelling develops in one or more mammary glands or in adjacent tissue. The mammary glands closest to the rear legs are most commonly affected. The number, size, and shape vary depending on the time of diagnosis. Some benign masses are only found when the dog is petted or during routine physical examinations.

Mammary masses that are severely inflamed and ulcerated or that cause a fever may resemble mastitis and are probably malignant (cancerous). With very advanced tumors, clotting disorders can develop, with bleeding from the gums, skin, vulva, or other superficial surfaces. Occasionally, lameness can occur if the tumor has spread to a bone.

Diagnostic Tests

Laboratory tests may be normal but are often recommended prior to biopsy or surgery. X-rays of the lungs and an ultrasound may be recommended to check for spread of the tumor, especially if a malignancy is suspected. X-rays or a specialized bone scan can be done to determine whether the tumor has spread to bone.

Aspiration of the mass with a fine needle often helps identify whether the tumor is benign or malignant. Similar aspirations of nearby lymph nodes (glands) may help to detect metastasis. If it is uncertain that the mass is really a tumor, small pieces may be removed for analysis by a pathologist. For small, well-defined tumors, your veterinarian may recommend proceeding directly to surgery to remove the mass, with subsequent submission of the tissue to a pathologist.

TREATMENT AND FOLLOW-UP

Treatment Options

A number of surgical procedures are available for treating these tumors. They range from a simple lumpectomy to a radical chain mastectomy (removal of all glands on one side), depending on the characteristics of the tumor and how many glands are involved.

- Lumpectomies are usually limited to small, well-defined nodules.
- Removal of one entire gland may be done when a single tumor is located in the center of the gland.
- A partial mastectomy (removal of 1-3 glands) or chain mastectomy is done when multiple glands are affected on one side.
- Removing both chains of mammary glands during the same surgery is not usually recommended, because it is difficult to get adequate closure of the surgical wounds and the procedure is hard on the dog.
- No particular surgical procedure is more effective than others, so the technique chosen is usually based on the clinical findings in each dog.

Removal of the ovaries (assuming the bitch is still intact) has not been proven to alter the prognosis following surgery; however, the remaining mammary tissues will usually shrink somewhat, which makes it easier for the owner and veterinarian to detect new tumors. Radiation therapy and chemotherapy have not been very effective for treatment of mammary tumors in dogs.

Follow-up Care

Most dogs do well following surgery for mammary tumors but may require hospitalization for a few days. In some cases, drains are inserted for a few days, and bandaging is required for some dogs. Periodic laboratory tests and x-rays may be done to monitor for metastasis if the tumor was malignant.

Prognosis

For benign mammary tumors, prognosis is good following surgery. Dogs with malignant tumors less than 1.5 inches (3 cm) in diameter have a better prognosis following surgery than those with larger tumors.

The presence of multiple tumors does not seem to affect prognosis. Survival for longer than 2 years may be possible with some low-grade cancers. Tumors that are large and invade deep tissues have a poor prognosis because of their higher potential for metastasis. Dogs that have been spayed prior to developing a mammary tumor have a better prognosis with some types of carcinomas than unspayed dogs.

SPECIAL INSTRUCTIONS:

Mastitis

Ronald M. Bright, DVM, MS, DACVS

BASIC INFORMATION
Description
Mastitis is inflammation and/or infection of one or more mammary glands (breasts). It is an uncommon condition in dogs and cats. It usually arises immediately after a pregnancy or during a pseudopregnancy. Pseudopregnancy occurs most often in the dog and is a condition in which the dog displays many features of being pregnant but is not.

Causes
Most cases of mastitis involve infections that arise when bacteria are introduced through the open teat of the breast or when bacteria spread to the mammary tissue from another site via the bloodstream. Lactation (production of milk) during the postpartum period (after giving birth) allows bacteria easier access to the mammary gland.

Mastitis can arise from abnormal collection of milk within the mammary glands and is sometimes associated with poor hygiene. Rarely, mastitis may occur from the trauma of kittens or puppies suckling. Conversely, young offspring with an infection may transfer the bacteria to the mother, who subsequently develops mastitis.

🔲 Clinical Signs
Mastitis can occur suddenly (acute mastitis) or develop slowly and become chronic. Signs of acute mastitis include the following:
- The involved glands are swollen, reddened in appearance, and tender to the touch.
- Some affected animals are lethargic, have a fever, and do not eat well.
- One or more glands may be involved, with the last pair of glands (closest to the rear legs) being the ones most commonly affected.
- When an affected gland is squeezed, discolored milk or secretions that contain blood or pus may be seen.
- Severely involved glands can become gangrenous or abscessed and may occasionally develop deep ulcerations (sores).
- The offspring may become sick or die in some cases.

Chronic mastitis may be an incidental finding, especially in older, nonlactating, intact (unspayed) cats. With chronic mastitis, minimal inflammation may be present, but thickened tissue or nodules are detected. These changes are similar to those seen with mammary tumors.

🔷 Diagnostic Tests
A tentative diagnosis can often be made based on physical examination findings consistent with mastitis. Laboratory tests may indicate the presence of an infection (high white blood cell count). Examination of a milk sample may show a high cell count that is consistent with an infection. Culture of the milk helps to confirm the type of bacteria present and to identify possible antibiotic choices.

TREATMENT AND FOLLOW-UP
🔳 Treatment Options
It is important that therapy be started shortly after confirmation of the diagnosis. Appropriate antibiotics are started immediately, even while the culture results are pending. It is important that the affected glands be kept empty of secretions, which can be done manually by some owners.

The offspring can continue to suckle mildly infected glands, but the nutritional value of the milk is poor. It is best not to allow suckling from severely infected glands or those glands that have gangrene or are abscessed. If only one or two glands are affected, they may be bandaged to prevent the neonates from suckling them. If nursing from healthy glands is not possible, then hand rearing is required.

In severely diseased (abscessed or gangrenous) glands, milk secretions may be stripped from each gland twice daily and warm, wet compresses applied to help with healing. Surgical drainage may be done in some cases. More radical surgery (mastectomy) may be recommended for glands that do not respond to treatment.

If the mother is systemically ill, hospitalization may be necessary to allow more intensive therapy (such as intravenous fluids or injectable antibiotics).

🐾 Follow-up Care
Recheck visits may be needed to monitor response to treatment and determine how long the antibiotics should be given. Notify your veterinarian if any clinical signs worsen or if more glands become involved once therapy has started.

Prognosis
Prognosis for most animals with mastitis is good, especially if treatment is begun without delay. Recovery may be slower or more complicated in animals that are seriously ill and require hospitalization.

SPECIAL INSTRUCTIONS:

Ovarian Remnant Syndrome

Ronald M. Bright, DVM, MS, DACVS

BASIC INFORMATION

Description

This condition arises when functional residual ovarian tissue is left in the abdomen following an ovariohysterectomy (OHE, OVH, "spay") or ovariectomy (OVE). Because the ovaries secrete estrogen, signs related to the continued production of estrogen can be observed in what was otherwise thought to be a sterilized animal.

Causes

Inappropriate surgical technique is the usual cause of this syndrome. Accessory ovarian tissue in an abnormal location has never been reported in the dog and only rarely in the cat. Usually the ovarian remnant is located on the right side, because the right ovary is more difficult to visualize and isolate during the sterilization procedure.

Clinical Signs

Most dogs and cats with retained ovarian tissue have signs that are similar to being in heat. The signs can arise soon after the "spay" or can be delayed, in some cases for years. A "false pregnancy" may also be seen and is more common in the dog than in the cat.

Diagnostic Tests

The easiest way to confirm the problem is to look at cells taken from a vaginal swab. The vaginal cells undergo changes that are a direct result of estrogen's influence.

A more sophisticated way to confirm that an ovarian remnant is still in the abdomen is to run hormone analyses. Measurement of estrogen compounds can be helpful, but the test is not always reliable. Measurement of progesterone levels is much more useful.

Lastly, confirmation can be made during an exploratory laparotomy (abdominal surgery to search for possible retained ovarian tissue).

TREATMENT AND FOLLOW-UP

Treatment Options

Surgery to remove the ovarian remnant tissue is the treatment of choice. It is usually done when the animal shows signs of being in heat, because the ovarian tissue is easier to identify during that time. The tissue removed is usually submitted for pathologic analysis to confirm that the tissue is actually ovarian in origin and not an estrogen-secreting tumor.

Follow-up Care

Clinical signs usually resolve within days after surgery. If the animal continues to demonstrate signs of heat at a later date, then remnant tissue probably still remains. Absence of signs confirms successful treatment of the problem. Postoperative care is similar to that recommended after a routine spay surgery.

Prognosis

Prognosis is good if the ovarian remnant is successfully removed. In some cases, these remnants are not easy to find, and recurrence of signs is possible if ovarian tissue is left in the abdomen.

SPECIAL INSTRUCTIONS:

Paraphimosis in Dogs

Russell W. Fugazzi, DVM

BASIC INFORMATION

Description

Paraphimosis is a condition in which the penis protrudes from the prepuce (sheath around the penis) and does not return to its normal position.

Causes

Paraphimosis can occur for many reasons in any dog, such as the following:

- German shepherd dogs and golden retrievers have a possibly inherited condition in which the opening of the prepuce is narrow or the sheath is shorter than normal, and the penis can become trapped outside the prepuce.
- The condition occurs most often when hair becomes wrapped around the base of the penis while an erection is occurring. The hair forms a ring that entraps the penis, prevents it from returning to a normal position, and can actually strangulate the penis.
- Trauma to the penis and infection or foreign bodies in the penis and prepuce may cause paraphimosis.
- Neurologic problems that allow the penis to hang out of the prepuce, such as paralysis involving the rear legs, may be a cause.
- Tumors (often cancer) of the penis and prepuce may be contributing factors.

Clinical Signs

Signs typically develop quickly. Initially, insistent licking of the genital area or the penis may be the only sign. After several hours, the penis may become terribly swollen and turn purple or black. This swelling can be very painful and often prevents normal urination.

Diagnostic Tests

Diagnosis is usually made by careful physical examination. The condition usually causes no direct changes in laboratory tests, although some testing may be recommended if an infection or cancer is suspected.

TREATMENT AND FOLLOW-UP

Treatment Options

Paraphimosis is considered an emergency. The immediate goal is to relocate the penis to its normal position within the prepuce. Your veterinarian may insert a urinary catheter into the penis and urethra if there is concern that the urinary tract is obstructed. Antibiotics may be recommended if an infection is present. Other therapy may involve the following:

- Lubrication of the penis with topically applied jellies or salves
- Application of special solutions to try and shrink the swelling
- Removal of foreign bodies, including matted or tangled hair rings
- Removal of any tumors present
- Surgical enlargement of the opening of the prepuce and manual replacement of the penis
- Surgical amputation of the penis if the penis is so severely affected that it is no longer healthy or if the prepuce is too short to cover the entire penis

Follow-up Care

Once the penis is returned to its normal position, the dog is usually isolated from any source of stimulation, such as female dogs in heat or excitable activities. The dog is also monitored constantly to make sure it can urinate normally. If surgery was done, postoperative medications may be prescribed, and rechecks are scheduled to evaluate the surgical site and remove the sutures. Notify your veterinarian if any signs recur, especially if the condition is associated with congenital problems of the penis and prepuce or is neurologic in origin.

Prognosis

Most affected dogs have a very poor prognosis for returning to normal breeding function. With early, successful medical or surgical management, prognosis for a comfortable life is fair to good in most cases.

SPECIAL INSTRUCTIONS:

Penile Tumors in Dogs

Ronald M. Bright, DVM, MS, DACVS

BASIC INFORMATION

Description

These tumors affect the surface of the penis. They may occasionally extend to the urinary tract (urethra) or the overlying prepuce (sheath). Some tumors (such as papillomas) are benign, whereas other tumors (such as squamous cell carcinomas) are malignant.

Causes

The most common tumor, transmissible venereal tumor (TVT) occurs worldwide and is a sexually transmissible tumor. It is seen in high concentrations in areas where large numbers of dogs roam free. It most often affects young, sexually active dogs. A viral cause is suspected. Other types of penile tumors occur spontaneously and are relatively rare.

Clinical Signs

Affected dogs usually show chronic signs of discomfort, licking of the penis and prepuce, and bloody or light-pink discharge from the prepuce. Swelling and inability of the penis to move beyond the opening of the prepuce are seen occasionally. A mass may be visible in the opening of the prepuce or on the penis, and a foul odor may sometimes occur in the area.

Diagnostic Tests

A presumptive diagnosis can be made based on the location of the tumor, clinical signs, and physical examination findings. A TVT may also be suspected based on the geographic location and habits of the dog. A sample obtained by aspiration with a fine needle often identifies the mass as being a tumor and sometimes positively identifies the tumor type. Occasionally, tissue biopsies or complete removal of the tumor, followed by microscopic examination, is necessary to confirm the diagnosis. Laboratory tests, x-rays, and sometimes an ultrasound may be recommended to determine whether the tumor has spread to other parts of the body (metastasized).

TREATMENT AND FOLLOW-UP

Treatment Options

Treatment depends on the type of tumor present. Numerous options are available for treating TVTs. Chemotherapy with a drug called *vincristine* is a common choice. The drug is given intravenously on a weekly basis for several treatments. Surgical removal can be tried in some cases, but recurrence is a common problem. To prevent recurrence, surgery may be combined with radiation therapy. Dogs with TVT should not be allowed to roam free, and your veterinarian may recommend castration to help decrease the desire to breed with other dogs.

Other types of tumors that arise on the tip of the penis may be treated by surgical removal and partial amputation of the penis. Tumors that develop near the base of the penis are more difficult to treat and may require complete removal of the penis and redirection of the urethra to another location (urethrostomy). In these cases, your veterinarian may refer your dog to a veterinary surgery or oncology specialist for further evaluation and treatment.

Follow-up Care

Recheck visits are scheduled at regular intervals while dogs are undergoing treatment for TVTs, and some laboratory testing may be recommended to monitor for side effects of the chemotherapy. If surgery was done, postoperative medications may be prescribed, and rechecks are scheduled to evaluate the surgical site and remove the sutures. Notify your veterinarian if the dog has any problems urinating or if bleeding is detected from the penis or the incision. Long-term monitoring (laboratory tests, x-rays, ultrasound) is often needed if the tumor was found to be malignant.

Prognosis

Prognosis is highly dependent on whether the tumor is benign or malignant. Many TVTs that are found when they are small can be treated successfully with chemotherapy and do not recur. In some cases, TVTs can behave in a malignant fashion and spread to other parts of the body. In these cases, the prognosis is often poor. Prognosis is good for other benign tumors that can be completely removed with surgery. Prognosis is often very poor with tumors that are malignant, cannot be completely removed, or are unresponsive to chemotherapy or radiation therapy.

SPECIAL INSTRUCTIONS:

Phimosis

Ronald M. Bright, DVM, MS, DACVS

BASIC INFORMATION
Description
Phimosis is the inability of the penis to protrude or extend beyond the prepuce (sheath). This condition is also known as *preputial stenosis*.

Causes
Phimosis can be a congenital (present from birth) problem, or it can arise later in life from scarring around the opening of the prepuce caused by a tumor or trauma. The congenital form may not be detected for weeks or months.

Clinical Signs
Signs related to the congenital form are dependent on the size of the opening of the prepuce. The prepuce may be distended, and the dog may be unable to urinate normally. A small stream of urine or drops of urine are often seen and may be accompanied by an infection of the prepuce, with discharge of pus from the prepuce. Some ulceration (raw sores) of the prepuce may be present.

The acquired form that develops later in a dog's life usually causes significant inflammation and swelling of the prepuce. Evidence of a tumor or wound to the prepuce may be present.

With either form of phimosis, licking of the area is a common sign. In severe cases, urine may build up within the prepuce, causing it to become distended. Animals with phimosis are unable to breed.

Diagnostic Tests
Close inspection of the prepuce usually defines the problem and allows an accurate diagnosis to be made. Sometimes, however, a poorly developed penis or the presence of hermaphroditism may be confused with phimosis, so these conditions must be ruled out. An animal that is an hermaphrodite has both ovarian and testicular tissues. Because conflicting sets of hormones are produced, the external sexual structures may be deformed or underdeveloped.

Specialized testing and/or exploratory surgery of the abdomen (to look for ovarian and testicular tissue) are needed to make the diagnosis of hermaphroditism.

TREATMENT AND FOLLOW-UP
Treatment Options
If phimosis is caused by inflammation or infection, it may respond to medical therapy, which can consist of antibiotics, warm compresses applied directly to the prepuce, and insertion of a urinary catheter for several days.

Phimosis caused by a stricture (narrowing of the preputial opening with scar tissue) or by a tumor is treated with surgery. Surgery consists of enlarging the opening of the prepuce and removal of any scar tissue or tumors. Without surgery, a severe and painful infection of the prepuce may become a chronic problem. A second surgery may be necessary as the dog matures and grows, if the original one was performed when the dog was very small. If a tumor is present, additional therapy may be recommended by your veterinarian.

Follow-up Care
Recheck visits and monitoring are usually needed for some time. If phimosis is caused by a tumor, then monitoring for recurrence of the tumor is necessary. Scarring of the preputial opening may also occur after surgery, and the size of the opening may slowly decrease. Sometimes, the size of the preputial opening allows the penis to be extruded but not retracted, and paraphimosis develops. Paraphimosis can occur if too much tissue is removed from the prepuce. (See the handout on **Paraphimosis in Dogs**.)

Prognosis
Animals undergoing surgery usually have a good prognosis. The need for a second surgery is low unless the original surgery was performed when the dog was a small puppy.

SPECIAL INSTRUCTIONS:

Pregnancy Loss in Bitches

Ronald M. Bright, DVM, MS, DACVS

BASIC INFORMATION

Description

Pregnancy loss can occur from early death (during the first half of the pregnancy) and subsequent resorption of the fetuses, which is indistinguishable from a failure to conceive. Pregnancy loss can arise with abortion during the second half of pregnancy. It may also involve the birth of stillborn pups or the presence of nonviable puppies in the uterus.

Causes

Bacterial infections, such as brucellosis, are potential causes. A *Brucella* infection typically causes abortion late in the pregnancy. It is possible that infected bitches can proceed to term and give birth to stillborn or weak pups. Other types of bacteria, including normal inhabitants of the vagina (*Mycoplasma*, *Ureaplasma*) have also been associated with pregnancy loss.

Some viruses, such as herpesvirus, canine distemper virus, and parvovirus, can result in loss of puppies during the last 3 weeks of pregnancy. Herpesvirus infection produces changes to the placenta that result in the birth of stillborn, disfigured, mummified, or weak pups that vary in size.

Toxoplasmosis, a protozoal disease, is a very rare cause. If loss of pregnancy occurs, the bitch is usually quite ill from the disease. Lack of the hormone *luteinizing hormone* can cause decreased progesterone levels, resulting in loss of pregnancy.

Clinical Signs

Most dogs suffering from interrupted pregnancies have no specific clinical signs but may exhibit lethargy, fever, and decreased appetite. Vaginal discharge (blood, pus, or both) may occur.

Diagnostic Tests

Your veterinarian may recommend testing of both the bitch and the dead pups to search for a cause. Such tests may include routine laboratory tests, bacterial cultures, viral assays, hormonal assays, x-rays, an abdominal ultrasound, and other specialized tests. The dead puppies may be submitted for pathologic examination (necropsy).

Measurement of progesterone levels on a weekly basis in the pregnant bitch for 6-8 weeks may be helpful. If progesterone levels fall below a certain level, then further testing, monitoring, or treatment may be necessary.

TREATMENT AND FOLLOW-UP

Treatment Options

The presence of brucellosis presents a real dilemma in how to proceed. Brucellosis is not curable, and even if it appears to be successfully treated, it often recurs weeks, months, or years later. Brucellosis is transmissible to humans and may require reporting to health authorities. If the bitch is in a kennel, euthanasia may be necessary to eradicate the disease and prevent exposure to other dogs. Spaying of the dog decreases shedding of bacteria in the urine and may help prevent transmission of the disease.

Treatment of a bitch for a bacterial infection at the time of abortion is not usually helpful in preserving any remaining fetuses. However, administration of antibiotics may be necessary to keep the bitch from becoming systemically ill. Some antibiotics are not safe for use during pregnancy.

Herpesvirus-infected bitches rarely need treatment, and they rarely lose more than one litter to this virus. If pups are thought to have the virus, keep them in a very warm environment to try and keep the virus from multiplying in the pups.

Bitches with very low progesterone levels can be treated with progesterone drugs. Some bitches may have poor milk production early in the lactation period if given progesterone while pregnant.

Follow-up Care

It is important to test all breeding bitches for brucellosis every 6 months, even if they are not being used in an active breeding program. Testing for herpesvirus is not very helpful in detecting the disease.

Repeated measurement of progesterone levels is often necessary in bitches with a history of low progesterone, so that the dosage and frequency of progesterone supplementation can be determined. Indiscriminate use of progesterone can result in nonviable pups or pups born with congenital abnormalities.

Prognosis

Some forms of pregnancy loss can be corrected, with subsequent pregnancies carried to term. If the pregnancy loss was related to a bacterial infection, a swab of material can be obtained from deep within the vagina for bacterial culturing early in the next heat cycle. If the culture is positive, appropriate antibiotics can be started. Improving the cleanliness of the environment and providing better nutrition may be helpful. It can take considerable effort and cooperation with your veterinarian to rectify pregnancy loss problems, so that the dog may be bred again successfully and give birth to normal puppies.

SPECIAL INSTRUCTIONS:

Pseudocyesis

Ronald M. Bright, DVM, MS, DACVS

BASIC INFORMATION

Description

Pseudocyesis occurs when an intact (unspayed) and nonpregnant female dog goes through a phase of mammary (breast) development, lactation (production of milk), and behavior similar to that of pregnant bitches. The affected bitch often allows nursing and displays mothering tendencies. This condition is sometimes referred to as a *false pregnancy* or a *false whelping*. Pseudocyesis occurs during the later stages (diestrus) of a heat cycle.

Causes

All bitches produce the hormone, progesterone, for 2 months after ovulation, which results in mammary development. When progesterone decreases abruptly near the end of the diestrus phase of the heat cycle, it stimulates release of another hormone (prolactin) that causes mothering behavior and lactation.

Pseudocyesis can also arise from withdrawal of progesterone therapy in an intact bitch or following an ovariohysterectomy (spay surgery) during the later phases of the heat cycle.

Clinical Signs

Mammary gland distention and the presence of a light-colored fluid or milk at the nipples are commonly seen. Common behavioral changes include mothering of inanimate objects in the household, nesting, and periods of aggression. Hair loss is sometimes seen but is uncommon. Inflammation of the mammary glands may also occur, because the breast tissue is enlarged and engorged. Glands with mastitis are often swollen, painful, and warm.

Diagnostic Tests

Diagnosis is often based on the presence of the clinical signs in a dog that was in heat approximately 2 months previously. If there is any chance the bitch was bred when it was last in heat, an abdominal ultrasound may be recommended to rule out a pregnancy.

TREATMENT AND FOLLOW-UP

Treatment Options

Most signs of pseudocyesis usually disappear spontaneously within 2-3 weeks. Mammary glands should not be massaged or milked out, which would result in even more mammary engorgement. Gently wrapping the mammary glands to apply direct pressure may decrease the release of prolactin hormone, with subsequent decrease in milk production. The wrap also provides some protection to the glands from trauma.

A drug called *megestrol acetate* can be tried for this condition, but clinical signs often return once the treatment is stopped. This drug may also cause changes in temperament and an increase in appetite. If the bitch has sugar diabetes, mammary tumors, or an infection of the uterus, this drug should not be used. For all these reasons, the drug is not often recommended for pseudocyesis.

Testosterone, which is a male hormone, can be given to decrease milk production. Some drugs (bromocriptine, cabergoline) that inhibit the release of prolactin (the hormone responsible for milk production) can also be tried. The most common side effect of these drugs is vomiting.

Spaying the dog does little for the current episode of pseudocyesis but prevents a recurrence in the future.

In aggressive animals, short-term use of a tranquilizer can be helpful. However, some commonly used sedatives can stimulate milk production and may worsen the clinical signs.

Follow-up Care

Continued monitoring and recheck examinations may be recommended over a 2- to 4-week period.

Prognosis

The age at which pseudocyesis occurs is variable, and it does not always occur with every heat cycle. The development of this condition may be an indicator of normal function of the ovaries and does not usually indicate a uterine disease. There is some evidence that repeated episodes of pseudocyesis may be associated with an increased incidence of malignant mammary tumors in the dog's later years.

SPECIAL INSTRUCTIONS:

Pyometra Complex

Ronald M. Bright, DVM, MS, DACVS

BASIC INFORMATION
Description

Pyometra is a term used to describe a pus-filled uterus. It occurs more often in dogs than in cats. The severity of this disease is influenced by whether the cervix is open (and draining pus) or closed. Most affected dogs and cats are 6 years of age or older and still have both their ovaries and uterus. Sometimes, spayed animals can get an infection of the remnant of the uterus that is left behind in the abdomen near the cervix; this is called a *stump pyometra*. Stump pyometra is more likely to occur if ovarian tissue was left behind during the original spay surgery and continues to produce hormones.

Causes

The hormone, progesterone, normally causes the lining of the uterus to produce a fluid-like secretion. When the uterus is idle for a long time, such as between the periods of heat (estrus), this fluid may accumulate and the lining of the uterus may become thickened. If inflammation and bacterial contamination occur, the secretions become infected. If the cervix is closed and the infected material cannot drain to the outside, the uterus may become very distended, and the infection can spread to other parts of the body, causing the animal to be seriously ill.

Dogs given estrogen treatments can also develop pyometra within 1-10 weeks after administration.

Clinical Signs

Signs in cats are usually seen within 4 weeks after the last heat cycle. In dogs, they often occur about 8 weeks after the last heat cycle. Because the infection can affect many other organs, the signs can vary:

- Many animals are very ill and often (but not always) have some vaginal discharge.
- Many dogs have decreased appetite, lethargy, increased thirst and urination, depression, vomiting, and diarrhea.
- Signs in cats are often not as obvious; depression and decreased appetite may be the only signs seen until the disease becomes advanced.
- When vaginal discharge does not occur, the diagnosis is more of a challenge.
- Most animals have a fever, but body temperature in some animals may be normal or even below normal.

Diagnostic Tests

It is helpful to know when the animal's last heat cycle occurred. Some animals have obvious uterine enlargement when the abdomen is palpated (felt by the veterinarian); however, this may be difficult to determine in obese animals.

Because pyometra affects other organs, laboratory tests are often recommended to look for evidence of infection, kidney disease, liver changes, and sometimes anemia. The white blood count is usually greatly elevated. X-rays of the abdomen often show tubular, fluid-filled structures in the area of the uterus. The uterus can have a similar appearance during early pregnancy, and occasionally x-rays are inconclusive, so an ultrasound may be recommended to determine uterine location, thickness, and size and the presence of fluid. Bacterial culture of the uterine fluid may be recommended, especially at the time of surgery.

TREATMENT AND FOLLOW-UP
Treatment Options

The treatment of choice is surgery to remove the uterus and the ovaries (ovariohysterectomy). Most animals require hospitalization with aggressive fluid therapy and antibiotics prior to surgery. In rare instances, the uterus ruptures prior to surgery, causing the animal to become very ill. These animals may require emergency surgery followed by intensive care. If the animal has already been spayed, the remaining stump of the uterus and any ovarian remnants left behind from the original spay surgery must be removed.

If the owner wishes to use the animal for future breeding, medical therapy may be considered. Medical therapy using a prostaglandin drug (*Lutalyse*) is limited to those animals that have an open cervix and are not critically ill. However, owners must be aware of the potential risks to the animal if surgery is delayed. If prostaglandin drugs are used when the cervix is closed, the uterus may rupture, with release of its contents into the abdomen. Medical treatment may allow some animals to be successfully bred during the following heat period.

Follow-up Care

Antibiotics are usually given, and laboratory tests may be repeated until the results return to normal. Animals treated medically are monitored for side effects of the drug, such as restlessness, vomiting, drooling, abdominal cramping, and repeated defecation. Repeated x-rays and ultrasounds may be needed to monitor uterine size.

Prognosis

The rate of recurrence of pyometra after medical therapy is 10-77% within 27 months. Animals surviving surgical correction of the problem have an excellent prognosis.

SPECIAL INSTRUCTIONS:

Subinvolution of Placental Sites in Dogs

Ronald M. Bright, DVM, MS, DACVS

BASIC INFORMATION

Description

Subinvolution of placental sites (SIPS) occurs when normal healing does not take place at the sites where the placentas of the fetuses attached to the wall of uterus. Normally, the lining of the uterus (endometrium) repairs itself once the placenta tears away from the wall as the puppy is born. Failure of this process may result in a pinkish-brown vulvar discharge 3 or more weeks after whelping.

Causes

The underlying cause is unknown.

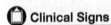 ### Clinical Signs

SIPS occurs most often in the young bitch, usually after the first pregnancy. The bitch usually appears to be healthy in all respects except for a pinkish vulvar discharge.

Diagnostic Tests

SIPS is considered the primary diagnosis when other causes of similar vulvar discharge are ruled out. Findings that rule out other diseases and help confirm SIPS include the following:

- Tests for brucellosis and infections of the uterus are negative.
- Examination of vaginal smears under the microscope (cytology) shows no evidence of inflammation.
- Culturing of the vaginal discharge does not show a growth pattern compatible with a bacterial infection.

Other diagnostic tests, such as x-rays, an abdominal ultrasound, and abdominal palpation, are done to assess the size of the uterus and rule out the possibility of retained fetuses or placental material. Excessive fluid within the uterus is more suggestive of an inflammation or infection of the uterus.

If the vulvar discharge is chronic and excessive, a blood count may reveal anemia in the bitch. A blood count with a significant increase in white blood cells is suggestive of an infection.

Definitive diagnosis of SIPS can be made when a pathologist examines a biopsy of uterine tissue, but uterine biopsies are seldom done.

TREATMENT AND FOLLOW-UP

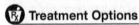 ### Treatment Options

If the bitch is to be bred again, the animal is usually monitored closely until the discharge is gone. If the bitch is not to be used again for future breedings, then surgical sterilization (spay surgery) is recommended.

Follow-up Care

Microscopic evaluation of the discharge is usually recommended on a weekly basis. If the discharge becomes pus-like, then a bacterial culture may be done. Results of the culture (if positive) are then used to select the best antibiotic therapy. The red blood cell count is also monitored frequently for any evidence of anemia, although the need for a transfusion is very rare.

Prognosis

In some instances, the pinkish discharge may persist until the onset of the next heat cycle. SIPS rarely occurs after subsequent pregnancies and deliveries.

SPECIAL INSTRUCTIONS:

Testicular Tumors in Dogs

Ronald M. Bright, DVM, MS, DACVS

BASIC INFORMATION

Description

In the intact (unneutered) male dog, tumors involving the testes are the second most common form of cancer. Most of these tumors are benign in nature, and they are not usually aggressive.

There are several types of cells within the testes that can, individually or in combination with other types of cells, form tumors. Forty percent of the time, multiple primary tumor types are present within the same testis. These include Sertoli cell tumors, seminomas, and interstitial cell tumors, which all occur with equal frequency.

Cryptorchid (retained) testes have a higher incidence of tumors and seem to be predisposed to the formation of tumors.

Testicular tumors are most often diagnosed in the older dog (median age, 10 years). Certain breeds, such as the German shepherd dog, Afghan hound, Weimaraner, and Shetland sheepdog, appear to have an increased risk of developing these tumors.

Causes

A retained testicle is one that is located in an abnormal position—the abdomen, the inguinal area (groin), or in front of the scrotum. A retained testicle has a higher risk of tumor formation, especially the Sertoli cell tumor and seminoma types. Increasing age, breed, and exposure to carcinogens may also influence the development of tumors.

Clinical Signs

Most signs are related to the actual presence of the mass within the testicle. Palpation (feeling the scrotum with the fingers) may reveal nodular enlargement of the testicle or pain.

Sertoli cell tumors can produce estrogen hormone, which results in feminizing signs such as enlarged nipples, a pendulous prepuce, attraction of other male dogs, symmetrical hair loss, and hyperpigmentation of the skin of the groin. Estrogen can also cause prostatic changes and can depress the bone marrow, resulting in anemia and platelet or white blood cell abnormalities.

In the rare case of a malignant tumor, signs may be related to other organs to which the tumor has spread. With testosterone-secreting tumors, an enlarged prostate may be present.

Diagnostic Tests

Palpation of the testicle initially raises concern that a nodule or enlargement of the testicle may represent a tumor. Signs of feminization in an intact male and an enlarged prostate may indirectly point to the possibility of a testicular tumor. A fine-needle aspiration of testicular tissue followed by cytologic evaluation by a pathologist may help confirm the presence of a tumor. A surgical biopsy can be done to help definitively diagnose the tumor type.

If spread of a malignant testicular tumor is suspected, a rectal examination is indicated to attempt to detect enlargement of lymph nodes in the vicinity. The prostate gland can also be palpated via a rectal exam. Laboratory blood work may confirm bone marrow involvement, which occurs primarily with the Sertoli cell tumors. An ultrasound of the abdomen may identify testicles that have not descended into the scrotum and may detect enlarged lymph nodes. An additional test to evaluate estrogen levels can be done to confirm the cause of feminization. Not all dogs have increased estrogen, however. Chest x-rays may also be recommended prior to surgery to make sure the lungs are clear.

TREATMENT AND FOLLOW-UP

Treatment Options

Most testicular tumors (85%) are locally confined, and castration with removal of the tumor is curative. Unilateral removal of the affected testicle can be done in a valuable breeding animal, if the remaining testicle is in its normal location.

When the tumor is malignant and has spread to other organs (lymph nodes, liver, lungs, skin, spleen), additional treatment modalities, such as chemotherapy and radiotherapy, can be considered. Overall, the number of dogs treated with these other modalities has been too small to judge their effectiveness. The survival time in a small number of dogs undergoing chemotherapy ranged from 5 to 31 months. Three of four dogs undergoing radiation therapy for enlarged regional lymph nodes (when the metastasis was confined to these lymph nodes) survived longer than 3 years.

Follow-up Care

Most signs of feminization resolve within approximately 3 weeks. Additional chemotherapy and/or radiotherapy may be an option for the more malignant forms of testicular tumors.

Prognosis

Prognosis in most animals with benign tumors is good. If the tumor has spread, the prognosis is guarded (uncertain) to poor.

SPECIAL INSTRUCTIONS:

Uterine Prolapse

Ronald M. Bright, DVM, MS, DACVS

BASIC INFORMATION

Description

Uterine prolapse is movement of a portion of the uterus through a dilated cervix and the vagina until it becomes visible at the vulva (opening of the vagina). Uterine prolapse can occur in cats after only one pregnancy, but in dogs it usually occurs after the animal has given birth to multiple litters of puppies.

Causes

The condition usually results from prolonged straining during the birth of kittens or puppies. It may also arise with forceful extraction of the fetus during a difficult delivery or with excessive traction on retained fetal membranes after the puppy or kitty has passed. Occasionally, uterine prolapse develops in association with a uterine infection. In cats it can occur without any predisposing conditions.

Clinical Signs

An animal with a prolapsed uterus usually has one or two tubular masses bulging from the vulva. Sometimes a mass is not visible but can be felt when the veterinarian performs a vaginal examination. In these latter cases, the animal often has some abdominal pain or restlessness, vaginal discharge, excessive licking of the vulva, or a swollen area near the vulva. The animal may strain as if trying to pass a fetus.

If uterine tissue is visible, it often has "doughnut" shape and can be swollen, very red in color, or encrusted with hair, feces, placental tissue, or kitty litter (cats). Occasionally, an animal may develop shock from rupture of a large uterine artery.

Diagnostic Tests

A prolapse that bulges through the vulva must be examined closely to determine whether the vagina or the uterus is prolapsed. A partial or hidden uterine prolapse may require digital examination (with a finger) or vaginoscopy (examination of the vagina with a special scope) to confirm the diagnosis. Laboratory tests, x-rays, and/or an ultrasound may be recommended to rule out infections, retained fetuses, and other conditions such as vaginal tumors or twisting of the uterus.

TREATMENT AND FOLLOW-UP

Treatment Options

If the animal is in shock, aggressive therapy with intravenous fluids and other medications is needed to correct the condition. Antibiotics are recommended in many cases.

Manual reduction of the prolapse (gently pushing the exposed tissue back into the abdomen) can be attempted if the animal is in good physical condition and the uterus appears healthy. General or epidural anesthesia is often necessary for the procedure, and sometimes the opening of the vulva must be surgically enlarged (episiotomy). The uterus is gently cleaned and coated with sterile lubricating jelly prior to replacement. Although replacement may be possible, recurrence is common, so the animal is often spayed after the uterus is back in the abdomen.

If only partial replacement is achieved and the owner wants to use the animal for future breeding, abdominal surgery is required to further return the uterus to its normal position. If the exposed uterine tissue is unhealthy and dying, then spaying (ovariohysterectomy) may be recommended once the uterus is back in the abdomen.

On rare occasions, the damage to the uterus is so severe that it must be amputated. Amputation is followed by abdominal surgery to remove the ovaries and any other associated tissues.

Follow-up Care

After manual replacement or surgery, watch the animal for any bleeding, weakness, problems urinating, failure to pass urine, or signs of infection (fever, vaginal discharge, lethargy, poor appetite). After manual replacement only, watch for the prolapsed tissue to reappear. Recheck visits and additional monitoring or testing depend on what procedure was used to correct the problem.

Prognosis

In most cases of simple, manual replacement there is a risk of recurrence. Prognosis is good following surgical removal of the uterus.

SPECIAL INSTRUCTIONS:

Vaginal Edema in Dogs

Ronald M. Bright, DVM, MS, DACVS

BASIC INFORMATION

Description

Vaginal edema is often referred to as a vaginal prolapse, because vaginal tissue can often be seen protruding from the vulva. *Edema* means that the vaginal tissue is swollen, and sometimes increased amounts of vaginal tissue actually form on the floor of the vagina.

Causes

Vaginal edema is thought to arise from an exaggerated response to the hormone, estrogen, by the lining of the vagina. Clinical signs are usually seen around the time of estrus (when the dog is in heat), when estrogen levels are at their highest. Vaginal edema occurs only in intact bitches (female dogs that are not spayed).

Vaginal edema occurs most often in young, large-breed female dogs. Breeds that may be affected more often include the boxer, English bulldog, mastiff, German shepherd dog, Saint Bernard, Labrador retriever, Chesapeake Bay retriever, Airedale terrier, and Weimaraner. It is not considered an inherited trait, however, and is not passed on to the offspring.

Rarely, vaginal edema may develop after the animal gives birth to a litter of pups.

Clinical Signs

The owners often observe a mass of tissue protruding from the vulva. The quantity of swollen tissue can vary, from a small amount that is shaped like a tongue or a doughnut to a large amount that involves the entire end of the vagina. The dog may lick the vulva excessively, have difficulty urinating, or urinate more frequently. A bulge may be seen around the vulva or between the vulva and the anus.

Dogs with this condition often have difficulty in mating. Vaginal edema tends to recur during future heat cycles.

Diagnostic Tests

A tentative diagnosis can be made based on the fact that the bitch is in heat and there is a swollen mass protruding from the vagina. A history of one or more previous episodes of the problem also supports the diagnosis. Palpation (feeling) of the mass and deter-mining that it arises from the floor of the vagina confirm the diagnosis. In older females, or when the possibility exists that the mass may be a tumor, a biopsy of the tissue may be recommended.

TREATMENT AND FOLLOW-UP

Treatment Options

Medical therapy may be tried and involves the following measures:

- Applying some form of lubricant to the exposed tissue helps keep the tissue from drying out.
- An Elizabethan collar is applied to the dog to prevent self-induced trauma to the tissue from excessive licking.
- The swollen tissue may be manually pushed back into the vagina and some sutures placed across the vulva to stitch it partially closed. This procedure may keep the vaginal tissue in place until the dog goes out of heat.
- Insertion of a temporary urinary catheter may be necessary to ensure that the dog can urinate.
- In some cases, hormonal therapy can be tried to shorten the time the dog is in heat, but often the problem is discovered too late in estrus for this to be tried.

Surgical therapy is often delayed until most of the swelling subsides, in order to avoid excessive bleeding.

- Once the dog goes out of heat, the vaginal swelling slowly decreases. When the swelling is gone, an ovariohysterectomy (spay) is often recommended. Spaying is considered the treatment of choice in the nonbreeding dog.
- Rarely, it may be necessary to amputate the exposed vaginal tissue, especially if it has dried out and become unhealthy. Amputation is somewhat risky, because the urethral opening must be preserved and can be difficult to find and work around.

Follow-up Care and Prognosis

Removal of the ovaries and uterus results in complete remission of the signs, and recurrences are not a problem. Use of medical therapy alone runs the risk of recurrence when the dog comes into heat again.

SPECIAL INSTRUCTIONS:

Vaginitis in Dogs

Ronald M. Bright, DVM, MS, DACVS

BASIC INFORMATION

Description

Vaginitis is inflammation that is often associated with an infection or irritation of the delicate lining of the vagina. The condition can occur at any age in female dogs that are either spayed or intact (still have their ovaries and uterus).

Causes

Numerous factors may encourage or contribute to vaginitis, such as the following:

- Anatomic abnormalities of the genital tract (vagina, vulva, cervix) or the urinary tract (urethra) can lead to a secondary bacterial vaginitis.
- Trauma at the time of mating or during the act of giving birth can predispose to this condition.
- Tumors of the vagina can be associated with bacterial infections.
- Some cases of juvenile vaginitis, where the cause is unknown, are seen in dogs less than 1 year of age.
- Urinary tract disorders (especially infections) can often affect of the vagina, because the urethra opens near the end of the vagina.
- Viral infections, such as herpesvirus, can cause inflammation of the lining of the vagina.

Clinical Signs

Most animals with vaginitis are presented to the veterinarian because of licking of the vulva or discharge from the vulva. Scooting the bottom along the floor is also common. Signs of a urinary tract problem may be seen, such as incontinence, frequent urination, or discomfort during or after urination. Intact females may be reluctant to mate. All affected females, regardless of the stage of their heat cycle, spay status, or age, may attract the attention of male dogs.

Diagnostic Tests

Digital examination (placement of the veterinarian's gloved finger into the vagina) often reveals a thick, stringy discharge and sometimes a congenital, structural abnormality of the vagina.

Looking at the vagina through a vaginal speculum with a light source may reveal areas of ulceration or redness and the presence of small, raised bumps or nodules. Sometimes, abnormalities of the structure and anatomy of the vagina are confirmed. Pooling of urine may be detected, which indicates urinary tract involvement. In some cases, masses may be seen, suggesting the presence of cancer.

Looking at a sample of the vaginal discharge under the microscope may demonstrate abnormal inflammatory cells and an increase in the number of bacteria. Examination of a urine sample (urinalysis) may help determine whether a urinary infection is present. Sometimes special stains of the vaginal discharge or cultures of the vagina and urine may be necessary to identify which specific bacterial are involved. A biopsy may be recommended in some cases.

Routine laboratory tests, x-rays, and possibly an ultrasound may be recommended, to rule out other conditions that produce similar signs or if involvement of the uterus is suspected.

TREATMENT AND FOLLOW-UP

Treatment Options

The form of vaginitis that occurs in young, intact female dogs (juvenile vaginitis) generally requires no treatment and usually resolves after the dog's first heat cycle. Medications do not appear to shorten the duration of signs and are not routinely used.

Correction of underlying anatomic or structural problems (either urinary or vaginal) may be necessary, as well as treatment of any secondary bacterial infections. When a bacterial infection is present and there are no known predisposing urinary or genital abnormalities, appropriate antibiotics are usually started. Treatment of viral vaginitis is not usually done, but the affected dog is separated from pregnant dogs and very young puppies, to avoid exposing them to the infection.

Some cases of vaginitis become chronic when they do not respond to the initial therapy. Local therapy applied directly to the vagina may help in these cases and can include antiseptic douches and anti-inflammatory drugs (cortisone preparations).

Follow-up Care

Recheck visits may be recommended to monitor response to treatment or to monitor cases of juvenile vaginitis for spontaneous recovery. Notify your veterinarian if the signs persist, because further testing may be needed.

Prognosis

In animals with predisposing causes involving the urinary or genital tract that are correctable by surgery, recovery is often complete. Prognosis for juvenile vaginitis is also good. Dogs with the viral form of vaginitis should never be used for breeding. Breeding of dogs with any type of active vaginitis is also discouraged.

SPECIAL INSTRUCTIONS:

SECTION 9

Hemolymphatic System

Section Editor: Kristi S. Lively, DVM, DABVP

Acute Lymphocytic Leukemia
Anemia in Dogs and Cats
Anticoagulant Rodenticide Toxicity
Aplastic Anemia
Babesia Infection in Dogs
Chronic Lymphocytic Leukemia
Coagulopathy Associated with Liver Disease
Disseminated Intravascular Coagulation
Fever of Unknown Origin
Hemobartonellosis in Cats
Hemophilia A
Hemophilia B
Hypercalcemia Associated with Cancer

Immune-Mediated Hemolytic Anemia
Immune-Mediated Thrombocytopenia
Lymphedema
Lymphoma in Cats
Lymphoma in Dogs
Mastocytosis
Primary and Secondary Polycythemia
Splenic Hemangiosarcoma
Splenic Torsion
Splenomegaly
Thrombocytopenia: Other Causes
Thrombosis
Von Willebrand Disease

Acute Lymphocytic Leukemia

Kristi S. Lively, DVM, DABVP

BASIC INFORMATION

Description

Acute lymphocytic leukemia (ALL) is a cancer of young lymphocytes, a type of white blood cell (WBC). The lymphocytes involved are formed in the bone marrow and other lymphoid organs. Malignant proliferation of the precursor cells, called *blast cells*, occurs and these cells are released into the bloodstream. Other types of blast cells are present in the bone marrow, so many different types of leukemia are possible, but this handout pertains only to ALL.

With ALL, so many blast cells are released into the blood that the WBC count becomes very elevated (leukocytosis). Leukocytosis can occur in response to infection, stress, or inflammation, but with these conditions the WBCs appear normal. Leukemia differs from these forms of leukocytosis in that the WBCs being produced are abnormal and represent a malignancy.

Lymphocytic leukemia may be acute (sudden in onset) or chronic (developing slowly). ALL forms from immature blast cells, whereas chronic leukemia involves more developed lymphocytes. In general, acute leukemia is a more aggressive disease than chronic leukemia. ALL is a dangerous, rapidly progressive cancer that most often affects young dogs and cats.

Causes

The cause of ALL has not been identified in dogs. Some viruses of cats, birds, and cattle can influence the development of leukemia and other cancers in those species.

Clinical Signs

Patients with ALL are typically sick but may have vague signs. The gums may be pale if anemia is present. Other common signs include lethargy, decreased appetite, weight loss, excessive drinking and urination, lameness, vomiting, and diarrhea. Enlargement of the spleen, lymph nodes (glands), and/or liver occurs in some animals.

Diagnostic Tests

The complete blood count (CBC) reveals a persistent, unexplained high lymphocyte count. The lymphocytes are often identified as immature blast forms. Sometimes the count is so elevated that the diagnosis of leukemia is obvious, but early in the course of the disease the WBC count may only be moderately elevated.

• Low blood counts of red blood cells (anemia), platelets, and neutrophils (another form of WBC) may also be detected. These cells are also formed in the bone marrow, and their production may be decreased if the marrow is taken over by the malignant lymphocytes.

• It may be necessary to submit a blood sample for further analysis if the diagnosis of leukemia is not definite. Special stains and tests may be performed to identify the cancer cells and their stage of development.

Bone marrow aspiration may be recommended to evaluate the various cells present in the marrow and to confirm the identity of the cancerous cells. A fine needle aspiration or biopsy of enlarged lymph nodes may be needed to differentiate leukemia from lymphoma, another form of cancer of lymphocytes.

Cats are usually tested for feline leukemia virus. Other laboratory tests, x-rays, and possibly an ultrasound may be recommended to assess the involvement of other organs, to rule out other causes of very high lymphocyte counts, and to differentiate ALL from lymphoma.

TREATMENT AND FOLLOW-UP

Treatment Options

Dogs and cats with ALL are generally quite sick at the time of diagnosis, and treatment should be started early and done aggressively. Chemotherapy is the treatment of choice. Protocols may include drugs such as vincristine, L-asparaginase, cyclophosphamide, doxorubicin, and prednisone. Other supportive care may be needed, such as intravenous fluids, nutritional support, antibiotics, and transfusions.

Follow-up Care

Blood counts and other laboratory tests are repeated periodically to assess response to treatment and to monitor for side effects from the chemotherapeutic medications. Drug doses are adjusted if the neutrophil counts become excessively low, because low neutrophil counts predispose the patient to infections. Antibiotics may be prescribed to help prevent infection if the neutrophil counts are low.

Prognosis

Prognosis is grave, and survival time depends largely on the response to chemotherapy. With aggressive chemotherapy, only about 30% of patients achieve remission (disappearance of the cancerous cells from the blood). Without chemotherapy, most patients die within a few weeks of diagnosis. Even with chemotherapy, most animals survive only a few months.

SPECIAL INSTRUCTIONS:

Anemia in Dogs and Cats

Kristi S. Lively, DVM, DABVP

BASIC INFORMATION

Description

Anemia is an abnormally low red blood cell (RBC) count. The primary function of the RBC is to transport oxygen to tissues, so inadequate RBC numbers cause decreased oxygenation of tissues. Anemia is not a specific disease but reflects an underlying disease process.

Causes

Anemia may be caused by decreased production of RBCs, increased destruction of RBCs (hemolysis), or loss of RBCs. Decreased RBC production arises secondary to chronic metabolic diseases, such as kidney disease, cancer, or malnutrition. RBCs are produced in the bone marrow, and infections or cancer of the marrow may also affect production.

Excessive RBC destruction is commonly immune mediated, although toxins, infections, blood parasites, cancer, drug reactions, and inherited RBC membrane defects can also cause hemolysis. Anemia secondary to blood loss may be overtly noted with trauma, but it may be hidden with other conditions, such as gastrointestinal tract bleeding, certain parasites (fleas, ticks, hookworms), and clotting disorders.

Clinical Signs

Clinical signs of anemia depend on both the severity of the anemia and the underlying cause. Clinical anemia typically causes weakness, lethargy, increased heart rate, poor appetite, and pale gums. Signs of the underlying cause may include fever, jaundice, enlarged spleen, pica (eating abnormal objects such as dirt), enlarged lymph nodes (glands), vomiting, diarrhea, weight loss, or depression.

Diagnostic Tests

Anemia is reasonably easy to diagnose, but diagnosing the underlying cause may be more difficult. Packed cell volume (PCV) is one measurement of the RBC count. Normal PCV values vary depending on the species of animal and the laboratory being used. An abnormally low PCV value confirms the diagnosis of anemia.

If anemia is diagnosed, other laboratory tests may be recommended to further characterize the cause of the anemia:

- Evaluation of a blood smear to identify potential blood parasites
- Biochemistry profile and urinalysis to evaluate organ function
- Fecal examination to identify internal parasites
- Reticulocyte count to determine whether the bone marrow is trying to replace lost RBCs
- Bone marrow aspiration and evaluation if there is no evidence that the RBCs are regenerating (low reticulocyte count)
- X-rays to evaluate for the presence of tumors, size of various organs, or evidence of trauma
- Clotting tests if excessive or persistent bleeding is present
- Other tests to screen for potential immune-mediated destruction of RBCs

TREATMENT AND FOLLOW-UP

Treatment Options

If the anemia is severe and life-threatening, hospitalization and blood transfusions may be recommended to stabilize the patient while the underlying disease is identified and potentially treated. Patients with severe anemia may also require oxygen therapy to compensate for decreased oxygen delivery to tissues. The treatment plan is then directed at the underlying cause and may include immunosuppressive drugs, antibiotics, parasite control, chemotherapy, or hormone injections. Not all underlying causes of anemia are treatable.

Follow-up Care

Follow-up depends on the underlying cause. Isolated events such as trauma may require monitoring of the PCV for a few days, whereas chronic conditions such as cancer or renal disease may require long-term monitoring. Immune-mediated anemia usually requires several months of therapy and monitoring.

Prognosis

The prognosis for anemia alone can be good with early intervention in reversible cases. Long-term prognosis depends on the severity of the underlying disease and whether the underlying disease can be treated.

SPECIAL INSTRUCTIONS:

Anticoagulant Rodenticide Toxicity

Kristi S. Lively, DVM, DABVP

BASIC INFORMATION

Description

Ingestion (eating) of certain rodent poisons (rodenticides) by dogs and cats can cause bleeding problems because they act as anticoagulants (prevent blood clotting). The pet may directly ingest rodent bait, may ingest food contaminated with the poison, or may even ingest a rodent that has died from the poison (especially cats).

Active ingredients in these rodenticides fall into two categories, *coumarin-based products* (warfarin, coumafuryl, brodifacoum, and bromadiolone) and *indanedione-based products* (diphacinone, pindone, yalone, and chlorophacinone). Coumarin-based products have a shorter duration of action.

Agents in these categories also fall into two generations, depending on when they were first developed.
- First-generation anticoagulants (warfarin, pindone, coumafuryl, coumachlor, isovaleryl-indanedione) are less toxic and often require ingestion of a larger amount to be problematic.
- Second-generation anticoagulants (brodifacoum, bromadiolone) are highly toxic after a single exposure.

Most of these poisons are bright blue-green pellets, and dogs and cats often confuse them for tasty kibble.

Causes and Toxicity

These products interfere with vitamin K activity in the body, which is required for blood to clot normally. When vitamin K–related clotting proteins are inactive, signs of bleeding occur. Coumarin-based products affect vitamin K for days, whereas the effects of indanedione-based products may last for weeks.

Clinical Signs

Signs can take several days to develop, because vitamin K stores must first be depleted. Signs are related to anemia or bleeding tendencies. External signs of bleeding are not always present if the bleeding is internal, so weakness and depression may be the only signs noted. Pale gums; bruising; nose bleeds; blood in the urine, feces, or eyes; or difficulty breathing may occur. Bleeding may be sudden and life-threatening.

Diagnostic Tests

If ingestion of the rodenticide is seen by the owner, the diagnosis is straightforward. Not all rat poisons are anticoagulants, so it is important to inform your veterinarian which product was ingested. If ingestion or exposure was not witnessed, other causes of bleeding must be ruled out through a series of laboratory tests that assess platelets, various aspects of blood clotting, and effects on other organs. A test to detect abnormally high levels of inactive vitamin K–dependent proteins (PIVKA test) may be submitted. Additional tests, such as x-rays and an ultrasound, may be recommended.

TREATMENT AND FOLLOW-UP

Treatment Options

If ingestion has just occurred, vomiting may be induced to minimize absorption of the toxin. Treatment involves providing adequate vitamin K1 so that blood clotting remains normal. Even if the poison is vomited and there is no external evidence of bleeding, treatment with vitamin K1 is usually instituted to ensure patient safety. Contact your veterinarian immediately if you suspect possible ingestion of rat poison, even if your pet seems fine, so that blood clotting can be assessed and preventive treatment can be started.

The duration and dosage of vitamin K1 required depend on the type of toxin ingested. Coumarin products are active for days, whereas indanedione products are active for weeks. First-generation products require lower doses of vitamin K1 than second-generation products. If the exact type of toxin is not known, treatment is often given at high doses for 4-6 weeks. Initially, vitamin K1 may be given by injection for 1-2 days, and then pills may be started. Oral vitamin K1 is given with food to maximize its absorption.

If bleeding and anemia are severe, hospitalization is often necessary. Whole blood or plasma transfusions and intensive supportive care needed to stabilize the patient.

Follow-up Care

Certain clotting and other laboratory tests are often repeated during therapy and 48 hours after stopping vitamin K to ensure that there is no more active toxin in the system. If clotting tests are abnormal after the drug is stopped, vitamin K treatment is usually continued for 2 more weeks. If the vitamin K is stopped for longer than 48 hours and the toxin is still active, bleeding may recur, so it is very important to precisely follow your veterinarian's instructions. Notify your veterinarian if any signs recur or any changes occur in the medication schedule.

Prognosis

Because vitamin K1 is the antidote for anticoagulant rodenticide toxicosis, prognosis is excellent if treatment is started in a timely manner and is carried out for an appropriate duration with adequate patient monitoring. In cases of severe anemia and bleeding, where aggressive hospitalization and transfusions are needed, prognosis is more guarded (uncertain). These rodenticides can be lethal to dogs and cats.

SPECIAL INSTRUCTIONS:

Aplastic Anemia

Kristi S. Lively, DVM, DABVP

BASIC INFORMATION

Description

The bone marrow is responsible for producing platelets, red blood cells (RBCs), and white blood cells (WBCs). These cells are formed from precursor cells that reside in the bone marrow, and many become mature while in the bone marrow. Diseases of the marrow can affect one or all of these cell lines, resulting in inadequate circulating numbers of mature cells. These cells are important for blood clotting (platelets), immune functions (WBCs), and oxygen delivery to tissues (RBCs). Aplastic anemia occurs when bone marrow function is so severely impaired that numbers of all three cell types diminish (called *pancytopenia*).

Causes

The cause of aplastic anemia is not always identified but may be related to infection with feline leukemia virus (FeLV) in cats, parvovirus in dogs or cats, or ehrlichiosis in dogs. Adverse reactions to drugs, such as estrogen, methimazole, azathioprine, griseofulvin, albendazole, captopril, phenylbutazone, trimethoprim-sulfa, and chemotherapeutic medications, may also cause pancytopenia. Tumors that secrete feminizing hormones (Sertoli cell and interstitial cell tumors) may be a cause. Immune-mediated destruction of precursor cells in the bone marrow is also a possible cause in some animals.

Clinical Signs

Clinical signs vary depending on the severity of the aplastic anemia. Signs often include weakness, pale gums, lethargy, blood in the feces or urine, nose bleeds, and abnormal bruising. If the WBCs are markedly affected, secondary infections may occur, because the immune system is compromised.

Diagnostic Tests

Aplastic anemia is usually recognized when a complete blood count (CBC) reveals a low platelet count (thrombocytopenia), a low WBC count (leukopenia), and a nonregenerative, low RBC count (anemia). A thorough history is then taken to determine possible exposure to ticks, toxins, or drugs that are potentially harmful to the bone marrow. Laboratory tests may be recommended to rule out infectious diseases and to determine the effects on other organs. A Coombs' test may be performed to identify an immune-mediated component to the disease.

Bone marrow aspiration or biopsy is an important diagnostic procedure because it provides further information on the status of the precursor cells in the bone marrow, as well as information on the production and maturation of the different cell lines. With aplastic anemia, the precursor cells of all three cell lines are decreased or absent. Occasionally, infectious organisms may be found in the marrow samples.

If a cancerous process is suspected, imaging (x-rays, ultrasounds) of the chest, abdomen, and reproductive tract, as well as biopsy of any abnormal masses, may be recommended.

TREATMENT AND FOLLOW-UP

Treatment Options

When a primary cause of the pancytopenia is identified, treatment is directed at that condition. Potentially toxic substances or drugs are withdrawn. Supportive care may be needed, including hospitalization, oxygen therapy, blood transfusions, intravenous fluids, and antibiotics for secondary infections. If an autoimmune disorder is suspected, immune-suppressive medications, such as prednisone, azathioprine, cyclosporine, cyclophosphamide, or intravenous immune globulin, may be tried. Medications that stimulate the bone marrow, such as erythropoietin or granulocyte colony-stimulating factor, have been tried in only a small number of patients, and it is uncertain whether they provide much benefit. Whereas people with aplastic anemia may undergo bone marrow transplantation, this procedure is not routinely available for animals.

Follow-up Care

The CBC is monitored approximately every 3 days at first, and then weekly to monthly if the patient improves. Other monitoring is based on the underlying cause.

Prognosis

Prognosis is guarded (uncertain) to poor, depending on the underlying cause. Some toxins and infections cause irreversible bone marrow damage, whereas the effects of others are reversible once treated or once exposure to the toxin is eliminated. Secondary infections may develop into life-threatening sepsis (widespread infection in multiple organs) because the immune system is compromised. Patients are also at risk for life-threatening bleeding from the low numbers of platelets. When recovery does occur, it requires weeks to months of therapy and monitoring, which can be expensive.

SPECIAL INSTRUCTIONS:

Babesia Infection in Dogs

Kristi S. Lively, DVM, DABVP

BASIC INFORMATION
Description
Babesia is a blood parasite that causes anemia (an abnormally low red blood cell count) in dogs all over the world. The anemia arises from destruction of red blood cells. *Babesia* rarely affects cats. It is spread by ticks and occurs most commonly in the southeastern United States and in the Great Lakes region. Babesial infections affect greyhounds and pit bulls more often than other breeds. Puppies younger than 8 months of age may be more susceptible.

Causes
Even though more than 100 species of *Babesia* species exist, currently *Babesia canis* and *Babesia gibsoni* are the only two species known to infect dogs. *Babesia* infection (babesiosis) occurs most commonly when a tick carrying the *Babesia* organism attaches to a dog (for at least 2 days) and releases the infection into the dog's bloodstream. The organisms multiply and infect red blood cells. New ticks pick up the infection from an infected dog and spread it to other dogs. Pregnant dogs can spread the infection to their unborn puppies. Infection may also be transmitted from dog to dog through bite wounds and via blood transfusion.

The dog's immune system recognizes the infected red blood cells and destroys them in an effort to kill the parasite. The resulting anemia may be mild to severe.

Severe inflammation may also arise in other body systems, including the liver, kidneys, eyes, neurologic system, and respiratory system.

Clinical Signs
The infection typically incubates 10-21 days before clinical signs develop. Most infected dogs clear the infection and never become ill, but they may become carriers. Signs may occur in carrier dogs when they are stressed. Babesiosis may be classified as uncomplicated or complicated.

In uncomplicated cases, dogs are acutely ill, with fever, loss of appetite, depression, pale gums, enlargement of the spleen, and dark urine. Signs may be mild to severe, depending on the extent of the anemia. Symptoms of the anemia include weakness, jaundice, fever, depression, sudden collapse, and red- or orange-colored urine.

Complicated babesiosis may manifest as acute kidney failure, neurologic or blood clotting disorders, liver or breathing problems, inflammation of the heart muscle, low blood pressure, inflammation of the pancreas or eyes, or swelling of the legs. Shock, severe weakness, vomiting, and death may also occur.

Diagnostic Tests
The best diagnostic test for babesiosis is demonstrating the parasite on a blood smear; however, the parasite may not always be present in the sample, so a negative blood smear does not rule out infection. Because the organisms are hard to find, alternative testing is often necessary and may require sending samples to a laboratory. Some tests to confirm the diagnosis do not differentiate well among the various *Babesia* species and may give false-negative results early in the infection. These false-negative results complicate the screening process for carriers of the disease.

Other laboratory tests may be needed to detect problems in other organs, to evaluate blood clotting, to rule out other causes of anemia, and to assess the immune system's reaction to the disease.

TREATMENT AND FOLLOW-UP
Treatment Options
Treatments are aimed at reversing the anemia and suppressing or clearing the infection. To stabilize the anemia, many dogs require a blood transfusion. A steroid (such as prednisone) may be given to decrease destruction of the red blood cells. Other complicating factors must also be addressed with appropriate therapy.

No known treatment clears all *Babesia* infections. Imidocarb dipropionate is the only drug approved in the United States for treatment of babesiosis. A single injection of the drug often clears *B. canis* and probably *B. gibsoni*. Side effects include pain at the injection site, tremors, elevated heart rate, fever, drooling, facial swelling, vomiting, and breathing problems. For *B. gibsoni* and the other small *Babesia* species, multiple injections may be needed.

A vaccine is available in France that is 89% effective against certain strains of *Babesia*. The best prevention is strict tick control.

Follow-up Care
All blood donors should be screened for babesiosis before donating, especially greyhounds and dogs from areas of the country where *Babesia* species are known to exist. Dogs that clear the initial infection but become carriers may have relapses when subjected to stress, such as surgery, pregnancy, or other illness. Females that test positive should not be used for breeding.

Prognosis
Prognosis is best when the infection is caught before the anemia becomes severe. Severe and complicated cases require more supportive care, and prognosis depends on the severity of anemia, severity of other organ involvement, and response to treatment.

SPECIAL INSTRUCTIONS:

Chronic Lymphocytic Leukemia

Kristi S. Lively, DVM, DABVP

BASIC INFORMATION

Description

Chronic lymphocytic leukemia (CLL) is a cancer of lymphocytes, a type of white blood cell (WBC). Lymphocytes are formed in the bone marrow and other lymphoid organs. When malignant proliferation occurs, these cells are released into the bloodstream.

With CLL, so many cancerous lymphocytes are released into the blood that the WBC count becomes very elevated (leukocytosis). Leukocytosis can occur in response to infection, stress, or inflammation but with these conditions the WBCs appear normal. Leukemia differs from other forms of leukocytosis in that the WBCs being produced are abnormal and represent a malignancy.

Lymphocytic leukemia may be acute (sudden in onset) or chronic (developing slowly), depending on the stage of the lymphocyte precursor involved. Acute leukemia forms when immature blast cells proliferate, whereas chronic leukemia involves more developed lymphocytes. In general, acute leukemia is more aggressive than CLL. CLL is a slowly progressive disease, often of older dogs and cats.

Causes

The cause of CLL has not been identified in either dogs or cats. CLL in dogs tends to involve a particular type of lymphocyte, called the *T cell*. CLL is rare in cats.

Clinical Signs

About 50% of patients with CLL have no clinical signs, and the disease is discovered when a blood count is done for another reason. Lethargy is the most common sign. Other signs include weight loss, loss of appetite, and enlargement of the spleen, liver, or lymph nodes (glands). Vomiting or diarrhea may be present if the gastrointestinal tract is affected.

A condition called *hyperviscosity syndrome* is a potential complication of CLL and arises when the lymphocytes produce a protein that builds up in the blood. The malignant lymphocytes all tend to form the same type of protein, which is a monoclonal antibody. Excessive levels of these proteins cause the blood to thicken and may cause small blood vessels to bleed. Signs of hyperviscosity syndrome may include nose bleeds, seizures, blurred vision, or blindness.

Diagnostic Tests

The complete blood count (CBC) reveals a persistent, unexplained, elevated lymphocyte count. Sometimes the count is so elevated the diagnosis of leukemia is obvious. However, CLL can be confused with leukocytosis from other causes if the lymphocyte count is only moderately elevated. Low blood counts of red blood cells (anemia) and neutrophils (another type of WBC) may also occur. It may be necessary to submit a blood sample for further analysis if the diagnosis of leukemia is not definite. Special stains and tests may be performed to identify the cancer cells and their stage of development.

A protein electrophoresis test may be done to confirm that blood protein is elevated and to determine whether the protein is a monoclonal antibody. A bone marrow aspiration may be recommended to evaluate the various cells present in the marrow and to confirm the identity of the cancerous cells. A fine-needle aspiration or biopsy of enlarged lymph nodes may be needed to differentiate leukemia from lymphoma, another cancer of lymphocytes.

Other laboratory tests, x-rays, and possibly an ultrasound may be recommended to assess involvement of other organs, to rule out other causes of leukocytosis, and to differentiate CLL from acute lymphocytic leukemia, other forms of lymphoma, and other types of leukemia.

TREATMENT AND FOLLOW-UP

Treatment Options

Since the course of this disease is very slowly progressive, treatment may not be indicated at the time of diagnosis. If the lymphocyte count is less than 60,000-75,000 cells per microliter (µL) and the patient has no abnormalities in other blood cells, treatment may be delayed. Treatment is usually started right away if clinical signs develop, if hyperviscosity syndrome is detected, if the lymphocyte count rises above 75,000/µL, or if anemia, low platelet counts, or low neutrophil counts occur.

Chemotherapy is the treatment of choice, and protocols may include drugs such as chlorambucil, prednisone, and vincristine. Occasionally other supportive treatments are needed, depending on the animal's clinical signs and the presence of other abnormal laboratory results.

Follow-up Care

If no treatment is started, the CBC is repeated periodically to monitor the lymphocyte count. During chemotherapy, CBCs are also rechecked to assess response to treatment and to monitor for side effects from the chemotherapeutic medications.

Prognosis

Prognosis for remission is good, with survival times of 2-3 years being common. Even without chemotherapy, patients may live 1-2 years beyond diagnosis. In some animals, chemotherapy may be stopped if remission lasts for longer than 1 year.

SPECIAL INSTRUCTIONS:

Coagulopathy Associated with Liver Disease

Kristi S. Lively, DVM, DABVP

BASIC INFORMATION

Description

The liver is responsible for producing many of the proteins involved in the normal blood clotting (coagulation) process, particularly factors VII, IX, X, and XI. When the liver is severely diseased, these proteins are not produced in normal amounts. If production of these proteins falls below 10% of normal, spontaneous bleeding may occur.

Causes

For liver function to be affected enough that the production of these proteins is diminished, the underlying liver disease must be widespread and serious. Diseases of the liver causing widespread damage include toxins, inflammation, vascular shunts, cancer, fatty infiltration, and terminal scarring (cirrhosis).

🗐 Clinical Signs

The underlying liver disease may cause decreased appetite, fever, weight loss, lethargy, vomiting, or diarrhea. Some patients with significant liver dysfunction become jaundiced, with yellow discoloration of the skin, the gums, and the white part of the eyes (sclera). If liver disease is significant enough to cause a bleeding tendency, the patient may have bruising of the skin, gums, and sclera. The urine may be a dark, yellow-orange color if jaundice is present, or it may be blood tinged.

🔬 Diagnostic Tests

In patients with liver disease, liver blood tests are usually elevated, and other laboratory tests, such as blood protein, glucose, and bilirubin, may also be abnormal. Your veterinarian may recommend additional liver function tests, such as measurement of blood ammonia levels or bile acids. If a bleeding disorder is suspected, a coagulation panel of several different clotting tests is often performed. X-rays and an ultrasound of the liver may be done to evaluate any structural changes. A liver biopsy may be performed to determine the underlying cause of the liver disease, but it may not be recommended until coagulation tests improve and the concern for secondary bleeding decreases. Other tests may be recommended to rule out other diseases that cause similar clinical signs, as well as other clotting disorders.

TREATMENT AND FOLLOW-UP

℞ Treatment Options

Treatment is aimed at correcting the underlying cause of the liver disease whenever possible. Such treatment may include antibiotics, steroids, intravenous fluids, nutritional support, plasma transfusions, blood transfusions, or chemotherapy, depending on the cause. Supplements that improve liver health or replace deficiencies caused by the liver disease may also be administered. These include vitamin B, vitamin K, SAM-e (S-adenosylmethionine), milk thistle, taurine, and carnitine. Seriously ill animals may require an extended hospital stay.

🐾 Follow-up Care

Laboratory testing of liver function and blood clotting is repeated every few days initially, to assess response to therapy and progression of the disease. Periodic laboratory monitoring and repeated x-rays and/or ultrasounds may be needed long term.

Prognosis

Liver disease that is so advanced that it causes significant clotting factor deficiencies has a guarded (uncertain) to poor prognosis. In some cases, however, the disease may be reversed with aggressive and intensive therapy. The reversibility of the disease depends largely on whether the underlying cause is treatable and the extent of liver damage present at the time of diagnosis.

SPECIAL INSTRUCTIONS:

Disseminated Intravascular Coagulation

Kristi S. Lively, DVM, DABVP

BASIC INFORMATION

Description

Disseminated intravascular coagulation (DIC) is a life-threatening condition caused by widespread, excessive activation of clotting proteins and the formation of microscopic blood clots. Widespread, extensive microclotting results in consumption of these proteins. Once the level of circulating clotting proteins falls, a severe bleeding tendency develops. DIC is sometimes called *consumptive coagulation* or *consumptive coagulopathy*.

Causes

DIC is not a primary disorder; that is, it does not arise spontaneously by itself. Rather, it is a secondary disorder that develops in association with serious underlying diseases. Underlying causes include infections such as bacterial, viral, tick-borne, and parasitic diseases. Severe inflammation associated with heat stroke, burns, cancer, trauma, shock, snake bites, autoimmune diseases, and other diseases may also predispose a patient to DIC.

🗎 Clinical Signs

Clinical signs are initially related to the primary disease condition. In severe or fulminant DIC, evidence of abnormal hemorrhaging is present, such as bruising of the skin, gums, inner aspect of the ear flaps, and sclerae (white part of the eyes). Bleeding may develop at sites where blood samples were drawn or in the urinary or intestinal tracts. Sudden respiratory distress and neurologic signs may occur but are less common. Life-threatening clot formation or bleeding, heart failure, or multiple organ failure may cause sudden death.

🔧 Diagnostic Tests

Thorough diagnostic testing is usually needed to identify the underlying disease. The presence of DIC is confirmed by performing a coagulation panel that includes a platelet count, various blood clotting assays, measurement of a blood protein called *fibrinogen*, and/or measurement of D-dimer levels in the blood. D-dimers are fragments of material produced during degradation of a blood clot. Results of the coagulation panel often reveal prolonged bleeding time, a decreased platelet count, and increased levels of D-dimers or fibrinogen degradation products.

TREATMENT AND FOLLOW-UP

℞ Treatment Options

Treatment is aimed at stabilizing or reversing the underlying disorder whenever possible. Extended hospitalization for intensive therapy and advanced supportive care may be required. Attempts may be made with medications, such as heparin, to minimize dangerous clot formation and maintain adequate circulation in tissues. Intravenous fluids may be administered to help support circulation, and plasma or blood transfusions are often indicated for significant blood loss.

🐾 Follow-up Care

Coagulation tests are repeated periodically to assess the effects of therapy and to monitor recovery from DIC. Other monitoring and testing are based on the underlying disease or condition.

Prognosis

Prognosis is guarded (very uncertain) to poor, depending on the severity of the underlying disease. If tiny blood clots (thrombi) form in single or multiple organs and organ failure ensues, the prognosis becomes grave. Treatment and ongoing monitoring can be intense and expensive.

SPECIAL INSTRUCTIONS:

Fever of Unknown Origin
Kristi S. Lively, DVM, DABVP

BASIC INFORMATION
Description
A fever is a body temperature higher than the normal range. In dogs and cats, normal body temperature is approximately 100-102.5° F (38-39.5° C). Fever of unknown origin (FUO) is diagnosed when the fever is chronic (lasting for 3 weeks or longer) or recurs frequently and physical examinations and routine laboratory tests have not identified the source of the fever.

Causes
The most common causes of fever are infection, immune disease, inflammation, and cancer. Infectious causes include, but are not limited to:
- Tick-related infections, such as Rocky Mountain spotted fever, ehrlichiosis, Lyme disease, and babesiosis in dogs
- Viruses such as feline immunodeficiency virus (FIV), feline leukemia virus (FeLV), and feline infectious peritonitis (FIP) virus in cats
- Bacterial or fungal infections from bite wounds, pneumonia, or infections of the heart valves, uterus, urinary tract, joints, or bones
- Infections with protozoal agents, such as toxoplasmosis (cats and dogs) and neosporosis (dogs), or blood parasites, such as hemobartonellosis (cats)

Inflammatory and immune-mediated causes include:
- Drug or vaccine reactions
- Immune-mediated anemia, thrombocytopenia, or joint disease

Any type of cancer can cause a fever from release of inflammatory chemicals or destruction of tissue by tumor cells.

Clinical Signs
Clinical signs depend largely on the underlying cause but are often vague and nonspecific. Many patients are lethargic and have a poor appetite; they may lose weight and may become dehydrated. These patients tend to be ill for several weeks as the fever persists and the underlying cause goes unidentified.

Diagnostic Tests
A very thorough history is needed to determine the cause of the fever, so be sure to relay to your veterinarian all the medications and supplements recently administered to your pet, its vaccine status and dates, travel history, and exposure to other animals. A detailed physical examination is done to look for potential sources of the fever. Numerous laboratory tests are usually needed to rule out the various causes of fever. Some of the most common tests are the following:
- Complete blood count, serum biochemistry panel, electrolytes
- Urinalysis, urine culture
- Viral testing for FIV, FeLV, FIP
- X-rays of the chest and abdomen, including the spine
- Specialized tests for the common tick-borne, fungal, and protozoal diseases in your geographic area

- Blood smear evaluation and specialized tests for blood parasites

If these screening tests come back negative or nondiagnostic, then additional, more advanced diagnostics may be recommended, such as the following:
- Abdominal ultrasound and echocardiogram (heart ultrasound)
- Needle aspiration of glands (lymph nodes), tumors, or any abnormal tissue
- Bone marrow evaluation
- Cultures of the blood and certain body tissues
- X-rays of bones and joints, as well as joint taps
- Specialized testing for unusual or rare bacterial infections, such as brucellosis or tuberculosis
- Spinal tap and analysis of cerebrospinal fluid
- Advanced imaging, such as magnetic resonance imaging (MRI) or computed tomography (CT scan)

Diagnosing the cause of an FUO requires time, patience, and many different tests and procedures, especially if the most common causes of fever are ruled out.

TREATMENT AND FOLLOW-UP
Treatment Options
Once the cause is identified, specific treatment is aimed at the underlying cause. In some cases of FUO, even after many diagnostic tests, a specific cause for the fever is not identified. In these cases, a trial may be started with broad-spectrum antibiotics, antifungal agents, or anti-inflammatory drugs. Sometimes a diagnosis is assumed, based on a positive response to treatment (the fever disappears), or a disease can be ruled out because of a lack of response (the fever continues).

In cases of prolonged illness or very high fever, the animal may also require hospitalization for nutritional support, intravenous fluid therapy, and administration of antifever medications. Never give medications that are designed to treat fevers in people to your pets! Some human medications, such as ibuprofen and acetaminophen (*Tylenol*), are toxic to pets and can cause life-threatening problems.

Follow-up Care
Follow-up visits and repeat testing depend on the underlying cause, the type of treatment instituted, and the response to that treatment. Some causes of FUO and certain infections require long-term or lifelong monitoring.

Prognosis
Prognosis is good if a treatable cause is identified and the animal responds to treatment. Certain causes of FUO are untreatable (such as some forms of cancer) or pose a health risk to humans.

SPECIAL INSTRUCTIONS:

Hemobartonellosis in Cats

Kristi S. Lively, DVM, DABVP

BASIC INFORMATION

Description

Hemobartonellosis is a relatively common bacterial infection of cats in North America and is also called *feline infectious anemia*. The infection causes anemia by destruction of red blood cells (RBCs). The *Hemobartonella* organism is most commonly spread by blood-sucking parasites such as mosquitoes, lice, fleas, and ticks. It may also be spread via bite wounds or transmitted to unborn offspring in pregnant females. Cats that are also infected with feline leukemia virus are at a higher risk for more severe infection.

Causes

Hemobartonella felis (newly renamed *Mycoplasma haemophilus*) is transferred via blood-sucking insects or by entry into the body through the mouth, in bite wounds, or through blood transfusions. The parasites are active in the blood 2-17 days after infection and can remain active for 3-8 weeks. The cat's immune system attempts to clear infected RBCs by destroying these cells in the spleen. The RBC destruction results in anemia that may be mild to severe.

Clinical Signs

Clinical signs appear within 7-30 days but may be cyclical, which sometimes makes the disease difficult to recognize. Signs may become worse during times of stress, such as illness or surgery. Signs of anemia vary, depending on whether the anemia is mild or severe, and may include lethargy, weakness, loss of appetite, cyclical fevers, jaundice, pale gums, and weight loss. Severe anemia can cause marked depression and even death.

Diagnostic Tests

The diagnosis of *Hemobartonella* infection can be difficult due to its cyclical nature. Occasionally the organisms are seen in a drop of blood examined under the microscope, but their absence does not rule out the infection. Because the organisms are hard to find, more sophisticated testing is often necessary and may require sending samples to a diagnostic laboratory. Cats diagnosed with hemobartonellosis are also tested for feline leukemia virus, because the latter infection may make the disease worse and recovery more difficult.

TREATMENT AND FOLLOW-UP

Treatment Options

Because diagnosis can be difficult, if hemobartonellosis is highly suspected, treatment may be started while laboratory tests are pending. The infection is susceptible to tetracycline-type antibiotics (such as doxycycline), with clinical improvement noted within just a few days. The parasite is never completely eliminated from the blood, however, so cats may become chronic carriers. Relapse of infection is uncommon but can occur.

In severe cases of anemia, blood transfusions may be indicated. Low-dose steroids (such as prednisone) may also be given if immune-mediated destruction of RBCs is also present. Healthy carrier cats usually are not treated.

Follow-up Care

Cats receiving tetracycline antibiotics are monitored for side effects to the drugs, including fever, decreased appetite, gastric upset, esophageal irritation, and liver disease. If oral tablets are administered, dosing is followed with several milliliters of water to prevent the tablets from sticking in the esophagus and causing inflammation. If tetracycline antibiotics are not well tolerated, other antibiotics may be tried. Periodic rechecks and monitoring of RBC levels are also needed. Strict external parasite control is a must for all cats.

Prognosis

Prognosis is good if the initial diagnosis is made before the cat becomes severely anemic. Severely affected cats may need a longer hospitalization and multiple transfusions to recover. Concurrent risk factors, such as leukemia virus infection, make the prognosis more guarded (uncertain).

SPECIAL INSTRUCTIONS:

Hemophilia A

Kristi S. Lively, DVM, DABVP

BASIC INFORMATION

Description

Hemophilia A is the most common inherited bleeding disorder of domestic animals. It arises from a deficiency in factor VIII, a protein necessary for the blood to clot. Normally, when a blood vessel is damaged, a complex interaction of several clotting factors takes place that starts and maintains a normal blood clot. Patients lacking one of these factors, such as factor VIII, cannot effectively activate this sequence of events, so excessive bleeding occurs.

Hemophilia A can affect dogs of any breed, but the German shepherd dog may be more commonly affected than other breeds. Males are also more commonly affected than females. Cats are rarely affected.

Causes

This is a sex-linked recessive disease, which means that it is linked to the X chromosome. Females have two X chromosomes, so, unless both X chromosomes are abnormal, females rarely exhibit signs of the disease. However, females that do not show any signs may still pass an abnormal X chromosome to their offspring, which makes them silent carriers of this disease. Males only have one X chromosome; therefore, if a male has the abnormal X chromosome, he will show clinical signs of disease. Affected males may also pass this disease on to their offspring.

Clinical Signs

The severity of signs depends on the level of factor VIII. Carriers or patients with mild forms of the disease may show no signs of bleeding and may never require treatment. More severely affected patients may show signs at a young age. Signs include prolonged bleeding when the baby teeth fall out, unexplained bruising, bloody bowel movements, painful joint swelling and lameness, and nose bleeds. Dangerous bleeding into the brain or spinal cord or into the chest cavity may cause neurologic signs or respiratory distress, respectively. Excessive bleeding may occur during elective surgery or following trauma and may even be life-threatening.

Cats and small dogs may develop mild signs such as depression, decreased appetite, or lethargy. It is thought that smaller animals tolerate the disease better because of their lighter body weight (less pressure and pounding on structures such as joints).

Diagnostic Tests

Several tests are needed to evaluate the degree of blood loss, the ability of the blood to clot, which part of the clotting sequence is abnormal, and the levels of clotting factors present in the blood. Such tests may include the following:

- Complete blood count, to check a platelet count and evaluate for possible anemia
- Biochemistry profile, to check for internal organ damage
- Coagulation panel, with tests such as prothrombin and partial thrombin time
- Specific assay for factor VIII (also used to test female carriers), with results reported as a percentage of normal

TREATMENT AND FOLLOW-UP

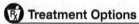 Treatment Options

Hemophilia A is a lifelong disorder with no cure. Patients with mild disease may never require treatment or may need treatment only in case of surgery or trauma. During episodes of more severe bleeding, hospitalization with cage rest and transfusions of plasma or blood products containing clotting factors are needed to replace factor VIII and control bleeding. Transfusions may need to be repeated every 8-12 hours until the bleeding stops. Red blood cell transfusions may be necessary if bleeding results in severe anemia.

Follow-up Care

Because this is an inherited disorder, it is a good idea to contact the breeder of the animal so that the parents and other littermates may be tested for the disease. Individuals that test positive, including carriers, should not be used for breeding.

It is important to control the activities of affected individuals, to minimize injury and the risk of bleeding. Drugs that affect platelet function and unnecessary surgeries are avoided, if possible. If surgery is required, transfusions are often performed before, during, and after the procedure to try and control bleeding. During severe bleeding episodes, laboratory tests may be recommended to monitor for evidence of continued blood loss and the development of anemia.

Prognosis

Prognosis is very poor for pets with severe disease. Recurring bleeding episodes require repeated transfusions, which can become quite expensive. Dogs with severe disease are often euthanized or die from a severe bleeding episode.

SPECIAL INSTRUCTIONS:

Hemophilia B

Kristi S. Lively, DVM, DABVP

BASIC INFORMATION

Description

Hemophilia B is the second most common inherited bleeding disorder of domestic animals. It arises from a deficiency in factor IX, a protein necessary for the blood to clot. Normally, when a blood vessel is damaged, a complex interaction of several clotting factors takes place that starts and maintains a normal blood clot. Patients lacking some of these factors, such as factor IX, cannot effectively activate this sequence of events, so excessive bleeding occurs.

Males are more commonly affected than females. Hemophilia B occurs in a number of purebred and mixed-breed dogs. The British shorthair and Siamese-cross breeds are the most commonly affected cats.

Causes

This is a sex-linked, recessive disease, which means that it is linked to the X chromosome. Females have two X chromosomes, so unless both X chromosomes are abnormal, females rarely exhibit signs of the disease. However, females that do not show any signs may still pass an abnormal X chromosome to their offspring, which makes them silent carriers of this disease. Males only have one X chromosome; therefore, if a male has the abnormal X chromosome, he will show clinical signs of the disease. Affected males may also pass this disease on to their offspring.

Clinical Signs

The severity of signs depends on the level of factor IX in the blood. Carriers or patients with mild forms of the disease may show no signs of bleeding and may never require treatment. More severely affected patients may show signs at a young age. Signs include prolonged bleeding when the baby teeth fall out, unexplained bruising, bloody bowel movements, painful joint swelling and lameness, and nose bleeds. Dangerous bleeding into the brain or spinal cord or into the chest cavity may cause neurologic signs or respiratory distress, respectively. Excessive bleeding may occur during elective surgery or following trauma and may even be life-threatening.

Cats and small dogs may develop mild signs such as depression, decreased appetite, or lethargy. It is thought that smaller animals tolerate the disease better because of their lighter body weight (less pressure and pounding on structures such as joints).

Diagnostic Tests

Several tests are needed to evaluate the degree of blood loss, the ability of the blood to clot, which part of the clotting sequence is abnormal, and the levels of clotting factors present in the blood. Such tests may include the following:

- Complete blood count, to check a platelet count and to evaluate for possible anemia
- Biochemistry profile, to check for internal organ damage
- Coagulation panel, with tests such as prothrombin and partial thrombin time
- Specific assay for factor IX (also used to test female carriers), with the results reported as a percentage of normal
- Assays of other clotting factors to make sure they are normal

Clotting factor IX is dependent on normal vitamin K levels in the blood. Other clotting factors are also affected by vitamin K availability, so testing may also be recommended to screen for vitamin K–related problems.

TREATMENT AND FOLLOW-UP

Treatment Options

Hemophilia B is a lifelong disorder with no cure. Patients with mild disease may never require treatment or may need treatment only in case of surgery or trauma. During episodes of more severe bleeding, hospitalization with cage rest and transfusions of plasma or blood products containing clotting factors are needed to replace factor IX and control bleeding. Transfusions may be needed every 8-12 hours until the bleeding stops. Red blood cell transfusions may be necessary if bleeding results in severe anemia.

Follow-up Care

Because this is an inherited disorder, it is a good idea to contact the breeder of the animal so that the parents and other littermates may be tested for the disease. Individuals that test positive, including carriers, should not be used for breeding.

It is important to control the activities of affected individuals, to minimize injury and the risk of bleeding. Drugs that affect platelet function and unnecessary surgeries are avoided, if possible. If surgery is required, transfusions are often performed before, during, and after the procedure to try and control bleeding. During severe bleeding episodes, laboratory tests may be recommended to monitor for evidence of continued blood loss and the development of anemia.

Prognosis

Prognosis is very poor for pets with severe disease. Recurring bleeding episodes require repeated transfusions, which can become quite expensive. Dogs with severe disease are often euthanized or die from a severe bleeding episode.

SPECIAL INSTRUCTIONS:

Hypercalcemia Associated with Cancer

Kristi S. Lively, DVM, DABVP

BASIC INFORMATION

Description

Certain cancers may cause calcium levels in the blood to become elevated (hypercalcemia). When calcium levels are excessive, problems can arise in the bones, kidneys, neurologic system, and muscular system. Regulation of calcium is controlled by the hormones, calcitriol and parathyroid hormone (PTH). Certain tumors secrete a substance called *parathyroid hormone–related peptide* (PTH-rp). This protein closely mimics normal PTH. The body responds to elevated PTH-rp by increasing calcium levels inappropriately. Normally, the kidneys would eliminate the excess calcium, but the PTH-rp tells the kidneys to conserve calcium instead of eliminating it.

Causes

Cancers that produce PTH-rp or destroy bones are the most likely cause of hypercalcemia. Examples include lymphoma, leukemia, bone tumors, anal sac carcinoma, stomach carcinoma, multiple myeloma, and mammary (breast) tumors. Lymphoma is the most commonly involved tumor in the dog. Tumors of the parathyroid gland tumor may secrete excessive amounts of PTH, which elevates calcium. Hypercalcemia associated with malignancies must be differentiated from noncancerous causes of high calcium.

Clinical Signs

Sometimes elevated calcium levels are found coincidentally on routine laboratory tests, and a search for the underlying cause can be started before any clinical signs develop. When clinical signs are present, they may include vomiting, lack of appetite, lethargy, excessive thirst and urination, slow heart rate, muscle weakness, and, rarely, mental depression, seizures, or coma.

Diagnostic Tests

If elevated calcium levels are identified, the laboratory test is usually repeated on a new blood sample to ensure that the finding is correct. If the second test confirms the presence of hypercalcemia, then your veterinarian will recommend a series of tests to look for an underlying cause, which can be difficult to find in some cases. Such tests often include the following:

- A thorough physical examination to search for small or hidden tumors, enlarged lymph nodes (glands), and other abnormalities
- Routine laboratory and urinalysis tests
- A blood panel that measures ionized calcium, PTH, and PTH-rp levels
- X-rays of the chest, abdomen, long bones, and spine
- An abdominal ultrasound to identify any tumors or changes in the spleen, liver, and kidneys
- Bone marrow aspiration to search for leukemia or lymphoma
- Fine-needle aspiration or biopsy of suspected tumors

Additional testing may also be needed to rule out noncancerous causes of hypercalcemia.

TREATMENT AND FOLLOW-UP

Treatment Options

Treatment depends largely on identification of the underlying tumor and the degree of hypercalcemia. Options for the cancer include surgery, chemotherapy, radiation therapy, or a combination of these, depending on the tumor type and location.

Mildly elevated calcium may be treated with fluid therapy to flush out excess calcium through the kidneys. Moderate to severe hypercalcemia often requires additional medications, such as diuretics (furosemide) and steroids (prednisone), to lower calcium levels more rapidly and aggressively. Kidney failure can develop with severe hypercalcemia, so hospitalization with intravenous fluid therapy and additional medications is often required.

Follow-up Care

Monitoring of kidney function and calcium levels is done in hospitalized animals and animals with chronically elevated calcium. Other laboratory tests may be repeated, depending on initial results and the treatments used.

Prognosis

Cancers causing hypercalcemia generally carry a more guarded (uncertain) prognosis than other cancers. Animals with hypercalcemia-induced kidney failure have a very poor prognosis.

SPECIAL INSTRUCTIONS:

Immune-Mediated Hemolytic Anemia

Kristi S. Lively, DVM, DABVP

BASIC INFORMATION

Description

Anemia is an abnormally low red blood cell (RBC) count. The RBC's primary function is to transport oxygen to tissues; when oxygen transport decreases to critical levels, clinical signs occur. Immune-mediated hemolytic anemia (IMHA) occurs when the RBCs are destroyed by the body's own immune system. Certain breeds of dogs are predisposed to IMHA, including the cocker spaniel, poodles, West Highland white terrier, Old English sheepdog, schnauzer, and Irish setter. In cats, IMHA is often associated with certain infections.

Causes

With *primary IMHA*, excessive RBC destruction is immune mediated. The targeted RBCs are coated with antibody; the immune system incorrectly recognizes these cells as foreign and destroys them (hemolysis). *Secondary hemolytic* anemia can be caused by toxins, infections, blood parasites, cancer, drug reactions, and inherited RBC membrane defects. In dogs, 60-75% of IMHA cases are primary and not related to an underlying cause. In cats, secondary hemolytic anemia is more common and is often associated with feline leukemia virus or *Hemobartonella* infection.

Clinical Signs

Clinical signs depend on the severity and the underlying cause of the anemia. Anemia typically causes weakness, lethargy, increased heart rate, poor appetite, and pale gums. Other signs may include fever, jaundice (elevated bilirubin), an enlarged spleen, pica (eating abnormal objects such as dirt), a heart murmur, enlarged glands (lymph nodes), vomiting, diarrhea, weight loss, or depression. Death can occur rapidly if the hemolysis is severe.

Diagnostic Tests

Anemia is diagnosed by measurement of the RBC count or packed cell volume (PCV). When anemia is diagnosed, other laboratory tests may be recommended to further determine whether it is immune-mediated and whether new RBCs are being produced. Additional testing is often needed to evaluate the function of other organs, measure bilirubin levels, detect internal parasites, and search for underlying causes. X-rays may be recommended to search for tumors and damage from trauma and to evaluate various organs.

TREATMENT AND FOLLOW-UP

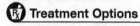 Treatment Options

If the anemia is severe and life-threatening, hospitalization with repeated blood transfusions (see handouts on **Transfusion Therapy in Dogs** and **Transfusion Therapy in Cats**), oxygen therapy, and intensive supportive care may be recommended to stabilize the patient while the cause of anemia is investigated. Treatment is then directed at the underlying cause and may include immune-suppressive drugs, antibiotics, parasite control, chemotherapy, or other measures.

For primary IMHA, the main treatment is immune suppression. Treatment is often required for months, with drug doses slowly tapered over time. High doses of steroids (prednisone, dexamethasone) are commonly given initially. Steroids can be combined with other medications (such as azathioprine or cyclosporine) to achieve a more rapid and complete immune suppression, and such combinations are often considered for more serious forms of the disease.

Once immune-suppressive drugs are started, improvement in RBC survival often occurs in 1-7 days, if the patient is going to respond to the medications. Patients with jaundice may be started on very aggressive therapy, because they often do not respond to steroids alone. In some resistant cases, splenectomy may be recommended to slow RBC destruction.

The formation of clots in blood vessels (thromboembolic disease) is a major complication of IMHA, causing death in 30-80% of cases in dogs. These clots can occur throughout the body, with life-threatening consequences. Heparin or low-dose aspirin therapy may be started to minimize clot formation.

Follow-up Care

Responsive cases may be hospitalized for 4-7 days, and longer hospital stays are often needed for severe cases. Steroids have many side effects, including excessive thirst and urination, panting, secondary urinary tract infections, liver enzyme alterations, and skin and hair coat changes. These effects slowly resolve as the steroids are tapered. When steroids are combined with other immune-suppressive medications, the steroids can be used at lower doses and tapered sooner.

Immune-mediated anemias require several months of therapy and monitoring of RBC counts as the medications are tapered. If medications are withdrawn too quickly, hemolysis may recur. Other laboratory tests are often used to monitor for side effects of the medications.

Prognosis

For patients that respond quickly to immunosuppression and do not need repeated transfusions, prognosis is good. IMHA can be a very dangerous disease, however, especially in patients with jaundice and thromboembolic disease. Animals that require repeated transfusions or quickly destroy transfused RBCs have a much poorer prognosis. Mortality rates of 20-80% have been reported with hemolytic anemia. Mortality rates dramatically increase if thromboembolic disease is present. Relapse rates (typically around 15%) in dogs are minimized with long-term use of steroids and azathioprine.

SPECIAL INSTRUCTIONS:

Immune-Mediated Thrombocytopenia

Kristi S. Lively, DVM, DABVP

BASIC INFORMATION
Description
Platelets (also called *thrombocytes*) are tiny cell fragments that circulate in the bloodstream and participate in the formation of blood clots. Excessively low platelet counts (thrombocytopenia) can lead to bleeding tendencies, because without platelets the blood cannot clot properly. Thrombocytopenia is not a common condition, but it can occur in any breed, age, or sex of dog or cat. Pets with cancer are at higher risk.

The normal platelet count in dogs and cats ranges from 200,000 to 500,000 per microliter (μL), although there are some breed variations in dogs. About 50,000 platelets/μL are needed to prevent spontaneous bleeding and bruising. Platelets are stored in the spleen and are removed from circulation by the spleen when they become old.

In immune-mediated thrombocytopenia (ITP), the immune system incorrectly identifies the platelets as foreign material and coats them with antibody. The spleen removes these coated platelets from the blood and destroys them. Antibody-coated platelets also do not function well while they are still circulating.

ITP occurs most commonly in middle-aged to older dogs, with poodles, cocker spaniels, and Old English sheepdogs overrepresented. In cats, ITP is very uncommon and is often associated with feline leukemia virus (FeLV) infection.

Causes
Immune-mediated destruction of platelets may develop in association with other conditions such as cancer, blood parasites, drug reactions, and infections; this is known as *secondary ITP*. Immune destruction of platelets can also arise spontaneously, for no apparent reason, and this is called *primary ITP*.

Clinical Signs
Signs do not typically develop until the platelet count falls below 50,000/μL. Signs can vary but include small bruises (petechiae and ecchymoses) on the skin, gums, and eyes; nose bleeds; blood in the urine; swollen and painful joints; and blood in the feces. Signs become more obvious with lower, more dangerous platelet counts. Life-threatening breathing difficulty and seizures may also occur. With secondary ITP, signs of the underlying illness may also be present.

Diagnostic Tests
A blood clotting problem may be suspected from the clinical signs. Thrombocytopenia is diagnosed by a blood platelet count. Other laboratory tests are needed to search for an underlying cause, to evaluate other organs, and to determine the presence of anemia. Additional procedures that may be recommended include x-rays, an ultrasound, other clotting tests, bone marrow aspiration, and certain immune tests. If signs of bleeding are noted but the platelet count is normal, other disorders of coagulation (clotting function) must be investigated.

TREATMENT AND FOLLOW-UP
Treatment Options
For primary ITP, the main treatment is immune suppression, usually with high doses of steroids such as prednisone or dexamethasone. Treatment is often required for several months, and drug doses are slowly tapered over time. Steroids can be combined with other medications (vincristine, azathioprine, cyclosporine) to achieve a more rapid and complete immune suppression. These medications may be reserved for more seriously affected animals.

Other treatments are based on any underlying cause of the thrombocytopenia that is identified and may include antibiotics, antiparasite therapy, withdrawal of certain drugs, and chemotherapy. If bleeding is severe enough to cause anemia, hospitalization and blood transfusions may be required. Platelet transfusions are rarely available for animals. In resistant cases, splenectomy may be recommended to slow platelet destruction, but its effectiveness in animals is controversial.

Follow-up Care
Once immune-suppressive drugs are started, platelet counts often increase in 1-7 days if the patient is going to respond to the medications. Steroids have many effects, including excessive thirst, excessive urination, panting, secondary urinary tract infections, liver enzyme alterations, and skin and hair coat changes. These side effects usually resolve slowly as the steroids are decreased. When steroids are combined with other immune-suppressive medications, the steroids can often be used at lower doses and tapered sooner.

ITP often requires several months of therapy, and repeated platelet counts are needed as medications are tapered. If medications are withdrawn too soon or too quickly, ITP may recur. Other laboratory tests are used to monitor for side effects from the medications and for the onset of secondary infections from the immune suppression.

Prognosis
Prognosis depends on the underlying cause and whether the patient responds well to therapy. Thrombocytopenia secondary to infections or drug reactions often has an excellent prognosis, whereas thrombocytopenia secondary to cancer may have a poor prognosis. Primary ITP has a variable prognosis, with some dogs responding very well and others having a minimal response.

SPECIAL INSTRUCTIONS:

Lymphedema

Kristi S. Lively, DVM, DABVP

BASIC INFORMATION

Description

The lymphatic system is a network of vessels and lymph tissue that carries a protein-rich fluid called *lymph*. Lymphoid tissue is found in many organs, including the spleen, bone marrow, tonsils, and lymph nodes (glands). These organs play a role in the production and circulation of antibody-producing cells called *lymphocytes*, which are an integral part of the body's immune system. Lymph is not pumped through the body like blood is pumped by the heart. The contraction of nearby muscles helps lymph slowly move through the lymphatic vessels.

In addition to its immune properties, the lymphatic system also helps to drain excess fluid from tissues and helps to transport a fatty liquid rich in lymphocytes, known as *chyle*, back to the bloodstream. Disorders affecting the lymphatic system can cause abnormal fluid accumulation and tissue swelling, which is called *lymphedema*. Lymphedema can arise as a congenital (primary) or an acquired (secondary) condition. It is more common in dogs than in cats. English bulldogs, poodles, Labrador retrievers, and Old English sheepdogs are predisposed to the condition.

Causes

Congenital lymphedema is caused by an inherited malformation of the lymphatic system. In these patients, normal lymph vessels or tissues may be completely absent or dramatically reduced. Secondary lymphedema can be caused by congestive heart failure, venous hypertension (high pressure in veins), trauma, inflammation, or infection. Some of these problems result in excessive fluid production that overwhelms the lymphatic drainage system. If damage occurs to the lymphatic system from trauma, surgery, radiation therapy, infection, or cancer, the ability to effectively transport fluid is also affected.

Clinical Signs

Congenital lymphedema is often present at birth or develops in the first few months of life. Secondary lymphedema can occur any time during the animal's life. Swelling typically starts in one or more of the legs and may progress to affect other areas of the body. The swelling "pits" when touched, which means that the swelling indents when pressure is applied to it, and the indentation may persist for several minutes. The swelling is not usually painful and does not cause a fever unless a secondary infection occurs. Eventually, the pitting quality of the swelling disappears as scarring develops within the tissue.

Diagnostic Tests

A number of diagnostic tests are needed to rule out more common causes of tissue swelling. A thorough history and physical examination may identify underlying heart disease, trauma, or evidence of infection. Laboratory tests are usually done to rule out diseases that cause loss of protein and to search for evidence of infection and cancer. Tests for heartworm disease, tick-borne infections, and other causes of vasculitis (vessel inflammation) may be recommended.

Fine-needle aspiration of the affected area or nearby lymph nodes reveals no cancerous or inflammatory cells, unless secondary infection has occurred. X-rays of the affected limb may be recommended if trauma is suspected. X-rays and/or ultrasound imaging of the abdomen and chest may be performed to evaluate the heart and screen for cancer.

If lymphedema is highly suspected, lymphangiography may be considered. In this procedure, dye is injected below the swollen areas, and the flow is observed through video x-rays (fluoroscopy) or a series of still x-rays. Lymphangiography is often performed at veterinary referral facilities.

TREATMENT AND FOLLOW-UP

Treatment Options

Unless a correctable underlying condition is diagnosed, lymphedema is not considered curable. Resting the animal and massage of the affected limb may improve lymph circulation. In some patients, the use of long-term pressure wraps and physical therapy are needed. Antibiotics are used to treat secondary infections. Surgery may be attempted in some cases, based on the results of lymphangiography. Medications, such as benzopyrones (coumarin, flavonoids, rutin), may be tried to reduce production of the protein-rich fluid. Diuretics, steroids, and other medications have little beneficial effect on lymphedema.

Follow-up Care

Long-standing lymphedema may predispose the animal to infections in the swollen area. The affected site also undergoes eventual scarring and fibrosis. With long-term bandaging, complications are possible if the bandages are not applied and changed correctly.

Prognosis

With respect to congenital lymphedema, generalized forms are usually lethal. Puppies, especially English bulldogs with severe lymphedema, often die soon after birth. Improvement or resolution of the edema may occur in those animals with involvement of only the rear legs.

Prognosis for secondary lymphedema depends on the underlying cause; it is not typically reversible. Focal lymphedema may be tolerated well, even without therapy.

SPECIAL INSTRUCTIONS:

Lymphoma in Cats

Kristi S. Lively, DVM, DABVP

BASIC INFORMATION
Description
Lymphoma (also called *lymphosarcoma, LSA*) is a common cancer of middle-aged and older cats. It is a cancer of the white blood cells known as *lymphocytes*, of which there are two main types—B cells and T cells. Lymphoma may affect the skin, eyes, central nervous system (spinal cord and brain), gastrointestinal tract, liver, and lungs. This cancer can be aggressive if left untreated but often responds favorably to chemotherapy, which adds months and sometimes years to the pet's life.

Causes
Even though this is a common cancer of people and pets, it is not known why it develops. In some cats, feline leukemia virus (FeLV) may play a role. This virus is becoming less common, however, as more cats are vaccinated or live indoors, thereby decreasing their risk of infection. Environmental factors such as cigarette smoke may increase the risk for LSA, and other environmental factors remain under investigation. There is no known breed or sex predilection in cats.

Clinical Signs
Clinical signs depend on the area of the body affected. Three common forms of LSA exist in cats: the widespread multicentric form, the mediastinal form, and the alimentary (gastrointestinal) form.

Widespread enlargement of the lymph nodes (glands) may be the only sign with the multicentric form. The mediastinal form develops in the front of the chest and may cause difficulty breathing. The alimentary form can affect any portion of the stomach or intestines and often causes signs such as weight loss, lethargy, loss of appetite, vomiting, and diarrhea. An abdominal mass may develop that can be felt on physical examination. Some cats have enlargement of the liver and spleen.

Other forms of LSA may cause skin lumps, sudden blindness, seizures, back pain, or shortness of breath. Fever, excessive drinking and urination, or abnormal bleeding can also occur.

Diagnostic Tests
Diagnosis of LSA can be easy if all external lymph nodes are enlarged or difficult if the tumor is in a less accessible organ. The tests performed depend on the location of the tumor, but the following may be recommended:
• A complete blood count, biochemistry profile, and urinalysis
• Fine-needle aspiration of a lymph node or mass, with examination of cells under the microscope (cytology)
• Biopsy of enlarged lymph nodes or other organs
• X-rays and/or an ultrasound to evaluate for internal organ involvement

• Bone marrow aspiration if bone marrow involvement is suspected
• FeLV test
• Endoscopy (passing a flexible tube into the stomach and upper intestines) and biopsy
• Specialized testing to determine the type of lymphoma (B cell versus T cell)

TREATMENT AND FOLLOW-UP
Treatment Options
Treatment of lymphoma depends on the organs involved, but most cases require chemotherapy because the disease is widespread. Surgery may be needed in some cases, such as the alimentary form, to relieve an intestinal obstruction caused by the tumor. A variety of chemotherapeutic protocols are available, consisting of combinations of oral and injectable medications. (See handout on **Chemotherapy and Your Pet**.)

Treatment is started when the disease is diagnosed, even if the cat does not seem ill, because waiting may drastically reduce long-term survival. The goal of cancer therapy is to achieve long-term remission and good quality of life. Remission is achieved when signs of disease have disappeared.

Follow-up Care
Frequent recheck visits are needed to administer some forms of chemotherapy and to monitor response to the medications. Laboratory tests are used to monitor for side effects of the medications and evidence of spread of the disease. Sometimes x-rays and ultrasound studies are also repeated periodically to check the internal organs.

Prognosis
Prognosis depends on several factors, including FeLV status, location of the cancer, cell type (B versus T; acute/aggressive versus low-grade/chronic), and how quickly the cancer is diagnosed and treated. Prognosis is better in cats that achieve complete remission, maintain remission, and tolerate the chemotherapy. In general, remissions of 2 years or longer can be achieved in 30-40% of cats that respond well to chemotherapy. About 70% of cats achieve at least an additional 4-6 months of good quality of life. Cats that are not treated may survive only 4-6 weeks after diagnosis.

Lymphoma eventually comes out of remission, with recurrence of clinical signs or spread of cancer to other organ systems. The cancer may become resistant to the drugs that have been used, so new drugs may be chosen to try and rescue the animal and put the disease back into remission.

SPECIAL INSTRUCTIONS:

Lymphoma in Dogs

Kristi S. Lively, DVM, DABVP

BASIC INFORMATION

Description

Lymphoma (also called *lymphosarcoma, LSA*) is a common cancer of middle-aged and older dogs. It is a cancer of the white blood cells known as *lymphocytes*, of which there are two main types— B cells and T cells. Lymphoma may originate in any lymph tissue, including the lymph nodes (glands), spleen, liver, bone marrow, and thymus. LSA is not restricted to certain organs and may also affect the skin, eyes, central nervous system, gastrointestinal tract, liver, and lungs. It may be the most common cancer in dogs. This cancer can be aggressive if left untreated, but it often responds favorably to chemotherapy, adding months and sometimes years to the pet's life.

Causes

Even though this is a common cancer of people and dogs, it is not known why it develops. A genetic predisposition may exist, because certain breeds, such as the golden retriever, boxer, basset hound, Scottish terrier, bulldog, Airedale terrier, and Saint Bernard, seem prone to the disease.

Clinical Signs

Clinical signs depend on the area of the body affected. Widespread enlargement of the lymph nodes may be the only sign in dogs with the common multicentric form of LSA, but some dogs may also have enlargement of the liver and spleen. Other forms of LSA may cause skin lumps, sudden blindness, seizures, back pain, or shortness of breath. Fever, excessive drinking and urination, or abnormal bleeding can also occur.

Diagnostic Tests

Diagnosis of LSA can be easy if all external lymph nodes are enlarged or difficult if the tumor is in a less accessible organ. The tests performed depend on the location of the tumor, but the following may be recommended:

- A complete blood count, biochemistry profile, and urinalysis
- Fine-needle aspiration of a lymph node or mass, with examination of cells under the microscope (cytology)
- Biopsy of enlarged lymph nodes or other organs
- X-rays and/or an ultrasound to evaluate for internal organ involvement
- Bone marrow aspiration if bone marrow involvement is suspected
- Specialized testing to determine the type of lymphoma (B cell versus T cell)

TREATMENT AND FOLLOW-UP

Treatment Options

Treatment of lymphoma depends on the organs involved, but most cases require chemotherapy because the disease is widespread. A variety of chemotherapeutic protocols are available, consisting of combinations of oral and injectable medications. The protocol recommended often depends on the type of lymphoma (B cell or T cell), which organs are affected, and the personal and financial choices of the owner. (See handout on **Chemotherapy and Your Pet**.)

Treatment is started when the disease is diagnosed, even if the dog does not seem ill, because waiting may drastically reduce long-term survival. The goal of cancer therapy is to achieve long-term remission and good quality of life. Remission is achieved when the signs of disease have disappeared.

Follow-up Care

Frequent recheck visits are needed to administer some forms of chemotherapy and to monitor response to the medications. Laboratory tests are used to monitor for side effects of the medications and for evidence of spread of the disease. Sometimes x-rays and ultrasound studies are also repeated periodically to check the internal organs.

Prognosis

Prognosis is best in dogs that achieve complete remission, maintain remission, and tolerate their chemotherapeutic medications. Patients with B-cell lymphoma often achieve and maintain remission more successfully than dogs with T-cell lymphoma. Treatment of multicentric lymphoma in dogs has a 75-90% response rate, with average survival times of 9-12 months. Patients treated before they are feeling sick usually have better response rates.

Lymphomas involving other organs, such as the skin, the intestines, or the respiratory system, have lower remission rates. When LSA is complicated by high calcium levels (hypercalcemia), success rates also tend to be lower. In dogs that do not receive chemotherapy, survival time may be as short as 4-6 weeks. In these patients, oral prednisone may be used temporarily to alleviate some of the clinical signs.

Lymphoma eventually comes out of remission, with recurrence of clinical signs such as lymph node enlargement or spread of the cancer to other organ systems. The cancer may become resistant to the drugs that have been used, so new drugs may be chosen to try and rescue the animal and put the disease back into remission.

SPECIAL INSTRUCTIONS:

Mastocytosis

Kristi S. Lively, DVM, DABVP

BASIC INFORMATION

Description

Mast cells usually reside in connective tissues but are occasionally found in the bloodstream. They contain granules that store histamine and other chemicals that activate inflammation. *Mast cell tumors* (MCT) represent the most common form of mast cell disease. These tumors usually arise in the skin and are sometimes called *cutaneous mastocytosis*. (See the handouts on **Mast Cell Tumors in Dogs** and **Mast Cell Tumors in Cats**.)

Mastocythemia is the presence of abnormal numbers of mast cells in the blood or bone marrow. Mastocythemia may indicate a form of disseminated mast cell cancer called *systemic mastocytosis*. Although cutaneous MCT is more common in dogs, cats develop systemic mastocytosis more often. *Mast cell leukemia* develops when malignant mast cells proliferate in the bone marrow and are released into the circulation (bloodstream).

Causes

Mast cells are normally produced in the bone marrow; from there, they circulate to other areas of the body. Why mast cells become malignant is unknown. A genetic predisposition or viral influence is suspected for MCT in dogs, but the cause of mastocytosis remains a mystery in cats. Cancerous mast cells may multiple in the spleen, skin, gut, liver, and other soft tissues.

Clinical Signs

Clinical signs depend on the organ system involved. Mast cells secrete histamine, a chemical that can cause stomach ulcers. Patients with systemic disease may exhibit vomiting, diarrhea, weight loss, and lack of appetite. Heparin may be released by mast cells and can cause bleeding tendencies, such as abnormal bruising or blood in the feces. If the spleen is involved, abdominal distention or a palpably enlarged spleen may be detected. Acute collapse may occur following a sudden release of histamine, perforation of a gastrointestinal ulcer, or bleeding from the spleen. Patients with liver involvement may be jaundiced.

Diagnostic Tests

Laboratory tests are usually recommended in patients with suspected mast cell disease. The complete blood count may reveal mast cells in the blood, as well as anemia and alterations in the white blood cell count. Blood clotting tests may be indicated if any abnormal bleeding or bruising is present. Affected cats may be tested for feline leukemia virus and feline immunodeficiency virus infection. Abdominal x-rays and an ultrasound are often performed to evaluate the spleen, liver, and other organs. Fine-needle aspiration may be done on accessible masses. Chest x-rays may be recommended to look for metastasis (spread of the cancer).

If bone marrow involvement is suspected, bone marrow aspiration may be performed to evaluate the degree of proliferation of mast cells. Any masses that are surgically removed are usually submitted for histopathologic examination to determine the degree of malignancy, which can help predict future tumor behavior and prognosis. Other tests may be recommended to rule out diseases that cause similar clinical signs.

TREATMENT AND FOLLOW-UP

Treatment Options

Aggressive treatment is recommended whenever mast cell disease is diagnosed. Whenever possible, surgical excision (removal) of the MCT is performed, followed by appropriate medical or radiation therapy. If the spleen is involved, surgical removal of the spleen is indicated.

For animals with systemic mastocytosis, especially in the gut or in multiple organs, about 50% respond to high doses of prednisone (steroid) for several months, followed by lower doses for 1 year. If no response is detected to steroids after the first 2-3 weeks, or for highly malignant cells, other chemotherapeutic agents may be considered. L-Asparaginase and vincristine may be recommended in dogs, and lomustine and vinblastine in cats. Supportive care with antacids and gut-protective agents may be used to prevent stomach ulcers. Antihistamines may also be recommended.

Follow-up Care

Laboratory tests and sometimes bone marrow aspirations are used to monitor the response to therapy and side effects of the medications. Tests may also be repeated with any evidence of recurrence of mast cell disease, such as new skin nodules, enlargement of the liver or spleen, or return of clinical signs.

Prognosis

Prognosis varies depending on the response to treatment and the organ systems involved. Patients with rapidly progressive disease have a poorer prognosis than patients with slow-growing tumors. Involvement of the liver and gut carries a more guarded prognosis than other forms. If the disease does not respond to steroids, prognosis is also poor.

Cats with splenic mastocytosis often have a good prognosis following splenectomy and may live for a few years. Even cats with mast cell disease in the liver and nearby lymph nodes often do well for up to 14 months following splenectomy.

SPECIAL INSTRUCTIONS:

Primary and Secondary Polycythemia

Kristi S. Lively, DVM, DABVP

BASIC INFORMATION

Description

Polycythemia is an elevated red blood cell (RBC) count that is accompanied by an increased packed cell volume (PCV) and increased hemoglobin level. Polycythemia may be *relative* or *absolute*. In relative polycythemia, the RBC count is not truly increased, but the PCV is elevated because there is less fluid (plasma) in the blood, which makes the relative amount of RBCs appear to be high. Absolute polycythemia occurs when more RBCs are produced than normal and their count is truly elevated.

Causes

Dehydration is a common cause of relative polycythemia. Absolute polycythemia may be *primary* or *secondary*. Primary polycythemia (polycythemia vera) is a spontaneous proliferation of RBCs in the bone marrow. Secondary polycythemia is induced by physiologic changes that increase the body's demand for oxygen, such as certain types of heart disease, living at high altitudes, lung disease, severe obesity, and defective oxygen transport.

Secondary polycythemia may also be caused by increased levels of erythropoietin, a hormone that stimulates RBC production. Erythropoietin levels may be increased with certain kidney diseases, and erythropoietin-like substances may be secreted by certain tumors.

Clinical Signs

With relative polycythemia, vomiting or diarrhea may be present and may result in dehydration. Absolute polycythemia usually occurs in older animals. Signs may include gums that are bright red, increased drinking and urination, seizures or other behavioral changes, weakness, hemorrhages within the eyes, retinal detachments, and blindness.

Diagnostic Tests

Once a high RBC count or high PCV is discovered, several additional tests are usually needed to look for evidence of dehydration and to determine whether the polycythemia is relative or absolute. Depending on the initial results, tests may be recommended to determine the cause of the dehydration, to differentiate primary from secondary polycythemia, and to look for underlying diseases. Erythropoietin levels may be checked, but in as many as half of patients with secondary polycythemia abnormally high levels are not detected.

X-rays and an abdominal ultrasound are often useful in searching for underlying conditions, such as lung disease, heart disease, and kidney problems. A bone marrow aspiration or biopsy may be recommended in cases of primary polycythemia.

TREATMENT AND FOLLOW-UP

Treatment Options

The goals of treatment are to correct any underlying dehydration and/or causes of secondary polycythemia and to remove contributing factors whenever possible. Phlebotomy and fluid therapy may be used in cases of absolute polycythemia to temporarily lower the PCV, thin the blood, and alleviate clinical signs. Phlebotomy is the removal of RBCs by drawing blood from a vein (similar to when a blood sample is taken for laboratory tests but in larger volumes). Phlebotomy may not be appropriate for patients with diseases that cause low oxygen levels.

A chemotherapeutic drug, hydroxyurea, may be recommended for primary polycythemia. Appropriate treatments for any heart and lung diseases are started. If possible, tumors or masses that may be secreting erythropoietin-like substances are surgically removed.

Follow-up Care

Periodic phlebotomy maybe required in patients with absolute polycythemia. The PCV is usually checked weekly until it is stable, and then periodically. Underlying diseases also require ongoing monitoring.

Prognosis

Prognosis depends largely on the severity of the underlying disease and response to treatment. Patients with polycythemia are more prone to complications but may survive for long periods of time (greater than 1 year).

SPECIAL INSTRUCTIONS:

Splenic Hemangiosarcoma

Kristi S. Lively, DVM, DABVP

BASIC INFORMATION

Description

Hemangiosarcoma is a highly malignant tumor of blood vessels. It commonly arises in the spleen, an organ in the abdomen. Growth of a mass on the spleen may go undetected until it becomes quite large or ruptures, which may result in life-threatening bleeding into the abdomen. Hemangiosarcoma has a high propensity to spread quickly to other organs, such as the heart, lungs, and liver. Dogs at risk include middle-aged to older, large-breed dogs, especially the German shepherd dog, Labrador retriever, and golden retriever. Splenic hemangiosarcoma is quite rare in the cat.

Causes

The reason this tumor develops is unknown. Hemangiosarcomas can form in any tissue that contains blood vessels. The most common sites include the skin, spleen, and heart. Less common sites include the central nervous system (brain and spinal cord), conjunctiva of the eyes, lungs, and liver.

Clinical Signs

Clinical signs are usually related to internal bleeding that arises from rupture of the splenic mass. Signs may include depression, weakness or collapse, pale gums, abdominal distention, and elevated heart and respiratory rates from shock. If bleeding stops spontaneously (on its own), the signs may subside. However, signs often soon recur due to repeated episodes of bleeding. The bleeding can be life-threatening and can result in death if untreated.

Diagnostic Tests

An abdominal mass may be discovered during a routine physical examination. Unexplained anemia found on a routine laboratory test may raise the suspicion of a hemangiosarcoma, especially in a dog of a compatible breed and age. X-rays and an ultrasound are often needed to confirm the presence of a mass and whether it involves the spleen, as well as to evaluate other abdominal organs for potential involvement or spread of the tumor.

Chest x-rays and an echocardiogram (heart ultrasound) may be recommended to check for evidence of tumors in the lungs and heart. Often, a biopsy is needed to confirm the diagnosis, since there are various tumors that may arise in the spleen, some of which are benign (such as hemangioma). It is not often possible to determine from routine tests whether the tumor is benign or malignant, so biopsies are commonly done at the time of surgery

to remove the mass. Further tests may be recommended to rule out other diseases that can cause anemia and clinical signs.

TREATMENT AND FOLLOW-UP

Treatment Options

If no evidence is uncovered that the tumor has spread, then removal of the mass and the spleen (splenectomy) may be a good treatment option to stop the bleeding episodes. The splenectomy is sometimes performed as an emergency procedure after the animal has been stabilized. Efforts to stabilize the animal usually require hospitalization and may include intravenous fluids and blood transfusions.

Surgery is not considered a cure for hemangiosarcoma, because it is a highly malignant disease and usually spreads to other sites in the body. If the mass is benign, surgery may be curative and eliminates the risk of ongoing blood loss.

Once a diagnosis of hemangiosarcoma is made by histopathology, chemotherapy may be considered to slow the spread of disease to other body systems. Current chemotherapy protocols include the drug, doxorubicin (*Adriamycin*), which is given intravenously every 3-4 weeks. Chemotherapy without surgical removal of the splenic mass is not usually done, because chemotherapy does not eliminate the ongoing risk of internal bleeding.

Follow-up Care

Most animals are hospitalized for a few days after surgery. Some develop irregular heart rhythms (cardiac arrhythmias) after splenectomy, so careful monitoring and additional medications may be required. Laboratory tests are often repeated to ensure that the anemia is resolving.

Laboratory tests are also periodically done to monitor for recurrence of anemia, which may indicate the tumor has spread. X-rays and ultrasounds may be repeated to search for evidence of metastasis (spread) of the tumor. Laboratory tests are also needed to monitor the side effects of the chemotherapeutic agents used.

Prognosis

Hemangiosarcoma is an aggressive cancer, with survival times of 1-4 months with surgery alone. Additional chemotherapy improves survival times over those achieved with surgery alone. Removal of the spleen spares the patient a sudden death from a bleeding episode, but almost all animals eventually succumb to the cancer.

SPECIAL INSTRUCTIONS:

Splenic Torsion

Kristi S. Lively, DVM, DABVP

BASIC INFORMATION
Description
The spleen is a large, tongue-shaped organ located in the abdomen, between the stomach and the left kidney. The spleen serves as a storage site for red blood cells and also clears old red blood cells from the bloodstream. The spleen is a component of the immune system, because antibody-producing lymphocytes (white blood cells) are located in the spleen. Because these functions are also carried out in other areas of the body (bone marrow and lymph nodes), an animal can live a normal life after having its spleen removed.

Splenic torsion occurs when the spleen rotates around the blood vessels entering the spleen or twists upon itself, thereby decreasing blood flow to the spleen. Torsion may occur as an isolated event or in conjunction with gastric dilation and volvulus (stomach bloating and twisting). Splenic torsion is more common in large-breed, deep-chested dogs, such as the Great Dane, German shepherd dog, and Labrador retriever.

Causes
The cause of splenic torsion is not always known, but twisting of the spleen may be affected by excessive exercise, rolling, running, or jumping behavior, gastric dilation and volvulus, or cancer of the spleen. Any problem that compromises the integrity of the ligaments supporting the spleen in the abdomen may also predispose to this condition.

Clinical Signs
Signs vary depending on whether the torsion arises suddenly or slowly. Acute torsion may cause sudden collapse and abdominal pain. Chronic torsion can produce more subtle or vague signs, such as intermittent lack of appetite, occasional vomiting, weight loss, weakness, and blood-tinged urine. Affected dogs may have pale gums, abdominal discomfort, and an irregular or elevated heart rate. Sometimes, an enlarged spleen can be felt in the abdomen during physical examination.

Diagnostic Tests
Laboratory tests may reveal an anemia, low platelet count, elevated white cell count, elevated liver tests, and hemoglobin in the urine. Abdominal x-rays or ultrasound may indicate an abdominal mass; an enlarged, deformed spleen; or a spleen in an abnormal location. Ultrasonography may also detect turbulent blood flow in the large vessels entering the spleen. An electrocardiogram (ECG) may identify an irregular heart rhythm (arrhythmia). Other tests may be recommended to rule out diseases that cause similar signs or to check for splenic cancer in other areas of the body.

TREATMENT AND FOLLOW-UP

Treatment Options
Surgery to remove the spleen is the treatment of choice. With acute splenic torsion, the animal is initially stabilized with intravenous fluids and other emergency medications. Surgery to remove the spleen is performed as soon as the patient is stable enough to undergo anesthesia. Following splenectomy, the animal may be hospitalized for several days for continued fluid therapy and cardiovascular monitoring. Serious postoperative arrhythmias may require treatment. Any predisposing conditions must also be addressed.

Follow-up Care
Cardiac arrhythmias can be life-threatening if they are severe and not adequately controlled, so continuous ECG monitoring and antiarrhythmic medications may be required for several days. Other monitoring and follow-up depends on the underlying cause.

Prognosis
Prognosis for recovery from uncomplicated splenic torsion is good if the problem is corrected before cardiovascular collapse (shock) occurs. If the torsion is associated with gastric dilation and volvulus, the prognosis may be guarded (more uncertain).

SPECIAL INSTRUCTIONS:

Splenomegaly

Kristi S. Lively, DVM, DABVP

BASIC INFORMATION

Description

The spleen is a large organ located in the abdomen, between the stomach and the left kidney. Splenomegaly is enlargement of the spleen. The spleen functions as a storage site for extra platelets and red blood cells, releasing them into the bloodstream in times of need or during a crisis. The spleen also clears old red blood cells from the circulation and serves as part of the immune system. Many antibody-producing lymphocytes are located in the spleen. Because these functions are also carried out by other body systems, such as the bone marrow and lymph nodes (lymph glands), an animal can live a normal life after removal of the spleen.

Causes

The four most common causes of splenomegaly are inflammation, hyperplasia (increased number of cells), congestion (increased blood retention), and infiltration of the spleen with tumor or certain infections. Inflammation of the spleen most often develops with infections, such as ehrlichiosis, brucellosis, feline infectious peritonitis, toxoplasmosis, and hemobartonellosis. Hyperplasia occurs when the spleen needs to support immune functions, to produce more red blood cells, or to clear more red blood cells. Congestion occurs when blood flow from the spleen is impaired; it may arise with splenic torsion (twisting of the spleen), certain medications, or heart disease. The most common cancers that infiltrate or involve the spleen are hemangiosarcoma, fibrosarcoma, leiomyosarcoma, mastocytosis, leukemias, and lymphoma. Sometimes enlargement of the spleen may be isolated to one area, causing a mass effect. This occurs with some types of tumor (hemangioma, plasmacytoma), infections, and hemorrhage resulting from trauma.

Clinical Signs

Clinical signs are usually caused by the underlying disorder and not the splenomegaly, so they can be extremely variable. The enlarged spleen may be palpable (felt) by your veterinarian during a physical examination. If the spleen is bleeding, free blood or fluid may be detected in the abdomen, and pale gums, increased or irregular heart rates, sudden weakness, collapse, and shock may occur. Some causes of splenomegaly are associated with fever, weight loss, decreased appetite, abdominal discomfort, or enlarged lymph nodes.

Diagnostic Tests

When splenomegaly is found, several tests are usually needed to search for the underlying cause. Routine laboratory tests, tests for certain infections and immune disorders, and blood clotting tests may be recommended. X-rays and ultrasounds of the chest and abdomen are often performed to evaluate for masses, metastatic disease, congested blood flow, bleeding into the abdomen, or abnormalities in other organs. Unfortunately, these tests cannot always differentiate between malignant and benign enlargement of the spleen.

Additional tests vary based on the suspicion of the underlying cause and may include further evaluation of the heart and aspiration of the spleen with a needle to collect cells for microscopic analysis.

TREATMENT AND FOLLOW-UP

Treatment Options

Treatment varies greatly depending on the underlying cause of the splenomegaly. Some causes are managed medically with chemotherapy, transfusions, immune-suppressive medications, or antibiotics. Other causes of splenomegaly are surgical problems that require removal of the spleen. Examples include splenic torsion, certain types of cancer, and bleeding splenic masses.

Follow-up Care

Follow-up plans are devised based on the underlying cause and whether medical or surgical therapy is undertaken. Some diseases are cured after surgery or medication, whereas others require repeated laboratory testing, x-rays, ultrasounds, and recheck visits. Your veterinarian will design a specific follow-up plan for your particular pet.

Prognosis

Prognosis is related to the underlying cause and the response to therapy. Disorders of the spleen that cause irregular heart rhythms, abnormal bleeding, or severe anemia carry a more guarded (uncertain) prognosis. Malignant tumors with high metastatic rates have a grave prognosis for long-term survival. Some infectious or inflammatory conditions may be cured with medical management.

SPECIAL INSTRUCTIONS:

Thrombocytopenia: Other Causes

Kristi S. Lively, DVM, DABVP

BASIC INFORMATION
Description
Platelets (also called *thrombocytes*) are tiny cell fragments that circulate in the bloodstream and participate in the formation of blood clots. Excessively low platelet counts (thrombocytopenia) can lead to bleeding tendencies, because without platelets the blood cannot clot properly. Thrombocytopenia is not a common condition, but it can occur in any breed, age, or sex of dog or cat. Pets with cancer are at higher risk.

Platelets are produced in the bone marrow. Once released into the bloodstream, they live an average of 10-12 days before being utilized. Normal platelet counts in dogs and cats range from 200,000 to 500,000 per microliter (μL), although there are some breed variations in dogs. Only about 50,000 platelets/μL are needed to prevent spontaneous bleeding and bruising. Platelets are stored in the spleen and removed from circulation by the spleen when they become old.

Causes
Immune-mediated destruction of platelets is discussed in the handout on **Immune-Mediated Thrombocytopenia**. This handout discusses other causes of thrombocytopenia, which include the following:
- Bone marrow cancer, scarring, or degeneration, with decreased production of platelets
- Infections that destroy platelets or decrease their production, such as ehrlichiosis or Rocky Mountain spotted fever in dogs and feline leukemia virus (FeLV) or feline immunodeficiency virus (FIV) in cats
- Inherited, congenital causes of low platelet counts
- Reactions to medications, such as estrogen, sulfonamides, chloramphenicol, and chemotherapeutic drugs
- Consumption of platelets following excessive clotting caused by inflammation of blood vessels (such as vasculitis from heartworm disease) or disseminated intravascular coagulation (a life-threatening clotting disorder)

Clinical Signs
Signs do not typically develop until the platelet count falls below 50,000/μL. Signs can vary but include small bruises (petechiae and ecchymoses) on the skin, gums, and eyes; nose bleeds; blood in the urine; swollen and painful joints; and blood in the stool. Signs become more obvious with lower, more dangerous platelet counts. Life-threatening breathing difficulty and seizures may also occur. Signs of the underlying illness may also be present.

Diagnostic Tests
A blood clotting problem may be suspected from the clinical signs. Thrombocytopenia is diagnosed by a blood platelet count. Other laboratory tests are needed to search for an underlying cause, to evaluate other organs, and to determine the presence of anemia. Additional procedures that may be recommended include x-rays, an ultrasound, other clotting tests, bone marrow aspiration, tests for infections and parasites, and certain immune tests. If signs of bleeding are noted but the platelet count is normal, other disorders of coagulation (clotting function) must be investigated.

TREATMENT AND FOLLOW-UP
Treatment Options
Treatments are based on the underlying cause of the thrombocytopenia and may include antibiotics, withdrawal of certain drugs, antiparasite therapy, chemotherapy, and sometimes immune-suppressive therapy. If bleeding is severe enough to cause anemia, hospitalization and blood transfusions may be required. Platelet transfusions are rarely available for animals.

Follow-up Care
As treatments are initiated, platelet counts are monitored every few days to assess the response to treatment. Other tests may be repeated to monitor for improvement in the underlying disease. Recheck visits may be needed for several months as medication doses are adjusted, depending on the underlying cause. It is very important to precisely follow your veterinarian's instructions, because, if medications are decreased or discontinued too soon, the thrombocytopenia may relapse. Notify your veterinarian if any signs recur or any changes are made in the medication schedule.

Prognosis
Prognosis depends on the underlying cause. Thrombocytopenia secondary to infections or drug reactions can carry an excellent prognosis, whereas thrombocytopenia secondary to cancer often has a much worse prognosis. Diagnostic tests and treatments can be expensive, depending on the underlying cause and how quickly the pet responds to therapy.

SPECIAL INSTRUCTIONS:

Thrombosis

Kristi S. Lively, DVM, DABVP

BASIC INFORMATION

Description

Thrombosis is the formation of a thrombus or an embolus within the heart or blood vascular system. A *thrombus* is a blood clot within a vessel or heart chamber. It may obstruct a vessel, or be attached to the wall of a vessel and cause turbulence or restricted blood flow. An *embolus* is a piece of clot that breaks off a thrombus, is carried to another location, and lodges at a distant site.

Causes

Certain diseases predispose cats and dogs to thrombosis. In cats, thrombus formation is most commonly associated with heart disease, especially dilated, hypertrophic, or restrictive cardiomyopathy. In dogs, thrombosis may be associated with elevated blood cholesterol, protein-losing diseases of the kidneys, hyperadrenocorticism (excessively high steroid production), hypothyroidism (low thyroid levels), surgery, trauma, and immune-mediated hemolytic anemia.

Both dogs and cats may develop thrombi from heartworm disease, severe bacterial infection of the blood, or serious widespread inflammation. Life-threatening conditions may lead to disseminated intravascular coagulation (DIC), in which microscopic thrombi form throughout the bloodstream. Emboli may also develop from air bubbles, fat particles, or pieces of catheters that enter the bloodstream.

Clinical Signs

Signs are related to the site of clot formation, whether vessel obstruction is complete or partial, and the underlying disease or condition. In cats with heart disease, an embolus may lodge where the end of the aorta branches into the arteries supplying blood to the rear legs. These cats may have a sudden onset of complete or partial rear limb paralysis, as well as dramatic pain, cool toes, pale or bluish claws, and lack of a pulse in the hind legs. They may also have clinical signs of the underlying cardiac disease.

The most common site of thrombosis in dogs is in the lungs. When a thrombus affects the lungs, it can cause sudden difficulty breathing, increased respiratory rate, and sudden death.

🔀 Diagnostic Tests

Diagnosis of thrombosis can sometimes be difficult. Initially, routine laboratory tests, including a heartworm test, are performed. X-rays of the chest and an echocardiogram (heart ultrasound) may be recommended to look for heart disease and for lung changes associated with pulmonary hypertension (elevated pressure in the blood vessels of the lungs), thrombosis, and heartworm disease. Measurements of oxygen levels in the blood (blood gas analysis) may show lower than normal oxygen levels. Blood pressure and

oxygen measurement may not be possible in areas of the body downstream from the clot, because of the lack of blood flow.

Specialized laboratory tests may be recommended to look for evidence of widespread microscopic blood clotting. Although they are uncommonly performed, advanced studies are sometimes done to confirm the presence of thrombosis. These tests may include angiography (injecting a dye into a blood vessel), ultrasonography of blood vessels, and nuclear or computed tomography (CT) scans. Other diagnostic tests are aimed at identifying the underlying disease.

TREATMENT AND FOLLOW-UP

℞ Treatment Options

Treatment is directed at correcting and controlling the underlying disease and starting supportive care for the organ system affected by the clot formation. Maintaining adequate circulation and oxygen flow to the tissues is crucial. Affected animals typically require hospitalization, with oxygen and fluid therapy. Medications (heparin, coumarin, tissue plasminogen factor, streptokinase) may be administered in an attempt to dissolve existing clots and prevent new clots, but often with mixed success. These medications require intensive monitoring, have potential side effects, and some can be very expensive. Other medications may be given to relieve pain and to lower blood or pulmonary pressures.

If cats are diagnosed with heart disease that increases their risk of clot formation, they may be started on low-dose aspirin or clopidogrel (*Plavix*) at the time of diagnosis to prevent future clot formation.

Follow-up Care

Patients maintained on long-term anticoagulant medications require repeated monitoring with blood clotting panels so that life-threatening bleeding tendencies can be avoided. Other monitoring and follow-up is based on the underlying disease.

Prognosis

Hospitalization to treat thrombotic disease often requires prolonged intensive care and can be expensive. Prognosis is guarded (uncertain), depending on the underlying cause, the site of the body affected by the clot, response to treatment, and the extent or severity of tissue damage. Prognosis is poor in cats with severe heart disease, and many die despite treatment, fail to regain rear limb function, or continue to develop more emboli. Those cats that do survive the initial crisis may recover the ability to walk after several weeks but have residual effects that affect their long-term mobility.

SPECIAL INSTRUCTIONS:

Von Willebrand Disease

Kristi S. Lively, DVM, DABVP

BASIC INFORMATION

Description

Von Willebrand disease (VWD) is an inherited bleeding disorder of the platelets that occurs in dogs, cats, and people. Platelets are responsible for helping blood clot. Von Willebrand factor is a protein produced by platelets that helps platelets stick together and form a clot. When this factor is abnormal or deficient, platelets do not effectively stick together, and the result is prolonged or inappropriate bleeding.

Causes

Three types of VWD exist, depending on the type and amount of factor present. In type I, the factor is normal but is present in very low amounts, and the severity of bleeding varies. Type I is most common in the Doberman pinscher, German shepherd dog, Shetland sheepdog, and standard poodle. In type II, the factor proteins are abnormal and decreased, which results in more severe bleeding episodes than in type I. Type II disease is typically seen in German shorthaired and wirehaired pointers. In type III, the factor is not made at all, and this is the most severe form. Type III is most commonly identified in the Scottish terrier, Chesapeake Bay retriever, and Shetland sheepdog.

Clinical Signs

Excessive or abnormal bleeding is the primary clinical sign of VWD. Because this is an inherited condition, signs may be seen early in life. Excessive bleeding from the gums occurs when baby teeth fall out. Nose bleeds, blood in the urine, dark or tarry stools, and swollen, painful joints may also occur. Sometimes excessive bleeding is not noted until after trauma or during surgery. Events that further affect platelet function, such as vaccination or use of nonsteroidal anti-inflammatory medications, may cause temporary bleeding and mild bruising.

Diagnostic Tests

In general, dogs with a suspected bleeding problem initially undergo routine laboratory testing, which may include a complete blood count, platelet count, biochemistry profile, and screening coagulation tests. If VWD is suspected, a test may be done in the clinic to assess platelet function; this is called the *buccal mucosal bleeding time*. This test is not specific for VWD, but an abnormal result increases suspicion for the disease.

To diagnose the presence of VWD, the amount of von Willebrand factor in the blood must be measured. The results can be labeled as normal, borderline, or abnormal. Dogs with abnormal amounts are at risk for increased bleeding tendency. Borderline results are sometimes rechecked, because the laboratory assay can be affected by many factors. The usual test for VWD does not identify the type (I, II, or III) present. If it is necessary to determine the type, further specialized tests must be run.

Some studies have shown a relationship between low thyroid hormone levels (hypothyroidism) and VWD, so your veterinarian may recommend thyroid tests to ensure that this is not a complicating factor.

TREATMENT AND FOLLOW-UP

Treatment Options

There is no cure for VWD. Treatment involves administration of normal von Willebrand factor during episodes of bleeding or when surgery is anticipated. Von Willebrand factor by itself cannot be purchased, but blood products containing the factor (such as plasma or cryoprecipitate) can be obtained from normal donors. Transfusions of these blood products are given during times of active bleeding and prior to surgery.

Injections of a drug called *DDAVP* (desmopressin acetate) may temporarily increase blood levels of von Willebrand factor for a few hours and is sometimes administered prior to surgery. There is some controversy as to whether this medication is effective. Dogs diagnosed with hypothyroidism are usually placed on a thyroid supplement.

Follow-up Care

Because there is no cure, prevention is aimed at eliminating affected dogs from the breeding pool. All dogs from breeds at risk for this disease and dogs with a history of VWD in their genetic line should be tested. Affected and carrier individuals should not be bred. Breeds routinely tested include the Doberman pinscher, golden retriever, Shetland sheepdog, Rottweiler, schnauzers, German shepherd dog, standard poodle, Scottish terriers, Pembroke Welsh corgi, German shorthaired and wirehaired pointers, and others.

Prognosis

Without treatment, severely affected dogs may bleed to death following injuries or surgeries not considered to be life-threatening. Dogs with borderline levels of von Willebrand factor may have increased bleeding tendencies that are not life-threatening but must be managed proactively with measures such as limiting the use of medications that affect platelet function, avoiding unnecessary invasive surgeries, and giving transfusions or DDAVP before planned surgeries.

SPECIAL INSTRUCTIONS:

SECTION 10

Immune System

Section Editor: Rhea V. Morgan, DVM, DACVIM (Small Animal), DACVO

Allergic Reactions
Extramedullary Plasmacytoma
Malignant Histiocytosis and Histiocytic Sarcoma

Multiple Myeloma
Systemic Lupus Erythematosus in Dogs: Systemic Aspects

Allergic Reactions

Rhea V. Morgan, DVM, DACVIM (Small Animal), DACVO

BASIC INFORMATION
Description

Allergic reactions occur when components of the immune system react to substances called *antigens*. Antigens are usually proteins. They may be introduced to the body through the skin, respiratory tract, or gut, or by injection. The systemic allergic reactions discussed here are anaphylaxis, urticaria, angioneurotic edema, and drug allergies. Allergic skin diseases, respiratory diseases, and adverse food reactions are discussed in other handouts.

Anaphylaxis is a severe, life-threatening hypersensitivity reaction. It is rare in both dogs and cats. *Urticaria*, or hives, are acute, focal swellings of the skin that are very itchy. *Angioneurotic edema* is sudden, soft swelling of tissues beneath the skin, especially the pinnae of the ears, lips, eyelids, and tissues of the face. Angioneurotic edema is not itchy or painful, but the skin overlying the swollen tissue may be red in color. *Drug allergies* are immune-mediated hypersensitivity reactions that are produced by antibodies formed by the immune system against some component of the drug.

Causes

Many different allergens can cause anaphylaxis, urticaria, and angioneurotic edema, including venoms from insects, drugs (usually injectable), vaccines, and blood or plasma transfusions. Urticaria and angioneurotic edema may occur after exposure to certain foods, and they can rarely arise with events that release histamine in the body, such as exposure to heat, cold, or pressure.

Drugs that can cause reactions include antibiotics and antibacterials (sulfonamides, penicillins, cephalosporins, tetracyclines), chemotherapeutic agents (asparaginase, doxorubicin), vaccines, and other medications (propylthiouracil, levamisole, aurothioglucose, methimazole, others). The drug dose, duration, formulation, and route of administration may all affect drug reactions. In some cases, genetics may influence the likelihood of a reaction; for example, the Doberman pinscher is more sensitive than other breeds to sulfonamide reactions.

Clinical Signs

In the dog, the target organ of anaphylaxis is the liver, so vomiting, diarrhea, respiratory distress, collapse, shock, and death can occur. In the cat, the target organs are the respiratory and gastrointestinal tracts, so facial itchiness, salivation, difficulty breathing, vomiting, diarrhea, shock, and collapse may be seen. Anaphylaxis may occur the first time an allergen is encountered.

Hives are localized or generalized red swellings or wheals in the skin. Dramatic sudden, soft, nonpainful swellings of the ears, eyelids, and face are typical findings with angioneurotic edema. If the edema affects the voice box area, the animal may have trouble breathing.

Drug allergies usually arise after the animal has been exposed to the drug for 5 or more days. A wide variety of signs may develop, including skin rashes, ulcerations, and scabby lesions; fever; joint swelling; pain in the muscles; weakness or wobbliness; kidney disease; hemolytic anemia; and decreased platelets.

Diagnostic Tests

Diagnosis is based primarily on the clinical signs. It is often difficult to identify the offending allergen in cases of urticaria or angioneurotic edema. Administration of a drug immediately before the onset of anaphylaxis is very suspicious. Diagnosis of drug reactions is often made by eliminating other conditions that could cause similar clinical signs and by improvement of the signs after the drug is withdrawn. Although drug reactions can be confirmed by a return of signs when the drug is reintroduced, this is not usually recommended for fear of a severe reaction.

TREATMENT AND FOLLOW-UP

Treatment Options

Anaphylaxis and severe drug reactions require immediate emergency treatment in the hospital, with intravenous fluids, supplemental oxygen, and administration of injectable steroids, epinephrine (adrenalin), and other drugs for shock. Urticaria, angioneurotic edema, and mild drug reactions are treated with injectable and oral antihistamines and steroids. For all allergic reactions, it is also important to withdraw or remove the antigen, if it is known.

Follow-up Care

Animals with severe allergic reactions are usually hospitalized for close monitoring for at least 24 hours. Monitoring may include measurements of heart and respiratory rates, blood pressure, and blood oxygen levels. Laboratory tests may be repeated to assess the effect of the reaction on liver and kidney function, blood sugar, blood cell counts, and blood clotting functions.

Most mild reactions are treated on an outpatient basis, but the animal may be rechecked daily if the signs do not respond quickly to treatment. Notify your veterinarian if the signs worsen or do not show steady improvement over the first 24 hours of therapy.

Prognosis

Anaphylaxis is a potentially life-threatening reaction that can be fatal if therapy is not started quickly and aggressively. Prognosis for urticaria, angioneurotic edema, and drug reactions are good to excellent. To prevent recurrences, exposure to the antigen should be avoided in the future.

SPECIAL INSTRUCTIONS:

Extramedullary Plasmacytoma

Rhea V. Morgan, DVM, DACVIM (Small Animal), DACVO

BASIC INFORMATION
Description
Extramedullary plasmacytoma is a tumor created by the proliferation of plasma cells, a type of white blood cell derived from B-cell lymphocytes. Most often, a solitary tumor develops and can be located in various areas of the body. Some plasmacytomas behave in a benign fashion; others exhibit more malignant behavior.

Unlike multiple myeloma, extramedullary plasmacytoma is not a widespread invasion of multiple organs by malignant plasma cells. (See the handout on **Multiple Myeloma.**)

Causes
It is not known why plasmacytomas develop. They are relatively common tumors in dogs but are rare in cats. In dogs, three forms of the disease have been described: tumors of the skin and mouth, tumors of the gastrointestinal (GI) tract, and solitary osseous plasmacytomas (SOP) of bone. Cocker spaniels appear to be predisposed to plasmacytomas. In cats, skin tumors occur most frequently, but the mouth, abdomen, eye, and brain may also be affected.

Under normal circumstances, plasma cells produce immunoglobulins (antibodies). Malignant plasma cells can produce large immunoglobulin proteins called *myeloma proteins* or *M proteins*. These proteins do not function like normal antibodies; instead they cause a variety of problems in different organs. In the dog, tumors of the skin and mouth do not usually produce these proteins but GI tumors may. SOP may progress over time to multiple myeloma, and these M proteins are always produced in multiple myeloma. In the cat, some plasmacytomas of soft tissue and bone produce immunoglobulins.

Clinical Signs
Plasmacytomas of the mouth and skin are often pink, hairless, round, and smooth or ulcerated masses. Skin tumors occur commonly on the head, ears, and feet. GI tumors may cause vomiting, diarrhea (with or without diarrhea), decreased appetite, and weight loss. SOP may cause bone pain or pathologic fractures (fractures caused by weakening of the bone rather than trauma).

Diagnostic Tests
Routine laboratory tests and x-rays are often recommended to investigate the clinical signs and to search for tumors elsewhere in the body. Fine-needle aspiration of the tumor may reveal plasma cells. Biopsy is often required to confirm the diagnosis. Extensive testing is then needed to rule out the presence of multiple myeloma.

TREATMENT AND FOLLOW-UP
Treatment Options
Surgical removal is the usual treatment for oral and skin tumors of the dog. In some cases, radiation therapy or cryotherapy (killing of the tumor by freezing) may be considered, especially if the tumor is located in an area that makes it hard to remove.

GI tumors are often treated by surgical removal. In some cases, surgery is followed by chemotherapy with prednisone and melphalan. Surgery and/or radiation therapy may be tried for SOPs initially, but chemotherapy is often required later in the course.

Antibiotics may be administered following surgery. Additional therapy may be needed if high levels of immunoglobulin are present in the blood. (See the handout on **Multiple Myeloma.**)

Follow-up Care
Periodic monitoring is needed after surgery for oral and skin tumors, to ensure they do not regrow and to watch for the development of new masses. Notify your veterinarian if any new masses are seen.

When chemotherapy is administered, follow-up visits and repeated laboratory tests are used to monitor response to treatment and side effects of the medications. Melphalan can decrease white blood cell and platelet counts.

Prognosis
Prognosis for dogs with plasmacytomas is better than for cats. Prognosis is good for most skin and oral tumors, because surgery is usually curative. For GI plasmacytomas, long-term survival can often be achieved with surgery and chemotherapy. SOPs often progress to multiple myeloma within 6 months, so long-term prognosis is poor.

Prognosis for affected cats is guarded (uncertain) to poor because metastasis (spread of the tumor) is common.

SPECIAL INSTRUCTIONS:

Malignant Histiocytosis and Histiocytic Sarcoma

Rhea V. Morgan, DVM, DACVIM (Small Animal), DACVO

BASIC INFORMATION

Description

Histiocytes are tissue cells that interact with white blood cells when tissues are inflamed. Malignant histiocytosis (MH) is the widespread proliferation of malignant histiocytes in various organs of the body. When the cancerous histiocytes form a solid tumor, it is called *histiocytic sarcoma* (HS). HS can metastasize (spread elsewhere in the body) and become disseminated. When this happens, HS is hard to differentiate from MH.

Causes

The cause of MH and HS in most animals is unknown; however, it is a genetic trait in the Bernese Mountain dog. The dog breeds most often affected include the flat-coated retriever, Bernese Mountain dog, Labrador retriever, and Rottweiler. Both conditions occur predominantly in male dogs 6-11 years of age, but any age and gender may be affected. These conditions are rare in the cat.

Clinical Signs

Signs of MH include loss of appetite, lethargy, fever, and dramatic weight loss. Other signs may be present, depending on the organs involved. On physical examination, the liver, spleen, and some lymph nodes (glands) may be enlarged.

Solitary HS are rapidly growing tumors that develop most often under the skin and within the soft tissues of the legs. HS may also arise in the spleen, lungs, brain, or nasal cavity and around joints. Unlike dogs with MH, those with HS do not often act ill, especially early in the clinical course. Surface tumors or growths under the skin may simply be discovered by the owner. Eventually, tumors in muscles and around joints may cause lameness, pain, and swelling. Internal tumors of the liver and spleen may cause signs similar to those of MH.

Diagnostic Tests

Routine laboratory tests and x-rays of the chest and abdomen are often performed to investigate the clinical signs. Common laboratory abnormalities include anemia, low platelet counts, low blood protein levels, abnormal liver function tests, and evidence of mild jaundice.

A fine-needle aspiration may be done on visible solitary tumors and may reveal abnormal histiocytes. Other tests that may be recommended include an abdominal ultrasound, aspiration of abdominal masses under ultrasound guidance, bone marrow aspiration or biopsy, and measurement of blood ferritin, which is often elevated in MH. It is important to evaluate the dog thoroughly to determine whether an HS has metastasized and what organs are involved with MH.

Biopsy of solitary tumors may be needed to reach a definitive diagnosis. Sophisticated immunohistochemical stains may be done on biopsy samples to confirm that the cells are actually histiocytes and not white blood cells.

TREATMENT AND FOLLOW-UP

Treatment Options

Chemotherapy is the main treatment option for MH and disseminated HS, but it is not often successful. Drugs such as lomustine, doxorubicin, cyclophosphamide, vincristine, prednisone, mitoxantrone, dacarbazine, and etoposide may be tried. Some drugs are used alone; others are used together in a specific protocol.

Solitary HS are treated by aggressive surgical removal, with incorporation of wide margins of apparently normal tissues that surround the tumor. Surgery may be followed by radiation therapy in some cases. Surgery for tumors on the legs may involve amputation of the entire limb. The benefit of follow-up chemotherapy has not been well defined in these cases.

Follow-up Care

Follow-up visits and repeated laboratory tests are used to monitor response to treatment and side effects of the medications. X-rays, abdominal ultrasounds, and bone marrow aspirations may also be repeated. Periodic monitoring is usually required for the rest of the life of the dog.

Prognosis

Dogs with solitary HS of the skin or underlying tissues that are treated with aggressive surgery have the best prognosis. Some of these tumors do not recur or metastasize. Metastasis can occur in as many as 60% of these cases, however. Prognosis for internal HS is poor. Dogs with tumors of the spleen, liver, or brain may succumb to their disease within a few weeks, and fewer than 20% survive for 1 year. Dogs with HS around the joint also have a poor prognosis, with average survival times of 6 months following amputation, and metastatic rates of about 90%.

Prognosis for MH is guarded (uncertain) to grave. Although remissions can be achieved with chemotherapy, they are often short (less than 100 days). Typical survival times are 3-5 months (range, 8-884 days). Only a few dogs with MH survive for 1 year or longer.

Because malignant histiocytic diseases are genetic and inherited in the Bernese Mountain dog, parents and offspring of affected dogs should not be bred.

SPECIAL INSTRUCTIONS:

Multiple Myeloma

Rhea V. Morgan, DVM, DACVIM (Small Animal), DACVO

BASIC INFORMATION
Description
Multiple myeloma is a malignant proliferation of plasma cells, which are white blood cells derived from B-cell lymphocytes. Under normal circumstances, plasma cells produce immunoglobulins (antibodies). Malignant plasma cells produce large proteins called *myeloma proteins* or *M proteins*. These proteins do not function like normal antibodies; instead, they cause a variety of problems in different organs.

Causes
The reason this cancer develops is unknown. Increased production of immunoglobulins such as M proteins can cause bleeding problems from altered platelet function, sludging of the blood, kidney failure, and deposition of an abnormal protein (amyloid) in numerous organs. Sludging of the blood decreases circulation in the smallest blood vessels and is known as *hyperviscosity syndrome.*

Malignant proliferation of plasma cells in the bone marrow can result in anemia, and low numbers of white blood cells and platelets. Because normal immunoglobulins are not produced, the animal is prone to infections. Plasma cells secrete a chemical that removes calcium from bone, causing blood calcium levels to increase (hypercalcemia). The malignant cells can also multiply directly in bone, liver, spleen, and other organs. Although multiple myeloma can occur in the cat, it is more common in the dog.

Clinical Signs
Nonspecific signs include lethargy, decreased appetite, increased thirst and urination, and weight loss. Bone pain may occur in the legs or along the spine. Bleeding tendencies and neurologic problems develop in some animals.

On physical examination, the liver and spleen are commonly enlarged in dogs. Cats may develop fluid in the chest or abdomen, with signs of respiratory distress or abdominal distention.

Diagnostic Tests
Routine laboratory tests, abdominal and chest x-rays, and an abdominal ultrasound are often recommended to investigate the clinical signs. Abdominal x-rays may reveal organ enlargement. About two thirds of affected dogs have small, "punched out" lesions in bones that may be seen on abdominal, chest, and bone x-rays. Hypercalcemia occurs in 5-20% of affected animals and indicates that further testing is needed to determine the cause.

Globulin proteins in the blood may be extremely elevated. A protein electrophoresis test is needed to better characterize which globulins are involved. Special urine tests can also be performed to look for Bence Jones proteins, which are secreted by the malignant plasma cells.

Bone marrow aspiration or biopsy is often needed to confirm the presence of malignant plasma cells. Sometimes the disease can be diagnosed by aspirations of the liver and spleen or biopsies of discrete masses.

TREATMENT AND FOLLOW-UP
Treatment Options
Chemotherapy is the main treatment. The goals of treatment are to kill the malignant cells, decrease blood protein and calcium levels, stabilize any weak areas in the bones, and relieve pain. The drugs most commonly used are oral prednisone and melphalan. Other chemotherapeutic agents may be tried if the animal does not respond well to these two drugs.

Mild elevations in calcium and blood protein levels may be treated with fluid therapy to flush excess calcium out through the kidneys and lessen the sludging of blood. Moderate to severe hypercalcemia often requires additional medications, such as diuretics (furosemide), to lower calcium levels more rapidly and aggressively. Kidney failure can develop with severe hypercalcemia, so hospitalization with intravenous fluid therapy and additional medications is often required.

Plasmapheresis may be considered to remove excess immunoglobulins. This procedure involves removing blood from the body, separating the blood into its various components, removing excessive protein, resuspending the blood in saline, and transfusing it back into the body. Plasmapheresis is performed only at certain veterinary referral facilities.

Antibiotics are commonly given until white blood cell counts improve. Pain medications may also be considered for animals with bone lesions. Occasionally, radiation therapy is used to alleviate specific areas of bone pain.

Follow-up Care
Follow-up visits and repeated laboratory tests are used to monitor response to treatment and side effects of the medications. Melphalan can decrease white blood cell and platelet counts. X-rays and bone marrow aspirations may also be repeated. A positive response is often seen in 1-2 months.

Prognosis
Prognosis varies in dogs. The average survival time for dogs is 540 days. Prognosis is poorest for dogs with hypercalcemia, high levels of Bence Jones proteins in the urine, kidney failure, pancytopenia (low numbers of all blood cells), and a poor response to therapy.

Prognosis is very poor in cats. The average survival time for cats on chemotherapy is 189 days, and some cats succumb to the disease within a few weeks of diagnosis.

SPECIAL INSTRUCTIONS:

Systemic Lupus Erythematosus in Dogs: Systemic Aspects

Rhea V. Morgan, DVM, DACVIM (Small Animal), DACVO

BASIC INFORMATION

Description

Systemic lupus erythematosus (SLE) is an autoimmune disease that arises when the body's immune system attacks multiple tissues or organs in the body, as if they were foreign. SLE may involve the joints, skin, kidneys, platelets, and red blood cells. Most affected dogs are young to middle-aged. Dogs of many breeds can develop SLE, but the German shepherd dog appears to be predisposed.

Causes

In SLE, antibodies are produced that form complexes with antigens (proteins) on or in the body's cells. These immune complexes become trapped in the blood vessels of certain organs, such as joints and kidneys, and cause an inflammatory reaction. The body's attempts to deal with the inflammatory reaction actually make the situation worse. It is not known why the body creates antibodies against its own tissues.

Clinical Signs

Vague signs may develop initially, such as weight loss, lethargy, poor appetite, and mild lameness. Dermatologic signs occur in about 33% of affected dogs. (See the handout on **Systemic Lupus Erythematosus: Dermatologic Aspects**.) Polyarthritis, which is inflammation in multiple joints, develops in about half of dogs with SLE and manifests as lameness, pain, and swelling of the joints. (See the handout on **Immune-Mediated Arthritis**.)

Dogs with kidney involvement may have no clinical signs initially. If significant kidney damage develops, then increased thirst and urination, muscle wasting, nausea, and vomiting may be seen. (See the handout on **Protein-Losing Nephropathy in Dogs**.) An immune-mediated hemolytic anemia occurs in about 30% of dogs with SLE, and platelets may also be affected. Associated signs include weakness and pale gums from anemia and widespread hemorrhages on the gums and skin from poor blood clotting. (See also the handouts on **Immune-Mediated Hemolytic Anemia** and **Immune-Mediated Thrombocytopenia**.)

Diagnostic Tests

Routine blood and urine tests are usually recommended and may show multiple abnormalities such as anemia, low platelet count, elevated protein levels in the blood and urine, and mildly altered kidney function. X-rays of the joints and abdomen may be indicated, depending on the clinical signs. An ultrasound of the abdomen is helpful to examine the kidneys. If excessive protein (proteinuria) is found in the urine, additional urine tests may be recommended. (See the handout on **Urine Protein Assays in Dogs**.)

Several immune assays may be performed, such as a lupus erythematosus (LE) clot test, antinuclear antibody assay (ANA), and Coombs' test. Immunologic tests may also be performed on biopsies of skin, kidneys, and joint tissues. Fluid may be aspirated from inflamed joints and sent for analysis and culture.

The diagnosis of SLE is difficult, because no single test is available that indicates the presence of the disease. Additional tests may be recommended to rule out other diseases that can cause similar signs and laboratory findings, which include infections, other immune diseases, drug reactions, and certain cancers. Making a diagnosis of SLE depends on eliminating these diseases and documenting at least one positive immunologic test and involvement of at least two different organ systems.

TREATMENT AND FOLLOW-UP

Treatment Options

Corticosteroid drugs, such as prednisone, are the most common treatment. High, immune-suppressive doses are usually needed to bring the disease under control, so it is important to rule out the presence of infectious diseases prior to starting therapy. Once clinical signs improve, the prednisone dosage may be tapered.

If the dog does not respond well to prednisone alone, stronger immune-suppressant medications, such as azathioprine, cyclosporine, and cyclophosphamide, may be added to the therapy. Other medications, supplements, and dietary changes may be recommended to help alleviate proteinuria, joint pain, vomiting, weight loss, and other signs.

Follow-up Care

Long-term monitoring is needed of both the disease and potential side effects of the medications used to treat it. Prednisone commonly increases appetite, thirst, and urinations and causes weight gain and secondary effects on the liver. The stronger immune suppressants can produce adverse effects on blood cells and on liver and kidney function. Periodic recheck visits and repeated laboratory tests are typically needed for the life of the dog.

Prognosis

SLE is a chronic, progressive disease that is difficult to control. Many pets do not respond to therapy or respond only partially (for example, the skin improves but the kidney disease does not). Sometimes response occurs early on but, as time goes by, the disease becomes harder to control. If kidney damage occurs and the kidneys begin fail, the prognosis is poor and survival times are usually short.

SPECIAL INSTRUCTIONS:

Musculoskeletal System

Section Editor: Mark C. Rochat, DVM, MS, DACVS

Angular Limb Deformities in Dogs
Bicipital Tendinopathy
Bone Tumors
Calcaneal Tendon Injury
Carpal and Tarsal Shearing Injuries
Cranial Cruciate Ligament Disease
Elbow Incongruency
Elbow Luxation, Traumatic
Fibrotic Myopathies
Fragmented Medial Coronoid Process Disease
Hip Dysplasia in Dogs
Hip Luxation
Hypertrophic Osteodystrophy in Dogs
Hypertrophic Osteopathy in Dogs
Immune-Mediated Arthritis
Juvenile Carpal Hyperextension/Hyperflexion Disorder

Legg-Calvé-Perthes Disease
Mandibular Fractures
Masticatory Myositis
Nutritional Bone Diseases
Osteoarthritis: Medical Management
Osteochondrosis (Osteochondritis Dissecans)
Osteomyelitis
Panosteitis
Patella Luxation
Sacroiliac Luxation
Scapular Luxation
Septic Arthritis
Shoulder Luxation
Stifle Luxation
Ununited Anconeal Process Disease

Angular Limb Deformities in Dogs

Mark C. Rochat, DVM, MS, DACVS

BASIC INFORMATION

Description

Angular limb deformities (ALDs) are a general class of bone growth disturbances that develop when the physis (growth plate) of a growing bone is damaged. The bones of the legs grow from physes at the ends of each bone. If a physis ceases to grow because of disease or trauma, the leg will be shortened (if the entire physis is damaged) or improperly angled (if a portion of the physis is damaged).

Causes

The cause of most ALDs is trauma. Sometimes even mild injuries can result in an ALD. In the dog, the most common ALD occurs when the ulna (the smaller bone of the foreleg) ceases to grow, forcing the radius (the larger bone of the foreleg) to deviate because the two are bound together by ligaments. Fractures, other bone diseases (such as hypertrophic osteodystrophy or retained cartilaginous cores), and breed-related conditions (such as pes varus in dachshunds) can cause ALDs.

Clinical Signs

Usually, a limb that was previously normal becomes bent or grows at an odd angle. Some breeds, especially the chondrodystrophic breeds (dachshunds, Pekingese, bulldogs, bassets hounds, and so on), have shortened, misshapen legs as part of their normal conformation, but ALD goes beyond what is considered normal. The opposite limb usually has a normal appearance for the breed.

Diagnostic Tests

An ALD may be suspected based on the clinical appearance of the leg. An orthopedic examination and x-rays are usually necessary to fully evaluate the extent of an ALD.

TREATMENT AND FOLLOW-UP

Treatment Options

If the ALD occurs in the foreleg (ulna and radius) and is detected early, before significant angling occurs, surgical removal of a small portion of the ulna is often curative. For more advanced deformities and deformities in other bones, various surgical techniques can be used to correct the malalignment. Such techniques can include removal of portions or wedges of bones, followed by insertion of a bone plate and screws into the bone, or use of external fixation devices. Other complicating factors, such as malalignment of the nearby joints, must be addressed as well.

Follow-up Care

Dogs that are still growing and sustain even mild trauma to the foreleg should be closely monitored for 4-6 weeks for the earliest signs of ALD. It is best to correct the condition early in the course, before it worsens. Postoperative care depends on the type of surgical procedure used but can involve bandage and splint changes, care of external pins, and restricted exercise until the surgery sites heals. Follow-up x-rays are performed periodically to monitor healing.

Prognosis

If the ALD in the foreleg is addressed early in its course, the prognosis is very good. For more advanced foreleg ALD, the prognosis varies from guarded (uncertain) to good. Concurrent malalignment and arthritis of the adjacent elbow and wrist (carpus) worsen the prognosis. ALD that affects other bones generally carries a favorable prognosis if the ALD can be corrected prior to the development of arthritis in the adjacent joints.

SPECIAL INSTRUCTIONS:

Bicipital Tendinopathy

Mark C. Rochat, DVM, MS, DACVS

BASIC INFORMATION

Description
Bicipital tendinopathy (BT) is a disease of middle-aged, large- and giant-breed dogs. The biceps tendon attaches the biceps muscle to the scapula (shoulder blade).

Causes
Most cases of BT result from chronic, repetitive injury, similar to human BT disease in athletes such as baseball pitchers or tennis players. The tendon is strained and torn in microscopic amounts, which leads to inflammation and pain. With time, osteoarthritis occurs and further increases pain and loss of mobility in the shoulder.

Clinical Signs
Variable degrees of lameness are observed. The lameness usually worsens with vigorous activity.

Diagnostic Tests
Manipulation of the shoulder may reveal loss of mobility and pain. Pain in the shoulder usually increases noticeably when pressure is placed on the biceps tendon while the leg is flexed.

TREATMENT AND FOLLOW-UP

Treatment Options
Injection of glucocorticoids (steroids that reduce inflammation) into or around the tendon may resolve the lameness, but strict rest for a minimum of 4-6 weeks is critical to allow the tendon time to fully heal. Repeated injections may be required. If an acceptable response is not observed after 3-4 injections, surgery is recommended. About 40% of affected dogs do not respond to steroid injections.

Surgical therapy involves releasing (cutting) the tendon so that it is not constantly irritated as the leg is used. Release of the biceps tendon can often be done easily by arthroscopy (involving passage of a tiny fiberoptic viewing scope into the joint). Your pet may be referred to a veterinary orthopedic surgeon for this procedure.

Follow-up Care
Steroid injections must be followed by strict restriction of exercise for a minimum of 4-6 weeks. If surgical release of the tendon is performed, exercise is restricted to short leash walks only for 4 weeks to allow the shoulder to fully heal. If signs of inflammation (excessive redness, pain, swelling, or discharge) are observed at the site of a surgical incision, notify your veterinarian. Sutures or staples are commonly removed 10-14 days after surgery.

Prognosis
Prognosis for return to full activity is very good.

SPECIAL INSTRUCTIONS:

Bone Tumors

Mark C. Rochat, DVM, MS, DACVS

BASIC INFORMATION
Description
Bone tumors are malignancies that either begin in bone (primary tumor) or spread to bone from other parts of the body (secondary or metastatic tumor). Primary tumors are by far the more common type. The most common primary tumor in dogs is osteosarcoma (85%), followed by chondrosarcoma.

Seventy-five percent of primary tumors occur in leg bones, but they can also occur in the skull, ribs, or spine. Primary tumors occur very rarely in cats, with osteosarcoma and related tumors being the most common types. Primary tumors commonly appear in only one location in one bone, whereas secondary tumors may occur in multiple sites.

Causes
Although tumors can develop at the site of a previous fracture or orthopedic surgical procedure, the cause of most bone tumors is unknown.

Clinical Signs
Bone tumors typically occur in older, male, large- and giant-breed dogs. Dogs with bone tumors usually become suddenly lame. The lameness typically is not associated with trauma, but sometimes minor events can result in a fracture of the diseased bone. The lameness associated with bone tumors progresses rapidly to non–weight-bearing lameness, with the animal holding the leg up. There may also be swelling of the limb at the tumor site and loss of muscle (atrophy) in the rest of the leg. Common sites for primary tumors are the shoulder, carpus (wrist), and stifle (knee).

Diagnostic Tests
Sudden onset of dramatic lameness with no known trauma in an older, large dog strongly suggests the possibility of a bone tumor. X-rays may show classic signs of a bone tumor, such as combined bone destruction and bone production. Other diseases, such as fungal infections, can cause similar x-ray changes, so a definitive diagnosis cannot usually be made from the x-rays alone.

A bone biopsy is usually recommended to confirm the presence of a tumor, to determine the tumor type, and to provide information that affects the treatment options. Laboratory tests and chest x-rays are done to look for tumors elsewhere and to assess the status of other organs. If a metastatic tumor is suspected, a thorough search is undertaken for the origin of the tumor.

TREATMENT AND FOLLOW-UP
Treatment Options
The main treatment of primary tumors is amputation of the affected leg. In the case of osteosarcoma, amputation is done to relieve the intense pain associated with the tumor. The surgery rarely cures the disease, because microscopic metastasis has usually occurred by the time of diagnosis. Chemotherapy is used after amputation to slow the progression of the metastatic cancer. (See also the handouts on **Limb Amputation** and **Chemotherapy and Your Pet**.) Other bone tumors, such as chondrosarcoma, may benefit more from amputation if metastasis has not already occurred.

When amputation is not an option, limb-sparing surgery, chemotherapy, or radiation therapy may reduce the pain caused by the tumor and improve the dog's quality of life for a short period of time. Limb-sparing surgery allows the dog to keep the leg but does not change the overall prognosis. The surgery is a very demanding procedure and significant complications can occur, so it is often performed by an experienced veterinary surgery specialist.

Follow-up Care
Following surgery, the incision is observed daily for signs of infection (excessive redness, swelling, pain, or discharge), and the sutures or staples are removed in 10-14 days. It is important to provide the animal with surfaces that allow a secure footing, especially for the first few days while it is adjusting to using three legs. Most dogs and cats do extremely well after amputation. Obese and very large dogs and dogs with other orthopedic or neurologic diseases are the least likely to do well as amputees.

Prognosis
Osteosarcoma is highly malignant, with most dogs surviving only 10-12 months after the initial diagnosis when treated with amputation and chemotherapy. Measurement of alkaline phosphate (ALP) levels in the blood is somewhat helpful in identifying dogs that may not live as long (elevated ALP before surgery) and dogs that may have longer survival times (ALP drops after surgery). Survival time following amputation alone is about 5 months. Amputation for osteosarcoma in cats is often curative, so prognosis is better.

Bone tumors are very painful, and euthanasia should be considered if specific treatment is not an option. Dogs with chondrosarcoma have longer survival times following amputation, especially if metastasis has not occurred at the time of diagnosis. Metastatic bone tumors, although uncommon, generally have a very poor prognosis because of the presence of tumors elsewhere in the body.

SPECIAL INSTRUCTIONS:

Calcaneal Tendon Injury

Mark C. Rochat, DVM, MS, DACVS

BASIC INFORMATION
Description
The calcaneal tendon is also known as the *Achilles tendon*. It is formed by the termination of several muscles and attaches to the calcaneus (heel). The calcaneal tendon is critical for normal walking.
Causes
The cause of calcaneal tendon rupture is usually a traumatic event, such as a fall from a height or laceration of the tendon. Chronic degeneration of the tendon may occur in sporting dogs. Parasitic diseases and other conditions can rarely result in calcaneal tendon rupture.

Clinical Signs
Rupture of the tendon causes the hock (ankle) to drop toward or almost touch the ground. The hock may be swollen. Swelling may also occur above the hock, with a thin, flat space visible between the hock and the swelling. When trauma is the cause, usually only one side is involved. In the more chronic form of tendon degeneration, both rear legs may be affected.

Diagnostic Tests
The diagnosis can often be made on the basis of physical examination. X-rays may reveal a fracture of the calcaneus bone where the tendon attaches. Ultrasound examination may be recommended to show where the rupture occurred.

TREATMENT AND FOLLOW-UP
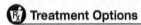 Treatment Options
If the injury is recent, reattachment of the tendon to the calcaneus bone or suturing of the torn ends of the calcaneal tendon is the preferred treatment. Following repair of the tendon, the hock must be prevented from moving by application of a cast (see the handout on **Fracture Repair: Casts and Splints**) or an external skeletal fixator device (see the handout on **Fracture Repair: External Skeletal Fixation**). Usually, the hock is immobilized (kept rigidly bent) for 6-8 weeks or longer, because tendons have a poor blood supply and heal very slowly.

If the injury is chronic and less likely to be successfully repaired, then fusion of the hock (see the handout on **Arthrodesis**) is an acceptable alternative treatment.

Follow-up Care
If the tendon is surgically repaired, the cast or external skeletal fixator requires special care for as long as it is in place. (See the appropriate handouts for details.)
Prognosis
If the injury is recent and properly repaired, prognosis is good for return to normal activity but may be somewhat guarded (uncertain) for return to full athletic function. As the tendon injury becomes more chronic, the chance of successful repair is less likely. Although arthrodesis results in a fused, rigid hock and loss of normal motion of the hock, it is often a better solution than attempting to repair a chronically damaged tendon.

SPECIAL INSTRUCTIONS:

Carpal and Tarsal Shearing Injuries

Mark C. Rochat, DVM, MS, DACVS

BASIC INFORMATION

Description

A carpal or tarsal shearing injury involves the loss of soft tissues (skin, muscle, tendons) over the carpus (wrist) or hock (ankle). Varying amounts of bone, cartilage, and ligaments that surround the joint can be lost as well. The tissues beneath the skin are visible and exposed to the external environment.

Causes

Carpal and tarsal shearing injuries occur when an animal is dragged behind or under a moving vehicle, often over pavement. Dragging of the leg destroys the soft tissues over the carpus (wrist) or hock (ankle), and sometimes the underlying bone as well.

Clinical Signs

Dogs and cats that sustain shearing injuries often have other serious injuries related to the traumatic event, so a variety of clinical signs may be observed. The skin and tissue over the involved joints and varying amounts of bone are usually missing and often grossly contaminated with debris and bacteria. Affected joints are often unstable, making the leg unusable. Non–weight-bearing lameness is common.

Diagnostic Tests

Routine laboratory tests, x-rays of the chest and abdomen, an electrocardiogram (to evaluate the heart rhythm), and an abdominal ultrasound may be recommended to identify and evaluate other injuries. X-rays of the affected joint are taken to identify fractures or dislocations associated with the shearing injury. Swabs and tissue samples of the injured joint may be submitted for bacterial culture.

TREATMENT AND FOLLOW-UP

Treatment Options

Initially, the wound may be splinted and bandaged while other injuries are treated and stabilized. Once the animal is stable, the wound is cleaned, and dead or excessively injured tissue is removed (débrided) under anesthesia. Fractures may be stabilized by various methods, and joint ligaments are reconstructed as needed.

The wound may be managed with multiple bandage changes until it heals on its own, or it may be closed by a number of different reconstructive surgical techniques. If injuries to the leg are severe, amputation of the limb may be the best method for resolving the problem and returning the animal to a pain-free, functional state. (See also the handout on **Limb Amputation**.)

Follow-up Care

Frequent recheck visits are usually needed for weeks following shearing injuries. The wounds are checked and cleaned, bandages are changed, and any orthopedic devices are evaluated. X-rays may be repeated to monitor healing of accompanying fractures and to check for signs of bone infection (osteomyelitis). Additional testing and monitoring may be needed for other accompanying injuries.

Prognosis

Prognosis varies from good to guarded (uncertain), depending on the extent of the injury to the carpus or tarsus, as well as other injuries sustained during the trauma. Owners must be prepared for the diligent therapy and nursing care, including frequent bandage changes and recheck visits, that are needed to resolve these shearing injuries.

SPECIAL INSTRUCTIONS:

Cranial Cruciate Ligament Disease

Mark C. Rochat, DVM, MS, DACVS

BASIC INFORMATION

Description

The cranial cruciate ligament (CCL) is the primary ligament that stabilizes the stifle (knee). CCL disease is a chronic process whereby the CCL degenerates and causes pain, instability, and osteoarthritis. Eventually the ligament ruptures, further increasing instability and pain in the joint. Usually, clinical signs of lameness are not readily appreciated until the ligament ruptures.

CCL disease most commonly affects middle-aged, large- and giant-breed dogs, but it occurs somewhat frequently in smaller dogs and occasionally in cats. The disease usually occurs in one leg, but rupture of the CCL in the other leg is common within 6-12 months following the first ligament tear.

Sometimes instability of the stifle results in injury to the medial meniscus. The menisci are two C-shaped cartilages in the knee. The medial meniscus (on the inside of the knee) is torn in about 50% of these cases.

Causes

The cause of CCL is greatly debated. The shape of the tibial plateau (the upper end of the tibia, which is the large bone just below the knee), combined with various other factors, has been implicated.

Clinical Signs

Although CCL disease is a chronic, progressive condition, in many cases sudden onset of lameness occurs in association with activity. If not immediately treated, the lameness often improves to some degree but does not completely resolve. Signs typical of arthritis (lameness that is worse with rest and improves with mild exercise, stiffness, and muscle wasting) are usually present and worsen with time.

Diagnostic Tests

Orthopedic examination reveals varying degrees of stiffness, fluid, pain, and crepitus (crunching sound) in the stifle. The inside edge of the stifle is often thickened as well. Thorough examination of the stifle with the animal under sedation often reveals excessive instability, particularly excessive movement of the tibia with respect to the femur (large thigh bone).

X-rays may reveal signs of osteoarthritis (degenerative arthritis) and malalignment of the tibia with the stifle, but they cannot show a ruptured ligament or torn meniscal cartilage. Sometimes the diagnosis is confirmed only at the time of surgery or with arthroscopy (passage of a fiberoptic viewing scope into the stifle).

TREATMENT AND FOLLOW-UP

Treatment Options

The best treatment for CCL disease is greatly debated. Medium, large- and giant-breed dogs recover quicker and regain the best function with surgery. Small dogs and cats are often treated initially with restricted exercise and medical therapy. (See the handout on **Osteoarthritis: Medical Management**.) In these latter animals, surgery is reserved for those that do not respond to medical therapy.

Numerous techniques are available for stabilizing the stifle. Keep in mind that the phrase "cruciate repair" is inaccurate, because in CCL disease the ligament is always beyond repair. Surgery is actually designed to improve stability of the joint. Available surgical techniques can be divided into three different types:

- Intra-articular techniques that create a new ligament and involve opening the joint, such as patellar tendon or biceps fascia grafting
- Extracapsular techniques that stabilize the stifle via surgery outside the joint, such as fibular head transposition and lateral suture placement
- Biomechanical techniques that change the angles and forces within the stifle, such as tibial plateau–leveling osteotomy (TPLO) and tibial tuberosity advancement (TTA).

Currently, no single technique has been proven to be superior. Biomechanical techniques are often favored for large and giant breeds, whereas extracapsular techniques are often used for smaller dogs and cats (and in some situations for larger dogs). Many of the described techniques can have good results in the hands of a capable veterinary surgeon. If the medial meniscus is damaged, it is removed.

Follow-up Care

Regardless of which technique is chosen, strict restriction of activity for at least 8-10 weeks after surgery is critical for ultimate success. The incision is observed daily for excessive redness, swelling, pain, or discharge. Physical rehabilitation and/or exercises at home also greatly improve the outcome of surgery.

Prognosis

Most dogs return to normal or near-normal function following surgery, appropriate activity restriction, and rehabilitation. Dogs with a torn meniscus have a slightly worse prognosis, but generally the outcome is still good. Dogs with osteoarthritis may require continued medical therapy if the signs do not completely resolve with surgery.

SPECIAL INSTRUCTIONS:

Elbow Incongruency

Mark C. Rochat, DVM, MS, DACVS

BASIC INFORMATION

Description

Elbow incongruency is abnormal alignment of the three bones that make up the elbow (the humerus of the upper arm and the radius and ulna of the forearm). When these three bones develop correctly, the force that comes from walking is evenly transferred from the radius and ulna to the humerus. If elbow incongruency occurs, excessive weight is usually carried by the largest part of the ulna, the medial coronoid, which results in damage to the coronoid and subsequent pain and arthritis.

Rarely, the radius protrudes upward against the humerus, causing similar problems. Two distinct diseases, fragmented medial coronoid process (FMCP) disease and ununited anconeal process (UAP) disease, are thought to occur largely because of this incongruency, but other conditions can arise as well. Elbow incongruency can also occur as a result of growth disturbances in the ulna near the carpus (wrist).

Causes

The cause is largely unknown, although with FMCP and UAP genetics play a role. Other contributing factors include breed of dog and nutrition. FMCP and UAP usually occur in young, growing, large- and giant-breed dogs, whereas other abnormalities occur in chondrodystrophoid breeds with short, curved bones, such as the dachshund, Pekinese, shih tzu, and basset hound. Ulnar growth disturbances can occur in any young, growing dog and usually result from some traumatic injury to the forearm.

🖐 Clinical Signs

The most common clinical sign is lameness of varying degrees that typically is worse after rest and heavy exercise. The lameness often gets better with stretching and mild exercise. Loss of muscle mass (atrophy), joint swelling, and pain are also common. When growth disturbances of the ulna are seen, both the elbow and carpus may be involved. The most severe changes may be observed at the carpus and consist of rotation and angling of the paw.

🔬 Diagnostic Tests

The diagnosis may be suspected following an orthopedic examination. X-rays confirm the diagnosis and further define the extent of the abnormality. Arthroscopic examination of the joint (via insertion of a tiny fiberoptic viewing scope) allows further characterization of the disease, provides an avenue for treating FMCP, and assists in the surgical treatment of other elbow conditions. Laboratory tests are usually normal but are commonly recommended prior to anesthesia.

TREATMENT AND FOLLOW-UP

℞ Treatment Options

Treatment options depend on the exact abnormalities present, and the best treatment is somewhat debated. FMCP can be treated via arthroscopic surgery, whereas other forms of elbow incongruency may require open surgery and cutting (osteotomy) the ulna below the elbow joint.

Elbow incongruency caused by growth abnormalities in the ulna is usually treated surgically, with correction of the abnormal angle in the bone at the carpus and cutting of the ulna just below the elbow at the same time. If the incongruency is severe or if severe degenerative arthritis is present in the elbow and is unresponsive to medical therapy, then arthrodesis (surgical fusion of the joint) or amputation may be indicated. (See the handouts on **Arthrodesis** and **Limb Amputation**.)

🐾 Follow-up Care

Oral analgesics (pain-relief) medications are commonly given before and after surgery. If signs of inflammation (excessive redness, pain, swelling, or discharge) are observed at the incision, notify your veterinarian. Sutures or staples are commonly removed from the incision at 10-14 days after surgery.

The dog's progress is checked again in 4-6 weeks, depending on the exact cause of the elbow incongruency. If cuts were made in the bone, x-rays are taken to evaluate the healing process. All dogs are restricted to short leash walks as their only activity for at least 4-6 weeks or until such time as bone healing occurs.

Prognosis

Prognosis is variable depending on the exact nature and cause of the incongruency. Prognosis is typically fair to good, but if severe incongruency or arthritis is present, prognosis is generally less favorable.

SPECIAL INSTRUCTIONS:

Elbow Luxation, Traumatic

Mark C. Rochat, DVM, MS, DACVS

BASIC INFORMATION

Description

Elbow luxation (dislocation) develops from a disruption of the normal alignment of the three bones that make up the elbow: the humerus (upper arm bone) and the radius and ulna (bones of the forearm). For a luxation to occur, the major ligaments (collateral ligaments) of the elbow must be torn.

Causes

Elbow luxation occurs in dogs and cats (rarely) as a result of severe trauma, such as being hit by a car or from a dog fight.

Clinical Signs

Elbow luxation makes the foreleg unusable, so a non–weight-bearing lameness occurs. The leg may be flexed (bent, held up) and the forearm outwardly rotated. The elbow is usually swollen and/or misshapen. Other signs of trauma (cuts, scratches, bruises) may also be present.

Diagnostic Tests

Palpation of the joint usually reveals malalignment of the elbow, loss of normal range of motion, and pain when the joint is manipulated (moved). X-rays confirm the diagnosis and help to identify fractures and any preexisting conditions (such as degenerative osteoarthritis) of the elbow. Routine preanesthetic laboratory tests are often performed, and additional tests may be recommended to evaluate other traumatized areas of the body.

TREATMENT AND FOLLOW-UP

Treatment Options

If the luxation is recent, it can often be reduced (manipulated back into normal position) with the animal under deep anesthesia. If the luxation is chronic or if other preexisting disease or bony abnormalities of the joint are present, surgical reduction must usually be performed. If significant damage to the elbow is present or the luxation is very chronic, arthrodesis (surgical fusion) of the joint or amputation of the limb may be the best solution. (See the handouts on **Arthrodesis** and **Limb Amputation**.)

Follow-up Care

Once reduction is complete, the leg (limb) is placed in a splint in a slightly extended (straightened) position for 2 weeks to allow fibrous (scar) tissue to develop. The toes and skin at the ends of the splint are observed twice daily for slippage of the splint and for any swelling, odor, pain, rub sores, or discharge around the toes and the upper end of the splint. Report any abnormalities to your veterinarian immediately.

If surgery is required, the bandage is observed daily for seepage of fluid through the bandage. After the bandage is removed, the incision is checked daily for excessive redness, discharge, swelling, or pain. Activity is limited to leash walking for at least 2 weeks after surgery or removal of the splint.

Prognosis

Although some degree of arthritis is likely to develop after an elbow luxation, prognosis for return to normal function is good following reduction of a recent luxation. Luxations that are chronic or associated with preexisting osteoarthritis or other abnormalities of the elbow carry a more guarded (uncertain) prognosis.

SPECIAL INSTRUCTIONS:

Fibrotic Myopathies

Mark C. Rochat, DVM, MS, DACVS

BASIC INFORMATION

Description

Fibrotic myopathies include several conditions in which normal, healthy muscle is replaced by fibrous (scar) tissue. The most common conditions are infraspinatus tendinopathy (IT) and quadriceps contracture (QC). Other muscles in the back leg (such as the gracilis, semitendinosus, and sartorius) may also be affected.

QC usually occurs in young, growing dogs. IT occurs most commonly in young and middle-aged dogs, especially in the spaniel, hunting, and working breeds.

Causes

The cause of most of the fibrotic myopathies, except for QC, is often unknown. QC usually arises as a result of trauma that leads to a break in the nearby femur (thigh bone) and subsequent treatment. Following the fracture, the quadriceps muscle and the periosteum covering the bone form adhesions if movement of the leg is limited for a prolonged period.

Other potential causes of fibrotic myopathies include chronic repetitive trauma, drug reactions, infections within the muscle, and neurogenic and vascular disorders.

Clinical Signs

Loss of the muscle results in lameness and joint immobility. Sometimes these myopathies are also painful. Dogs and cats with QC hold their hind leg out straight and the stifle (knee) and hock (ankle) cannot be bent. In severe cases, muscle contracture may even dislocate the hip.

The lameness that results from IT is classic for this condition. The dog outwardly rotates the front leg and flips the carpus (wrist) as it walks. Less common myopathies of the back leg result in an odd lameness that jerks the leg up suddenly with each step, as if it is being pulled upward by a string.

Diagnostic Tests

Diagnosis is often made by a thorough physical examination and observation of the lameness. With myopathies of the hind leg, a tense band of muscle can often be felt. Ultrasound examination of the muscle and tendon also helps identify the condition. Laboratory tests and x-rays are normal except for abnormalities caused by prior trauma.

TREATMENT AND FOLLOW-UP

Treatment Options

QC is a condition that must be prevented by proper surgical management of a fractured bone and rehabilitation (physical) therapy after surgery. Once QC occurs, no effective treatment is available to restore leg function, and amputation is usually required. In rare cases, arthrodesis (fusion of the stifle or knee joint) may be considered. (See the handouts on **Limb Amputation** and **Arthrodesis**.)

The treatment for IT involves surgically cutting the tendon as it crosses the shoulder joint.

The treatment for other hind leg myopathies is removal of the affected muscles and their tendons.

Follow-up Care

Activity after surgery for IT or the uncommon hind leg myopathies is limited to short leash walks for 2 weeks. The incision is inspected daily for signs of infection (excessive redness, pain, swelling, or discharge) and seroma (pocket of fluid buildup under the skin at the incision site) formation. Physical rehabilitation can help improve mobility of the shoulder.

Prognosis

Prognosis for return to full activity following treatment of IT is excellent. Prognosis for the uncommon hind leg myopathies is poor to guarded (uncertain), because these conditions often recur. Although QC may require amputation, most dogs and cats do very well after amputation. Use of the leg after arthrodesis of the stifle ranges from guarded to good.

SPECIAL INSTRUCTIONS:

Fragmented Medial Coronoid Process Disease

Mark C. Rochat, DVM, MS, DACVS

BASIC INFORMATION

Description

Fragmented medial coronoid process (FMCP) disease is a condition of young, large-breed dogs. FMCP is somewhat unique for a developmental, "juvenile" disease, in that it may not become apparent until the dog is several years old. It is more common in male dogs. It is also called *ununited coronoid process disease, jump-down syndrome, elbow dysplasia,* and *medial compartment disease.*

Causes

FMCP is thought to occur because uneven growth or alignment of the three bones around the elbow (humerus, radius, and ulna) leads to excessive pressure against the larger, medial coronoid process on the inside of the ulna. This uneven growth leads to fragmentation of the coronoid process, pain, arthritis, and lameness. The coronoid is not fractured in the traumatic sense of the word, but it is broken off due to the constant, uneven pressure placed upon it.

Clinical Signs

The clinical signs are the same as for any joint condition, namely lameness, pain, and joint stiffness after rest that initially improves with activity but then worsens with further activity.

Diagnostic Tests

Examination of the elbow reveals loss of range of motion and pain with movement of the joint. Muscle shrinkage (atrophy), joint stiffness, and thickening of the joint may be detected. Fluid (effusion) may also be felt in the joint. Direct pressure against the inside aspect of the elbow may cause a painful response.

X-rays often show signs of secondary arthritis but rarely reveal the fragment, because it is surrounded by normal bone, making it hard to see with most angles of the x-ray beam. If (after x-rays) doubt still exists regarding the diagnosis, computed tomography (CT) scanning can be done and has a high degree of accuracy. It is important to identify other developmental diseases in or around the joint as well.

TREATMENT AND FOLLOW-UP

Treatment Options

Although some debate exists regarding the best treatment, removal of the fragment and associated unhealthy cartilage is generally considered the best treatment. Fragment removal is ideally done by arthroscopic surgery (through a small fiberoptic viewing scope), but traditional open-joint surgery can also be effective. Medical treatment alone can be tried by administering drugs for arthritis, sometimes with acceptable results.

Follow-up Care

Dogs that undergo surgery are restricted from full activity for 8 weeks to allow the cartilage in the joint to completely heal. Physical rehabilitation therapy can also significantly improve the function of the elbow following surgery. Medical management (see the handout on **Osteoarthritis: Medical Management**) is pursued aggressively to slow the progression of the osteoarthritis.

Prognosis

Prognosis for FMCP is generally guarded (uncertain) but varies greatly from dog to dog. Many dogs have some degree of secondary arthritis; in some cases it is severe, and in others it is mild.

SPECIAL INSTRUCTIONS:

Hip Dysplasia in Dogs

Mark C. Rochat, DVM, MS, DACVS

BASIC INFORMATION

Description

The hip joint consists of the femoral head (ball) of the thigh bone and the acetabulum (socket) on the side of the pelvis. These two bony structures are held together primarily by the ligament of the head of the femur and the capsule that surrounds the joint. In canine hip dysplasia (CHD) the ligament and joint capsule are too loose, and the ball does not sit securely in the socket.

Because CHD develops in puppyhood, the socket does not form properly. The laxity (looseness) stretches the joint capsule, which is painful and results in inflammation. With time, scar tissue and osteoarthritis (degenerative joint disease) develop. The dog may actually improve for a period of time, but often the lameness gets worse as the osteoarthritis worsens and the joint is slowly destroyed. Even young dogs may have severe destruction of their hips, requiring surgery. CHD occurs most commonly in young large and giant breeds of dogs but can also occur in smaller dogs and occasionally in cats. CHD usually develops in both hips, but sometimes only one hip is affected.

Causes

CHD is caused by multiple factors, including genetics, nutrition (especially intake of high energy and calcium), and activity.

Clinical Signs

Sometimes CHD does not result in lameness or pain, but signs of osteoarthritis (lameness that is worse after rest and strenuous activity) are typical. Signs are often present as early as 4-6 months of age. The lameness may improve for a while as scar tissue builds up and stabilizes the joint, but arthritis and destruction of joint cartilage continues, and the dog often becomes progressively lame with time.

Diagnostic Tests

Orthopedic examination reveals pain and loss of mobility in the affected hip, especially when the hip is extended (stretched out behind the dog). A test called the Ortolani maneuver may show looseness of the hip joint. X-rays and a thorough orthopedic examination while the dog is anesthetized are often needed to evaluate the hip joint and to determine what treatment option may be best for your pet.

Because of the inherited tendency of CHD, x-rays are also used to evaluate dogs for hip dysplasia prior to breeding. Two different x-ray methods are available and the results may be submitted to the Orthopedic Foundation for Animals (OFA) for review. For more information, visit the websites *www.offa.org* and *www.pennhip.org*.

TREATMENT AND FOLLOW-UP

℞ Treatment Options

Medical therapy (see the handout on **Osteoarthritis: Medical Management**) may be effective for older dogs that are mildly affected or when financial limitations eliminate the surgical options.

Very young dogs (less than 16 weeks) with signs or genetic tendencies for CHD can be treated with a simple procedure called *juvenile pubic symphysiodesis* (JPS). This procedure uses heat to destroy the growing cartilage of part of the pelvis so that the acetabulum rotates to better cover the femoral head. The procedure is only effective when done at a very early age.

If the dog is lame, still growing (5-12 months), and has appropriate physical and x-ray findings (such as minimal to no osteoarthritis), a triple pelvic osteotomy (see the handout on **Triple Pelvic Osteotomy for Hip Dysplasia**) can be performed to rotate the acetabulum and achieve the same purpose as the JPS.

If the dog is a mature adult and does not respond well to medical therapy, then femoral head and neck ostectomy or total hip arthroplasty (see the handouts on **Femoral Head and Neck Ostectomy** and **Total Hip Arthroplasty**) may be considered to resolve the pain associated with CHD and improve hip joint mobility.

🐾 Follow-up Care

Follow-up examinations and repeated testing depend on what treatment plan is chosen. When medical therapy is used, the dog is periodically evaluated to identify subtle deteriorations and adjust the plan. Following JPS, the incision is examined daily for excessive redness, swelling, pain, or discharge. Exercise restriction is generally unnecessary. Specific postoperative care is discussed in the handouts for the **Triple Pelvic Osteotomy for Hip Dysplasia, Femoral Head and Neck Ostectomy,** and **Total Hip Arthroplasty**.

Prognosis

Prognosis varies, depending on the severity and progression of the disease. Some dogs have CHD and never develop significant signs of lameness or stiffness. X-rays are a useful tool but should not be the sole criterion used to judge the severity of the disease. Dogs that are appropriately treated with JPS, triple pelvic osteotomy, femoral head and neck ostectomy, or total hip arthroplasty generally do well. More details on prognosis and complications are covered in the respective handouts for these procedures.

SPECIAL INSTRUCTIONS:

Hip Luxation

Mark C. Rochat, DVM, MS, DACVS

BASIC INFORMATION
Description
Hip luxation or dislocation occurs with separation of the femoral head (ball of the thighbone) from the acetabulum (cup of the hip socket).
Causes
Hip luxation almost always results from a serious traumatic event, such as being hit by a car, a dog fight, falling from a height, or a malicious act. Hip luxation should not be confused with hip subluxation, such as occurs with hip dysplasia. Subluxation is a partial dislocation, whereas luxation is a complete dislocation. For luxation to occur, the major stabilizing ligament and surrounding tissues must be torn. Hip subluxation occurs when these structures are stretched but not torn.

Clinical Signs
Animals with a hip luxation typically stand with their leg outwardly rotated and the toes placed underneath them. The leg with the luxation is usually shorter. Pain, crepitus (grinding sound made when the hip is moved), and swelling may be appreciated when the hip joint is manipulated.

Diagnostic Tests
Physical examination reveals that the prominent bony features of the hip are not properly positioned. X-rays confirm the diagnosis and help to identify any accompanying fractures or underlying disease of the hip that might make treatment difficult. Other tests, such as laboratory assays and chest and abdominal x-rays, may be recommended to identify other injuries and factors that might make anesthesia dangerous.

TREATMENT AND FOLLOW-UP

Treatment Options
If the hip is normal in all other respects (no underlying disease such as hip dysplasia or arthritis) and the luxation is recent, then closed reduction is usually performed. Closed reduction is manipulation and manual replacement of the thighbone (femur) back into the hip socket without making an incision. It requires general anesthesia and is successful about 50% of the time.

Numerous surgical techniques can be used to keep the ball in the socket after the ball is manually replaced. Surgery may also be performed if the closed reduction fails or is not appropriate. If factors such as hip dysplasia or arthritis are present, then the femoral head may be removed surgically (see the handout on **Femoral Head and Neck Ostectomy**) or replaced (see the handout on **Total Hip Replacement**).

Follow-up Care
If closed reduction is performed, a special bandage called an *Ehmer sling* is applied once the hip is back in place. Ehmer slings are prone to slipping and may cause skin sores or loss of blood supply to the lower leg, so great diligence is required to quickly identify problems associated with the sling. Notify your veterinarian immediately if you have any concerns about the sling.

If surgery is performed, a bandage may or may not be applied, depending on the specific procedure that was performed. Regardless of the corrective procedure, the animal is usually confined to a cage for at least 4 weeks and gradually returned to full activity over the following 4 weeks.

Prognosis
Prognosis depends on the nature of the luxation, associated injuries, and the specific treatment used to correct the luxation. Recent traumatic luxations that are not complicated by other joint disease and are repaired quickly have a good prognosis for return of full function. Secondary arthritis may develop in some affected joints over time.

SPECIAL INSTRUCTIONS:

Hypertrophic Osteodystrophy in Dogs

Mark C. Rochat, DVM, MS, DACVS

BASIC INFORMATION

Description

Hypertrophic osteodystrophy (HOD) is a disease of the ends of the bones (metaphyses) of growing dogs that occurs between the ages of 2 and 8 months. It affects large-breed dogs. The disease is more common in males. It is also known as *canine scurvy, skeletal scurvy, Mueller-Barlow disease, osteodystrophy types 1* and *2, metaphyseal dysplasia,* and *metaphyseal osteopathy*. Weimeraners may be more susceptible to this disease than other breeds.

Causes

The cause is unknown. Bacterial and viral infections, insufficient vitamin C, and excessive dietary calcium have been suggested as causes, but none are proven.

Clinical Signs

Lameness, ranging from mild to severe, is usually observed in all four legs. Palpation of the ends of the bones reveals warmth, swelling, and pain. The changes may be most obvious at the end of the radius (large bone in the forearm). The initial (acute) phase of the disease may last 7-10 days. Signs include diarrhea, fever, depression, poor appetite, and weight loss. The dog may be in such pain that it is reluctant or unable to rise or walk.

Diagnostic Tests

The age and breed of dog, as well as finding pain around the ends of the bones, suggest HOD as the cause of the lameness. X-rays are usually diagnostic when they show a loss of bone adjacent to the normal growth plate (physis). Laboratory and other tests may be recommended to rule out other causes of diarrhea, fever, and weight loss.

TREATMENT AND FOLLOW-UP

Treatment Options

Supportive care, consisting of rest, good nursing care, and administration of nonsteroidal anti-inflammatory drugs designed for use in dogs, usually results in a successful outcome. Occasionally, the pain may be severe enough to warrant more potent pain-relief medications, such as opioid drugs or tramadol.

Follow-up Care

Most dogs recover within 7-10 days, but relapses are possible. Notify your veterinarian if the signs do not resolve within this time period or if they recur. In rare instances, HOD can result in disturbances of bone growth, with subsequent deformity and angling of the bones. If the deformity is severe, corrective surgery may be required.

Prognosis

Prognosis is generally good, because the disease usually resolves with symptomatic treatment.

SPECIAL INSTRUCTIONS:

Hypertrophic Osteopathy in Dogs

Mark C. Rochat, DVM, MS, DACVS

BASIC INFORMATION

Description

Hypertrophic osteopathy (HO) is a disease of older and sometimes middle-aged dogs. HO usually accompanies cancerous conditions, such as lung, esophageal, and bladder tumors. It may also arise with other conditions, such as heartworm disease, heart valve infection (endocarditis), congenital heart defects (patent ductus arteriosus), and granulomatous diseases. The condition begins in the paws and lower legs and progresses upward over time. The disease was formerly known as *hypertrophic pulmonary osteoarthropathy* (HPOA). When it occurs in the presence of cancer, it is termed a *paraneoplastic syndrome*.

Causes

The cause of HO is unknown but is suspected to be an increase in nerve-controlled blood supply to the outer covering of the bone (periosteum). The increased blood flow to the periosteum results in the production of new bone and stretching of the periosteum. Stretching of the periosteum is very painful.

Clinical Signs

Lameness in one or more legs is the most common sign. Often, all four limbs are involved to one degree or another. The legs are often swollen, warm, and painful. The dog may be lethargic and may have other signs associated with the primary, underlying condition.

Diagnostic Tests

Palpation (pressing with the fingers) of the shafts (diaphyses) of the bones results in a marked pain response. X-rays of the bones demonstrate production of new bone along the diaphyses and swelling of the nearby soft tissues. The process begins on the paws (metacarpal and metatarsal bones) and progresses up the legs. Chest x-rays often reveal a lung mass (commonly a tumor). Other tests may be recommended to search for a cause, including laboratory tests, tests for heartworm disease, abdominal x-rays, and an abdominal ultrasound. In some affected dogs, the platelet count is elevated.

TREATMENT AND FOLLOW-UP

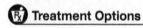

Treatment Options

Treatment is directed at the primary cause and can involve surgery to remove lung or bladder masses, chemotherapy, drugs for heartworm disease, and other measures. Analgesic (pain-relief) drugs are indicated until bony changes resolve.

Follow-up Care

The frequency of subsequent visits and testing is determined based on the treatment used for the primary (initiating) cause. X-rays of the bones may be repeated to monitor resolution of the bony changes.

Prognosis

Prognosis depends on the underlying cause and is often poor in the long term, because many cases of HO are associated with malignant tumors. Prognosis for resolution of HO bony changes is excellent if the underlying cause can be successfully treated (such as heartworm disease). With successful treatment of the underlying cause, the pain that occurs with HO quickly improves within 1-2 weeks, but the changes in the bone may take several months to resolve.

SPECIAL INSTRUCTIONS:

Immune-Mediated Arthritis

Rhea V. Morgan, DVM, DACVIM (Small Animal), DACVO
Mark C. Rochat, DVM, MS, DACVS

BASIC INFORMATION

Description

Immune-mediated arthritis develops when the immune system attacks joint tissues, causing inflammation. This type of arthritis commonly involves multiple joints (polyarthritis) and comes in two forms. In the milder form, x-ray evidence of bony destruction is not present early in the disease. Common examples include idiopathic polyarthritis, drug-induced polyarthritis, systemic lupus erythematosus (SLE or lupus), and polyarthritis of chronic disease.

In the more severe form (erosive arthritis), destruction of joint surfaces and bone occurs throughout the disease. Examples include rheumatoid arthritis (RA), erosive polyarthritis of greyhounds, and chronic polyarthritis of cats. With the exception of the last disease, all forms of immune-mediated arthritis occur more commonly in dogs.

Causes

In many of these diseases, the precipitating cause of the condition is unknown (idiopathic). In RA, the body's own immunoglobulins are involved and are deposited on the lining of the joints. In some cases, the immune system is activated by bacterial or viral infections, such as in Lyme disease, staphylococcal infections, and L-form bacterial infections. Sulfonamides may cause drug-induced polyarthritis. Polyarthritis of chronic disease may arise with discospondylitis, bacterial endocarditis, certain intestinal problems, various cancers, and other conditions.

Clinical Signs

Lameness, stiffness, loss of appetite, fever, pain, and joint swelling in one or more joints are common signs. Signs can be intermittent or constant and can shift from leg to leg. The joints most often involved are the carpus (wrist), hock (ankle), and feet. Other clinical signs may be present in animals with SLE or polyarthritis of chronic disease. SLE commonly affects other organs, including the kidneys and skin.

Adult, small-breed dogs develop RA most often. Erosive polyarthritis of greyhounds usually occurs in young dogs (younger than 3 years). Feline polyarthritis may affect cats 1-5 years of age.

Diagnostic Tests

Diagnosis of polyarthritis can often be achieved by a thorough physical examination, but x-rays and joint fluid analysis are needed to determine what type of polyarthritis is present. Erosive arthritis produces the most visible joint damage on x-rays, especially early in the disease. Laboratory tests may be performed for SLE, RA, and other potential underlying causes. Other organ tests may be indicated in cases of chronic illness or SLE.

TREATMENT AND FOLLOW-UP

Treatment Options

Glucocorticoids (steroids), such as prednisone, are commonly given in high doses initially and then tapered once the signs improve. In mild cases, nonsteroidal anti-inflammatory drugs (NSAIDs) may be sufficient for long-term control of the signs, once the steroids have been discontinued. Steroids and NSAIDs are not used together, because they can cause severe gastrointestinal irritation and even ulceration.

Examples of NSAIDs that are used in dogs include carprofen (*Rimadyl*), deracoxib (*Deramaxx*), firocoxib (*Previcox*), meloxicam (*Metacam*), tepoxalin (*Zubrin*), and etodolac (*Etogesic*). Meloxicam is most commonly used in cats. It is important to note that NSAIDs designed for people are often toxic to animals and should not be used.

In some dogs, these conditions do not respond well to prednisone alone, so more potent immune-suppressive drugs (such as azathioprine, cyclophosphamide, or methotrexate) must be added to the therapy. Response to therapy is evaluated by repeated joint fluid analysis. Injectable aurothioglucose (gold salt therapy) has been used with success in dogs with RA. Surgical fusion of the joint (see the handout on **Arthrodesis**) may be considered in cases of severe destruction and collapse of the joint.

Other treatments may be indicated based on concurrent illnesses or infections. Drugs that may be implicated in triggering the polyarthritis (such as sulfonamides) are withdrawn.

Follow-up Care

Immune-mediated arthritis is commonly a chronic disease that requires long-term treatment and follow-up. Signs associated with severe erosive arthritis may take 3-6 months to resolve. Periodic physical examinations and joint fluid analyses are often needed to monitor progression of the disease and the response to therapy. Periodic laboratory tests are required to identify bone marrow suppression, bladder inflammation (cystitis), hepatitis, and pancreatitis, which are occasionally associated with cyclophosphamide or azathioprine therapy. Testing for feline leukemia virus may be done yearly in cats on immune-suppressive therapy because they are more likely to contract the disease while taking these medications.

Prognosis

Prognosis is good for cases of mild, nonerosive arthritis with no evidence of joint destruction, especially if they respond well to an initial course of steroids. Periodic flare-ups can occur, so therapy is often continued long term. Prognosis is poor for cases of severe erosive polyarthritis with joint destruction (especially in multiple joints) and for greyhound polyarthritis.

SPECIAL INSTRUCTIONS:

Juvenile Carpal Hyperextension/ Hyperflexion Disorder

Mark C. Rochat, DVM, MS, DACVS

BASIC INFORMATION

Description

Juvenile carpal hyperextension/hyperflexion disorder is a condition of very young, large-breed puppies that results in either bowing (hyperflexion) or dropping (hyperextension) of the carpi (the wrists).

Causes

The cause of juvenile carpal hyperextension/hyperflexion disorder is unknown, but the condition is suspected to be influenced by poor nutrition and/or lack of activity.

Clinical Signs

The carpi of the puppy are either bowed, so that the paws are pulled backward and under, or dropped, so that the dog walks on the back of its feet and wrists. The condition is not painful.

Diagnostic Tests

Physical examination of the puppy usually identifies the problem. X-rays usually show that the bones are normal and help to exclude other abnormalities, such as growth disturbances and other developmental conditions.

TREATMENT AND FOLLOW-UP

Treatment Options

Most experts agree that institution of a normal diet and encouragement of exercise on surfaces with good traction will resolve the condition. Surgery is rarely, if ever, indicated.

Follow-up Care

Periodic examinations are commonly used to monitor progress and check for improvement in the condition.

Prognosis

With proper treatment, prognosis is excellent when no other abnormalities are present.

SPECIAL INSTRUCTIONS:

Legg-Calvé-Perthes Disease

Rhea V. Morgan, DVM, DACVIM (Small Animal), DACVO
Mark C. Rochat, DVM, MS, DACVS

BASIC INFORMATION

Description

Legg-Calvé-Perthes disease, or avascular necrosis of the femoral head, is an unusual disease of young, toy- or small-breed dogs. In these dogs, the head of the femur (the part of the thighbone that fits into the hip socket) dies from a disturbance in its blood supply. The affected bone eventually weakens, tiny fractures develop, and the bone collapses. Osteoarthritis (degenerative joint disease) of the hip joint then occurs over time, leading to progressive dysfunction and pain.

Causes

The disease is inherited in the Manchester terrier and may be inherited in other small breeds. The exact cause of interruption in blood flow to the femoral head is unknown.

Clinical Signs

Lameness in a rear leg that is not associated with injury in a young dog is the most common sign. The lameness often worsens over several weeks and may eventually cause the dog to carry the leg (non–weight-bearing lameness). As the leg is used less and bears less weight, the muscles near the hip shrink (atrophy). Manipulation of the hip often causes pain. Occasionally, acute (sudden) lameness develops if the bone collapses.

The average age at onset is 5-8 months, with a range of 3-13 months. Both legs are affected in only 12-17% of the dogs.

Diagnostic Tests

Physical examination findings of pain and decreased mobility of the hip joint in a young, small-breed dog allows a tentative diagnosis. X-rays are needed to confirm the diagnosis and usually show changes characteristic of the disease.

TREATMENT AND FOLLOW-UP

Treatment Options

If collapse and osteoarthritic changes have occurred in response to the disease, the treatment of choice is surgical removal of the femoral head and neck. This procedure is called a *femoral head ostectomy* (FHO). (See also the handout on **Femoral Head and Neck Ostectomy.**) Total hip replacement surgery may be considered in large and small dogs. If both legs are affected, the worst leg is usually operated first, followed by the second leg 4-6 weeks later.

Postoperative anti-inflammatory drugs and/or pain-relief medications may be prescribed. On rare occasions, the disease may be identified early in its course, before collapse of the femoral head occurs. In this instance, putting the limb in a sling to prevent collapse while the bone heals may avoid the need for surgery.

Follow-up Care

Following surgery, the dog is rested for 1-2 days, after which physical rehabilitation exercises and/or low-impact exercises (such as leash walking or swimming) are started. It is critical that the dog begin to use the leg early and often, to avoid a stiff hip joint that is not very functional.

Prognosis

Most small dogs do very well without a normal ball-and-socket joint at the hip, although refinements in total hip replacement surgery may offer better function. If an FHO is performed, the muscles of the thigh hold the leg and hip together, and, over time, the dog often returns to near-normal weight-bearing activity. Obesity should be prevented in these dogs throughout life, to decrease stress on the hip. Affected dogs should not be used for breeding.

SPECIAL INSTRUCTIONS:

Mandibular Fractures

Mark C. Rochat, DVM, MS, DACVS

BASIC INFORMATION

Description

The mandible is the jaw bone. Fractures of the mandible are common in dogs and cats. The fracture is often open, which means that the bone is exposed (usually to the inside of the mouth).

Causes

Mandibular fractures usually result from a traumatic event, such as being hit by a car, being kicked by a horse, a fall from a great height, or a dog fight. Fractures can also occur in young and old animals when their mandible becomes soft from chronic kidney or nutritional disease. Mandibular fractures can also occur as a result of severe dental disease (sometimes during removal of diseased teeth) or cancer of the jaw.

Clinical Signs

Animals with mandibular fractures usually salivate (drool) excessively and are reluctant to move their mouth. The jaw may be slightly dropped, and the animal may be unable to close its mouth. Blood may be seen around the mouth. Other signs related to the trauma, such as a concussion or loss of consciousness, difficult or labored breathing, and broken legs, may be seen. Other traumatic injuries (such as abnormal heart rhythms or rupture of the bladder) may not be as immediately obvious, so diligent veterinary care is required to identify and properly treat these conditions.

Diagnostic Tests

Because other injuries may have occurred during the trauma that created the broken bone, extensive evaluation of the animal is often done prior to surgery. As a part of the presurgical evaluation, laboratory tests, x-rays of the chest, an electrocardiogram (to identify abnormal heart rhythms), and an ultrasound of the abdomen may be recommended. When the animal can be safely anesthetized, x-rays or computed tomography (CT) scans are performed to evaluate the broken mandible and the rest of the skull. Although a CT scan is more expensive and less available, some mandibular fractures are complicated and hard to fully evaluate with only x-rays.

TREATMENT AND FOLLOW-UP

Treatment Options

If the fracture is simple and likely to heal quickly, use of a muzzle created from medical tape may be sufficient. Tape muzzles cannot be easily be applied to cats and dogs with short, flat faces so other methods must be used. The muzzle keeps the jaw in place and prevents the mouth from being opened widely.

When open fractures are present, the break is usually repaired as soon as possible, and antibiotics are given. If both sides of the mandible are split apart where they join at the front of the mouth (a common injury in young dogs and cats), a single wire may be placed around the front of both pieces of the jaw and anchored behind the lower canine teeth.

Other repair methods, such as acrylic splints and internal fixation with bone plates and screws (see the handout on **Fracture Repair: Internal Fixation**) may be used for more complicated fractures. Regardless of the repair method chosen, proper alignment of the teeth is critical to avoid future dental problems.

Follow-up Care

Dogs treated with tape muzzles must have their face frequently and gently cleaned. Soft food is fed in gruel or meatball form, or a temporary feeding tube is inserted into the esophagus (the tube that connects the mouth to the stomach) or into the stomach. Oral analgesic (pain-relief) medications are usually given. An Elizabethan collar (plastic cone) is also worn at all times. If signs of inflammation (excessive redness, pain, swelling, or discharge) are observed, notify your veterinarian.

Until the fracture has healed, the animal is restricted from chewing on anything other than soft food. X-rays are taken every 4-6 weeks to evaluate the healing process. After healing of the bone is complete, tape muzzles, wires, and acrylic splints are removed. If a feeding tube was placed, it can be removed at this time also. If a bone plate and screws were used, they are usually left in place unless a specific problem occurs with the implants.

Prognosis

With proper care, simple fractures resulting from trauma usually heal well. Complicated fractures and fractures that develop because of an underlying disease are often more difficult to get to heal without complications. Complications of these fractures include persistent osteomyelitis (bone infection), malocclusion (abnormal alignment of the teeth), sequestra formation (in which pieces of bone die), failure to heal, and loosening of the surgical implants (mainly acrylic devices or wires).

SPECIAL INSTRUCTIONS:

Masticatory Myositis

Rhea V. Morgan, DVM, DACVIM (Small Animal), DACVO

BASIC INFORMATION
Description

Masticatory myositis is inflammation of the muscles of the head that are used for chewing (mastication). These muscles include the temporalis muscles, which are located in the forehead region above and beside the eyes, and the masseter muscles, which are located in the cheek area. The inflammation may be sudden in onset (acute) or chronic. It usually affects large-breed dogs. Other names for this disease are *eosinophilic myositis, atrophic myositis,* and *masticatory myopathy.*

Causes

Masticatory myositis is an immune-mediated disease. The dog's own immune system attacks various components of the muscles. This group of muscles has a unique origin in the embryo and is different (contains type 2 M muscle fibers) from other skeletal muscles. This difference may explain why only these muscles become inflamed.

Clinical Signs

Acute myositis usually causes symmetrical swelling and pain of the muscles. If the muscles become terribly swollen, one or both eyes may bulge. Rarely, this bulging may result in permanent damage to the eye and blindness. The dog may be in pain and reluctant to open the mouth. Fever, lethargy, decreased appetite, and enlargement of nearby lymph nodes (glands) may also occur. Signs may last 2-3 weeks.

With the chronic form of the disease, the muscles shrink (atrophy) and become scarred (fibrosis). Fibrosis prevents the muscles from working well, and the dog may not be able to voluntarily open its mouth. Scarring can be so severe that the mouth becomes locked in one position and cannot easily be manually opened. These dogs have difficulty taking in food and may lose weight. Shrinkage of the muscles may allow the eyes to rest deeper in the socket than normal (enophthalmos).

Diagnostic Tests

Clinical evidence of painful swelling of the masticatory muscles in a large-breed dog may allow a tentative diagnosis. Laboratory tests may be performed to rule out infection and to look for evidence of increased eosinophils (a type of white blood cell) in the blood. Muscle enzyme levels in the blood may also be elevated. A specific test exists for this disease that detects type 2 M antibodies

in the blood. Samples are sent to an outside laboratory, and results take several days to return.

X-rays of the head may be recommended to rule out problems with the bones and joints of the skull and jaw. A biopsy of the muscles may also be done and usually identifies both acute and chronic changes in the muscles. Occasionally, electrodiagnostic tests are performed on the muscles and other immunologic laboratory tests are submitted.

TREATMENT AND FOLLOW-UP

Treatment Options

Because this is an immune-mediated disease, therapy is designed to suppress the immune reaction. Steroids, such as prednisone, are started at high doses for 2-4 weeks and then slowly tapered over several months. Other immune-suppressive drugs may be added if the disease does not respond well to the prednisone, if the dog does not tolerate side effects of the prednisone, or if the signs return as the prednisone is decreased. Immune-suppressive drugs that may be considered include azathioprine, cyclophosphamide, and cyclosporine.

If the dog cannot eat, a feeding tube may be inserted. If the dog cannot open its mouth very far, then the mouth may be manually forced open with the animal under general anesthesia. Fracture of the jaw is a potential side effect of this procedure.

Follow-up Care

Frequent examinations are needed initially to monitor muscle swelling, ability to open the mouth and chew food, and any loss in body weight. High doses of prednisone may cause increased appetite, thirst, and urination, and urinary accidents in the house. Laboratory tests are often repeated periodically to check for adverse effects on the blood and liver from the prednisone and other immune-suppressive drugs. Modifications may be needed in the therapy if side effects occur. Therapy is usually required for weeks to months.

Prognosis

Prognosis is best when the disease is diagnosed in the acute phase and aggressive therapy is started. Excessive scarring of the muscles that causes an inability to open the mouth has a poorer prognosis. Once muscles have atrophied (shrunk), they rarely return to a normal size or shape. In these cases, the bones of the head may remain very prominent.

SPECIAL INSTRUCTIONS:

Nutritional Bone Diseases

Rhea V. Morgan, DVM, DACVIM (Small Animal), DACVO

BASIC INFORMATION
Description

Nutrition-related bone diseases are rare in animals fed commercially prepared diets, because most commercial diets are balanced and comply with guidelines set by the Association of American Feed Control Officials (AAFCO). Many commercial foods are also subjected to feeding trials that follow AAFCO procedures to substantiate they are complete and balanced for the targeted life stage. Foods that comply with AAFCO standards are identified on the label.

Causes

Three nutritional bone diseases that can occur in both dogs and cats are the following:

* *Nutritional secondary hyperparathyroidism* arises when diets low in calcium and high in phosphorus are fed, especially to young, growing animals. This condition is most likely to develop when the animal is fed an all-meat or all-grain diet. Low dietary calcium levels, an inappropriate calcium/phosphorus ratio in the diet, low circulating vitamin D levels, and increased activity of the parathyroid gland all lead to loss of calcium and weakening of the bones (osteopenia).
* *Hypovitaminosis D* can occur rarely from inadequate intake and absorption of vitamin D or decreased formation of the active form of vitamin D (D3) because of lack of sunlight. Young animals with hypovitaminosis D develop rickets, which is the production of weak, abnormal bones. In mature animals, the bones become soft.
* *Hypervitaminosis A* develops from prolonged, excessive intake of vitamin A. This may occur with diets that contain large amounts of raw liver and milk, so the condition is more common in cats. It can also arise from feeding vitamin A supplements. This condition adversely affects bone growth and results in misshapen, shorter bones and abnormal bone growth, especially of the spine, breast bone, and ribs.

Clinical Signs

Signs of nutritional hyperparathyroidism and hypovitaminosis D include loose teeth, a soft jaw bone ("rubber jaw"), and problems chewing. As the bones weaken, folding fractures may occur, resulting in pain, lameness, and difficulty walking. These pathologic fractures may develop with normal activity and may involve multiple legs or the spine.

Cats with hypervitaminosis A may be depressed and reluctant to move or groom themselves because it can be painful for them to bend their spine. The head and neck may be bent toward the chest, and the cat may seem to have pain in the neck region. Lameness or weakness may be detected in one or more legs.

Diagnostic Tests

Tentative diagnosis of these conditions can sometimes be reached from a history of feeding a poor, unbalanced diet or excessive intake of vitamin supplements. With nutritional hyperparathyroidism and hypovitaminosis D, blood calcium and phosphorus levels are sometimes abnormal, and levels of parathyroid hormone are increased. X-rays usually reveal loss of calcium in the outer portion (cortex) of the bones and one or more fractures. Fractures may be recent or old (healed) and may involve multiple bones.

With hypervitaminosis A, blood levels of this vitamin are usually elevated, and x-rays show characteristic bony changes. Changes in the vertebrae of the spine can be severe and can include scoliosis (abnormal curvature) and fusion. Abnormal bony nodules may be seen on the surfaces of some bones.

TREATMENT AND FOLLOW-UP

Treatment Options

The primary treatment is to provide the animal with a well-balanced diet. With nutritional hyperparathyroidism, calcium and phosphorus supplements are given while the bones are healing and then stopped. With hypervitaminosis A, all extra supplements are stopped immediately.

Animals with folding fractures must be kept quiet in a crate or cage for several weeks. Anti-inflammatory drugs or pain-relieving medications may be recommended. Gentle handling and extra care must be taken to prevent new injuries to the bones. Animals that develop angular limb deformities from premature fusion of bone growth plates may require corrective surgery. (See also the handout on **Angular Limb Deformities in Dogs**.)

Follow-up Care

Periodic recheck visits are needed to monitor the animal's progress. Laboratory tests and x-rays are usually repeated every 4-8 weeks until laboratory abnormalities resolve and bony changes improve. Folding fractures may take 3 months or more to heal.

Prognosis

With nutritional hyperparathyroidism and hypovitaminosis D, bone strength may return to normal. If severe bony changes are not present initially, prognosis is good. Spinal fractures may cause permanent weakness or paralysis.

With hypervitaminosis A, bony changes stop as soon as vitamin A levels return to normal, but they do not often improve significantly. Euthanasia may be considered for seriously affected cats that remain in pain despite appropriate therapy.

SPECIAL INSTRUCTIONS:

MORGAN • *Small Animal Practice Client Handouts*   Osteoarthritis: Medical Management   **295**

Osteoarthritis: Medical Management

Rhea V. Morgan, DVM, DACVIM (Small Animal), DACVO
Mark C. Rochat, DVM, MS, DACVS

BASIC INFORMATION

Description

Osteoarthritis (OA) or degenerative joint disease (DJD) is a chronic degenerative condition of one or more joints that results in decreased mobility and pain. OA is categorized as primary (very rare in dogs and cats) when it occurs with aging or an unknown cause or secondary when it results from another condition. Secondary OA is extremely common in dogs and is increasingly diagnosed in cats. OA can affect any joint, but the hip, stifle (knee), elbow, and shoulder joints are most commonly involved in dogs. In most cases, OA develops slowly over months to years and worsens with time.

Causes

Any event that injures, damages, strains, or causes a joint and its surrounding structures to become inflamed may eventually lead to OA. It is a common consequence of hip dysplasia, cranial cruciate ligament disease, osteochondritis dissecans, and other developmental or degenerative joint diseases in dogs. It may also occur after septic or immune-mediated arthritis, prolonged immobilization of a joint, joint surgery, direct trauma or dislocation of a joint, and certain metabolic bone diseases.

Clinical Signs

Lameness, stiffness, and pain are the most common signs. Stiffness is often worse after periods of rest and improves as the animal becomes more active. Lameness may be constant or sporadic and may worsen after exercise, especially if the exercise is followed by a rest period. Affected joints may crackle, pop, or grate and have decreased range of motion. Manual movement of the joint or affected leg may cause obvious pain. As the OA worsens, the animal may be reluctant to get up and move around.

Diagnostic Tests

OA may be suspected based on the history and clinical signs. X-rays of affected joints are needed to confirm the diagnosis, but the radiographic signs of OA often do not correlate with clinical signs and historical findings. In some cases, fluid can be retrieved to confirm the diagnosis by analysis and culture. With OA, joint fluid is not actively inflamed or infected.

TREATMENT AND FOLLOW-UP

Treatment Options

Medical therapy is the most commonly used treatment. Surgery may be needed in cases of joint instability (such as cranial cruciate ligament rupture or joint dislocation) or severe, debilitating disorders (such as hip dysplasia) to provide permanent fusion (arthrodesis) of selected joints. (See the handouts on these surgical options.)

Medical therapy involves measures to decrease stress on the joint, improve the health of cartilage and joint surfaces, improve mobility, and decrease pain. Weight loss decreases stress on joints. Consistent, frequent, low-impact exercise (such as walking or swimming) can help facilitate weight loss and improve joint mobility and muscle mass in the affected legs. High-impact forms of exercise, such as running and jumping, are avoided. When available, physical rehabilitation can also significantly improve your pet's quality of life.

A variety of supplements, such as glucosamine, chondroitin sulfate, and omega-3 fatty acids, appear to decrease chronic degenerative processes within joints and may also alleviate some pain. These supplements are safe and can be used for years if needed. As an alternative to glucosamine/chondroitin sulfate, injectable polysulfated glycosaminoglycans can be administered by your veterinarian.

Nonsteroidal anti-inflammatory drugs (NSAIDs) are commonly administered for acute episodes of clinical signs and may be needed in some animals for long periods. Examples of drugs that are used in dogs include carprofen (*Rimadyl*), deracoxib (*Deramaxx*), firocoxib (*Previcox*), meloxicam (*Metacam*), tepoxalin (*Zubrin*), and etodolac (*Etogesic*). Meloxicam is most commonly used in cats. It is important to note that NSAIDs designed for people are often toxic to animals and should not be used.

Acupuncture has provided relief to some animals. Steroid medications are usually given only as a last resort because of their serious side effects and generally destructive effects on joint cartilage.

Follow-up Care

Periodic rechecks are advised to monitor response to therapy and progression of the disease. X-rays are not much help for monitoring the progression of OA but may be useful when surgery is planned. Laboratory tests are often performed prior to and during long-term NSAID therapy, because these drugs can cause or aggravate existing liver and kidney disease.

Prognosis

OA is a chronic, progressive disease whose course is difficult to predict. Even when an acceptable treatment regimen is achieved initially, modifications are usually required as the disease progresses. When medical therapy is unsuccessful and cannot be further adjusted, surgical alternatives such as joint fusion, arthroplasty, or joint replacement may be considered.

SPECIAL INSTRUCTIONS:

Copyright © 2011 by Saunders, an imprint of Elsevier Inc. All rights reserved.

Osteochondrosis (Osteochondritis Dissecans)

Mark C. Rochat, DVM, MS, DACVS

BASIC INFORMATION

Description

Osteochondrosis (OC) and osteochondritis dissecans (OCD) are two forms of a developmental orthopedic disease. OC typically affects young, male, large- and giant-breed dogs. It very rarely occurs in small dogs and cats. The ends of normal leg bones grow joint cartilage that covers the end of the bone. The cartilage is programmed to gradually turn into bone as the bone matures.

OC occurs when the cartilage fails to change into bone and becomes thickened in a single spot. This area of thickened cartilage is poorly nourished by joint fluid and prone to fragmentation (break apart or come loose) with normal activity. The disease is referred to *OC* until the fragmentation leads to the creation of a flap, and then the term *OCD* is used. When the flap of cartilage develops, clinical signs of joint pain occur.

Common sites affected in the dog include the head of the humerus (shoulder), the termination of the humerus (elbow), the talus of the hock (ankle), and the end of the femur at the stifle (knee).

Causes

Numerous factors have been implicated in OC, including nutritional excesses (primarily protein, calcium, and calories), genetic factors, and environmental factors. Because OC has a genetic component, dogs affected with OC should not be bred.

Clinical Signs

Dogs with OCD show signs typical of joint disease. They are stiff after resting, but the stiffness subsides as the joint warms up with activity. The joint becomes stiff and sore again after exercise. Lameness can vary from mild to severe. Signs of secondary osteoarthritis occur early in life and progress at a variable rate over time. (See also the handout on **Osteoarthritis: Medical Management**.)

Diagnostic Tests

Physical and orthopedic examinations often reveal pain in the joint that is made worse by flexing (bending) and extending (unbending) the joint. X-rays demonstrate a defect in the bone in specific locations on the joint surface, depending on the joint involved. Also depending on the specific joint involved, significant numbers of dogs have a similar bone defect in the opposite joint. Other developmental conditions may be found when OC occurs in the elbow.

TREATMENT AND FOLLOW-UP

Treatment Options

Medical management is typically ineffective. In general, surgery is considered only if signs of pain are identified and a cartilage flap is present, because OC without these signs may resolve on its own without surgical intervention. Removal of the flap can be done by either an arthrotomy (surgically opening the joint) or arthroscopy (done through a tiny incision using a viewing scope).

Follow-up Care

Limited activity for 4-6 weeks is usually recommended after surgery. Rest allows the defect in the bone (where the flap was) to properly heal in with fibrocartilage. Ancillary therapy may involve nonsteroidal anti-inflammatory drugs, cartilage-protective agents, and a weight reduction program. Because OC has a genetic component, dogs affected with OC should not be bred.

Prognosis

Prognosis for OCD of the shoulder is excellent. Prognosis for OCD in the elbow is also good unless the flap is very large or significant osteoarthritis is already present. OCD of the stifle and hock, although much less common, carries a generally guarded (uncertain) to poor prognosis for good long-term function, even with appropriate therapy.

SPECIAL INSTRUCTIONS:

Osteomyelitis

Rhea V. Morgan, DVM, DACVIM (Small Animal), DACVO
Mark C. Rochat, DVM, MS, DACVS

BASIC INFORMATION

Description

Osteomyelitis is bone inflammation caused by infection. Infection most commonly arises from external sources of contamination, such as puncture wounds, openings in the skin over a fracture, or shearing injuries that result in loss of skin and muscle (with exposure of underlying bone). Osteomyelitis can also occur as a consequence of surgery. Infections in nearby tissues may spread to bone, and, occasionally, infections can spread to bone via the bloodstream from other areas of the body.

Causes

Bacteria are the most common cause of osteomyelitis. Bacteria commonly involved include staphylococci (staph), streptococci (strep), and coliform bacteria (such as *Escherichia coli*). Anaerobic bacteria (those that thrive in the absence of oxygen) are also important causes of osteomyelitis. Brucellosis, a disease most often present in breeding dogs, may infect bone. Other bacterial agents are involved less often.

A number of fungal infections, such as blastomycosis, coccidioidomycosis, cryptococcosis, histoplasmosis, and aspergillosis, which ordinarily enter the body through the nose and lungs, can spread to bone.

Clinical Signs

Some cases of osteomyelitis develop suddenly (acute osteomyelitis), with signs arising within 5-21 days after an injury, surgery, or other illness. The bone affected may be swollen, painful, and warm to the touch. Lameness, fever, lethargy, and decreased appetite usually occur. Other signs may be present, depending on the underlying cause and primary location of the infection.

Chronic osteomyelitis develops months to years after an injury, surgery, or previous illness. The affected leg is often lame and painful. If the infection has broken through to the skin surface, a draining hole or tract may be seen. Other systemic signs are uncommon, although intermittent fever and lethargy may be observed.

Diagnostic Tests

Diagnosis often requires a combination of clinical signs, x-ray findings, and laboratory test results. Most x-ray changes do not appear in bone for at least 2 weeks after the onset of the infection. A complete blood count may reveal evidence of infection and chronic anemia. Samples from the affected tissues may be submitted for culture.

When the diagnosis is not confirmed by these tests, bone scans and/or surgical exploration of the site may be recommended. With surgery, biopsies can be submitted for bacterial culture and histopathology. Other tests may be required to determine the underlying cause of the infection and to rule out other diseases that cause similar clinical signs.

TREATMENT AND FOLLOW-UP

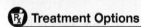 Treatment Options

Acute bacterial osteomyelitis is usually treated with 4-6 weeks of antibiotics. Some cases require more long-term treatment. For fungal osteomyelitis, antifungal drugs are usually needed for months. (See also the handout for each fungal disease.) In addition to medical therapy, contaminated injuries are cleaned, débrided (removal of dead tissue), and allowed to drain. Fractures are repaired, and the leg is stabilized. Shearing injuries may require frequent, sterile bandage changes.

Long-term antibiotics are administered for chronic bacterial osteomyelitis. Many cases also require surgery to remove dead bone, remove contaminated surgical implants (plates, screws, pins, wires), and stabilize the leg. Bone grafts may be used to stimulate bone healing when the infection is resolved, and special techniques may be performed that concentrate antibiotics at the site. Amputation may be considered for severe cases that do not respond well to these treatments. Some of these procedures may require your pet be referred to a veterinary surgery specialist.

Follow-up Care

Frequent examinations are usually needed to monitor response to treatment and to change bandages and assess healing. X-rays are often repeated every 4-6 weeks until bone healing is complete. Blood tests may be repeated to determine whether the infection is resolving. Some cases require monitoring for many months.

Prognosis

Prognosis depends on the severity of the condition and the response to therapy. Fungal osteomyelitis is difficult to treat but may resolve with months of therapy. Surgical débridement and appropriate antibiotic therapy may achieve cure rates close to 90% for acute bacterial osteomyelitis. Early diagnosis combined with aggressive, appropriate therapy provides the best chance for a cure.

SPECIAL INSTRUCTIONS:

Panosteitis

Mark C. Rochat, DVM, MS, DACVS

BASIC INFORMATION
Description
Panosteitis is a bone disease that affects young dogs. It is most common in large-breed, male dogs. It is also called *juvenile osteomyelitis, enostosis,* and *eosinophilic panosteitis.* The disease tends to affect the shafts of the bones (diaphyseal and metaphyseal regions) more than the ends (near the joints). The disease is most common in the ulna (a bone in the forearm) but can affect other long bones of the limbs, such as the humerus, femur, tibia, and radius.

Causes
The cause is unknown, although recent evidence suggests the possibility of a link between the disease and high-calorie, high-protein diets.

Clinical Signs
Lameness in one or more legs is the most common sign. The lameness can often shift from one leg to another over time. Lameness can range in severity from mild to moderate and is not associated with the time of day or any period of rest. The degree of lameness may worsen with activity and exercise. No general signs, such as depression, fever, or loss of appetite, are typically observed.

Diagnostic Tests
Deep palpation (feeling or pressing) of the shafts of the long bones usually results in a marked pain response. X-rays may be normal in the early stages of the disease but usually demonstrate changes in the marrow cavity of the affected bones. Other diseases of growing dogs that might benefit from surgical correction (such as elbow disorders and osteochondritis dissecans) can exist simultaneously with panosteitis, so a thorough examination is advisable. The diagnosis is usually made by a combination of compatible clinical signs and x-ray findings.

TREATMENT AND FOLLOW-UP
Treatment Options
Rest and nonsteroidal anti-inflammatory drugs specifically intended for use in dogs help alleviate the pain associated with panosteitis. The disease usually resolves with time.

Follow-up Care
The disease may develop in other long bones after signs subside in the original bone. Rarely, panosteitis can occur in young adult dogs. Notify your veterinarian if lameness fails to resolve in a few weeks or occurs in other limbs.

Prognosis
Prognosis is excellent, because the disease usually resolves on its own and secondary complications are extremely rare.

SPECIAL INSTRUCTIONS:

Patella Luxation

Mark C. Rochat, DVM, MS, DACVS

BASIC INFORMATION

Description

The patella is the kneecap. Patella luxation is dislocation of the patella from the groove (trochlear sulcus) in the femur (thigh bone) in which the patella normally rides. Patella luxation occurs most commonly in small-breed dogs but can occur in large dogs and cats. In most cases, the patella dislocates toward the inside of the knee (medial luxation), but dislocation toward the outside of the knee (lateral luxation) can also occur, especially in large dogs.

Causes

Patellar luxation is usually a developmental disease but can also occur as a result of trauma. Multiple causes have been suggested, including genetic influences. Several abnormalities can occur in the leg anatomy of affected dogs, beginning at the hip and progressing down to below the stifle (knee). The muscles of the legs may be malaligned and the major bones somewhat deformed. Patella luxation is the most obvious abnormality and the one that causes pain and dysfunction, but the other abnormalities must be addressed for the patella to properly ride in the trochlear sulcus.

Clinical Signs

The most commonly reported sign is a variable degree of intermittent lameness. Classically, the dog suddenly stops, may cry out, picks up the leg for several steps, stretches the leg out behind it, and then resumes normal activity. This sequence of signs occurs because the patella dislocates and then returns to its normal position when the leg is stretched backward. With time, the stifle develops osteoarthritis from abnormal movement of the patella.

Diagnostic Tests

The luxation can usually be detected during a physical examination, and other anatomic abnormalities may also be detected. The extent of the luxation is often graded on a scale of 1 to 4, as follows:

- Grade 1 is the mildest form. In these cases, the patella can be manually luxated during the examination, but then it returns to a normal position. Dogs with grade 1 luxations may have no clinical signs.
- With grade 2 cases, the patella spontaneously luxates and returns to its normal position. A "skipping" gait or lameness is common.
- With grade 3 cases, the patella is dislocated constantly but can be manually returned to a normal position momentarily. Lameness is commonly present but varies in severity.
- Grade 4 is the most severe form. In these cases, the patella is dislocated continuously and cannot be manually replaced, and lameness is significant.

X-rays may reveal the luxation, show other anatomic abnormalities in the leg, and help decide what specific measures should be taken to correct the condition.

TREATMENT AND FOLLOW-UP

Treatment Options

Dogs with patellar luxations that have no clinical (outward) signs (an uncommon event) generally do not benefit from surgery. Young dogs and dogs with patellar luxation and lameness should have the luxation corrected. A number of techniques are commonly used to achieve proper alignment of the patella. Which specific procedure is chosen depends to some degree on the x-ray findings and the results of the initial orthopedic examination. Your dog may be referred to a veterinary orthopedic surgeon for evaluation prior to surgery.

Techniques that may be considered include the following:

- If the trochlear sulcus is too shallow, it can be deepened by either a block or wedge recession trochleoplasty.
- In most situations, the attachment of the patellar tendon to the tibia (shin bone) is cut, moved laterally (toward the outside of the stifle), and secured to the tibia with a single, small, stainless steel pin.
- Dogs that have grade 4 luxations often require additional procedures to cut and straighten the femur (thigh bone) and tibia, thereby straightening the leg and resolving the luxation.

Follow-up Care

After surgery, activity is limited to short leash walks. Other activities such as running, jumping, stair climbing, and playing are prohibited. Physical rehabilitation therapy can greatly improve the recovery of stifle function. X-rays of the stifle are taken every 4-6 weeks until the osteotomy in the tibia is healed. The pin may be left in place indefinitely. Normal exercise and full activity are allowed after all tissues, including the bone, have healed.

Prognosis

Prognosis is favorable for most dogs. After surgery, about 25% of the dogs have an improvement in their luxation by 1-2 grades, with the rest of the dogs becoming normal. Dogs with grade 4 luxations often have a more guarded (uncertain) prognosis but can still improve substantially with proper treatment.

SPECIAL INSTRUCTIONS:

Sacroiliac Luxation

Mark C. Rochat, DVM, MS, DACVS

BASIC INFORMATION

Description
The sacroiliac (SI) joint is the connection between the pelvis and the sacrum of the lower spine. SI joints are present on both sides of the pelvis, and they have very limited motion. Luxation means that the joint is dislocated and the pelvis is no longer connected to the sacrum on the affected side. Many SI luxations are accompanied by fractures of the pelvis, often through the floor of the pelvis.

Causes
Major trauma, such as being hit by a car, can result in dislocation of the SI joint. One or both joints may be dislocated, and any animal can be affected.

Clinical Signs
Significant lameness and other signs of trauma are usually present. The pelvis is often malaligned and painful when felt (palpated). If both sides are affected or additional spinal trauma has occurred, the animal may be unable to walk. Adjacent vertebral fractures may cause paralysis of the tail and loss of bladder and anal function.

Diagnostic Tests
X-rays of the pelvis are needed to confirm the diagnosis and to help identify fractures or other injuries. Nerve damage can occur in conjunction with the luxation, and nerve function must also be carefully evaluated. Laboratory tests, x-rays of the abdomen and chest, an electrocardiogram (to identify abnormal heart rhythms), and an ultrasound of the abdomen may be recommended to identify and assess other injuries.

TREATMENT AND FOLLOW-UP

Treatment Options
Medical therapy is usually indicated if only one side is dislocated, there is minimal malalignment of the pelvis, and the remainder of the pelvis is intact (with no other fractures or dislocations). SI luxations treated medically heal by the formation of scar tissue, which can take a long time. Medical therapy consists of cage confinement, vigilant nursing care, physical rehabilitation exercises, and pain-relief medications for at least 3 weeks. The animal is then allowed restricted, controlled activity for another 4 weeks, until healing is complete. Full return to function may take as long as 3 months.

Surgical stabilization of the SI luxation may be done with a screw or other techniques. Surgery may be required if both SI joints are dislocated, the joint separation is wide, the pelvis is fractured and the pelvic canal is narrowed, or other pelvic injuries are present. Surgical intervention usually results in quicker healing and a faster return to normal activity.

Follow-up Care
Periodic follow-up visits are usually scheduled to monitor the animal's progress. If surgery is performed, x-rays are taken every 4-6 weeks to assess healing. Other tests may be repeated to monitor other injuries associated with the SI luxation.

Prognosis
Prognosis for return to normal function is generally excellent for luxations that are not complicated by spinal trauma or nerve damage. Prognosis can be guarded if the SI joint luxation is accompanied by neurologic abnormalities, severe trauma to the abdominal organs, or multiple fractures of the pelvis.

SPECIAL INSTRUCTIONS:

Scapular Luxation

Mark C. Rochat, DVM, MS, DACVS

BASIC INFORMATION

Description

Scapular luxation is the separation of the scapula (shoulder blade) from the body wall and ribs. The scapula is normally attached to the body by several muscles.

Causes

The cause of scapular luxation is always a traumatic event, such as a fall from a great height or being hit or dragged by a car.

Clinical Signs

Initially, the animal may carry the leg and be unwilling to put weight on it. With time, the pain subsides and the animal will bear weight, but the shoulder rides up above (higher than) the back bone of the chest area, and lameness is obvious.

Diagnostic Tests

The diagnosis is often made by observing the abnormal position of the shoulder. Because other injuries might have occurred during the trauma that created the scapula luxation, extensive evaluation of the animal is often done prior to surgery. As part of the presurgical evaluation, laboratory tests, x-rays of the chest, an electrocardiogram (to identify abnormal heart rhythms), and an ultrasound of the abdomen may be recommended. X-rays of the scapula may be taken and compared with those of the opposite side.

TREATMENT AND FOLLOW-UP

Treatment Options

Bandaging alone may be sufficient for affected cats, if the injury is recent. Scapular luxation in dogs is treated by placing wires or heavy suture through the scapula and around the nearby ribs. The leg is placed in a bandage while scar tissue forms that will anchor the scapula to the body wall.

Follow-up Care

The bandage is maintained for 2-3 weeks, followed by another 3-4 weeks of exercise limited to short leash walks only. Running, jumping, and playing are avoided.

Prognosis

Prognosis for return to normal activity, especially with early treatment, is very good.

SPECIAL INSTRUCTIONS:

Septic Arthritis

Rhea V. Morgan, DVM, DACVIM (Small Animal), DACVO
Mark C. Rochat, DVM, MS, DACVS

BASIC INFORMATION

Description

Septic arthritis occurs when one or more joints become infected, usually with bacteria. The infection may spread to the joint via the bloodstream from some other area in the body (hematogenous or blood-borne infection). More commonly, the joint may become contaminated from an external source of infection during surgery, joint fluid sampling or injections, or following trauma. Young animals that do not have well-developed immune systems and animals that are immunocompromised or have arthritic joints are more likely to develop bacterial arthritis. Septic arthritis is a serious condition that requires immediate and aggressive therapy to avoid destruction of the joint cartilage by enzymes released by bacteria and white blood cells.

Causes

The bacteria that most commonly cause septic arthritis are staphylococci (staph), streptococci (strep), and coliform bacteria (such as *Escherichia coli*). Certain generalized fungal infections may infect bones and secondarily invade joints. The bacterium that causes Lyme disease, *Borrelia burgdorferi*, can also infect joints. In some cases of Lyme disease, however, joint inflammation arises more from an immune-mediated response rather than direct damage from the bacteria. Likewise, arthritis can be a component of ehrlichiosis and Rocky Mountain spotted fever, which are acquired from ticks. Other bacterial agents are less commonly involved.

Clinical Signs

Joint swelling, lameness, and severe pain in the joint are the most common signs. The skin over the joint may feel warm and may be reddened. The animal may be lethargic and may have a fever and decreased appetite. If the infection has spread through the bloodstream, several joints are commonly involved, and other signs of infection are often present. External sources of infection typically affect only one joint and uncommonly produce systemic signs.

Diagnostic Tests

A tentative diagnosis may sometimes be based on the history and clinical signs. Laboratory tests and x-rays may be recommended to evaluate the joints and other organs and to search for evidence of infection. Definitive diagnosis requires analysis of fluid retrieved from the joint. Cultures of joint fluid, blood, and other sites may be recommended if a widespread infection is suspected. Special laboratory tests may be needed to test for tick-borne diseases and to determine the specific bacteria or fungus involved.

TREATMENT AND FOLLOW-UP

Treatment Options

For bacterial infections, antibiotic therapy is started as soon as laboratory samples have been submitted, because some tests take several days to return. Some animals initially require hospitalization for administration of injectable antibiotics. Oral antibiotics may be continued for several weeks. Antifungal drugs are started for fungal infections. Other treatments and supportive care may be needed for widespread infections. Nonsteroidal anti-inflammatory drugs and medications for pain may also be considered.

Severely affected single joints may be opened and drained surgically, particularly those contaminated during surgery or from bite wounds, and in cases that do not respond to antibiotics within 2-3 days. The joint may be irrigated, with all abnormal tissue removed, and then left open to drain or closed after placement of a surgical drain. Joints that are not surgically closed require daily, sterile bandage changes until the infection resolves and the joint can be surgically closed. Alternatively, the joint may be irrigated using large needles or arthroscopic methods. Surgery is generally not indicated when multiple joints are affected.

Follow-up Care

Antibiotics are commonly given for at least 4 weeks, or for 2 weeks past resolution of all clinical signs. Once pain and swelling have subsided, physical therapy exercises may be recommended to prevent stiffness and encourage healing. Frequent rechecks are needed initially to monitor response to treatment and to make adjustments in therapy. Other methods of monitoring treatment progress, such as laboratory tests and repeated x-rays, depend on the underlying cause and whether the infection is affecting other organs.

Prognosis

Prognosis with septic arthritis is variable. If it is discovered early and treated aggressively, bacterial arthritis may respond well to therapy. Fungal infections, in general, are more difficult to treat. Widespread, severe bacterial infections (sepsis) have a poor prognosis.

Septic arthritis that requires surgery has a poorer prognosis, because chronic osteoarthritis (degenerative joint disease) is more likely to result. Osteoarthritis can develop as a long-term consequence of septic arthritis in any joint and may cause joint deformity, decreased joint mobility (restricted range of motion), and lameness. (See also the handout on **Osteoarthritis: Medical Management**.)

SPECIAL INSTRUCTIONS:

Shoulder Luxation

Mark C. Rochat, DVM, MS, DACVS

BASIC INFORMATION
Description

Shoulder luxation (dislocation) occurs in one of two forms: traumatic or congenital/degenerative. In the traumatic form, the ligaments that maintain alignment of the shoulder are ruptured during a severe traumatic event, and the shoulder dislocates. In the congenital form, the ligaments never properly develop. The neck of the scapula (shoulder blade) may also be misshapen. Traumatic luxation can occur in any age or breed of dog, but it is rare in cats. The congenital form usually occurs in small-breed dogs.

Causes

Traumatic shoulder luxation results from serious accidents, such as blunt force trauma (such as being hit by a car or kicked by a horse or a fall from a height). Congenital luxation occurs as the dog grows, but clinical signs may not be apparent until young adulthood.

Clinical Signs

The most common clinical sign is lameness of varying intensity. Other signs of trauma may accompany traumatic shoulder luxation. Congenital luxation may occur in both shoulders, whereas traumatic luxation generally occurs only on one side. Depending on the direction in which the joint is dislocated, the leg may be held at an odd angle in a number of different directions. If the luxation is traumatic and chronic, lameness and pain may be less than expected.

Diagnostic Tests

Orthopedic examination usually identifies the luxation, along with pain and crepitus (a crunchy or "bubble-wrap" sound) in the area of the joint. X-rays reveal the dislocation and any other fractures or injuries that may be present in cases of traumatic luxation. Malformation of the scapula is seen in cases of congenital luxation.

TREATMENT AND FOLLOW-UP

Treatment Options

Recent traumatic luxations can often be reduced (put back in place) while the dog is under anesthesia. A splint or Velpeau bandage is placed on the leg for 10-14 days to allow scar tissue to form and stabilize the shoulder. More chronic luxations and those that are very unstable must usually be surgically stabilized, using methods that reconstruct the supporting ligaments of the joint.

Congenital luxations are also stabilized by surgical reconstruction of the shoulder ligaments. If the scapula is misshapen, removal of the end of the glenoid, which is the bone closest to the joint (excision arthroplasty), generally resolves the pain associated with the luxation. A mild alteration in gait may persist after this procedure. Fusion of the shoulder joint also alleviates pain but results in a somewhat awkward gait. Joints that are surgically stabilized may be placed in a special bandage called a *Velpeau bandage* to protect the surgical repair.

Follow-up Care

The dog is confined to a cage for 2-6 weeks after application of a splint or surgical repair, depending on the type of luxation and treatment used. Dogs also benefit from physical therapy exercises to maximize range of motion and function of the affected shoulder joint.

Prognosis

Prognosis for recent traumatic luxations is generally good. Chronic traumatic and congenital luxations are more difficult to successfully resolve. Excision arthroplasty or fusion may be considered for those joints that are very unstable or remain unstable despite conventional therapy.

SPECIAL INSTRUCTIONS:

Stifle Luxation

Mark C. Rochat, DVM, MS, DACVS

BASIC INFORMATION

Description

Stifle luxation is a severe, traumatic derangement of the ligaments that support the stifle (knee). Tearing of the ligaments causes the stifle to become unstable, so that the leg cannot be used properly.

Causes

Stifle luxation almost always is caused by some severe, traumatic force applied to the stifle, such as being hit or dragged by a car (dogs, cats) or caught in a car engine fan or fan belt (cats).

Clinical Signs

Signs of trauma to other parts of the body may be observed. The stifle may have lacerations around it, or the skin may be intact. The stifle itself is often severely distorted or misshapen. The animal is unable to bear weight on the leg.

Diagnostic Tests

Testing may sometimes be delayed until the animal is stabilized and more critical injuries are treated. Prior to anesthesia, laboratory tests and x-rays of the chest are commonly recommended. Orthopedic examination while the dog or cat is anesthetized helps determine what specific ligaments have been damaged. X-rays of the leg further define the extent of the injuries.

TREATMENT AND FOLLOW-UP

Treatment Options

In small dogs or cats, a pin is sometimes placed across the stifle joint (transarticular pin) to immobilize it at a functional angle while scar tissue builds up around the stifle that will permanently hold it in place. For larger dogs or at the surgeon's discretion, the individual ligaments are repaired or reconstructed and the limb placed in a splint or external skeletal fixator (see handouts on **Fracture Repair: Casts and Splints** and **Fracture Repair: External Skeletal Fixation**) to keep the joint from moving during the healing process.

Follow-up Care

The splint, external skeletal fixator, or transarticular pin is inspected at frequent (often weekly) intervals and removed when the stifle has healed (typically 2-6 weeks). Any incisions are inspected daily for evidence of infection (excessive redness, swelling, pain, or discharge), and the sutures or staples are removed in 10-14 days.

Prognosis

Prognosis for smaller dogs and cats is good. For larger dogs, the prognosis is more guarded (uncertain), but good function can usually be restored with aggressive therapy.

SPECIAL INSTRUCTIONS:

Ununited Anconeal Process Disease

Mark C. Rochat, DVM, MS, DACVS

BASIC INFORMATION

Description

The anconeal process is the portion of the ulna (one of the three bones that make up the elbow joint) that fits into the groove in the humerus (large bone of the foreleg) and helps to keep the structures of the elbow aligned. The anconeal process develops from a secondary growth center and should be permanently fused to the rest of the ulna by about 20 weeks of age. If the anconeal process is not fused by that time, it is considered ununited (UAP).

Although a UAP is not freely moveable, it is loose and continues to irritate the elbow joint, which leads to osteoarthritis, joint stiffness, and pain. UAP can occur with other developmental diseases of the elbow. (See also the handouts on **Fragmented Medial Coronoid Process Disease** and **Osteochondrosis [Osteochondritis Dissecans]**.)

Causes

Although the specific cause of UAP is unknown, it is common in certain breeds (such as the German shepherd dog and Saint Bernard) and may be inherited to some degree. Failure of the anconeal process to fuse may occur from uneven growth of the three bones around the elbow, which leads to excessive pressure against the growth center. UAP is fairly uncommon.

Clinical Signs

Clinical signs are the same as for any joint condition, namely lameness, pain, and joint stiffness after rest that initially improves with activity and then worsens with further activity. Circumduction (swinging the limb in an outward circle) may also be observed. UAP usually is present in young, large- or giant-breed dogs; however, older dogs may become lame because of the secondary arthritis that occurs with UAP. UAP may affect one or both elbows (11-43% of cases are bilateral).

Diagnostic Tests

Examination of the elbow may reveal loss of range of motion and pain with movement. Effusion (fluid in the joint), thickening of the joint, and crepitus (a crunchy or "bubble-wrap" sound) may also be felt on palpation and manipulation of the joint. X-rays confirm the diagnosis. X-rays of the opposite elbow are often taken for comparison.

TREATMENT AND FOLLOW-UP

Treatment Options

If the UAP is identified early, before secondary osteoarthritis has occurred, the condition is best treated by surgical insertion of a screw across the ulna into the anconeal process. This is followed by an ulnar osteotomy (cutting of the ulna) immediately below the joint.

If osteoarthritis is present or the anconeal process is very misshapen, surgical removal of the process is generally performed. Osteoarthritis will develop to some degree no matter what treatment approach is used, so additional medical therapy is often required. (See also the handout on **Osteoarthritis: Medical Management**.)

Follow-up Care

Activity is restricted to short walks on a leash for the first 2 weeks following removal of the process, or for 6 weeks if a screw was inserted. The incision is observed daily for signs of infection, and if a screw was placed, x-rays are taken every 4-6 weeks until the process has completely fused to the ulna.

Prognosis

If the disease is identified early and treated by screw fixation and ulnar osteotomy, the prognosis for satisfactory function of the elbow is usually good. If secondary osteoarthritis is present or the anconeal process has been removed, the prognosis is more guarded (uncertain) for full return to function.

SPECIAL INSTRUCTIONS:

SECTION 12

Dermatologic System

Section Editor: Emily Rothstein, DVM, DACVD

Acne in Cats
Acute Moist Dermatitis in Dogs
Alopecia X
Atopic Dermatitis in Dogs
Atypical Mycobacteriosis
Benign Skin Tumors in Dogs
Cheyletiellosis
Claw (Toenail) Disease, Asymmetrical
Claw (Toenail) Disease, Symmetrical
Cutaneous or Discoid Lupus Erythematosus
Cutaneous (Epitheliotropic) T-Cell Lymphoma
Cyclical Flank Alopecia
Deep Bacterial Pyoderma and Furunculosis
Demodicosis in Dogs
Dermatophytosis
Eosinophilic Granuloma Complex in Cats
Exfoliative Cutaneous Lupus Erythematosus
Flea Allergic Dermatitis
Food Reactions, Adverse
Juvenile Cellulitis

Lipomas in Dogs
Malassezia Dermatitis
Mast Cell Tumors in Cats
Mast Cell Tumors in Dogs
Nasal Depigmentation
Notoedric Mange
Pemphigus Complex
Pinnal Seborrhea
Plasma Cell Pododermatitis in Cats
Primary Seborrhea
Sarcoptic Mange
Sebaceous Adenitis in Dogs
Skin Fold Pyoderma (Intertrigo)
Sporotrichosis
Subcutaneous Abscesses and Cellulitis
Superficial Bacterial Folliculitis in Dogs
Systemic Lupus Erythematosus: Dermatologic Aspects
Vaccine-Associated Vasculitis in Dogs
Vitamin A–Responsive Dermatosis
Zinc-Responsive Dermatosis

Acne in Cats

Emily Rothstein, DVM, DACVD

BASIC INFORMATION

Description and Causes

Feline acne is obstruction of the hair follicles on the chin. The underlying cause and reason the problem develops are unknown.

Clinical Signs

Early lesions consist of blackheads and black debris on the chin. Sometimes mild scabbing, red bumps, and pimples occur. Lesions may also involve the skin of the upper and lower lips. After time, the pimples can get larger and cause the hair follicles to rupture (furunculosis), which leads to discomfort and bloody drainage.

Diagnostic Tests

Diagnosis is based on the presence of compatible clinical signs and elimination of other possible skin conditions of the chin.

TREATMENT AND FOLLOW-UP

Treatment Options

Secondary bacterial infections are treated with systemic antibiotics for 2-4 weeks. The hair may be clipped and the skin gently washed with a shampoo that contains benzoyl peroxide or ethyl lactate until the lesions have dried out and healed. Gentle washes can then be continued as needed. Topical antibacterial ointments or creams, such as 2% mupirocin, 0.75% metronidazole gel, or products containing clindamycin or tetracycline may also be helpful.

Follow-up Care

If lesions recur and are painful, or if bleeding pimples come back, a recheck visit should be scheduled with your veterinarian. Notify your veterinarian if any other clinical signs arise.

Prognosis

The prognosis for improvement is good, but affected cats may require lifelong topical therapy. Permanent hair loss and scarring are common after the lesions heal.

SPECIAL INSTRUCTIONS:

Acute Moist Dermatitis in Dogs

Emily Rothstein, DVM, DACVD

BASIC INFORMATION

Description

Acute moist dermatitis is a local skin irritation that arises when some primary problem leads to self-trauma, which initiates an itch-scratch cycle. It can occur in any breed and at any age. The lesion is commonly called a "hot spot."

Causes

Acute moist dermatitis is common in animals with flea allergic dermatitis and ear infections. Other underlying problems include other parasites (such as skin mites), environmental allergy, food allergy, contact dermatitis, anal sac conditions, and problems that cause pets to rub their eyes. Hot spots occur most often in hot and humid weather. Predisposed animals tend to have a dense undercoat, as in the golden retriever, Labrador retriever, German shepherd dog, and Saint Bernard.

Clinical Signs

Acute moist dermatitis is an intensely itchy to sometimes painful irritation of the skin surface. It develops rapidly and has the following features:

- There is hair loss, redness to the skin, and a moist skin surface.
- Lesions typically affect the tail base area, the outer thighs, neck, and face.
- Lesions are often solitary, although multiple lesions can occur.
- The area affected may be related to the underlying cause. Lesions associated with flea allergy or anal sacs disease often occur on the rump and at the base of the tail. Lesions associated with ear infections occur on the neck and head (near the ear).

Diagnostic Tests

Diagnosis is based on the typical appearance of the lesion, a history of a very rapid onset, and extreme itchiness. It is usually a single lesion. The location of the lesion may help narrow down the suspected cause.

TREATMENT AND FOLLOW-UP

Treatment Options

It is important to identify and treat the underlying cause. Hair is clipped from the affected area to allow removal of all surface debris by gentle cleansing with a dilute antimicrobial solution (such as chlorhexidine or povidone-iodine). Clipping and cleaning may require sedation, because these lesions can be quite painful.

Topical astringents such as aluminum acetate 2% (Domeboro solution) may be helpful to dry the area. Sometimes systemic steroids are used (see handout on **Atopic Dermatitis in Dogs**) to break the itch cycle. If there is evidence of a secondary bacterial infection caused by the itching, systemic antibiotics are used. Often, an Elizabethan collar is applied to prevent further trauma and allow the area to heal.

Follow-up Care

Even when the underlying reason for the hot spot is addressed, some dogs repeatedly develop the lesions. Careful attention must be paid to regular grooming, hygiene, flea control, and ear cleaning, especially during hot and humid weather conditions. If systemic antibiotics are instituted, a recheck is often performed to be sure the infection is gone.

Prognosis

The prognosis is excellent for recovery, but diligence is required to prevent or lessen future episodes.

SPECIAL INSTRUCTIONS:

Alopecia X

Emily Rothstein, DVM, DACVD

BASIC INFORMATION

Description

Alopecia X is a disorder of the hair follicles that most likely reflects a defect in the ability of the hair follicle to cycle properly through its growing and resting stages. Alopecia X may be a component of *atypical Cushing's disease*. It occurs in plush-coated breeds, most commonly Pomeranians and Samoyeds, but can occur in any breed of dog. It can also occur at any age.

Causes

One study proposed that the disease results from an adrenal steroid hormone imbalance, but no other systemic signs of hormonal problems have been associated with this disease. In addition, not all animals with this syndrome have classic hormone abnormalities on blood testing.

Clinical Signs

Symmetrical hair loss occurs on both sides of the trunk, around the neck (especially the collar area), backs of the thighs, and under the tail. The underlying skin frequently turns dark with time. The hair coat has a "puppy coat" appearance.

Diagnostic Tests

Initially, some routine skin and laboratory tests are performed to rule out the more common causes of hair loss. A skin biopsy may be performed to document findings consistent with this disease. Specialized hormone tests may be submitted after other diseases that resemble alopecia X have been eliminated.

TREATMENT AND FOLLOW-UP

Treatment Options

Controversy exists as to whether this disease requires treatment, because it is mainly a cosmetic problem. The best choice of therapy is also debated. Drugs such as melatonin, mitotane, and trilostane have been used for this condition. Melatonin can cause hair regrowth in some animals, but the mechanism of action is unknown. It is considered quite safe but can rarely cause an upset stomach in some dogs. Mitotane (Lysodren) causes hair regrowth in some cases, but this treatment is not always recommended, because the drug has potentially serious side effects. Trilostane has been effective in some cases and often has fewer side effects than mitotane.

The decision whether to treat this condition in your dog requires a thoughtful discussion with your veterinarian, as well as careful weighing of the pros and cons of treatment.

Follow-up Care

If a medication other than melatonin is used, follow-up blood tests are needed to monitor for drug side effects.

Prognosis

This is a cosmetic disease only. Even dogs that are treated for the condition often fail to grow normal hair coats again.

SPECIAL INSTRUCTIONS:

Atopic Dermatitis in Dogs

Emily Rothstein, DVM, DACVD

BASIC INFORMATION

Description

Atopic dermatitis is a genetically inherited, recurrent, itchy skin disease that is associated most commonly with an allergy to environmental allergens. The average age at onset is 1-3 years. Predisposed breeds include the boxer, Chihuahua, Gordon setter, Yorkshire terrier, cairn terrier, Boston terrier, Chinese shar-pei, Labrador retriever, golden retriever, West Highland white terrier, English setter, Irish setter, English bulldog, American cocker spaniel, pug, Dalmatian, Scottish terrier, wire fox terrier, miniature schnauzer, Belgian tervuren, Shiba inu, and Beauceron. There is no sex predilection in dogs.

Causes

Allergens are substances in the environment that cause allergic reactions. These can be pollens, house dust and house dust mites, mold spores, even feathers. Allergens cause reactions by sticking to the skin and thereby alerting the skin to that allergen. That is often why a dog will rub its face, lick its feet, and so on.

Clinical Signs

Mild to severe itchiness of the ears, face, axillae (armpits), feet, and belly occurs. Ear infections are common, as are bacterial and yeast infections caused by the scratching. Signs occur either during a specific pollen season or year round, depending on what the pet is allergic to. Common areas affected in the dog are face, the back of the front legs, and where the front legs and chest meet.

Diagnostic Tests

Diagnosis is often based on a history of itching, scratching, licking, and/or biting the body. Itchiness may occur seasonally or year round, depending on what the animal is allergic to. Your veterinarian also must eliminate other itchy skin diseases, such as parasites. Allergy testing can be supportive of the diagnosis and can be done by intradermal skin testing or blood testing. Both tests can give false-positive and false-negative results, however.

TREATMENT AND FOLLOW-UP

Treatment Options

Treatment is designed to make the pet more comfortable. It is not possible to cure environmental allergy, and dogs do not typically outgrow their allergies as humans do. Components of therapy involve the following:

- Allergy shots (immunotherapy) may be formulated based on results of allergy testing. Usually, the owner is taught by the veterinarian, and the shots are given by the owner at home. Initially, a low dose of dilute allergens is given, and then concentration and dose are increased. The rate of increase is scheduled to fit each patient. It may take up to 1 year to see beneficial results.
- Antihistamines can be used long term to control the itch. Sometimes these drugs are used alone, sometimes in conjunction with allergy shots or other therapy (such as fatty acids or steroids).
- Omega-3 fatty acids help reduce skin inflammation, are very safe, and are usually given in conjunction with other therapies.
- Glucocorticoids (steroids, cortisone) can be used in the short tem to control the itch.
- Cyclosporine (*Atopica*) may control clinical signs in some dogs.
- Topical therapy may also be tried. Routine bathing removes allergens. Lime sulfur dips can help reduce the itch. Rinses containing anti-itch medications help some pets but must be applied 1-3 times per week to be effective. Sprays containing steroids and other anti-itch medications can be used frequently to control the itch.
- Treatment of bacterial and yeast infections is often indicated.
- Strict flea control is important, because fleas worsen the problem, especially if the pet is also flea allergic.

Follow-up Care

Atopic dermatitis is a lifelong disease and requires long-term management. Recheck examinations are warranted to minimize flare-ups and to monitor response to treatment. As the seasons rotate and time goes on, modifications to therapy are often needed, so good communication between owner and veterinarian is essential. Occasionally, retesting for new allergies may be needed.

Prognosis

Atopic dermatitis is not curable but is manageable. The many therapeutic options can be tailored to fit different dogs and the abilities of their owners.

SPECIAL INSTRUCTIONS:

Atypical Mycobacteriosis

Emily Rothstein, DVM, DACVD

BASIC INFORMATION

Description

Atypical mycobacteriosis is an uncommon nodular disease of dogs and cats caused by fast-growing mycobacteria that are commonly found in the environment.

Causes

Mycobacteria are a special group of bacteria that have a waxy-type compound in their wall. This family of bacteria includes agents such as tuberculosis and leprosy bacteria. The bacteria involved in atypical mycobacteriosis in animals are related but different from these agents. The bacteria are introduced into the skin by trauma or contamination of a wound.

Clinical Signs

In the cat, skin nodules are most commonly found on the belly. Draining tracts and red-purple bumps that ooze material may be seen. The condition often becomes chronic or returns after attempted treatment.

Lesions in dogs usually develop after trauma or dog bite wounds. Recurrent abscesses, draining tracts, and large bumps that may ooze are the most common findings. In the dog, the bacterial infection may spread to other areas of the body, including the lungs.

Diagnostic Tests

A biopsy is usually needed to confirm the diagnosis. Samples of the skin and deeper tissues are submitted for microscopic examination and often for culture. The bacteria can be difficult to find, so multiple biopsies may be needed.

TREATMENT AND FOLLOW-UP

Treatment Options

Antibiotic treatment is started with drugs commonly effective against mycobacteria. The medication may be changed based on culture and susceptibility tests. It takes a very long time for these infections to resolve, so antibiotics are often given for months. Some animals are never cured, and the infection relapses once antibiotics are discontinued.

Surgical removal of the affected area is helpful, although poor healing is common if all affected tissue is not removed. Sometimes more than one surgery is needed.

Follow-up Care

Frequent rechecks are often needed to monitor the response to treatment and to determine how long to continue the antibiotics.

Prognosis

This disease is not curable, but remissions can occur, meaning that the infection clears up for a time. The prognosis for remission with medical and surgical treatment is better for dogs than for cats. These can be very stubborn and troublesome infections.

SPECIAL INSTRUCTIONS:

Benign Skin Tumors in Dogs

Emily Rothstein, DVM, DACVD

BASIC INFORMATION
Description
Several types of benign skin tumors can develop from skin structures in the dog. *Sebaceous adenomas* are growths involving the sebaceous glands (those glands that produce sebum or a waxy substance for the skin and coat) and the ducts. *Sebaceous epitheliomas* are growths that develop from only a part of the gland, called *basal cells. Sebaceous gland nodular hyperplasia* is a small bump that occurs when the entire gland grows larger and pushes up through the surface of the skin.

Another group of benign tumors, called *hair follicle tumors,* can arise within the hair follicle or hair shaft.

Causes
It is not known why these normal skin structures develop into benign skin tumors.

Clinical Signs
Sebaceous growths are common in older dogs, especially in the cocker spaniel, Siberian husky, miniature poodle, black and tan coonhound, beagle, and dachshund. Sebaceous tumors are uncommon in the cat, but Persian cats may develop them more often than others. These tumors can occur alone or in small groups, are often yellow-pink in color, and are shaped like a cauliflower. They often have a wart-like appearance. Adenomas are small to medium in size (usually less than ½ inch). Epitheliomas are often larger; they may be fingerlike projections or flatlike adenomas. They vary in size from quite small to inches across.

Nodular hyperplasia bumps can resemble sebaceous adenomas or epitheliomas. They usually have a greasy scab on the surface but rarely bother the pet unless they are located between the toes, under the collar, or in some area where they can become irritated. Sometimes, the waxy substance produced may be irritating if it sits on the surface for a while. Some dogs develop dozens of these bumps over their entire body.

Benign hair follicle tumors can range from less than 1 inch to the size of a golf ball or an orange. They often are partially hairless, and if one looks closely, a central depression can usually be seen on the surface. Some of these lesions rupture, exuding gray-white, thick material that may resemble pus but is really material from the hair follicle. The tumors usually occur in middle- to older-aged pets. Some commonly affected breeds are the German shepherd dog, poodles, Kerry blue terrier, Old English sheepdog, and keeshond.

Diagnostic Tests
Removal and biopsy of the tumor allows the exact type to be identified but may not be recommended if the tumor is causing no signs. An aspirate of the mass may be recommended to rule out other skin tumors of similar appearance.

TREATMENT AND FOLLOW-UP

Treatment Options
There may be no need to remove many of these tumors unless they bother the pet or the owner, especially since they usually only cause cosmetic problems. If the tumor bothers the pet, becomes irritated and inflamed, ruptures, or bleeds often, removal may be recommended. Removal may also be recommended for certain sebaceous epitheliomas.

Follow-up Care
Usually, if the tumor is completely removed, no follow-up is required. Most dogs continue to develop more of these tumors throughout their adult lifetime.

Prognosis
The prognosis is good for most of these tumors, because they are benign growths. In rare instances, the sebaceous epithelioma can behave more aggressively and recur at the surgery site or spread elsewhere.

SPECIAL INSTRUCTIONS:

Cheyletiellosis

Emily Rothstein, DVM, DACVD

BASIC INFORMATION

Description
Cheyletiellosis is an infestation of the skin and fur with a surface-dwelling mite. Variable amounts of itching and flakiness occur. The condition is also known as *walking dandruff*.

Causes
Cheyletiella yasguri is the species that affects dogs, and *Cheyletiella blakei* affects cats.

 Clinical Signs

These mites readily pass among dogs, cats, and humans, so the condition is very contagious. Moderate to marked dandruff and hair loss are the classic signs. Cats may develop red skin and small red bumps with scabs. Other cats may only lick lots of hair off their backs without developing dandruff or bumps.

 Diagnostic Tests

Hair and dandruff are collected with the use of acetate tape (such as Scotch tape), a flea comb, or a dull scalpel blade and placed on a glass slide with mineral oil. The mites and/or their eggs can be seen under the microscope. The mites are also sometimes identified in a fecal laboratory test and may be seen without magnification on the skin because they look like "walking dandruff."

TREATMENT AND FOLLOW-UP

 Treatment Options

All dogs and cats in contact with the infected animal are treated. Several topical therapies are available:
- Lime sulfur dips applied weekly for 6 weeks
- Topical antiparasite powder, dip, shampoo, or spray applied weekly for 4 weeks
- Fipronil (*Frontline*) spotted or sprayed on monthly for 2 treatments
- Selamectin (*Revolution*) applied topically every 30 days; response may possibly be improved by applying every 2 weeks for 3 treatments

Other medications not specifically approved for this condition may be tried, either orally or by injection. The environment must also be treated with an insecticide spray or fogger that is effective against fleas.

 Follow-up Care

The pet is checked after 3-4 weeks of therapy to be sure the dandruff and itchiness are improving.

Prognosis
Prognosis is very good as long as all animals in the household and the local environment are treated.

SPECIAL INSTRUCTIONS:

Claw (Toenail) Disease, Asymmetrical

Emily Rothstein, DVM, DACVD

BASIC INFORMATION

Description

The disease is an abnormality in one claw or multiple claws on one paw. The claws or toenails on the other paws are normal. It occurs in both dogs and cats.

Causes

Secondary bacterial infections are the most common cause. This disease can be caused by trauma to the claw, which often leads to infection. Examples of trauma included bite wounds, crush injuries, torn claws, exposure to chemicals, and burns from heat. Fungal infections are less common causes. Tumors of the foot may also affect the claws.

Clinical Signs

Lameness, pain, and licking or biting of the claw occur in varying degrees, depending on the cause. The skin around the claw can be swollen, red, scabbing, and/or oozing. The hair may be lost around the claw. Swollen glands (nearby lymph nodes) are possible, and occasionally fever, depression, and decreased appetite are seen.

Diagnostic Tests

A known traumatic event to the claw can suggest the cause. Examination of debris from the fold of skin at the base of the claw under the microscope may be helpful, especially if evidence of bacterial or fungal infection or cancer cells are found. Sometimes bacterial and fungal cultures are submitted. X-rays of the area are sometimes needed. Biopsy of the skin and claw may be done in certain cases.

TREATMENT AND FOLLOW-UP

Treatment Options

A common treatment is removal of any broken, loose, or painful claws. Sometimes the claws are so loose that they can simply be pulled off. More often, the toe is too sore to allow this, so the animal must be sedated and the claw removed. Foot soaks may make the pet more comfortable. If bacterial infection is present, appropriate antibiotics are given for at least 4-8 weeks and 2 weeks beyond clinical cure. If there is a fungal infection, antifungal agents are typically given for up to 3-6 months. Rarely, treatment may require amputation of the end of the toe for tumors or to resolve difficult fungal infections.

Follow-up Care

Recheck visits are needed for those pets with infection, because the infection can be difficult to resolve. Some dogs with certain tumors are monitored for metastasis (spread) by checking lymph nodes and performing chest x-rays periodically (depending on the tumor).

Prognosis

Prognosis is usually very good for bacterial infection, as long as antibiotics are given long enough. Fungal infections can be very difficult to cure. Some cancers are cured by removal, and some require long-term monitoring.

SPECIAL INSTRUCTIONS:

Claw (Toenail) Disease, Symmetrical

Emily Rothstein, DVM, DACVD

BASIC INFORMATION

Description

This disease includes any abnormalities that affect multiple claws on multiple paws.

Causes

Widespread claw disease often develops because of other underlying diseases. Examples include:

- Inherited disorders of the skin, such as dermatomyositis of the Shetland sheepdog and collie and acrodermatitis of bull terriers
- Hormonal disorders, such as hypothyroidism (low thyroid hormone levels) and Cushing's disease (high cortisone levels) in the dog, hyperthyroidism (high thyroid hormone levels) in the cat, and sugar diabetes (diabetes mellitus)
- Allergic skin disease
- Zinc deficiency in the dog
- Parasitic skin diseases, such as demodicosis (mites) in the dog
- Feline immunodeficiency virus (FIV) and feline leukemia virus (FeLV) infections in the cat
- Immune-mediated skin disorders, such as pemphigus foliaceus (especially in the cat) and pemphigus vulgaris
- Miscellaneous conditions of unknown cause

Clinical Signs

Lameness, pain, and licking or biting of the claws may be seen, depending on the cause. The skin around the claws can be swollen, red, scabby, and/or oozing. Hair loss around the claws is common. Glands (lymph nodes) nearest the affected claws may be swollen, and occasionally fever, depression, and decreased appetite are seen. Signs of the underlying disease process are also present.

Diagnostic Tests

Debris from the skin folds around the claws and scrapings of the skin can be examined under the microscope for infection, mites, and cells that are seen with immune diseases. Laboratory tests are usually needed to look for possible underlying diseases and causes. Biopsy of the claw and skin can also be helpful.

TREATMENT AND FOLLOW-UP

Treatment Options

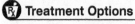

Treatment of secondary bacterial infections is important. Immune-mediated diseases require aggressive therapy to suppress the immune system, which often involves steroids and other medications.

Other therapies may be tried depending on the underlying cause and whether a specific cause can be determined. For example, if a food allergy is suspected, a food elimination trial may be done for at least 8 weeks. Omega-6 and omega-3 fatty acid supplements can be tried for a minimum of 3-4 months. Oral vitamin E can be tried. Oral tetracycline and niacinamide or pentoxifylline may be helpful in some cases. Gelatin (Knox) or biotin may be given to strengthen the claws.

If the disease does not respond to conventional therapy and affects only a few claws, a declaw procedure with removal of the tip of the toe and claw may be considered. If a tumor is suspected or confirmed based on x-rays and a biopsy, then a toe amputation is often performed.

Follow-up Care

Claws grow very slowly, so it is important to monitor them every few months for improvement. Typically, rechecks are performed every 2-3 months until the disease is controlled, which can take a long time. Many cases are not cured, so rechecks may be needed every 6-12 months.

Since all of the medications used to treat the immune-mediated diseases have potential side effects, blood and urine tests are monitored, sometimes every 2 weeks. The dosages of medication are tapered as the pet's signs improve, and the animal is monitored for worsening of the signs, which may require increasing the medication again. With certain underlying causes or conditions (such as pemphigus, allergy, inherited disorders), therapy is lifelong.

Prognosis

Usually, unless the diseased claw is removed, treatment is for life. It is hard to predict which pets will do well. Most of diseases that cause claw problems can be managed (such as allergies, hormonal diseases, or pemphigus foliaceus), and the pet remains comfortable. Some diseases are more serious (such as pemphigus vulgaris or acrodermatitis of bull terriers), and eventually the pet is euthanized.

SPECIAL INSTRUCTIONS:

Cutaneous or Discoid Lupus Erythematosus

Emily Rothstein, DVM, DACVD

BASIC INFORMATION

Description

Cutaneous lupus erythematosus is an ulcerative skin disease that involves the hairless, "button" part of the nose of dogs and cats. In severe cases, the skin around the nose, lips, and parts of the mouth may be affected.

Causes

Discoid lupus is likely caused by a combination of genetic factors and the effects of sunlight on the skin, which may induce a destructive immune response. The condition occurs most often in the collie, Shetland sheepdog, German shepherd dog, and Siberian husky. The immune system attacks the bottom layer of the skin (epidermis) with secondary erosions and ulcerations.

Clinical Signs

Early lesions include redness and loss of pigment of the skin and nose. As lesions worsen, the cobblestone architecture of the tip of the nose is lost. Later, skin may become quite raw, and scabs can be seen.

Diagnostic Tests

The clinical appearance can suggest the diagnosis, but a biopsy is needed to absolutely determine the presence of this condition, since several other diseases create a similar appearance. Specialized examination of the biopsy specimens may be needed to determine the presence of an autoimmune reaction in which the immune system is attacking the skin cells. Other laboratory tests may be recommended prior to starting therapy to determine whether it is safe to start certain medications.

TREATMENT AND FOLLOW-UP

Treatment Options

Avoiding exposure to the sun and using sunscreens are important measures to protect the skin from ultraviolet light. Topical therapy (applied directly to the skin) with steroids or immune-modulating drugs may be successful in mild cases. Systemic therapy with oral vitamin E, steroids, and other immune-suppressive drugs is indicated if topical therapy is ineffective and for severe cases. Numerous drug options are available for this disease, and some of them have potential side effects that require careful monitoring.

Follow-up Care

After treatment has been started, recheck visits are usually scheduled about every 2-4 weeks to evaluate the response to therapy. Once clinical remission has been achieved, the visits are often continued at 1-month intervals as the drug dosages are being tapered, and then every 6 months during maintenance therapy. If systemic therapy is used, laboratory tests are periodically needed to monitor for side effects from the medications and to make sure no secondary infections are starting.

Prognosis

This disease can usually be successfully controlled, but a cure is not expected. Prolonged treatment and monitoring are typically required, with periodic adjustment of medications and their dosages.

SPECIAL INSTRUCTIONS:

Cutaneous (Epitheliotropic) T-Cell Lymphoma

Emily Rothstein, DVM, DACVD

BASIC INFORMATION
Description and Causes

This disease is an uncommon skin cancer and a form of lymphoma. It is a malignancy of a particular type of white blood cell, the T-cell lymphocyte. It affects both dogs and cats. In the past, the disease was known as *mycosis fungoides*.

Clinical Signs

In dogs, four different clinical presentations have been described:
- A red, scaling, flaking, and itchy form
- A form involving the junction between mucous membranes (the smooth, hairless tissues of the lips, eyelids, ears, vulva, and so on) and skin that causes redness, loss of pigment, and ulceration
- A form of single or multiple raised nodules or bumps
- A form in which red, thickened, raw lesions develop in the mouth and thickening of the foot pads occurs, with loss of pigment

Cats often develop well-defined bumps within the skin of the head and neck that are surrounded by hair loss, redness, and dandruff. In both dogs and cats, the glands (lymph nodes) may be enlarged, and the animal may not feel well.

Diagnostic Tests

Because this disease is so rare, it is not very high on anyone's list of suspicions. It is common for routine tests to be performed first for the more common skin diseases and for laboratory tests to be submitted looking for the cause. If these do not reveal a cause, skin biopsy is often recommended. Examination of the biopsy reveals the presence of skin lymphoma, although special testing may be required to confirm that it involves T cells. Once the diagnosis is made, further testing may be needed to prove that the cancer involves only the skin.

TREATMENT AND FOLLOW-UP

Treatment Options

Treatment of this disease involves chemotherapy. The most common drug chosen is lomustine (CCNU), but several other drugs (such as prednisone, cyclophosphamide, vincristine, chlorambucil, doxorubicin, and methotrexate) have shown some success. Some of the chemotherapeutic drugs are given orally, whereas others must be given intravenously. Each is given at a different frequency, in a strict protocol that will be outlined by your veterinarian. Throughout chemotherapy, blood tests must be run to monitor for the side effects of these drugs.

Follow-up Care

Recheck visits are needed in some cases to administer the chemotherapy and in all cases to monitor the skin for response to treatment. Blood samples are also drawn at the recheck visits to monitor for side effects from the chemotherapy.

Prognosis

Prognosis is variable. Animals diagnosed late in the course may survive only 5-10 months. Mildly affected dogs may survive for longer periods. This disease is not usually cured; the primary goal of treatment is to maintain a good quality of life for as long as possible.

SPECIAL INSTRUCTIONS:

Cyclical Flank Alopecia

Emily Rothstein, DVM, DACVD

BASIC INFORMATION

Description

This disorder is also called *seasonal flank alopecia* or *canine recurrent flank alopecia*. It is a hair follicle abnormality that causes hair loss (alopecia) on the trunk of the body. The hair loss is usually symmetrical (same pattern on both sides of the trunk) and seasonal. It is not itchy, and increased darkening (pigmentation) of the skin often occurs in the area of hair loss.

It is most common in the English bulldog, French bulldog, boxer, and Airedale terrier. It also has been seen in the miniature schnauzer, miniature poodle, Doberman pinscher, Bouvier de Flandres, Scottish terrier, Staffordshire bull terrier, Affenpinscher, and a few other breeds.

Causes

The underlying cause of this condition is poorly understood. Because of a higher incidence in certain breeds, a genetic influence is suspected. Since the hair loss happens most commonly in fall and spring and occurs more often at certain latitudes of the world, the seasons of the year probably also influence the condition.

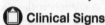 Clinical Signs

Typically, a symmetrical hair loss occurs on both sides of the dog in the "saddle region" of the trunk, with subsequent darkening of the underlying skin. Rarely, it occurs on one side only or along the top of the dog's back. The hair loss usually has a well demarcated border that may resemble a map. Spontaneous regrowth of hair usually occurs within 3-8 months.

The condition often occurs every year at about the same time (either spring or fall), yet some animals (20%) lose their hair only once. Sometimes the hair loss skips a year. The extent of the hair loss can vary from year to year.

Diagnostic Tests

Diagnosis is based on the following factors: classic clinical signs occurring in a dog of a compatible breed, a seasonal history, elimination of other possible causes of the hair loss, and a biopsy of the skin. Timing of the biopsy can be important, because a biopsy taken late in the seasonal cycle of hair loss can show normal skin since the hair is about to grow in.

TREATMENT AND FOLLOW-UP

Treatment Options

The hair typically regrows on its own at the end of the season. Since this hair loss is only a cosmetic condition, no therapy is usually needed. Melatonin therapy is effective in some dogs if started before hair loss begins; therefore, it must be started before the typical start of the seasonal cycle.

Follow-up Care

No follow-up is necessary for those dogs whose seasonal hair loss is predictable. Dogs that do not regrow hair in 3-8 months should be evaluated for other diseases that mimic this one.

Prognosis

Prognosis is excellent, because the disorder does not affect the rest of the skin or dog, and the hair loss is cosmetic only.

SPECIAL INSTRUCTIONS:

Deep Bacterial Pyoderma and Furunculosis

Emily Rothstein, DVM, DACVD

BASIC INFORMATION

Description

This disease involves the deeper tissues of the skin and is usually caused by a bacterial infection. Furunculosis is inflammation and infection that arises after a hair follicle ruptures. A furuncle is an infected swelling that involves a hair follicle and is commonly known as a *boil*.

Causes

Deep pyoderma most often begins as a superficial bacterial skin infection, especially one that involves the hair follicles of the dog. After a hair follicle fills with infection, it ruptures and creates a more widespread reaction under the surface of the skin. This reaction is very irritating and causes further inflammation and infection. These conditions usually arise secondary to other skin diseases such as demodicosis or hypothyroidism.

Clinical Signs

The condition may be restricted to only a certain area on the surface of the body, or it may be generalized. Red bumps, pimples, hair loss, lesions resembling blood blisters, and bleeding, scabbing, and tenderness of the skin are often seen. Sometimes the pet is itchy. Lymph nodes (glands) are often enlarged, especially those closest to the infection.

Diagnostic Tests

A presumptive diagnosis can often be made based on typical physical examination findings. More specific tests, such as examining skin material under the microscope on a slide or skin biopsy, are helpful to confirm the diagnosis. Bacterial culture of the skin helps to identify the specific bacteria involved and aids in selection of the proper systemic antibiotic. Other testing may be needed to search for an underlying or contributing cause.

TREATMENT AND FOLLOW-UP

Treatment Options

Any underlying cause must be identified and treated. Antibiotics are given for a minimum of 4 weeks or for 2 weeks or more after complete resolution of all clinical signs. Antibiotics are often given for a total of 6-12 weeks.

Antiseptic shampoos (such as those containing benzoyl peroxide, chlorhexidine, or ethyl lactate) may be used once or twice weekly to aid in removal of scabs and debris as the animal heals.

Follow-up Care

Monitoring of both the infection and any underlying cause is done via recheck visits. If the problem comes back shortly after discontinuation of medication (within 2-4 weeks), notify your veterinarian, because this may indicate that the infection was not cleared, and many months of therapy may be needed.

Prognosis

If the underlying cause can be corrected, then the prognosis is good, and the infection often resolves with prolonged antibiotic therapy. If the underlying cause cannot be identified or treated, then the condition usually recurs. Scarring and permanent hair loss can result from these infections.

In some dogs, the infections recur soon after therapy is finished, and they must be retreated. Some animals may be treated on and off for life whenever clinical signs recur.

SPECIAL INSTRUCTIONS:

Demodicosis in Dogs

Emily Rothstein, DVM, DACVD

BASIC INFORMATION
Description and Causes

Demodicosis is the proliferation of *Demodex canis* mites in hair follicles. Dogs that develop clinical signs may have localized or generalized lesions. *Demodex* mites are passed from the mother to the puppy within the first few days of birth, so dogs that are born by cesarean section and not allowed to nurse do not have these mites. The presence of very low numbers of *Demodex* mites on dogs is considered normal.

Clinical demodicosis occurs when the number of mites increases to excessive levels. Dogs that develop juvenile-onset, generalized disease appear to be genetically predisposed to the condition. Adult-onset demodicosis is frequently associated with poor immune function (immunosuppression) resulting from underlying conditions such as Cushing's disease, hypothyroidism, immunosuppressive drugs, or cancer.

Clinical Signs

Demodicosis is called *localized* when hair loss occurs only in isolated, patchy areas. Comedones (blackheads) may also be present. Pimples and small red bumps may occur and indicate a secondary bacterial infection. Localized demodicosis is rarely itchy.

With generalized demodicosis, hair loss and lesions may occur over the body and be extensive. Blackheads, pimples, red bumps, and bleeding areas may be present. Scabs often indicate secondary infection, which can cause itchiness.

Diagnostic Tests

Diagnosis is based on finding *Demodex canis* mites in samples taken from the skin. Samples are taken by scraping the skin or plucking hairs and are examined under the microscope. Rarely, a skin biopsy is needed to identify the mite. Other laboratory testing may be indicated in dogs with adult-onset demodicosis.

TREATMENT AND FOLLOW-UP

Treatment Options

Localized and demodicosis are treated differently:

- For localized disease, rotenone ointment (*Goodwinol*) can be applied to one or two lesions; however, areas of hair loss may become larger, because the hair may be rubbed off during the application process.
- Benzoyl peroxide gel (*Pyoben, Oxydex*) can be applied once daily to areas of hair loss. It does not kill or remove the mites from the follicles but helps to limit secondary infection and

unplugs hair follicles. This product bleaches fabric, so make certain that the product dries completely after application.
- Many cases of localized demodicosis are self-limited and require only monitoring. Because localized demodicosis may progress to a generalized form, be sure to watch for new areas of hair loss or the development of blackheads.

For dogs with generalized demodicosis of juvenile onset, all secondary bacterial infections are treated, and efforts are made to improve the overall health of the animal. Measures that your veterinarian may discuss with you include deworming, vaccinations, nutrition, and spaying or neutering. The demodicosis is specifically treated with amitraz (*Mitaban*) dips, as follows:

- The hair must be trimmed very short, after which the dog is bathed in a benzoyl peroxide–based shampoo and towel dried.
- Mix one bottle of Mitaban with 2 gallons of warm water.
- Sponge the mixture onto the dog, making sure to wet all skin surfaces.
- Allow the dog to air dry, and keep it from getting wet between dips.
- Repeat dips every 2 weeks until two negative skin scrapings occur 2 weeks apart; follow with one more dip.
- Sedation is a likely side effect, but occasionally a dog has more serious signs such as vomiting, severe itching, or seizures. Small dogs are more susceptible to these side effects, and sometimes it is best to dip small dogs in the hospital and closely monitor them for 24 hours afterward. Notify your veterinarian if any of these signs occur.

In cases of adult-onset generalized demodicosis, all secondary bacterial infections are treated. Sometimes infections are so severe that they must be treated first, with amitraz dips delayed for awhile. Any underlying cause must also be addressed. Several other products are available for treating demodicosis but have not been specifically approved for this disease. Your veterinarian may discuss these options if the amitraz treatment is unsuccessful.

Follow-up Care

Successful management of demodicosis can be difficult. Localized cases are rechecked every few weeks until the dog outgrows the disease. Dogs with juvenile-onset generalized disease are usually rechecked monthly until secondary infections are resolved, then every 4-8 weeks throughout the course of therapy. Some animals with generalized disease are not cured and must be treated periodically for life to control the lesions.

Prognosis

Prognosis is very good for puppies with localized demodicosis. Eighty-five percent of dogs with juvenile-onset generalized demodicosis are cured. Resolution of adult-onset cases varies based on the overall health of the animal.

SPECIAL INSTRUCTIONS:

Dermatophytosis

Emily Rothstein, DVM, DACVD

BASIC INFORMATION

Description

Dermatophytosis is a fungal skin infection of dogs and cats that targets the growing hairs and the surface of the skin. The common name for this infection is *ringworm*, because the lesions often have a ring or round shape in people.

Causes

The most common causes are *Microsporum canis* (obtained from animals such as cats), *Microsporum gypsum* (obtained from the soil), and *Trichophyton mentagrophytes* (obtained from animals such as cattle or horses). These fungi are called *dermatophytes*.

All dermatophytes are contagious to humans. Dermatophytes infect only growing hairs, so when the hair stops growing or falls out, the infection resolves. Drugs and diseases that suppress immunity increase the risk of persistent dermatophytosis. Trauma and skin irritation (even bathing or grooming) may help establish a dermatophyte infection.

Clinical Signs

Hair loss is the most common sign but is variable. Dandruff, crusty scaling, and itchiness can occur and are also variable. Pimples, red bumps, scabs, scrapes or hair loss from licking, and increased pigmentation of skin can be seen.

Diagnostic Tests

Definitive diagnosis is made by fungal culture, which allows identification of the genus and species of the dermatophyte. The growth of the fungus on a culture typically takes 2-4 weeks and can be performed at the veterinarian's office or at an outside laboratory. Some cultures can be completed in a few days, but their accuracy is considered poor. Wood's lamp examination can be done in the examination room and involves using a cobalt-blue light to identify dermatophytes that fluoresce. However, it only identifies some varieties of *Microsporum canis*. False-negative results are common, and false-positives can also occur.

TREATMENT AND FOLLOW-UP

Treatment Options

Topical therapy is used for focal lesions. Drugs with good antifungal activity include clotrimazole, ketoconazole, and miconazole. Lime sulfur dip can also be used, and it is applied weekly until two negative fungal cultures are achieved 1 month apart. Precautions associated with lime sulfur include the following:

- Do not allow cats to self-groom while the product is still wet.
- The product can tarnish jewelry and stain fabric.
- The strong sulfur odor is somewhat offensive.

Agents that have less activity against dermatophytes and have limited use include thiabendazole, iodine products, and chlorhexidine products.

Oral medications are commonly used for widespread or persistent infections. Examples include griseofulvin, ketoconazole, itraconazole, fluconazole, and terbinafine. These medications are usually continued for 2 weeks after a negative fungal culture is achieved. Precautions associated with these drugs include the following:

- Griseofulvin has potential adverse effects on the bone marrow (where many types of blood cells are produced).
- Ketoconazole is preferred in the dog but must be used with caution in cats. Side effects include vomiting, decreased appetite, and, in rare cases, liver disease.
- Itraconazole and fluconazole are similar to ketoconazole; however, cats tolerate itraconazole better. Vomiting, loss of appetite, and liver disease can still occur with itraconazole. Fluconazole is typically used in dogs that do not tolerate ketoconazole.
- Terbinafine is costly and is infrequently used in dogs or cats to treat ringworm, but there may be fewer adverse effects on the liver with this drug.
- Be sure to notify your veterinarian and stop the medication if any of these side effects are encountered.

Environmental control is also important. Affected cats should be isolated from other animals, and all furred pets in the home should be treated. The environment must be cleaned of hairs and spores, which can harbor the ringworm for months. Cleaning with a 1:10 bleach solution can be effective but is not appropriate for all surfaces. Infected animals should not be allowed to infect other animals, especially at kennels, shows, and dog parks.

Follow-up Care

Repeated cultures must be performed to monitor response to therapy, because therapy is recommended until two negative cultures are obtained 1 month apart. Laboratory tests are often needed to monitor for the side effects of these medications.

Prognosis

Prognosis is very good for a cure; however, some purebred cats can be difficult to treat. Some cats look worse early in the therapy as infected hairs fall out, but new hair usually begins to grow after 1-2 months. Follow-up cultures are essential when deciding when therapy can be stopped, because the pet may looks better weeks before the fungus is actually gone.

SPECIAL INSTRUCTIONS:

Eosinophilic Granuloma Complex in Cats

Emily Rothstein, DVM, DACVD

BASIC INFORMATION

Description

Eosinophilic granuloma complex derives its name from the classic finding of white blood cells called *eosinophils* in these skin lesions. A granuloma is a firm nodule of inflammation. The word "complex" was added to the name when it was discovered that flat lesions and ulcerated lesions may also occur. The flat lesions are often called *eosinophilic plaques,* and the ulcerated lesions have been called *indolent, rodent,* or *eosinophilic ulcers.* Although eosinophilic granulomas can occur in other species, this particular complex of lesions occurs only in the cat.

Causes

The underlying cause of this condition is believed to be a form of an allergic reaction; that is, the immune system overreacts to something to which the cat is exposed. Possible inciting agents include the following:

- Environmental allergens
- Foods
- External skin parasites, such as fleas, mites, or lice
- Bacterial skin infections
- Fungal infections of the skin, such as ringworm
- Viral infections, such as feline leukemia virus or feline immunodeficiency virus

🗋 Clinical Signs

The three types of lesions of this complex cannot always be differentiated based on their appearance, but some features are classic for each:

- *Eosinophilic granulomas* may be round or linear (oblong). The lesions are typically red, hairless, and raw (ulcerated). Most granulomas are not itchy. The most common lesion is a swelling of the chin area ("pouty chin"). Linear red, raised lesions may be found on the backs of the legs. The foot pads may also be affected.
- *Eosinophilic plaques* are often hairless, raised, raw sores within the skin. Lesions are commonly located on the belly, the insides of the thighs and armpits, and on the neck and back. Itchiness is a common feature of the plaques.
- An *indolent eosinophilic ulcer* occurs as a raw depression or erosion in the skin of the lips. It is typically found on the upper lip, but the roof of the mouth or back of throat may be involved.

These lesions are not usually itchy or painful. Nearby glands (lymph nodes) may be enlarged.

Diagnostic Tests

The general appearance of these lesions is frequently suggestive of the diagnosis, but testing is often needed to confirm the diagnosis. Sometimes eosinophils are found when smears of the lesions are examined under the microscope. Eosinophil numbers are occasionally elevated in a blood count. A skin biopsy usually confirms the diagnosis.

TREATMENT AND FOLLOW-UP

℞ Treatment Options

Treatment involves several different steps. It is important to decrease exposure to and control any underlying allergies. Antibiotics may be administered in some cases for 2-4 weeks. Steroid medications are needed to shrink the lesions, and several different types of steroids are available.

If the lesions do not respond to the steroids or if steroids become less effective over time, other drugs may be tried that modify the immune response. Small unresponsive lesions may also be treated by surgical removal, laser therapy, cryotherapy (freezing of the tissue), or radiation therapy.

🐾 Follow-up Care

It may take your pet 2, 4, or 6 weeks to show a response to therapy. It is very important that the underlying allergy be managed, as well as the actual lesions. Therapy is needed as long as allergy control is inadequate; when allergy control is good, recurrences are uncommon. If immune-suppressive drugs are given, monitoring of body weight, appetite, and certain blood values is required.

Prognosis

With adequate control of the underlying allergy, the prognosis is good; however, some allergies are difficult to identify and control. If the lesions are a result of food allergy or flea allergy, changing the food to a special diet or eliminating fleas usually prevents a recurrence. Since environmental allergies are more difficult to control, lesions associated with them are more likely to recur.

SPECIAL INSTRUCTIONS:

Exfoliative Cutaneous Lupus Erythematosus

Emily Rothstein, DVM, DACVD

BASIC INFORMATION

Description
Exfoliative lupus erythematosus is a generalized (widespread) skin disease that produces a lot of dandruff or flakiness. It was initially reported as a hereditary disease in the German shorthaired pointer and was called *lupoid dermatosis*. So far, this breed is the only one affected.

Causes
Why the disease arises is poorly understood, although a hereditary component is suspected. The skin lesions probably develop secondary to an immune reaction, but the triggering event is unknown.

Clinical Signs
Young, female dogs may be affected more often. Severe dandruff, hair loss, scabs, and occasionally oozing from the skin are seen. These lesions can vary in severity and occur on the muzzle and ear flaps and along the back. Lesions may also become widespread. Enlarged glands (lymph nodes), pain or discomfort, itchiness, and fever may also be seen in some cases.

Diagnostic Tests
The breed and age of dog, together with the clinical signs listed, usually are suggestive of the diagnosis. It is important to rule out other causes of dandruff, such *Demodex* mites, ringworm, and bacterial infections, so testing may be performed for these other conditions. Results of a skin biopsy usually confirm the diagnosis, but specialized stains may be required to document the immune reaction. Other laboratory tests may be recommended prior to starting therapy, to determine whether it is safe to start certain medications.

TREATMENT AND PROGNOSIS

Treatment Options
The disease does not respond well to any current treatments. Antiseborrheic shampoos (which often contain sulfur or salicylic acid) help to remove excess dandruff and skin scales. Oral treatments may be tried, such as fatty acid supplements, steroids, and other immune-suppressive medications. Monitoring of blood tests is needed when immune-suppressive medications are used.

Prognosis
Therapy may help the symptoms, but a waxing-and-waning course is typical. Many dogs are eventually euthanized because of the disease.

SPECIAL INSTRUCTIONS:

Flea Allergic Dermatitis

Emily Rothstein, DVM, DACVD

BASIC INFORMATION
Description and Cause

Flea allergic dermatitis arises from an adverse immunologic response to flea saliva. It is an extremely itchy dermatitis that follows exposure to fleas. It arises most often in dogs and cats aged 6 months to 5 years. In the northern United States, is often a seasonal disease, occurring from May until the first freeze, but it can occur all year round in warmer areas.

Clinical Signs

Dogs have moderate to severe itchiness, papules (little red bumps), redness, and self-trauma from biting and scratching in the affected areas. Most commonly affected locations in dogs are the base of the tail, over the back, the backs of the thighs, and the front legs. Hair loss, scratched skin, increase in skin pigmentation (blackening), and scaling (dandruff) are commonly seen.

In cats, head and neck itching, very red lesions on the belly, and tiny bumps with scabs can be seen.

Diagnostic Tests

The diagnosis is often made from circumstantial evidence, such as suspicious history and physical examination findings, particularly lesion distribution, response to flea control, and presence of fleas and flea "dirt" (especially with use of a flea comb). Flea dirt is actually flea feces. They are small black flecks that resemble dirt, but, when a drop of water is added, they reconstitute to a bloody liquid.

TREATMENT AND FOLLOW-UP

Treatment Options

Flea control on the individual animal and any house mates must be aggressively pursued and can involve the following:

- Topical agents include baths and sprays. (See the **Flea Product Chart** that accompanies this handout.) Note that some products made for dogs *must not* be applied to cats.
- Oral agents kill fleas immediately or help reduce their reproduction.
- Many of these agents can be used together. Your veterinarian will help you pick the best program for your pet or pets.

Environmental flea control is also extremely important, and your veterinarian may choose from the following options:

- Adulticides kill adult fleas. These products are synthetic pyrethrins and have a quick killing action. They (especially permethrin) are toxic to cats in any concentration stronger that 0.5%. They are stable for use indoors and out and are available from veterinarians, pet stores, and home supply stores.
- Juvenile hormone analogues kill eggs and immature or larval forms. Methoprene is for indoor use only. Pyripoxiyfen and fenoxycarb may be used indoors or outdoors.
- Outdoor organic control can be accomplished by using nematodes, called *Steinernema carpocapsae,* that kill the immature forms of fleas. Nontoxic indoor control can be accomplished with sodium borate products made for flea control.
- Fleas like humid environments and moist, organic matter. It is important to clean any of these areas that may be in the yard (such as under porches or decks).
- Severe itchiness may require temporary treatment with steroids and baths.

Follow-up Care

If the pet does not improve, it should be re-evaluated. Problems with administration of flea products, environmental control, or the presence of an additional allergy could explain a poor response.

Prognosis

Prognosis is good to excellent with good flea control, but it is important to apply the products exactly as instructed, for the sake of both your pet and the environment. Because it only takes the saliva from one flea bite to exacerbate the problem, complete flea control is essential.

SPECIAL INSTRUCTIONS:

Food Reactions, Adverse

Emily Rothstein, DVM, DACVD

BASIC INFORMATION

Description

Adverse food reactions, also known as *food allergy*, cause a year-round, itchy skin condition in dogs and cats. The reaction is associated with ingestion of a substance found in the animal's diet.

Causes

Beef, fish, chicken, eggs, and dairy products are the allergens to which dogs and cats most commonly develop adverse reactions. However, anything the pet eats on a regular basis can cause the allergic reaction.

🗋 Clinical Signs

No breed or gender is predisposed, and reactions can occur at any age. When the onset is in dogs younger than 6 months or older than 6 years of age, food allergy is a more likely possibility than environmental allergies. The itching is nonseasonal, because the pet typically eats the allergenic substance every day. The itchiness can be mild to very intense. The pet may develop small pimples or reddened areas that eventually become scrapes and scabs. Often, the itching leads to secondary infections of the skin and ears. Gastrointestinal signs (vomiting, diarrhea, increased frequency of bowel movements) can be seen in 10-15% of affected pets.

🔬 Diagnostic Tests

The only way to accurately diagnose the condition is through a food trial:

- The trial is done either by preparing a home-cooked diet containing a protein the pet has never eaten and a specially chosen starch (usually white potatoes) or by feeding a hypoallergenic prescription diet (available through a veterinarian).
- Proteins chosen for the trial may include venison; rabbit; goat; pinto, navy, or garbanzo beans; ostrich; or alligator.

- The food trial usually lasts 8-10 weeks and does not allow *any* treats, chew toys (other than rubber or plastic) and not even chewable heartworm medications. Any accompanying bacterial infections must be treated and resolved by the end of the trial.

Clinical improvement is suggestive of the diagnosis; however, to confirm the diagnosis, the original diet must be fed again, to prove that the itchy skin condition will return and is associated with the original diet.

TREATMENT AND FOLLOW-UP

℞ Treatment Options

Food allergy is the easiest allergy to manage, because the offending food can almost always be avoided through the feeding of special foods. Strict control of every item that enters a pet's mouth will avoid relapses.

If needed, additional medications, baths, or rinses can be used (similar to the treatments for atopic dermatitis) until the skin and hair coat return to normal and all itchiness subsides.

🐾 Follow-up Care

Periodic rechecks are done until the animal has returned to normal and may be repeated with any return of the symptoms.

Prognosis

The prognosis is excellent as long as the offending protein is avoided. Everyone in contact with the pet must be educated as to which food or foods the pet must avoid. Care must be taken not to give the pet treats or chew toys that contain the allergen (such as beef-basted rawhide chews). Food allergy is more difficult to control in dogs and cats that roam free and may receive treats or food away from home or are allowed to raid the garbage at the neighbors' houses. The condition can also be harder to combat in households with small children who drop foodstuffs on the floor or surreptitiously feed the pet.

SPECIAL INSTRUCTIONS:

Juvenile Cellulitis

Emily Rothstein, DVM, DACVD

BASIC INFORMATION
Description
Juvenile cellulitis is an uncommon form of inflammation of the skin tissues in young puppies, usually 3-16 weeks of age. It most commonly occurs in purebred dogs. It has also been called *puppy strangles,* because the glands (lymph nodes) under the jaw may become enlarged and appear to be strangling the dog.

Cause
The cause is unknown. It may represent an abnormal immune response.

Clinical Signs
A sudden onset of pimples and discharge occurs on the lips and eyelids, in the ear canals, and on the muzzle. The lesions can burst and drain or ooze. Lymph nodes (glands) in nearby areas are commonly enlarged. Most puppies seem to feel ill with this condition. They may act as if they are uncomfortable, have a fever, lose their appetite, or become depressed, and some exhibit joint pain.

Diagnostic Tests
A presumptive diagnosis is often made from the typical clinical signs and age of the dog. A definitive diagnosis can be made by skin biopsy, when needed. Some testing may be required to rule out other causes of enlarged glands or other skin diseases that can occur in puppies of this age.

TREATMENT AND FOLLOW-UP

Treatment Options
Secondary bacterial infections can occur in this condition, and they are treated with antibiotics. Wash affected areas gently each day (if the area is not too tender) to remove the scabs. An antibacterial shampoo that contains chlorhexidine or benzoyl peroxide may be used. Steroid medications are usually given for 1-4 weeks until the condition is controlled, and then the dosage is decreased slowly over several weeks.

Follow-up Care
Some cases can be hard to control at first, and various steroid medications may be tried to find which one works the best. Recheck visits are often needed to monitor progress, especially as the steroids are decreased.

Prognosis
The prognosis for a complete cure is good. In severe cases, healing may be associated with permanent scarring of the skin of the face.

SPECIAL INSTRUCTIONS:

Lipomas in Dogs

Emily Rothstein, DVM, DACVD

BASIC INFORMATION

Description

Lipomas are benign tumors that arise from the growth of fat cells. They are more common in overweight, middle-aged to older dogs. The breeds most often affected are the Labrador retriever, Doberman pincher, miniature schnauzer, cocker spaniel, dachshund, and Weimaraner. Although only one tumor may be present, more often several of them develop over time.

Cause

The exact cause is unknown. It is not well defined what impact obesity has on these tumors, but in both conditions the numbers of fat cells in the body are increased.

Clinical Signs

Lipomas are well-defined, oval or round growths that can be felt under the skin (subcutaneous area). They usually feel smooth, soft or rubbery, and can be easily moved around under the skin. Most occur on the trunk (body) of the dog, especially under the chest. They can also occur on the legs and occasionally in the neck region. Lipomas start out small but can become quite large (several inches in diameter). Most lipomas do not cause any clinical signs and are discovered by petting or feeling the dog. Some lipomas can cause problems with walking if they develop in areas where the legs join the body, especially if they become very large.

In rare instances, lipomas can develop in areas other than the skin, such as in the abdomen, around the heart, or behind the eye. If lipomas develop in these areas, they may cause serious clinical signs.

Diagnostic Tests

Lipomas can mimic other, more malignant tumors, so obtaining a sample with a small needle (fine-needle aspiration) can be helpful in identifying them. When the sample is examined under the microscope (cytology), oily material is seen, and often fat cells can be identified. Biopsy of the tumor confirms that it is composed of only fat cells and that the tumor is benign. Malignant lipomas (liposarcomas) are rare but can occur.

TREATMENT AND FOLLOW-UP

Treatment Options

Many lipomas require only monitoring (once the tumor is identified as a lipoma by cytology), since most of them are benign and slow growing. However, tumors that are more deeply attached, are rapidly growing, or are very large are usually removed. Some lipomas penetrate or invade deeply into the surrounding muscle tissues. These are called *infiltrative lipomas,* and they can cause more problems and be more difficult to remove. This type of lipoma may recur after surgery, whereas recurrence is uncommon for most other lipomas. Strict weight control can be tried to prevent the development of more lipomas. Some lipomas shrink in size with weight loss, but others do not change much.

Follow-up Care

Monitoring the size and growth rate of any bump on a dog is important and should be done at regularly scheduled intervals (for example, every 3, 6, or 12 months), depending on the advice of your veterinarian. Report any changes in tumor size, shape, or firmness and any changes in the skin overlying the tumor to your veterinarian. If other lumps or bumps develop, schedule a recheck with your veterinarian. Regular monitoring is also indicated for dogs on a weight-reduction program.

Prognosis

Prognosis is generally good with benign lipomas. Infiltrative lipomas often recur and cause destruction of underlying tissues.

SPECIAL INSTRUCTIONS:

Malassezia Dermatitis

Emily Rothstein, DVM, DACVD

BASIC INFORMATION
Description
The yeast *Malassezia pachydermatis* commonly lives on the skin of dogs but may grow excessively and cause a skin infection. Breeds that are predisposed to the condition, possibly because they have significantly more yeast on their skin, include the basset hound, West Highland white terrier, dachshund, American cocker spaniel, English springer spaniel, and German shepherd dog.
Causes
Certain conditions encourage the overgrowth of this yeast in dogs:
*   Seborrhea and disorders that cause dandruff
*   Hormonal diseases such as hypothyroidism and canine Cushing's disease
*   Environmental allergies

Generalized *Malassezia* dermatitis in cats is usually associated with some sort of underlying (systemic) disease, such as metabolic diseases or cancer, but may also occur in cats with allergies.

 ### Clinical Signs
Itchiness is a major and consistent sign. Face-rubbing, head-shaking, foot-licking and chewing, and scooting may occur in dogs. The affected areas may be localized (ears, around the anus, muzzle, around the eyes, feet) or generalized.

Cats may have waxy ears, chin acne, dark debris on their claws, and/or generalized dandruff. Common skin changes include redness, thickening, increased pigmentation (darkening), dandruff, and greasiness. Hair loss is common in both dogs and cats. A strong, rancid odor may be detected on the skin, particularly in dogs.

Diagnostic Tests
Material is collected from the pet's skin, ears, and/or claws with a cotton swab, special tape, or scalpel blade and then applied to a glass slide. The material is treated with a special stain that allows the yeast to be seen under the microscope. This is the easiest way to make the diagnosis. Occasionally, skin biopsies are helpful.

TREATMENT AND FOLLOW-UP

 ### Treatment Options
Topical therapy involves the application of substances directly to the pet. Frequency of application varies depending on the severity of the condition, with applications 1-3 times weekly being common. Topical products include the following:
*   Selenium sulfide 1% (*Selsun Blue*) is recommended if the skin is greasy, waxy, and scaly, but it is irritating to some animals and should not be used in cats.
*   Certain shampoos kill or reduce the number of yeast on the skin, including ketoconazole (*Nizoral, KetoChlor*), 3-4% chlorhexidine shampoo, 2% chlorhexidine with 1% miconazole (*Malaseb*), and 1% miconazole (*Miconazole, Resizole*).
*   Rinses composed of vinegar and water (1:5 or 1:10 dilution) are inexpensive and effective long-term treatments that help prevent relapses in some dogs (such as swimmers).
*   Lime sulfur dips (2%) can be used to relieve the itching and have mild antiyeast properties. Lime sulfur can be very drying to the skin and hair coat and temporarily stains light-colored coats. It also has a fairly strong sulfur odor when applied, which remains (to a degree) once the pet is dry.

Systemic therapy involves giving antifungal medications orally, usually for 4 weeks:
*   Ketoconazole is helpful in dogs but can cause nausea, vomiting, decreased appetite, and liver problems. It is avoided in cats because it causes vomiting and loss of appetite.
*   Itraconazole is effective but often more expensive.
*   Fluconazole can be used when concerns exist about liver toxicity. It can cause nausea, vomiting, abdominal discomfort, decreased appetite, and liver problems, however.
*   Terbinafine may be considered but has the same potential side effects.

Often topical therapy helps speed the resolution of *Malassezia* dermatitis and is used in conjunction with systemic therapy. The underlying disease or allergy must also be managed to prevent or decrease recurrences.

 ### Follow-up Care
Clinical signs can take 3-4 weeks to improve. Recheck visits and re-examination of skin samples are important to assess the amount of yeast present prior to finishing or stopping the therapy.
Prognosis
The chances of clearing the yeast infection are good, but managing the underlying causative condition requires adequate treatment as well. Some animals need long-term topical therapy a few times a month and/or intermittent systemic therapy to keep the yeast counts under control.

SPECIAL INSTRUCTIONS:

Mast Cell Tumors in Cats

Emily Rothstein, DVM, DACVD

BASIC INFORMATION

Description

These tumors are composed of a white blood cell called a *mast cell*. Mast cell tumors (MCTs) are the second most common skin tumor of cats. Unlike in the dog, skin MCTs in cats are often benign.

Cause

The cause is unknown.

Clinical Signs

MCTs occur most often in middle-aged to older cats. Siamese cats may develop the tumors when they are young, however. Skin MCTs in cats are usually well-defined, firm, tan, hairless, small to medium-sized bumps. The most common areas affected are the head, neck, and upper regions of the body. Cats may develop only one MCT or several tumors separated by months or years. Rarely, numerous widespread tumors are found. Isolated skin MCTs are usually benign, but widespread MCTs may indicate spread of an internal MCT that is malignant. Occasionally skin MCTs are malignant and behave aggressively.

Diagnostic Tests

Taking a sample of the tumor with a needle (fine-needle aspiration) and examining the material under a microscope (cytology) is often helpful, because mast cells are unique. However, a biopsy of the tumor is needed to determine its aggressiveness (malignancy). If multiple tumors are discovered, then other tests may be recommended to evaluate the rest of the body for the presence of tumor. These may include:

- Checking nearby glands (lymph nodes) for mast cells
- Examining blood cells and the bone marrow for mast cells

- Performing an abdominal ultrasound to check the liver, spleen, and other organs
- Obtaining x-rays of the chest

TREATMENT AND FOLLOW-UP

Treatment Options

Surgical removal is the most common therapy if only one or several skin tumors are present. In this instance, it is best to remove and submit all tumors for biopsy. Most benign skin MCTs can be completely removed and do not recur. If multiple tumors are present or tumors cannot be completely removed with surgery, radiation therapy or chemotherapy with drugs such as steroids, or lomustine can be tried. Chemotherapy may also be considered when skin MCTs are associated with internal mast cell disease, but results have been mixed.

Follow-up Care

If the tumor is benign and has been completely removed, no follow-up may be required after surgery. Because cats can develop other MCTs over a period of months to years, periodic monitoring is recommended. If the tumor was malignant and chemotherapy was used, then recheck visits are scheduled at frequent intervals to monitor the response to treatment and side effects from the drugs. Always report the development of any new lumps to your veterinarian.

Prognosis

Prognosis for cats with isolated, benign MCTs of the skin is good. When skin MCTs are associated with internal mast cell disease, the prognosis is poor to guarded.

SPECIAL INSTRUCTIONS:

Mast Cell Tumors in Dogs

Emily Rothstein, DVM, DACVD

BASIC INFORMATION
Description and Causes

These tumors are composed of a white blood cell called a *mast cell*. Mast cell tumors (MCTs) are the most common malignant skin tumor of dogs. The cause is unknown, but a virus that causes mutations has been proposed, because many dogs with MCTs have mutations in a specific gene that may be responsible for the creation and/or progression of MCTs.

MCTs usually develop in middle-aged to older dogs but are occasionally found in dogs as young as 4 months. They occur commonly in the boxer, Boston terrier, bull terrier, bullmastiff, Staffordshire bull terrier, fox terrier, English bulldog, dachshund, Labrador retriever, golden retriever, beagle, pug, Chinese shar-pei, Rhodesian ridgeback, and Weimaraner. All MCTs in the dog are considered potentially malignant.

Clinical Signs

These tumors are generally hairless, red, swollen bumps that vary in size (less than 1 inch up to several inches). They often occur on the trunk (body), head, and legs. Sometimes, tumors on the legs and lips look only like areas of swelling. Rarely, if substances such as histamine and heparin are released from the tumors all at once, generalized swelling, poor blood clotting, low blood pressure (weakness, lethargy), and even death can occur.

Diagnostic Tests

Taking a sample of the tumor with a needle and examining the material under a microscope (cytology) is often helpful, because mast cells are unique. The grade or stage of tumor (severity of malignancy) can be determined only if the tumor is biopsied. Biopsy can be done in some tumors prior to removal, or the entire tumor can be removed and submitted for biopsy. MCTs are classified as stage I, II, or III. Stage III is the worst (most malignant).

Once a diagnosis of MCT is confirmed, other tests are needed to look for spread (metastasis) of the tumor. Examples include:
- Checking nearby glands (lymph nodes) for mast cells
- Examining blood cells and the bone marrow for mast cells
- Performing an abdominal ultrasound to check the liver, spleen, and other organs
- Obtaining x-rays of the chest

TREATMENT AND FOLLOW-UP
Treatment Options

Surgery is the most common treatment option and is done early as possible. If possible, a large area of normal tissue around the tumor is removed to try and prevent the tumor from coming back. All of this tissue is examined by the pathologist to determine whether the MCT has been completely removed.

If complete removal is not possible with surgery, radiation therapy or chemotherapy may be recommended. These treatments are used for some stage II and many stage III MCTs. Occasionally, certain antihistamine medications may be given to control the problems associated with histamine release.

Follow-up Care

Recheck examinations every 3-4 months are used to monitor the dog for new bumps and to check for metastasis to regional glands or internal organs. Laboratory tests (as often as every 1-3 weeks) are needed to monitor for the side effects of chemotherapy drugs.

Prognosis

Survival rates of dogs are about 83% with stage I tumors, 44% with stage II tumors, and 6% with stage III tumors. A bad prognosis is associated with tumors that grow rapidly, are located in deeper tissues, or cause the skin to be raw or ulcerated and when other signs are present.

SPECIAL INSTRUCTIONS:

Nasal Depigmentation

Emily Rothstein, DVM, DACVD

BASIC INFORMATION
Description and Causes
Acquired loss of pigment or lightening of the "button" part of the nose is known as *nasal depigmentation*. The condition has also been called *Dudley nose* or *snow nose*. The cause is usually unknown. It typically occurs in golden retrievers, yellow Labrador retrievers, Siberian huskies, and Alaskan malamutes.

Clinical Signs
Affected dogs are born with pigmented noses, but the black color of the "button" gradually lightens to a light brown or pinkish color. The changes may be permanent, or they may wax and wane. The condition is typically worse during the winter months (hence the name *snow nose*), with some increase in pigmentation in spring and summer. No rawness, itching, or scabbing occur. The normal cobblestone (bumpy) texture of the nose is preserved.

Diagnostic Tests
Diagnosis is based on the history and clinical findings. If a biopsy is done, it shows only a loss of pigmented (dark) cells.

TREATMENT AND FOLLOW-UP

Treatment Options
There is no known treatment; it is only a cosmetic problem. However, the condition is considered a defect in show dogs.

Follow-up Care
No specific follow-up is indicated.
Prognosis
The prognosis is good, because it does not affect the skin around the nose or the rest of the dog.

SPECIAL INSTRUCTIONS:

Notoedric Mange

Emily Rothstein, DVM, DACVD

BASIC INFORMATION
Description and Cause

Notoedres cati (known as *feline scabies*) is a highly contagious mite that primarily infects cats. Dogs, foxes, and rabbits can also be infected. The mite is also contagious to people.

Clinical Signs

Notoedres is a surface-dwelling mite that causes small, red bumps; thickening of the skin; and tightly adherent yellow-gray crusts. Scabs (yellow-gray) and thickened skin first appear on the edges of the ears and rapidly spread to the rest of the ear, face, eyelids, and neck. The feet and the area under the tail may also be affected, and lesions can become widespread.

Intense itching is caused by the mite, and severe scratching by the cat may cause secondary bacterial infections and enlarged lymph nodes.

Diagnostic Tests

Removing scabs with a dull scalpel blade and examining the material under a microscope usually reveals the mite. A skin biopsy can also be used to identify the mite on the surface of the skin.

TREATMENT AND FOLLOW-UP

Treatment Options

All cats in the household are treated. One treatment option involves removing the scabs and debris with a mild shampoo, then applying a 2-3% lime sulfur dip weekly for 6-8 treatments.

Two other therapies are also available, but the drugs have not been approved for this particular condition. Selamectin (*Revolution*) can be applied topically for two applications, 4 weeks apart. Ivermectin is a similar medication that is available for large animals in an injectable form. It can be very effective for *Notoedres* when given in a small dose to a cat. It must be given by your veterinarian every 2 weeks for a total of three shots.

Follow-up Care

The itch and scabs will go away with adequate treatment. If the signs persist, the pet should be re-evaluated, and other pets in the home should also be examined.

Prognosis

Prognosis is very good once the infected cat and all other cats in the house are treated and any secondary bacterial infections are resolved. Rarely, humans can contract this mite, become very itchy, and develop small red bumps. If treatment of the cat does not improve the owner's lesions, the problem should be discussed with the owner's medical provider.

SPECIAL INSTRUCTIONS:

Pemphigus Complex

Emily Rothstein, DVM, DACVD

BASIC INFORMATION

Description

The term *pemphigus complex* is used to describe an uncommon group of autoimmune skin diseases in the dog and cat. Five forms have been identified:

- *Pemphigus foliaceus* is the most common form in dogs and cats, and the dachshund, schipperke, Finnish spitz, bearded collie, chow chow, Akita, and Newfoundland are predisposed.
- *Pemphigus erythematosus* is a mild form of pemphigus foliaceous that affects primarily the Shetland sheepdog, collie, and German shepherd dog.
- *Pemphigus vulgaris* is the second rarest and most severe form.
- *Pemphigus vegetans* is the rarest form and is considered to be a benign variant of pemphigus vulgaris.
- *Paraneoplastic pemphigus* has been described in dogs with cancer.

Causes

An autoimmune problem occurs when the body's own immune system attacks normal body tissues. In pemphigus complex, the "glue" that holds the skin cells together is attacked and destroyed.

Clinical Signs

Pemphigus foliaceus usually causes pimples and honey-colored to brown scabs, which often begin on the face and ears.

- Loss of pigment (the dark color) on the nose is common; involvement of the mouth is rare.
- Feet, foot pads, nail beds, and the groin may be affected.
- Cats tend to have lesions of the toenails and adjacent skin, as well as the nipples.
- The disease generally progresses over 6 months but may wax and wane and may be accompanied by secondary bacterial skin infections (pyoderma), enlarged glands (lymph nodes), loss of appetite, and fever.
- Severe pain and itch can occur in some cases.

Pemphigus erythematosus often produces redness and pimples on the skin of the face and ears.

- Loss of pigment of the nose may be the initial lesion.
- Occasionally, the foot pads, scrotum, or vulva may be involved.
- Pain and itch are variable.

Pemphigus vulgaris is a blistering disease that often progresses to raw, ulcerated patches of skin. Lesions may be present in the mouth (most cases), armpits, and groin.

- Claws that are loose and fall off, or infection and inflammation of the skin around the claws, may be the only presenting sign.
- Secondary bacterial infection and enlarged lymph nodes may be present.
- Pain and itch are variable.

- Fever, poor appetite, and depression may occur in severely affected animals.

Pemphigus vegetans is a pimply-to-blistering disease in which the spots may develop into warty-like skin lesions that ooze liquid.

- Affected animals generally feel well otherwise.
- Pain and itch are variable.

Paraneoplastic pemphigus resembles pemphigus foliaceus but occurs in dogs with certain tumors.

Diagnostic Tests

Examination of the contents of a pimple or the debris under the scab of a lesion may reveal cells called *acantholytic cells*, which are highly suggestive of pemphigus complex. Skin biopsies confirm the diagnosis and often determine which form is present. Other tests may be needed to rule out similar-appearing skin diseases and to evaluate the general health of the animal prior to starting therapy.

TREATMENT AND FOLLOW-UP

Treatment Options

For pemphigus foliaceus and vulgaris, initially high doses of oral steroids are given to turn the immune system down. If oral steroids do not control the disease or cause unacceptable side effects, other immunosuppressive drugs may be tried.

For pemphigus erythematosus and vegetans, topical steroids are usually started, and exposure to the sun is limited, especially between 10 AM and 4 PM. This combination may resolve the problem; if needed, sunscreens that have an SPF value of 15 or greater and contain titanium dioxide may be beneficial when applied two to three times daily. Topical or systemic vitamin E may also help. If these measures do not achieve a satisfactory result or the signs recur, oral steroids may be added.

For paraneoplastic pemphigus, treatment is directed at the underlying cancer.

Follow-up Care

Since all of the medications used to treat pemphigus have potential side effects, blood and urine tests are monitored, sometimes every 2 weeks. Animals on potent topical steroids are monitored similarly to those on oral steroids, because topical steroids can be absorbed into the system. The medication doses are tapered as the pet's signs improve.

Prognosis

Prognosis is fair to good for control of pemphigus foliaceus, erythematosus, and vegetans, depending on the severity of the disease. The disease is never cured but can often be controlled; therapy may be required for life, and signs may wax and wane.

For pemphigus vulgaris, the prognosis is poor. The chances of managing the disease and keeping the pet comfortable are not good.

SPECIAL INSTRUCTIONS:

Pinnal Seborrhea

Emily Rothstein, DVM, DACVD

BASIC INFORMATION
Description
The pinna is the flap or erect part of the ear. The pinna stands up in some dogs and hangs down in others. Seborrhea is an overactivity of certain glands and/or increased production of skin cells that results in either greasy or flaky deposits on the surface of the skin. Pinnal seborrhea is a scaling disorder of the ear margins. Dachshunds seem to be predisposed, but it occurs in many different dogs with ears that hang down. It rarely occurs in dogs with upright ears.

Cause
The cause is unknown.

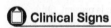 Clinical Signs
Ear margins are the only site affected. The margins can lose hair or develop scabbing, splitting, and raw areas. Dry heat makes the condition worse.

Diagnostic Tests
Diagnosis is often made based on the presence of typical clinical signs in a dog of compatible breed. Certain tests may be recommended to eliminate other skin diseases that affect the pinna of the ear. Laboratory tests may be needed to eliminate other causes of seborrhea. A biopsy is helpful in some cases to rule out those other causes.

TREATMENT AND FOLLOW-UP
Treatment Options
Symptomatic care is important. The main treatment is washing the ear margins with a shampoo that contains salicylic acid, sulfur, or benzoyl peroxide daily or a few times a week until all debris is removed. Once all the debris is gone, then the ears are shampooed as often as needed to keep the debris from building back up. Moisturizer is applied after shampooing. If the response to shampooing is unsatisfactory, then topical retinoid ointments (human acne medication) and/or oral fatty acid supplements may be tried. If topical therapy does not reduce the amount of buildup or if raw areas do not heal, then oral pentoxifylline may be considered. Severe cases may require surgical removal of the affected areas of the pinna.

Follow-up Care
Initial improvement is often noted within 4-6 weeks after treatment is started. If pentoxifylline is used, it may take 4-8 weeks for improvement to occur. Once the ear margins are back to normal (which may take 4-12 months), pentoxifylline can be decreased, from three times daily to once or twice daily, and eventually stopped if there is no worsening of the condition.

Prognosis
Most dogs respond to consistent therapy with shampooing, with or without moisturizers. Since this is a lifelong problem, long-term maintenance therapy is usually needed.

SPECIAL INSTRUCTIONS:

Plasma Cell Pododermatitis in Cats

Emily Rothstein, DVM, DACVD

BASIC INFORMATION
Description
This is a rare disease of the foot pads of cats. The foot pads become inflamed, and within the inflammation is an accumulation of plasma cells, a type of white blood cell involved in immune responses.

Cause
The cause is unknown but is thought to be immune-mediated; that is, the immune system causes or aggravates inflammation rather than quieting it down.

Clinical Signs
Initially soft, nonpainful swelling of the foot pads develops. More than one pad on more than one foot is typically involved. Lightly pigmented (pink) pads may look purple. The pads appear streaky, with white scaly material on the surface. Later, the pads can become bloody and painful. Rarely, kidney disease and inflammation of tissues in the mouth may also occur.

Diagnostic Tests
The appearance of the foot pads is suggestive of the disease. Removing cells with a small needle and examining them under the microscope can reveal reveals numerous plasma cells. Blood tests may be recommended to look for infection, kidney problems, or evidence of immune responses, but results are variable. Biopsy of the foot pad usually confirms the diagnosis.

TREATMENT AND FOLLOW-UP
Treatment Options
No treatment may be needed if the inflammation is mild and the foot pad changes do not bother the cat. In some cats, the condition spontaneously regresses (disappears). In other cats, medications are needed to turn down the immune system. Steroids or immune-suppressive medications may be recommended. Surgery can be done to remove lesions that affect only one foot pad, but this is uncommon.

Follow-up Care
If no treatment in started initially, the cat should be monitored repeatedly to ensure that the pads do not worsen and other clinical signs do not develop. Those cats receiving medications often need periodic blood tests to monitor for adverse effects of the medications.

Some cats respond very well to treatment; in those cases, the medication can be slowly decreased and eventually stopped, and the disease does not recur. Many pets require some medication for life, and recheck visits may be needed every 6-12 months, depending on the pet's condition and the potency of the medication. When any medication is used, the dose is tapered every month or so, and recheck visits are used to monitor worsening of clinical signs. Some cats never return to 100% normal, even with medication.

Prognosis
Prognosis can be excellent if the signs spontaneously resolve. Prognosis may only be fair, however, if long-term immune-suppressive drugs are needed or if the kidneys and mouth are involved.

SPECIAL INSTRUCTIONS:

Primary Seborrhea

Emily Rothstein, DVM, DACVD

BASIC INFORMATION
Description and Cause
Primary seborrhea is an inherited skin disease in which the surface cells of the skin multiply and turn over (shed) three times faster than normal. This rapid growth and shedding results in visible scaliness and dandruff on the surface of the skin.

Primary seborrhea occurs most commonly in the American cocker spaniel, West Highland white terrier, English springer spaniel, and basset hound. Other breeds that may be affected include the Jack Russell terrier (Parson Russell terrier), Cavalier King Charles spaniel, Wheaton terrier, Chinese shar-pei, dachshund, Doberman pinscher, German shepherd dog, Irish setter, and Labrador retriever. The condition may also be seen in Persian, Himalayan, and exotic shorthaired cats.

Clinical Signs
In dogs, itchiness is common, since the abnormal skin surface develops infections easily. Signs develop early in life and progress with age. Some breeds have skin that becomes quite greasy, especially in the neck fold, below the tail, and on the feet. Some breeds have a dry, flaky hair coat. Waxy and thickened ears are common. Foot pads may look thicker than normal.

Most cats develop signs within the first 2-3 days of life. The hair appears dirty and sticks together. Eventually the whole body becomes greasy and scaly, and the hair coat becomes very thin. Waxy material may accumulate in the ears and around the folds on the face. A rancid odor may be detected on the skin.

Diagnostic Tests
Primary seborrhea is usually suspected when the disease arises at a very early age. Certain tests, such as skin scrapings and skin cultures, may be recommended to eliminate other skin diseases that produce a similar clinical appearance. Laboratory tests may be needed to rule out other causes of seborrhea. Diagnosis is confirmed with a skin biopsy, which shows the subtle thickening of the skin surface.

TREATMENT AND FOLLOW-UP

Treatment Options
Treatment of dogs involves the following:
- Secondary bacterial and yeast infections on the skin and in the ears are treated with appropriate drugs.
- Antiseborrheic shampoos are helpful, and emollients (softening, soothing agents) may be used on dogs with dry skin. Initially, bathing may be required several times a week until the seborrhea is controlled; it is then decreased to several times a month.
- Most shampoos that are effective contain sulfur, salicylic acid, or both.
- Fatty acid supplements may help control the scaliness.
- Daily oral vitamin A is often helpful, and severe cases may respond to oral vitamin D3 therapy.

For cats, no effective treatment is known, but periodic clipping, bathing, and grooming may keep the cat comfortable.

Follow-up Care
When vitamin D3 is given, calcium levels in the blood must be monitored closely. Recheck visits are needed to monitor the condition of the skin and to determine when changes in therapy may be needed. Rechecks are also needed any time a change in the skin is detected at home (such as more odor from the skin, increased greasiness, or more itching).

Prognosis
The long-term outlook for the pet depends on the severity of the seborrhea. Seborrhea is a lifelong condition and is not curable. Affected cats are often euthanized.

SPECIAL INSTRUCTIONS:

Sarcoptic Mange

Emily Rothstein, DVM, DACVD

BASIC INFORMATION
Description and Causes

Sarcoptic mange is an itchy disease of dogs, coyotes, and foxes that is caused by the superficial burrowing mite *Sarcoptes scabiei* variety *canis*. The disease is sometimes called *scabies*. *Sarcoptes* mites can transiently infect humans and cats.

 Clinical Signs

Scabies causes nonseasonal, intense itchiness in dogs that is often accompanied by secondary skin signs. Hair loss, redness, small red bumps, scabs, and dandruff are commonly found on the edges of the ears, elbows, ankles, and underside of the trunk (belly). With long-term infestations, skin changes may become widespread, but the top of the dog is usually unaffected.

Well-groomed animals may have intense itchiness, with minimal to no skin lesions. Enlarged lymph nodes may be present, along with weight loss and lethargy secondary to the chronic itching and discomfort.

Humans in contact with infected dogs may develop an itchy patch of small red bumps (papules).

 Diagnostic Tests

Sarcoptic mange is suspected in any dog that is intensely itchy. Finding the mite, mite eggs, or mite fecal material on skin scrapings from affected areas confirms the diagnosis, but this evidence is found only 10-50% of the time. Sometimes the diagnosis is made even if mites are not found, by having a positive response to treatment for the mite.

TREATMENT AND FOLLOW-UP

 Treatment Options

All dogs in contact with the infected dog must be treated, and in severe cases the environment must also be treated with antiparasite sprays.

Topical therapy involves the application of medications such as the following:
- Lime sulfur dips may be done weekly for 6-8 treatments.
- Selamectin (*Revolution*) is licensed for use once monthly, but it is more effective if applied every 2 weeks for a total of three treatments.
- Fipronil spray (*Frontline*) may be applied every 2 weeks for a total of three treatments.

Systemic therapy involves use of oral medications to kill the mites. Several products are not licensed for use against this mite but have been shown to be very effective, and the decision on whether to use them requires discussion with your veterinarian. The breed of dog infested must be considered, because some oral medications are not safe in certain breeds.

Secondary bacterial infections must be appropriately treated also.

Environmental treatment is easily accomplished with sprays available from your veterinarian or pet store, often with the same products used for treating flea infestations.

 Follow-up Care

If your pet's itchiness has not decreased after 21 days of treatment, further diagnostic tests and re-evaluation are needed.

Prognosis

The prognosis is very good with adequate treatment of the mite and control of any secondary bacterial infections. All dogs in contact with the infested dog (including play companions) must be treated to prevent recurrence.

Rarely, humans exposed to these pets become slightly to very itchy from the mite, because it is contagious to humans. Evidence of the mite in people is usually small, itchy, red bumps, especially in areas that are in contact with the pet (such as hands, arms) or in areas that are tightly covered (such as pant lines near the waist). Some people need specific treatment for the mites and should discuss the situation with their medical provider.

SPECIAL INSTRUCTIONS:

Sebaceous Adenitis in Dogs

Emily Rothstein, DVM, DACVD

BASIC INFORMATION

Description

Sebaceous adenitis is an uncommon disease affecting certain glands of the skin that secrete an oily (sebaceous) material. Sebum (a waxy substance) builds up on the surface of the skin and the hair.

Cause

The cause is unknown, but it may be inherited in the standard poodle. Inflammation and destruction of the sebaceous glands, blockage of the ducts of the glands, and abnormal production of sebum may all contribute to the clinical signs.

Clinical Signs

Middle-aged dogs of several different breeds are affected most often. These breeds include the standard poodle, vizsla, Samoyed, Akita, German shepherd dog, Belgian shepherd, and some mixed-breed dogs. Both sides of the head, face, ear flaps, and trunk are usually affected. Lesions initially develop on the top of these locations, with the underside areas less commonly affected. Lesions can also develop on the tail, causing hair loss and waxiness, giving it a "rat tail" appearance. Secondary bacterial infections may cause large scabs and itchiness. Some common signs in particular breeds are as follows:

- In short-coated breeds (such as the vizsla), lesions do not seem to bother the dog and only appear as expanding areas of hair loss and dandruff. The dandruff is typically fine and does not stick to the surface of the dog. Swelling of the eyelids and muzzle can occur.
- In the standard poodle, lesions start as patches of thickened skin that eventually lose hair. Silver-white dandruff occurs, along with a dull, dry coat. Small clumps of firm skin may surround the hair shafts and are called *hair* or *follicular casts*. In some cases, a change in the color of the hair coat and straightening of the hair may be the first signs. Lesions typically start on the head and ear flaps and eventually involve the neck and top of the dog.
- Akitas usually develop widespread reddened and greasy changes to their coats. Matting of the hair; scaliness; yellow-brown, greasy debris; small bumps; and hair casts are common. The undercoat may be lost. Secondary bacterial infections are common.
- Lesions in German shepherd dogs usually start on the tail and move toward the head.
- Samoyeds have dull, brittle, and broken hairs in their coats. Follicular casts are common, and moderate to severe dandruff and hair loss may occur on the trunk.

Diagnostic Tests

A combination of classical clinical findings in a predisposed breed is suggestive of the diagnosis. Certain tests, such as skin scrapings and cultures, may be recommended to eliminate other skin diseases that produce a similar clinical appearance. Laboratory tests may be needed to rule out other causes of seborrhea. Diagnosis is confirmed with a skin biopsy.

TREATMENT AND FOLLOW-UP

Treatment Options

It is important to treat secondary infections to help resolve the scabs and itchiness. Mild cases may respond to shampoos (containing salicylic acid and/or sulfur) that decrease the buildup of sebum on the skin surface, followed by emollient (softening, soothing) rinses. Propylene glycol diluted with water may be used as a rinse once daily until signs are controlled, then decreased to once every few days. Baby oil solution (1:1 mixture with water) can be applied to the skin for several hours, then shampooed off. Both of these preparations are messy, however.

Drug therapy can help some dogs. Oral tetracycline and niacinamide given together can improve the inflammation and decrease the destruction of the sebaceous glands. Some dogs respond to omega-3 and omega-6 fatty acid supplements. Some dogs may respond to oral cyclosporine. Spontaneous remission, in which the disease resolves without any therapy, is rare.

Follow-up Care

Since the inflammation of the sebaceous glands cannot usually be stopped, treatment is aimed at controlling the signs. Recheck appointments are needed whenever the signs change, such as when more dandruff, more hair loss, more scabs, or itching is detected. All of these signs can indicate the presence of an infection. If cyclosporine is used for the disease, monitoring is needed to assess the response to treatment and any side effects associated with the drug.

Prognosis

Signs in some animals are controlled fairly well; their hair (although not all hair) grows back, and they have less dryness of the skin. Some dogs require intensive topical therapy for life with shampoos and rinses. Since this disease is probably inherited in some way, no affected dog should be used for breeding, because it could pass the faulty gene to its offspring.

SPECIAL INSTRUCTIONS:

Skin Fold Pyoderma (Intertrigo)

Emily Rothstein, DVM, DACVD

BASIC INFORMATION

Description and Causes

Intertrigo arises from an overgrowth or colonization of skin folds by normal skin bacteria and sometimes by yeast. Skin folds are considered normal in many animals. For example, facial and nasal folds occur in short-nosed, flat-faced breeds. Lip folds are common in spaniels and many water dogs. Tail and vulvar folds are common in some breeds and can also arise with obesity. Moisture, secretions (tears, saliva), and skin cells accumulate in these folds, which also have poor air circulation. Bacteria and yeast love to grow in this type of environment, which leads to inflammation and the typical clinical signs.

Clinical Signs

Hair loss, redness, accumulation of debris, and discoloration of adjacent skin are common findings. A foul odor may be detected in the area, and pimples sometimes develop in the skin of the folds.

Diagnostic Tests

A possible diagnosis may be made in the examination room, based on the presence of an infection located in skin folds. Swabs may be used to collect material from the area and examine it under the microscope. Finding bacteria and yeast helps to confirm the diagnosis.

TREATMENT AND FOLLOW-UP

Treatment Options

If possible, it is best to remove the fold surgically, especially if the infection does not respond well to treatment or recurs. Surgery of lip, facial, or vulvar folds is often very successful. Removal of facial or nasal folds dramatically affects the appearance of the dog, so discuss this option carefully with your veterinarian.

In overweight animals, weight reduction helps minimize folds in the armpit and belly regions, and sometimes around the vulva. Weight-reduction programs also benefit other organs of the body.

As far as medical treatment of the infected folds, folds that are not near the eyes may be cleaned every 1-3 days with an antiseptic shampoo or cleanser that contains chlorhexidine, benzoyl peroxide, or ethyl lactate. These agents are irritating to the eyes and should not be used near them. Special medicated pads or lid wipes may be used to clean facial and nasal folds. A topical antibiotic or antiseptic ointment, cream, or spray may also be applied (not near the eyes) once or twice daily to the folds. Rarely, oral antibiotics may be needed.

Follow-up Care

Rechecks are periodically needed as long as the pet has folds, because infections in these areas are common. Careful cleaning of the folds daily or several times a week with a gentle damp cloth, baby wipes, or medicated pads for dogs (Malaseb, Malacetic, Chlorhexidine 3% PS) helps keep the folds free of debris. If a foul odor, itchiness, redness, or persistent buildup of debris is noticed, consult with your veterinarian. Rechecks are also needed to monitor animals on weight-reduction programs.

Prognosis

Prognosis for improvement is excellent with adequate treatment, but the animal may need lifelong topical maintenance therapy if the folds are not removed surgically.

SPECIAL INSTRUCTIONS:

Sporotrichosis

Emily Rothstein, DVM, DACVD

BASIC INFORMATION
Description and Causes

Sporotrichosis is a skin infection caused by a fungus that develops in the fatty layer of the skin and creates swellings or nodules. *Sporothrix schenckii* is the fungus. It exists naturally in soil and organic plant matter.

Clinical Signs

In dogs, skin lesions consist of many firm bumps, often on the head, ear flaps, and trunk. Bumps can occur anywhere, however. Nodules may burst open, with drainage from the open holes. Nearby glands (lymph nodes) and their drainage channels can be involved and form bumps or become enlarged.

In cats, skin lesions consist of draining puncture wounds, abscesses, and widespread swelling of the skin. Lesions are often found on the head, legs, and base of the tail and are sometimes associated with cat fight wounds. Affected areas may ooze foul debris and scab over. Cats can spread the fungus around to other areas through normal grooming.

Diagnostic Tests

Diagnosis can often be made by examination of the draining material or a biopsy specimen under the microscope. In the cat, large numbers of the fungal organisms can often be found, but very low numbers occur in lesions from dogs, which can make the diagnosis more difficult. Tissue may also be submitted for culture in an attempt to grow the fungus. In dogs, if the fungus is not found, blood testing may be needed to establish the diagnosis.

Laboratory tests and x-rays may be recommended to rule out other fungal infections. Certain laboratory tests may also be needed to make sure treatments for the infection can be used safely.

TREATMENT AND FOLLOW-UP

Treatment Options

Oral antifungal medications must be used for 2-6 months or longer. A few different drugs are available, and you can discuss these with your veterinarian. The fungus can be passed to humans through the discharge, so all individuals handling animals with suspected sporotrichosis should wear gloves and properly dispose of contaminated material.

Follow-up Care

Recheck visits and follow-up laboratory tests are needed to follow the progress of treatment and to monitor for side effects associated with the medications.

Prognosis

Prognosis is guarded. These infections are often serious and difficult to treat.

SPECIAL INSTRUCTIONS:

Subcutaneous Abscesses and Cellulitis

Emily Rothstein, DVM, DACVD

BASIC INFORMATION

Description

A subcutaneous abscess is a collection of pus and infected material within the tissues beneath the skin. Cellulitis is an infection or inflammatory reaction that has spread out within these tissues, rather than being confined to one pocket.

Causes

The most common cause is a bacterial infection, although fungal infections and even sterile processes can cause similar signs. Bacteria are introduced into the deeper tissues through a wound or injury or by rupture of a hair follicle. (See also the handout for **Deep Bacterial Pyoderma and Furunculosis**.) Some of the more common causes are cat and dog bite wounds, punctures from thorns, and injuries that cause a break in the skin.

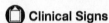 Clinical Signs

A painful swelling is commonly detected under the skin, and sometimes open, draining tracts or holes are seen in the skin. The skin overlying the abscess is usually red, but over time it may die, turn blue or black, and begin to slough (come off). The pet may have a fever, loss of appetite, and lethargy, and these may be the only signs detected at home. In these cases, the abscess or cellulitis is discovered by the veterinarian when the animal is examined.

Diagnostic Tests

A tentative diagnosis is based on the clinical signs described. The diagnosis is supported by the following:

- Examination of material from the infected site under the microscope shows pus and bacteria.
- A bacterial culture of the pus can be done and sometimes shows that more than one type of bacteria is present.
- Lancing of a swollen area suspected to be infected often determines whether an abscess is present.

If the animal is seriously ill, other laboratory tests may be recommended to determine what effects the infection is having on other organs in the body.

TREATMENT AND FOLLOW-UP

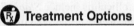 Treatment Options

An abscess must often be surgically opened to provide drainage, and this usually requires general anesthesia or heavy sedation. Sometimes dead tissue is removed, the cavity is flushed with an antiseptic solution, and a drain is left in place to allow continued drainage from the site. Cellulitis may be treated with warm, wet compresses initially. In some instances, an abscess will form (even with appropriate treatment) that requires surgical drainage. In both situations, antibiotics are given, usually for about 14 days.

Warm, wet compresses are often recommended postoperatively to encourage drainage and provide comfort. Additional nursing and supportive care may be needed for animals that are seriously ill from the infection.

Follow-up Care

Complete healing of an abscess usually occurs within 2 weeks but it can take longer if the cause of the deep infection (such as bite wounds, porcupine quills, or plant foreign material) is difficult to identify and treat. If the source of infection is not adequately identified and removed, a recurrence can be expected. In some cases, signs of infection begin soon after the antibiotics are finished; in others, signs of infection may return days to months later.

Prognosis

Prognosis is often very good with adequate treatment, but some lesions heal with a scar. Cases that are complicated by infestations of maggots or by kidney, liver, or blood changes have a poorer prognosis and require more intensive therapy.

SPECIAL INSTRUCTIONS:

Superficial Bacterial Folliculitis in Dogs

Emily Rothstein, DVM, DACVD

BASIC INFORMATION

Description

Folliculitis is a bacterial skin infection that leads to hair loss and inflammation of the hair follicles.

Causes

Common bacteria associated with folliculitis include *Staphylococcus* species, occasionally *Streptococcus* species, and others. Infections have a tendency arise in the presence of several abnormalities:

- Skin problems: allergy, seborrhea, excessive moisture
- Hormonal disorders: low thyroid levels, Cushing's disease with high cortisol levels, diabetes mellitus (sugar diabetes)
- Immunologic abnormalities
- Drugs given or applied to the pet that make the skin more susceptible to the bacteria

Clinical Signs

Circular areas of hair loss occur. Pimples and red bumps are usually seen, along with scabs, sometimes moist skin, and increased pigmentation. In inflamed areas, hair pulls out very easily. Sometimes after the lesions heal, there is a blackened circle that disappears over time. These lesions can occur anywhere on the body, but involvement of the head, ears, or feet is unusual.

Diagnostic Tests

Identification of bacteria and certain white blood cells (neutrophils) is often possible when a direct impression sample is made onto a glass slide and examined under the microscope. Occasionally a biopsy of the skin is necessary to make the diagnosis and to rule out other skin problems with similar appearances. Bacterial culture and antibiotic susceptibility testing may be needed to determine the best antibiotic for treatment. Laboratory testing to identify underlying causes may also be needed.

TREATMENT AND FOLLOW-UP

Treatment Options

Oral antibiotics are given for at least 3 weeks and occasionally for 4-6 weeks. Shampoo therapy is helpful to both remove the scabs and decrease the surface bacteria so that they cannot re-invade the skin. Any underlying or associated conditions should also be controlled.

Follow-up Care

The infection is treated for at least 1 week after all clinical signs resolve, so recheck visits are often needed prior to stopping the medications.

Prognosis

Prognosis is very good for a cure if the correct antibiotic is chosen and therapy is continued for a long enough time. Use of cortisone or steroids during this time makes the antibiotic treatment much less effective. Relapses can occur until the underlying cause is properly treated or managed or if the initial bacterial infection is resistant to the antibiotic.

SPECIAL INSTRUCTIONS:

Systemic Lupus Erythematosus: Dermatologic Aspects

Emily Rothstein, DVM, DACVD

BASIC INFORMATION

Description

Systemic lupus erythematosus (SLE) is a rare autoimmune disease that can affect not only the skin, but also the kidneys, joints, and blood system of the dog or cat. It affects the skin in 20-54% of cases. This handout pertains to only the skin component of the disease.

Causes

An autoimmune problem occurs when the body's own immune system attacks normal body tissues. In SLE, tissues of the skin, kidneys, joints and other organs may be attacked. The attack on the skin can be worsened by exposure to sunlight. SLE is more commonly seen in the Finnish spitz, collie, Shetland sheepdog, German shepherd dog, and poodles, as well as in Himalayan, Siamese, and Persian cats.

Clinical Signs

Clinical signs in dogs are as follows:

- Very irritated gums are commonly seen.
- Blisters and ulcerations often arise at the junction where haired skin meets the mucous membranes (non-haired tissue) of the mouth.
- Ulcers may also develop on the foot pads.
- Hives, redness, dandruff, scabs, and loss of pigment (the dark color in the skin) may occur.
- The face, ears, and lower aspect of the legs are commonly affected.
  Clinical signs in cats are as follows:
- Generalized dandruff and peeling of the skin, reddening of skin, hair loss, and scabs are commonly seen.
- The foot pads, face, neck, and legs are commonly affected.

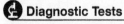 Diagnostic Tests

Because SLE can affect many different organs, laboratory, urine, and sometimes joint tests are recommended. A special test called an *antinuclear antibody assay* (ANA) is positive in 85-90% of cases, and other immune test results may also be abnormal. Skin biopsies typically show many changes suspicious of SLE but can be similar to other autoimmune skin diseases, which makes the diagnosis difficult. A diagnosis of SLE often requires that numerous tests be run, with results compatible with SLE in more than just one test.

TREATMENT AND FOLLOW-UP

Treatment Options

Immune-suppressive drugs are needed to attempt to control the skin disease and problems in other organ systems. This disease can be difficult to control, and often treatment starts with steroids (cortisones). If steroids are not effective or if the side effects (excessive drinking and urinating, weakness, panting) are too great, other immune-suppressive drugs (such as azathioprine or cyclosporine) may be tried. It may take 4-8 weeks to see a response to therapy. Once a response is seen in the skin and/or other systems, drug therapy is tapered. This is not a curable disease, so management is the goal.

Follow-up Care

Monitoring involves frequent blood tests because of the medications used. After treatment has been started, recheck visits are usually scheduled about every 2-4 weeks to evaluate the response to therapy. Once clinical remission has been achieved, the visits are often continued at 1-month intervals as the drug dosages are being tapered, and then every 4-6 months during maintenance therapy. Laboratory tests are periodically needed to monitor for side effects from the medications and to make sure no secondary infections are starting.

Prognosis

Prognosis is guarded to poor. Many pets do not respond to therapy or respond only partially (for example, the skin improves but the kidney disease does not). Sometimes response occurs early on, but as time goes on, the disease becomes harder to control.

SPECIAL INSTRUCTIONS:

Vaccine-Associated Vasculitis in Dogs

Emily Rothstein, DVM, DACVD

BASIC INFORMATION

Description and Cause

Vasculitis is an inflammation of blood vessels. In this condition, affected dogs develop an expanding area of hair loss at the site of a vaccination, especially after a rabies vaccination. Lesions may not develop for 2-4 months after vaccination, and the reaction can lead to permanent scarring and hair loss.

Clinical Signs

Usually a focal, round area of complete hair loss is the major finding. The skin may become thin or more pigmented (turn dark). The lesion is not itchy and does not bother the dog.

Diagnostic Tests

The diagnosis is usually made based on a history of prior vaccination in the same spot and typical clinical findings. Biopsy is often helpful in eliminating other causes of focal hair loss.

TREATMENT AND FOLLOW-UP

Treatment Options

During the acute phase of the reaction (when the vasculitis is first occurring), a drug called *pentoxifylline* may be used to decrease the inflammation and allow blood to flow more easily through the irritated vessels. Often, however, the problem is not discovered early enough for pentoxifylline to be effective. If the lesion is cosmetically disfiguring, it may be surgically removed.

Follow-up Care

The advantages and disadvantages of vaccination must be considered when future vaccinations are chosen. Reactions can worsen when vaccines of any sort are given in any area on the body. State veterinarians, in conjunction with your veterinarian, can assess the pros and cons of skipping or decreasing the frequency of vaccinations, such as rabies vaccinations (which are required by state law).

Prognosis

There is no cure, and the lesion is often permanent, but the problem is usually only a cosmetic issue.

SPECIAL INSTRUCTIONS:

Vitamin A–Responsive Dermatosis

Emily Rothstein, DVM, DACVD

BASIC INFORMATION

Description

This is a rare disease affecting the surface layer of the skin. It occurs most commonly in American cocker spaniels but it is also seen rarely in other breeds, such as the Gordon setter, miniature schnauzer, and Labrador retriever.

Cause

The actual cause of this disease is unknown, but it may be an inherited problem in the cocker spaniel. Vitamin A levels in the blood are normal, so it does not arise from a deficiency of vitamin A.

Clinical Signs

Unlike primary seborrhea, this disorder starts in adulthood. Lesions most commonly occur on the sides and underside of the chest and the belly. Mild to moderate itching may occur if a secondary bacterial infection is present. The hair coat is dull and dry, and the hair pulls out easily. Small, reddish bumps or pimples, scaliness, and dandruff are common. A large amount of waxy debris accumulates on the surface of hairs or in small clumps on the skin. The external ear canals are usually very waxy.

Diagnostic Tests

The diagnosis may be suspected when the clinical signs occur in an adult dog, especially in a cocker spaniel. Certain tests, such as skin scrapings and skin cultures, may be recommended to eliminate other skin diseases that produce a similar clinical appearance. Laboratory tests may be needed to rule out other causes of seborrhea and hair loss. Diagnosis is confirmed with a skin biopsy.

TREATMENT AND FOLLOW-UP

Treatment Options

Oral vitamin A is administered with a fatty meal. It can take 4-6 weeks of therapy for the skin to improve, and 8-10 weeks for the signs to disappear. Lifelong therapy is usually needed to maintain remission. Antiseborrheic shampoos and moisturizers may be used several times weekly until remission to speed up the rate of recovery. They may be used 2-4 times per month for maintenance care.

Follow-up Care

Rechecks visits are used to monitor the response and make adjustments in therapy. Notify your veterinarian if your pet's itchiness increases or returns, because it usually indicates a skin infection that needs treatment. Also notify your veterinarian if decreased appetite or weight loss, joint pain, or worsening of the skin condition occurs, because these can sometimes be side effects of vitamin A therapy.

Prognosis

Chronic vitamin A and topical therapy usually control the signs well. Signs usually relapse if the vitamin A is stopped.

SPECIAL INSTRUCTIONS:

Zinc-Responsive Dermatosis

Emily Rothstein, DVM, DACVD

BASIC INFORMATION
Description
This disease is associated with thickening and scaling of the skin that responds to zinc supplementation. At least two forms of the disease exist:
- Syndrome I occurs in Alaskan malamutes and Siberian huskies and is not associated with a zinc-deficient diet. Lesions usually arise in young, immature dogs (often younger than 2 years of age), and signs may worsen with illness, during pregnancy, or when the dog comes into heat.
- Syndrome II arises when a diet deficient in zinc is fed to the dog or when absorption of zinc (from the intestines) is altered from excessive calcium or phytates (substances found in high-cereal foods) in the diet. This form of the disease occurs most often with generic dog foods. Any breed of dog may be affected, and lesions may vary among pups within a litter.

Cause
Syndrome I may be inherited in malamutes and huskies and may arise from decreased absorption of zinc in the intestines. Syndrome II may arise for different reasons, such as insufficient levels of zinc in the diet, excessive supplementation with other minerals and vitamins, and poorly balanced diets.

Clinical Signs
General clinical signs are possible with this disease, such as poor appetite, poor or slow growth, poor wound healing, lethargy, fever, and enlarged lymph nodes (glands). Skin lesions of syndrome I have this appearance:
- Focal hair loss and redness occur early and progress to dandruff and scabbing.
- Lesions are typically seen around the eyes, mouth, foot pads, and anus, and at pressure points where skin overlies bone (such as the elbows and hocks).
- The hair coat may be dull and dry and may have a waxy feel.
- Secondary bacterial and/or yeast infections are common, which lead to itching.

Lesions of syndrome II are similar but occur primarily on the head and over pressure points.

Diagnostic Tests
The diagnosis is suspected when the clinical signs occur in a young dog, especially in a breed known to be predisposed. Certain tests, such as skin scrapings and cultures, may be recommended to eliminate other skin diseases that produce a similar clinical appearance in young dogs. A skin biopsy is important in making the diagnosis. Zinc analysis of the blood or hairs has not been very helpful in diagnosing this condition.

TREATMENT AND FOLLOW-UP
Treatment Options
Syndrome I requires lifelong supplementation with elemental zinc. If no response occurs within 4 weeks, the zinc dosage is often increased by 50% and a low dose of oral prednisone may be started to enhance zinc absorption. Sometimes, the addition of a fatty acid supplement to the therapy also improves zinc metabolism. Dogs that do not respond to these therapies may need injections of zinc sulfate, which are given weekly for a minimum of 4 weeks. Maintenance injections may be needed every 1-6 months to prevent relapses.

Syndrome II requires correction of nutritional imbalances, and zinc supplementation helps speed resolution of the symptoms. Once there is resolution of clinical signs in dogs with syndrome II, zinc supplementation is discontinued.

In all cases, secondary bacterial or yeast infections must also be treated.

Follow-up Care
In syndrome I, rechecks are needed to assess the response to therapy and to make adjustments in the dosage of zinc. Once the signs are controlled, rechecks are done if any signs worsen or recur. If prednisone is used, even at low doses, blood tests may be recommended periodically to check for possible changes in the liver or kidneys from the drug.

For dogs with syndrome II, once the problem is resolved and the dietary problem is corrected, rechecks are usually not needed.

Prognosis
Some cases of syndrome I are very difficult to control, and these dogs can relapse. In general, however, the outlook is good with lifelong zinc supplementation. The prognosis is good to excellent for resolution of syndrome II.

SPECIAL INSTRUCTIONS:

SECTION 13

Diseases of the Eye

Section Editor: Rhea V. Morgan, DVM, DACVIM (Small Animal), DACVO

Anterior Uveitis
Cataracts
Chorioretinitis and Optic Neuritis
Collie Eye Anomaly
Conjunctivitis
Corneal Ulceration
Distichiasis and Ectopic Cilia
Ectropion
Entropion
Eyelid Tumors
Feline Corneal Sequestration
Feline Eosinophilic Keratitis
Feline Herpesvirus Keratoconjunctivitis
Glaucoma in Cats
Glaucoma in Dogs
Horner's Syndrome
Hypertensive Retinopathy
Hyphema

Intraocular Tumors
Iridociliary Cysts
Iris Melanosis of Cats
Keratoconjunctivitis Sicca (Dry Eye)
Lens Luxation and Subluxation
Lipid Keratopathy
Orbital Cellulitis and Abscessation
Orbital Tumors
Pannus
Persistent Corneal Erosions
Pigmentary Keratitis
Progressive Retinal Atrophy
Prolapse of the Gland of the Third Eyelid
Proptosis of the Eye
Retinal Detachment
Retinal Dysplasia
Sudden Acquired Retinal Degeneration
Taurine Retinopathy

Anterior Uveitis

Rhea V. Morgan, DVM, DACVIM (Small Animal), DACVO

BASIC INFORMATION
Description
The anterior uvea is composed of the iris (tissue around the pupil) and the ciliary body. The ciliary body sits directly behind the iris and is not usually visible. Any inflammation of these tissues is called *anterior uveitis*.

Causes
Uveitis can arise as an isolated eye problem, but it is more commonly a sign of some illness elsewhere in the body.
• Eye problems that cause uveitis include corneal ulcers, cataracts, trauma, and tumors.
• More than 25 different infections can cause uveitis, including fungal, tick-borne, bacterial, viral, protozoal, and parasitic infections. Some types of infections occur more often in dogs, whereas others are more common in cats.
• In rare instances, the immune system may attack the uvea. In these cases, other parts of the body may also be affected.
• Tumors that arise elsewhere in the body may metastasize to the eye.
• Hypertension (high blood pressure), elevated circulating levels of protein or fat, and other blood disorders may cause uveitis.
Sometimes uveitis occurs for unknown reasons (such as pigmentary uveitis in golden retrievers) or the cause is never found (called *idiopathic*). In these cases, all laboratory test results are normal.

Clinical Signs
Uveitis can begin suddenly, or it can develop slowly and remain undetected for a long time. The eye is often red and painful. Squinting (especially in bright light), cloudiness, or discoloration of the eye may be noted. If only one eye is affected, the size and mobility of the pupils may be different. Vision may be decreased, and blindness is possible in severely affected eyes. If glaucoma occurs, the eye may be enlarged. If a generalized infection is the cause, the animal may act ill and show other clinical signs.

Diagnostic Tests
The presence of uveitis is confirmed by an eye examination, which may involve tear testing, fluorescein staining of the cornea, and glaucoma testing. If these tests cannot be performed or are inconclusive, your veterinarian may refer your pet to a veterinary ophthalmologist. A general physical examination is usually performed to search for any other changes that may signify the presence of a generalized (systemic) illness.

Laboratory tests are frequently done to rule out infections and look for underlying causes. Chest and abdominal x-rays and an abdominal ultrasound are sometimes recommended. If hypertension is suspected, blood pressure can be measured. In cloudy eyes that cannot be examined well, an ultrasound may be performed. The cause of uveitis can be difficult to find and may require numerous tests.

TREATMENT AND FOLLOW-UP
Treatment Options
Treatment involves administering medications for the eye problem and for any underlying causes. Typical eye medications include topical anti-inflammatory drugs (usually steroids), pupil dilators/pain relievers (such as atropine), and sometimes antibiotics and anti-glaucoma drugs. The severity of the inflammation often dictates how frequent and intense the therapy must be.

Once an underlying cause is determined, appropriate treatment is started for that condition. Examples include antibiotics, antifungal agents, and drugs for hypertension and blood disorders. Oral anti-inflammatory agents may also be used, but the administration of steroids is often delayed until infectious diseases are ruled out.

Removal of the eye may be recommended in cases of suspected intraocular tumors, blind eyes that remain painful, eyes with unresponsive glaucoma, or concern that an infection may persist in the eye and spread to other parts of the body (especially certain fungal infections).

Follow-up Care
Some cases of uveitis respond quickly to medications and resolve within days. Other cases of uveitis are more stubborn and require months of therapy. Prolonged therapy is often needed in cats with chronic uveitis, in dogs with fungal infections, in eyes with severe inflammation, and when the underlying cause is difficult to treat.

Recheck visits are done to assess response to treatment and to monitor for complications, such as glaucoma. Certain laboratory tests may also be repeated to monitor for side effects associated with the oral drugs used to treat uveitis.

Report any worsening of signs, particularly increased pain (squinting) or cloudiness, to your veterinarian immediately.

Prognosis
Whether uveitis will successfully resolve often depends on the underlying cause, the severity of the inflammation, and the diligence of the treatments. Many cases resolve with adequate therapy, but the animal must be monitored closely for recurrence of the inflammation as medications are tapered and stopped. Some cases of uveitis do not respond well and result in blindness or loss of the eye. Chronic uveitis in cats may require prolonged therapy (months to years).

SPECIAL INSTRUCTIONS:

Cataracts

Rhea V. Morgan, DVM, DACVIM (Small Animal), DACVO

BASIC INFORMATION

Description

A cataract is an opacity within the lens of the eye. Cataracts can be classified by their severity, age at onset, or underlying cause. *Incipient* cataracts are the mildest type, involve only a small portion of the lens, and do not affect vision. *Immature* cataracts affect 25-90% of the lens, may be severe enough to affect vision, and may be visible to owners. When the lens is completely opaque, a *mature* cataract is present, and vision is substantially decreased. Some cataracts shrink a little over time and become wrinkled. These *hypermature* cataracts may cause inflammation within the eye.

Based on the age at onset, a cataract may be described as congenital (present at birth), juvenile (onset at a few months to several years of age), adult, or senile (older animals). Cataracts are less common in cats than in dogs.

Causes

Congenital cataracts may arise from abnormal development of the lens or other ocular defects. Inherited cataracts are the most common type in dogs; they affect more than 40 different breeds and can arise at any age.

Other causes of cataracts include diabetes mellitus (sugar diabetes) in dogs, nutritional deficiencies (especially in the newborn), trauma to the eye, inflammation within the eye (such as uveitis), low blood calcium (rare), retinal degeneration, radiation therapy, and exposure to certain toxins or drugs (rare).

As they grow old, all animals develop a hardening of the center of the lens, which turns the lens a milky, gray-white color. This aging change is called *nuclear* or *lenticular sclerosis*. It is not the same as a cataract and is rarely treated.

Clinical Signs

Cataracts are often quite cloudy before vision is affected. Cloudiness in the eye may be detected first. Redness may also occur if the eye is inflamed. If the dog has sugar diabetes, then increased thirst and urination may be noted.

Diagnostic Tests

A complete eye examination is needed to confirm the diagnosis and may involve glaucoma testing and dilation of the pupil. Laboratory tests are usually performed to look for underlying causes. Simple lenticular sclerosis must also be ruled out.

TREATMENT AND FOLLOW-UP

Treatment Options

To date, there is no effective medical therapy for cataracts. Products available on the Internet have had minimal beneficial effects.

Cataracts that are small and do not affect vision may require no treatment. Not all cataracts progress, so monitoring may be the only initial recommendation.

For cataracts that are progressing and have reached the immature stage, surgical removal of the lens remains the most effective treatment. Not all eyes are candidates for surgery, however. In order for the eye to be operable, it must be free of inflammation, have a healthy retina, and have no evidence of glaucoma. In addition, any sugar diabetes must be well regulated prior to surgery, and the animal must be able to withstand general anesthesia.

Cataracts that are secondary to uveitis or retinal degeneration, associated with retinal detachments or other ocular defects, or complicated by other eye diseases (such as corneal edema, glaucoma, or tumors) are not often operable.

Your pet may be referred to a veterinary ophthalmologist to assess the cataract and determine what treatment options are available. If the eye is a potential candidate for surgery, two preoperative tests are usually recommended: an electroretinogram (ERG) to measure retinal function and an ultrasound of the eye to ensure that no retinal detachments are present. Anti-inflammatory medications may be given prior to surgery.

Most operable cataracts can be removed via phacofragmentation surgery. This is not laser surgery. It involves use of ultrasound to shatter and remove lens material through a small incision. If both eyes are affected and otherwise healthy, they are often operated at the same time, to avoid two general anesthetic procedures. If the lens bag (capsule) that is left behind is healthy, then an intraocular lens implant (IOL) may be inserted to improve close-up vision.

Follow-up Care

Postoperatively, medications must be administered several times daily for weeks to months, and numerous recheck visits are needed. Close monitoring for complications, such as postoperative uveitis, glaucoma, and retinal detachments, is important. Often the animal must wear an Elizabethan collar for 3-4 weeks while the incision is healing.

Prognosis

For uncomplicated cataracts in healthy eyes, the success rate of cataract surgery is quite high (85-90%). Success rates are lower in eyes that have been inflamed or affected by glaucoma and for cataracts that are hypermature. Cataract surgery is considered an elective surgery, because most animals do quite well with diminished or no vision.

SPECIAL INSTRUCTIONS:

Chorioretinitis and Optic Neuritis

Rhea V. Morgan, DVM, DACVIM (Small Animal), DACVO

BASIC INFORMATION
Description

Inflammation of the tissues of the back of the eye (choroid, retina) is called *chorioretinitis*. The choroid is part of the uvea of the eye, so inflammation of the choroid may be called *posterior uveitis*. Involvement of the nerve leading from the eye to the brain is called *optic neuritis*. These conditions may occur alone or together and are inherently serious because they affect vision.

Causes

With the exception of trauma to the eye, these conditions are usually manifestations of a systemic or generalized problem. The choroid and retina are commonly affected by other diseases within the body, and optic neuritis may arise with certain disorders of the brain. Numerous causes must be considered:

- More than 25 different infections can cause this inflammation, including fungal, tick-borne, bacterial, viral, protozoal, and parasitic infections. Some types occur more often in dogs, whereas others are more common in cats.
- In rare instances, the immune system may attack the uvea, and other parts of the body may also be affected.
- Tumors may arise within the eye or metastasize to the eye from elsewhere in the body.
- Hypertension (high blood pressure), anemia, kidney disease, sugar diabetes, elevated blood protein levels, and other blood disorders may be causes.

Clinical Signs

Inflammation confined to the back of the eye may not be visible and may not be discovered until the animal is examined for other signs of illness. Inflammation that also affects the front of the eye can cause the eye to be red, cloudy, and painful (squinting). Vision may be affected, resulting in pupils of different sizes. If both eyes are inflamed, the animal may act blind. The onset of blindness can be quite sudden (within days).

Diagnostic Tests

Diagnosis of these conditions can be difficult without specialized instruments to examine the back of the eye. If the diagnosis cannot be confirmed, your veterinarian may refer your pet to a veterinary ophthalmologist or neurologist for further evaluation. A complete physical examination is usually performed to search for any other changes that may signify the presence of a generalized (systemic) problem.

Laboratory tests are frequently done to search for infections and underlying causes. Chest and abdominal x-rays and an abdominal ultrasound are sometimes recommended. If hypertension is suspected, blood pressure can be measured. In eyes that are cloudy and cannot be examined well, an ultrasound may be performed. If a brain disorder is suspected, computed tomography (CT scan) or magnetic resonance imaging and a spinal tap may be recommended. The cause of chorioretinitis and/or optic neuritis can be difficult to find and may require numerous tests.

TREATMENT AND FOLLOW-UP

Treatment Options

Treatment involves administering medications for the eye problem and for any underlying causes. Medications applied to the eye do not reach the retina and choroid but topical anti-inflammatory drugs (usually steroids), pupil dilators/pain relievers (such as atropine), and antibiotics may be used for inflammation in the front part of the eye.

Once an underlying cause is determined, appropriate treatment is started for that condition. Examples include antibiotics, anti-fungal agents, drugs for hypertension and blood disorders, and chemotherapy for certain tumors. Oral anti-inflammatory agents can reach the retina, choroid, optic nerve, and brain, but the administration of steroids is often delayed until infectious diseases are ruled out and a specific cause is determined.

Removal of the eye may be recommended in cases of suspected intraocular tumors, blind eyes that remain painful, eyes that develop unresponsive glaucoma, or concern that an infection may persist in the eye and spread to other parts of the body (especially certain fungal infections).

Follow-up Care

Chorioretinitis and optic neuritis often indicate the presence of a serious underlying disease. If treatable, these diseases usually require prolonged therapy (months), periodic recheck visits, and careful monitoring. Certain laboratory tests may be repeated to monitor for side effects associated with the oral drugs used to treat these conditions.

Report any worsening of signs, particularly the onset of pain (squinting) or decreased vision, to your veterinarian immediately.

Prognosis

Whether chorioretinitis or optic neuritis will resolve often depends on the underlying cause, the severity of the inflammation, and the diligence of the treatments. Many cases improve with adequate therapy, but permanent scarring within the retina may result in blindness. Some forms of optic neuritis improve with treatment but are not cured, so therapy must be continued for the life of the animal. Some of the causes of these conditions are life-threatening.

SPECIAL INSTRUCTIONS:

Collie Eye Anomaly

Rhea V. Morgan, DVM, DACVIM (Small Animal), DACVO

BASIC INFORMATION
Description
Collie eye anomaly (CEA) is abnormal development of the retina and the sclera (the white, firm, outer coating of the eyeball). CEA affects both eyes and occurs most often in rough and smooth collies. It is also found in the Shetland sheepdog, Australian shepherd, Lancashire heeler, and border collie.

Causes
CEA is inherited as an autosomal recessive trait. Dogs that inherit an abnormal gene from each parent (homozygous) will develop CEA. Dogs that inherit an abnormal gene from only one parent (heterozygous) will be carriers of the disease.

Clinical Signs
The following lesions are components of CEA:
- Choroidal hypoplasia is the most common lesion of CEA and represents underdevelopment of a portion of the retina and its background layer (the choroid). Lesions of choroidal hypoplasia may range from small to large. They do not often affect vision.
- A coloboma is a pit or hole in the back of the eye. It may affect the optic nerve as it leaves the retina or some nearby area. Small colobomas are not usually associated with vision abnormalities, but large colobomas may cause decreased vision and predispose the retina to detachment.
- The retinal vessels may be tortuous in some dogs, meaning that they twist and turn in an abnormal fashion. These vessel changes do not affect vision unless they predispose the eye to retinal hemorrhages.
- Retinal detachments can occur and may be partial or complete. Complete detachment results in total blindness, often by 6-12 months of age.
- Retinal hemorrhages may occur spontaneously, or they may be associated with retinal detachment.

Diagnostic Tests
The diagnosis of CEA is made by examination of the retina using an ophthalmoscope. Since most lesions of CEA are present at birth, CEA can be seen in puppies as early as 6 weeks of age. Retinal examination is facilitated by the application of drops to dilate the pupils. It is common for entire litters of puppies to be examined at 6-7 weeks by a veterinary ophthalmologist.

Examination at an early age helps to determine which puppies may potentially be used for breeding in the future and which puppies may develop vision abnormalities. Early examination is also important to identify all affected puppies. Puppies with only mild choroidal hypoplasia may be hard to recognize by 10-12 weeks of age, because mild hypoplasia lesions may fill in with pigment and disappear from view. Although these puppies look normal (and are called *go normals*), they are actually affected with CEA.

A genetic test for CEA has also been developed that can identify affected, carrier, and normal dogs. The test is performed on a blood sample and is available from OptiGen (*www.optigen.com*).

TREATMENT AND FOLLOW-UP
Treatment Options
No treatment exists for CEA. To date, no effective treatment is available to prevent the retinal detachments associated with this condition. Laser therapy may be tried for partial retinal detachments, if they are discovered early. To eliminate CEA from collies and other affected breeds, it is recommended that only normal animals be used for breeding. Because CEA is so widespread in the collie breed, homozygous normal dogs are hard to find. In collies, it is common for dogs with only choroidal hypoplasia to be used for breeding. Dogs with only the mildest form of the disease may still produce puppies with more severe lesions, if they are bred to another affected or carrier dog.

Follow-up Care
With the exception of the development of a retinal detachment, CEA is not a progressive disease. Puppies at risk for retinal detachments may be monitored periodically. Notify your veterinarian if any decrease in vision is noted.

Prognosis
Prognosis for puppies with choroidal hypoplasia or mild colobomas is good, because these lesions do not usually affect vision. Vision may be affected by larger colobomas. Retinal detachment invariably results in blindness in the affected eye. Retinal detachment can occur in one or both eyes.

SPECIAL INSTRUCTIONS:

Conjunctivitis

Rhea V. Morgan, DVM, DACVIM (Small Animal), DACVO

BASIC INFORMATION

Description

Conjunctivitis is inflammation of the tissues lining or covering the eyelids and eyeball.

Causes

Numerous factors can lead to conjunctivitis, including infection by bacteria or viruses (especially herpesvirus in cats), irritants, and trauma. Irritants can include chemicals, smoke, dust, soap, foreign bodies, abnormal hair, and many others. Young dogs (less than 1 year of age) may develop follicular conjunctivitis, which appears to be an excessive immune response to environmental irritants.

Certain forms of conjunctivitis may develop with allergies or accompany immune disorders. Conjunctivitis often occurs in eyes with dry eye (keratoconjunctivitis sicca). It can occur in association with many systemic or generalized illnesses, such as upper respiratory tract infections and generalized viral or bacterial infections. Rarely, parasites, fungal infections, and tumors of ocular tissues can cause conjunctivitis.

Clinical Signs

Redness of the conjunctiva is a common sign. Ocular discharge often develops and may be watery, mucoid (gelatinous, gray), or pus-like (thick, yellow-green). Swelling of the conjunctiva may occur in some cases. Follicular conjunctivitis in dogs receives its name from the small white swellings (follicles) that develop on the third eyelid and conjunctiva. Some forms of conjunctival inflammation (such as eosinophilic conjunctivitis in cats) can cause small pink growths to develop on the conjunctiva. With widespread or severe conjunctivitis, inflammation of the eyelids (*blepharitis*) or of the cornea (*keratitis*) may also occur.

Most eyes with mild conjunctivitis are not painful. Eyes with conjunctivitis associated with trauma, chemical burns, corneal ulceration, or foreign bodies may be painful (indicated by squinting, pawing, and so on).

Diagnostic Tests

Conjunctivitis must be differentiated from other causes of a red eye, including glaucoma, corneal ulceration, scleritis (inflammation of the deeper white tissue covering the eyeball), and uveitis (inflammation inside the eye). Other conditions, such as skin diseases and tumors of the eyelids that can affect the conjunctiva secondarily, may also be involved. A thorough eye examination with a tear test, fluorescein staining for a corneal ulcer, and glaucoma testing (intraocular pressure measurement) is often performed to rule out some of these other conditions.

To identify potential causes, further testing may include a conjunctival scraping and examination of the cells under the microscope (cytology), submission of a bacterial culture, or special assays for viruses. Biopsies are sometimes done in severe, unusual, or unresponsive cases.

TREATMENT AND FOLLOW-UP

Treatment Options

Specific treatment is directed at the underlying cause.

- For example, if irritants are thought to be the cause, then removal of the source of irritation is important. Local foreign bodies or exposure to chemicals is usually treated with flushing of the eye.
- Antibiotics are given for bacterial infections, and antiviral medications may be given for viral infections. These medications may be administered topically and orally (systemically).
- Conjunctivitis associated with dry eye often improves with therapy for that condition.
- Topical antihistamines and steroids are often used when conjunctivitis occurs in association with allergies or is thought to be an immune disease.
- The rare parasitic infestations are treated by removal of the parasite and ant-inflammatory medications.

Symptomatic treatment for conjunctivitis of unknown or uncertain origin may involve the administration of a topical antibiotic or steroid preparation, installation of soothing lubricant agents, and possibly the use of other anti-inflammatory drugs.

Follow-up Care

Some forms of conjunctivitis respond very quickly, whereas others are stubborn and require prolonged therapy. Recheck visits are frequently needed to evaluate the eye's response to treatment and to decide whether further diagnostic tests or other therapies are needed. Recheck visits also allow other associated problems (such as corneal ulceration or blepharitis) to be assessed.

Any eye with conjunctivitis that becomes painful (squinting, pawing at the eye) warrants re-examination as soon as possible; in the meantime, all steroid medications being administered are stopped.

Prognosis

Many forms of conjunctivitis, including those caused by one-time exposure to irritants, trauma, or corneal ulcers, resolve completely. Other forms of conjunctivitis can recur intermittently or become chronic. Examples of these include herpesvirus or eosinophilic conjunctivitis in cats and conjunctivitis associated with dry eye or allergic skin disease.

SPECIAL INSTRUCTIONS:

Corneal Ulceration

Rhea V. Morgan, DVM, DACVIM (Small Animal), DACVO

BASIC INFORMATION

Description

A corneal ulcer occurs when the protective surface layer of the cornea is lost. The deeper layers of the cornea are exposed and become prone to infection and injury. These deeper layers contain many nerves, and irritation of these nerves is very painful. Corneal ulcers range from superficial abrasions and small circular lesions to deep craters that may perforate. Ulcers may be complicated by secondary bacterial infections and by severe inflammation of the eye.

Causes

Many different causes exist, including trauma (such as cat scratches or foreign bodies), abnormalities of the eyelids (entropion, extra or abnormal eyelashes), decreased blinking (during sedation or general anesthesia, neurologic problems), and exposure to irritants (chemicals, soaps, heat or flame). Infections with bacteria, viruses, or fungal agents can cause ulcers. The presence of dry eyes or calcium infiltrates and edema (water retention) in the cornea can also predispose to ulceration.

Dogs with short, flat faces and prominent eyes are very prone to corneal ulcers, because their eyes are large and protrude beyond the eyelids. These dogs also have poor sensation (feeling) in the central cornea and blink less often than other dogs.

🖥 Clinical Signs

Pain is a hallmark sign of corneal injuries and ulceration. It is manifested by tearing, squinting, blinking, and sometimes pawing at the eye. The animal may also be quiet and withdrawn.

The eye is usually red. Thick discharge may develop with infection. The cornea may be cloudy or have visible irregularities. Other signs, such as swelling of the eyelids, inward rolling of the eyelid, protrusion of the third eyelid, or bruising around the head, may occur depending on the cause. Signs of upper respiratory tract infection may be noted in cases of herpesvirus infection in cats or distemper virus infection in dogs.

🔬 Diagnostic Tests

The presence of a corneal ulcer is confirmed by close examination and fluorescein staining of the cornea. Installation of a local anesthetic drop to numb the eye may be needed prior to examination. Other ocular testing, such as a Schirmer tear test, testing of reflexes, examination of the eyelids and interior of the eye, and glaucoma testing, may also be indicated. If a bacterial infection is suspected, a culture of the eye may be submitted.

TREATMENT AND FOLLOW-UP

℞ Treatment Options

Many ulcers can be treated on an outpatient basis, but hospitalization may be recommended for severe ulcers. Treatment can involve medications, surgery, and other measures, depending on the type and severity of the ulcer. Medications are applied to all ulcers:

- Topical antibiotics are administered to treat active infections and/or to prevent infections. If the ulcer is deep and there is concern about infection within the eye, then oral or injectable antibiotics may also be given.
- Topical atropine (pupil dilator) or other pain medications (nalbuphine, morphine) may be given, as needed.
- Topical and/or oral antiviral and antifungal medications are given for those infections.
- Oral nonsteroidal anti-inflammatory drugs may be considered for marked inflammation and discomfort, especially in dogs.

Ancillary measures include application of an Elizabethan collar to prevent self-trauma, application of soft contact bandage lenses, placement of a third eyelid flap to protect the cornea, and administration of the pet's own serum (used mainly for soft, melting ulcers). Surgical correction of any underlying causes, such as entropion correction or removal of foreign bodies or abnormal lashes, is also beneficial.

If the ulcer is deep enough to weaken the cornea, then supportive surgical techniques are often performed. These include various types of grafting techniques that use either conjunctival tissue from the animal's eye or harvested tissue from another animal. Small, deep lesions can sometimes be directly closed by suturing the edges together.

🐾 Follow-up Care

Recheck visits are needed to assess healing and response to treatment. Visit frequency can range from every 24-48 hours to every 7-14 days, depending on the severity. Fluorescein staining of the cornea is done at most visits to highlight the ulcer and to determine when it has healed.

Prognosis

Most superficial ulcers and abrasions heal quickly, with minimal scarring. Deep ulcers and ulcers that are infected are more difficult to treat, and secondary changes such as inflammation within the eye or scarring and pigmentation of the cornea can decrease vision. Certain bacteria produce substances that can melt the cornea, sometimes resulting in perforations and loss of vision and the eye. Ulcers that require surgical grafting often must be treated and monitored diligently for several weeks.

SPECIAL INSTRUCTIONS:

Distichiasis and Ectopic Cilia

Rhea V. Morgan, DVM, DACVIM (Small Animal), DACVO

BASIC INFORMATION

Description

Normal eyelashes develop from hair follicles on the skin surface of the eyelid. Distichia and ectopic cilia are eyelashes that grow from small glands in the middle layer of the eyelid. *Distichia* grow out the duct of the gland and point downward or upward from the smooth edge of the eyelid. These cilia may brush against the cornea as the lids open and close. *Ectopic cilia* exit from the conjunctival or inner surface of the lid and point directly at the cornea. Ectopic cilia most often develop on the central upper eyelid and may occur alone or in combination with distichia. Ectopic cilia may arise in just one eye, but it is common for distichia to be found in both eyes.

Causes

Distichiasis may be inherited. It is common in certain breeds of dogs, such as the American cocker spaniel, shih tzu, Bedlington terrier, boxer, Weimaraner, Shetland sheepdog, collie, Pekingese, and others. Purebred dogs are affected more often than mixed-breed dogs and cats. Ectopic cilia are less common but may be found in all types of dogs, usually before 1 year of age.

Clinical Signs

Signs associated with *distichiasis* often depend on the number and character of the lashes present. American cocker spaniels often have numerous distichia, but they are short and fine and often cause no clinical signs. In other dogs, watery tearing, increased mucus production, blinking or squinting, or conjunctivitis may be noted. Corneal ulcerations may occur in some dogs.

Ectopic cilia often cause corneal ulcers, marked squinting, and pain. Signs may improve for awhile if the conjunctiva grows over the eyelash, but invariably they return when the cilia grows longer and becomes exposed again. The resulting corneal ulcer does not respond well to medical therapy.

Diagnostic Tests

Distichia can often be seen with the naked eye and a light beam focused on the eyelid, but ectopic cilia can be very difficult to see. Magnification is often needed to locate ectopic cilia. The cornea is often stained with fluorescein to determine the presence of an ulcer. The eyelids and surface of the eye are also examined for other defects.

TREATMENT AND FOLLOW-UP

Treatment Options

No treatment of distichiasis is needed in dogs that are asymptomatic (including most American cocker spaniels). If only a few distichia or only minor signs are present, then topical lubricant ointments may be used to coat the cilia in oil and protect the cornea. If signs resolve, then this therapy may be continued indefinitely. Temporary plucking of the eyelashes is not usually performed, because they invariably grow back.

Multiple distichia are often treated with cryotherapy, which is the application of a freezing agent to the underside of the eyelid, over the affected gland. Affected glands may also be cauterized, but the heat generated by cautery often damages surrounding tissues more than freezing does. Surgery to remove the hairs is not often performed unless only one or two clusters are present.

Ectopic cilia are best treated by surgical removal of the cilia and the associated eyelid gland. Because these lashes are so small, surgery may be performed under an operating microscope. It is important to remove these cilia as soon as possible, so that the cornea is no longer irritated and pain is relieved.

Follow-up Care

Following distichia surgery, a topical antibiotic or lubricant may be applied to protect the cornea, because eyelid swelling is common for several days. An Elizabethan collar may also be applied to prevent self-trauma. Dark eyelid margins may turn pink after they are treated with cryotherapy, but the black color typically returns in 6-8 weeks.

After surgery for ectopic cilia, topical antibiotics and pain relievers may be used for corneal ulcers, and an Elizabethan collar may be applied until the ulcer heals. Dogs are periodically monitored postoperatively until the corneal ulcer and surgery site have healed.

Prognosis

No single procedure is effective for removing all distichia, because hair follicles are very difficult to kill. Some distichia can be expected to persist or return. In addition, more distichia may grow in new locations over the course of months to years. Periodic monitoring for regrowth is warranted, and repeated treatments may be needed.

Many dogs with ectopic cilia are cured with one surgery, if the entire hair follicle and associated glands are removed completely. Any recurrence of clinical signs (especially pain and squinting) requires re-examination for regrowth or eruption of new cilia.

SPECIAL INSTRUCTIONS:

Ectropion

Rhea V. Morgan, DVM, DACVIM (Small Animal), DACVO

BASIC INFORMATION
Description
Ectropion is outward rolling of the eyelid and usually involves the central part of the lower eyelid. It may also affect the upper lid. It occurs predominantly in the dog.

Causes
Ectropion may be inherited and may develop early in the American cocker spaniel, basset hound, bloodhound, Clumber spaniel, Great Dane, Newfoundland, mastiff, Saint Bernard, boxer, and other breeds. The Saint Bernard often has ectropion of the central eyelids, entropion of the outer portion of the eyelids, and excessive lid length, giving the opening of their eyes a "pagoda" or "diamond" shape. Individuals in other breeds may have a similar eyelid conformation.

Acquired ectropion may occur after eyelid trauma (especially lacerations or bite wounds) or eyelid surgery (such as overzealous entropion repair or removal of large lid tumors). Acquired ectropion may also develop in older dogs from decreased muscle tone of the eyelids and may be noted temporarily in hunting dogs when they become tired. Ectropion may also occur with paralysis of the seventh cranial nerve, which activates the eyelid muscles.

Clinical Signs
Many dogs have no clinical signs except for increased visibility of the conjunctiva of the lower eyelid. If the eyelid does not protect the nearby cornea or if ectropion is combined with entropion, then signs of corneal inflammation or ulceration (squinting, discharge, redness) may occur. Debris sometimes collects in the gap between the affected portion of the eyelid and the cornea and may be irritating to the eye.

Diagnostic Tests
Diagnosis is usually made by close examination of the eyelids. The eyelids may also be assessed for entropion, before and after local anesthetic drops are applied. The cornea is often stained with fluorescein to determine whether an ulcer is present.

TREATMENT AND FOLLOW-UP
Treatment Options
Dogs with minimal clinical signs may be treated conservatively by flushing debris from the eye with eye-irrigating solutions and applying a protective ophthalmic lubricant (usually an ointment or gel).

Surgical treatment is usually reserved for those cases with corneal irritation or inflammation, persistent conjunctivitis, or concurrent entropion. A variety of surgical procedures have been developed to correct ectropion, including simple wedge resection of the affected area. More complicated procedures are indicated if entropion and/or excessive lid length are also present.

Follow-up Care
For dogs treated conservatively with medical therapy, periodic rechecks may be indicated to monitor for ocular inflammation. Following surgery, it is common for an Elizabethan collar to be used. Topical antibiotics may also be applied to the eye. Sutures are usually removed in 10-14 days.

Prognosis
Simple ectropion may cause very few problems throughout the lifetime of the dog. Most forms of symptomatic ectropion are helped considerably by surgery.

SPECIAL INSTRUCTIONS:

Entropion

Rhea V. Morgan, DVM, DACVIM (Small Animal), DACVO

BASIC INFORMATION
Description
Entropion is inward rolling of the eyelid and may involve part or all of one or more eyelids. Entropion may be inherited and develop soon after birth, or it may be acquired.

Causes
Inherited entropion occurs in many different breeds of dogs, including the mastiff, American bulldog, Chinese shar-pei, Great Dane, Doberman pinscher, Labrador retriever, Rottweiler, Saint Bernard, boxer, and others. Because of their excessive facial folds, entropion may develop in shar-pei puppies soon after their eyelids open. In other breeds, the condition becomes obvious over several weeks to months.

Acquired entropion may develop following inflammation, trauma, or chronic eye pain. Acquired entropion is more common in the cat and may arise after ocular infection with feline herpesvirus. Some forms of eye pain cause spastic entropion, which often resolves when the pain subsides.

Clinical Signs
Clinical signs are quite variable and may include mild tearing, squinting and blinking, and production of large amounts of thick discharge. Some animals find it hard to keep their eyes open and may paw or rub at the eyes. The eye may be red, and the cornea may be ulcerated, inflamed, and cloudy. In shar-pei puppies, the eyes may barely be visible.

Diagnostic Tests
Entropion can usually be diagnosed by close examination of the eyelids, before and after local anesthetic drops are applied to the eye. The cornea may be stained with fluorescein to determine whether an ulcer is present.

TREATMENT AND FOLLOW-UP

Treatment Options
Temporary tacking can be performed for entropion in very young puppies. Sutures or staples are placed in the skin above and/or below the eyelids and pulled tight enough to cause the eyelids to roll out. This procedure allows time for the puppy to grow into the facial skin and may prevent the need for permanent entropion surgery. Temporary tacking is also occasionally used for spastic entropion and in animals that cannot undergo general anesthesia.

Spastic entropion usually resolves once the underlying problem has been corrected. Ocular ointments and a soft contact lens may be applied to protect the cornea until the problem resolves.

Most other cases of entropion require permanent corrective surgery. Simple entropion is often corrected by making parallel elliptical incisions in the skin of the affected portion of lid. The skin between the incisions is removed, and when the defect is sutured closed, the eyelid rolls outward. Other surgical techniques may be used if entropion affects the inner or outer corners of the lids or is accompanied by excessive lid length, ectropion, or other defects. In Chinese shar-pei and chow chow dogs that have persistent, excessive skin folds of the forehead, a permanent brow-tacking procedure may be considered after the dog is fully grown.

Follow-up Care
Temporary tacking sutures are sometimes removed by the mother dog as she cleans the puppies' faces, or they may fall out on their own. If the sutures are retained, they may be removed in 2-3 weeks.

Following permanent corrective surgery, an Elizabethan collar is often applied to prevent trauma to the suture line. Topical antibiotics may also be applied to both eyes, and sutures are usually removed in 10-14 days.

Prognosis
Simple entropion is often corrected with one surgery, and clinical signs usually resolve quickly. Complicated entropion may require more than one surgery or may be treated with staged surgeries, with two techniques performed several weeks or months apart.

SPECIAL INSTRUCTIONS:

Eyelid Tumors

Rhea V. Morgan, DVM, DACVIM (Small Animal), DACVO

BASIC INFORMATION

Description

Eyelid tumors are growths that occur within or near the eyelids. Most eyelid tumors in the dog are benign, whereas most in the cat are malignant. Older animals are affected most often. The growth rate of eyelid tumors ranges from very slow to very rapid.

Causes

Many eyelid tumors arise from the cells or tissues within the eyelid, but some originate in other locations and spread to the eye or invade the eyelid from adjacent structures.

In the dog, the most common tumor types are the sebaceous adenoma and the papilloma. Tumors that occur in both dogs and cats include the melanoma, mast cell tumor, basal cell carcinoma, squamous cell carcinoma, fibrosarcoma, lymphoma, and others. In most cases, it is not known why these tumors develop.

Clinical Signs

A mass is visible at the edge or within the eyelid. It may be smooth, irregular, nodular, or ulcerated. The color of these masses is quite variable. The eyelid may be deformed and inflamed. Conjunctivitis, ocular discharge, and corneal ulceration may also occur. Most tumors are not painful unless they cause ulceration, in which case the animal may paw or rub the eye and squinting may be noted.

Diagnostic Tests

The presence of a tumor can usually be determined by close examination of the eyelid and eye. Aspiration and cytology of larger masses may provide a tentative diagnosis as to the type of tumor present, but usually a definitive diagnosis requires biopsy and pathologic examination. Other tests may be performed to search for tumors elsewhere in the body if the eyelid tumor is suspected to be malignant or to have originated in another location. Preoperative laboratory tests and chest x-rays may also be recommended prior to anesthesia and surgery.

TREATMENT AND FOLLOW-UP

Treatment Options

Small, benign eyelid tumors can often be removed by a full-thickness resection, which involves taking out a wedge of the eyelid that includes the tumor. The eyelid is then sutured back together. Occasionally, these small tumors are removed with a laser and the defect is not sutured. Larger tumors require more involved surgeries, with formation of a new eyelid margin.

Other treatments that may be tried for particular types of tumors include cryotherapy (freezing), chemotherapy (especially for lymphoma and metastatic tumors), and radiation therapy. In severe cases in which the tumor is malignant and invading the eye or the tissues immediately around the eye, surgery to remove the eye and all affected tissues may be necessary.

Follow-up Care

Following surgery, it is common for the patient to be sent home with an Elizabethan collar in place to keep the animal from bothering the sutures. Topical antibiotics may be administered to the eye. The sutures are usually removed in 10-14 days. Signs of postoperative problems include squinting, tearing, and increased ocular discharge; if any of these signs occur, immediately notify your veterinarian.

Prognosis

Benign tumors that are completely removed are usually cured by surgery. Prognosis is particularly good when the tumors are still small at the time of surgery and the eyelid margin can be reformed as normally as possible. Following extensive surgery to remove large tumors, it may be necessary to monitor for growth of hairs that rub on the cornea and for corneal inflammation.

Malignant tumors often recur at the surgery site and may spread to other areas of the body. Following removal of these tumors, additional treatment and monitoring are usually needed. The long-term prognosis with many of the malignant tumors is poor.

SPECIAL INSTRUCTIONS:

Feline Corneal Sequestration

Rhea V. Morgan, DVM, DACVIM (Small Animal), DACVO

BASIC INFORMATION
Description
A corneal sequestrum is an area of dead tissue that arises following some sort of injury or irritation of the cornea. The reasons why a focal area of the cornea dies and becomes discolored are not well understood. The sequestrum appears as a dark brown, almost black spot.

Corneal sequestra can occur in any age of cat, but they usually develop in adult cats (average age, 5.5 years). Persian, Himalayan, British colorpoint, Burmese, Siamese, and American domestic shorthair cats appear to be predisposed. The lesion can occur in one (most commonly) or both eyes. Corneal sequestration has also been called *corneal nigrum, corneal mummification,* and *necrotizing keratitis.*

Causes
Numerous sources of irritation may result in a sequestrum, including prior corneal ulceration, entropion (in-rolling of the eyelids), abnormal eyelashes or hair rubbing on the eyes, chronic conjunctivitis, chronic exposure of the cornea, and dry eye from poor tear production. Feline herpesvirus (FHV) infection has also been incriminated as a contributing factor in this disease.

Clinical Signs
A round to oval, black spot develops in the cornea, often near the center. The spot looks very out of place and can be mistaken for a foreign body. The surrounding cornea may be red and cloudy. In some cats, the sequestrum causes no pain. If corneal ulceration is present, the eye may be painful, and the animal may exhibit squinting, tearing, and redness. Although they are rare, severe ulceration and corneal perforation may occur.

Diagnostic Tests
Diagnosis can usually be made by close examination of the cornea, sometimes with magnification. A complete ocular examination often involves tear testing, fluorescein staining of the cornea, and a thorough search for underlying causes. In some cases, cell samples may be submitted for FHV testing. Other causes of dark spots in the cornea, such as foreign bodies and melanoma tumors, must be ruled out.

TREATMENT AND FOLLOW-UP

Treatment Options
For the corneal sequestrum, two main treatment options exist:

- *Medical therapy* may be tried in cats that do not exhibit pain, especially if the sequestrum is close to the surface of the cornea. Over time, the cornea attempts to reject this dead tissue, and the sequestrum may fall off on its own. This process can be quite slow and may take many months (average, 11 months). The medications used include topical antibiotics, protective lubricants, and sometimes topical or oral antiviral agents.
- *Surgery* to remove the sequestrum is often chosen for cats that are in pain. Several techniques are available, depending on the size and depth of the lesion. Most involve removal of a portion of the cornea (keratectomy). Because some of these surgical procedures require magnification, such as an operating microscope, your cat may be referred to a veterinary ophthalmologist for the procedure. Healing after simple keratectomy is usually rapid (7-21 days), but it may take a few weeks if a grafting procedure was needed. Postoperative medications may include topical antibiotics, lubricants, pain medications, and antiviral agents.

Any underlying problems must also be addressed. Medications may be started to treat dry eye, FHV infection, or corneal ulcerations. Surgery may be needed to correct entropion or other eyelid problems.

Follow-up Care
Recheck examinations are often performed every 3-4 weeks if medical therapy is tried. Rechecks may be scheduled more frequently if the cornea is ulcerated and inflamed. Examinations often involve fluorescein staining of the cornea and monitoring of the opposite eye.

When surgery is performed, postoperative examinations are usually done every 7-14 days until the cornea is healed. If the sequestrum was quite deep and corneal grafting was required after its removal, then recheck visits may be needed for several weeks.

Prognosis
Corneal sequestra recur in 10-20% of affected eyes and can develop at a later date in the opposite eye. The reasons for recurrence are not well defined but may include failure to adequately address contributing factors; inability to remove the entire sequestrum (too deep), or poor healing responses on the part of the cornea. In most cases, successful treatment is possible and the affected cornea may be left with only mild scarring. Good vision is maintained in most eyes.

SPECIAL INSTRUCTIONS:

Feline Eosinophilic Keratitis

Rhea V. Morgan, DVM, DACVIM (Small Animal), DACVO

BASIC INFORMATION

Description

Eosinophilic keratitis is the development of a pink, white, or gray film in the cornea of cats. This film often contains white blood cells called *eosinophils* (hence, the name). The condition may be accompanied by calcium deposition in the cornea and may also involve the third eyelid and the outer eyelids.

Eosinophilic keratitis may be diagnosed in one or both eyes. The disease arises in cats of all ages but is most common in cats 4 years or younger. Neutered (castrated) male cats are affected more often than females. The condition occurs in domestic shorthaired and longhaired cats more often than in purebred cats.

Causes

The exact cause of the disease is unknown. Feline herpesvirus (FHV) infection may be present in many affected cats (up to 76%), but whether this is a cause or only an opportunistic infection is unknown.

Clinical Signs

A pink, white, or gray film begins at the upper-outer edge of the cornea, or sometimes at the lower edge of the cornea, behind the third eyelid. This film slowly spreads across the cornea, and firm, gritty, white calcium plaques may develop on the surface. If the condition is left untreated, the cornea becomes thickened, irregular, and opaque. Corneal ulcerations may also occur.

The underside of the eyelids and the entire third eyelid may become red and thickened. Squinting and pain can occur from the eyelids blinking over the gritty, calcified areas or from corneal ulceration. Although tearing may be seen, usually a thick discharge is present on the surface of the eye. In severe cases, the cornea becomes infected and vision is decreased.

Diagnostic Tests

A tentative diagnosis can often be reached by finding the classic changes in the cornea. The diagnosis is confirmed by taking cell samples from the eye and finding eosinophils or mast cells (another type of white blood cell) in the samples. Samples may also be submitted for FHV testing. Other causes of corneal inflammation are eliminated by a thorough examination that may include tear testing, fluorescein staining, and glaucoma testing.

TREATMENT AND FOLLOW-UP

Treatment Options

Eosinophilic keratitis usually responds to topical steroid medications. In severe cases, injectable steroids may also be placed in the conjunctiva of the eye, or oral steroids may be given. Steroid therapy may be delayed if a corneal ulcer is present, because the steroids may make the ulcer worse. In these cases, the eye may be treated with topical antibiotics and/or antiviral medications until the ulcer has healed.

Additional treatment for FHV may be considered, including oral lysine and antiherpes drugs such as famciclovir. Topical cyclosporine has been used with success in a small number of cats. For cats that do not respond or do not tolerate these medications, oral megestrol acetate may be tried. This medication requires careful monitoring because of its potential serious side effects, including diabetes mellitus (sugar diabetes), weight gain, and behavioral changes.

Once the corneal film has receded, the medications are slowly tapered to the lowest dose that keeps the condition in remission. In some cases, long-term oral lysine may be recommended to try and suppress the FHV infection.

Follow-up Care

Recheck visits are needed to assess response to treatment and to check for complicating factors, such as corneal ulcers. Examinations are performed until the cornea is clear and then periodically thereafter to monitor for recurrences. Report any worsening of the signs or any onset of pain (squinting or increased tearing) immediately to your veterinarian. If the eye becomes painful while a topical steroid is being given, stop the drug until the eye can be re-examined.

Prognosis

This condition can be easy or difficult to control. The disease is more difficult to treat when active herpesvirus infection and corneal ulcers are also present. Medications must often be given consistently for several weeks to months to bring the condition under control.

The condition can often be controlled but may not be cured. Recurrences (as high at 64%) are possible as the medications are tapered and can also develop months to years later. If only one eye is affected originally, the second eye may be affected at a later date.

Mildly affected corneas often return to normal. In moderate to severe cases, some cloudy corneal scarring or crystalline fatty deposits may remain in the corneas. Good vision is usually maintained in most adequately treated eyes.

SPECIAL INSTRUCTIONS:

Feline Herpesvirus Keratoconjunctivitis

Rhea V. Morgan, DVM, DACVIM (Small Animal), DACVO

BASIC INFORMATION

Description and Cause

Feline herpesvirus (FHV) infection is a common upper respiratory infection of cats. Most cats are exposed at some point during their life. In some cats, the virus is not cleared but only goes into remission (becomes latent) and can become reactivated during times of stress or illness. The virus often infects the surface tissues of the eye, affecting the cornea and conjunctiva. FHV may be the most common cause of chronic keratoconjunctivitis (corneal-conjunctival inflammation) in the cat. FHV has also been incriminated in the development of corneal sequestration, eosinophilic keratitis, bullous keratopathy, and dry eye in cats. These ocular conditions may occur even in cats that have been vaccinated for the virus.

Clinical Signs

Signs are highly variable and range from mild conjunctivitis to life-threatening illness. In severe cases, signs of upper respiratory infection, fever, loss of appetite, lethargy, conjunctival swelling, corneal ulceration and rupture, and copious ocular and nasal discharge may all occur. Secondary bacterial infections are also common in these cases. Signs are usually the most severe in kittens and unvaccinated cats. Kittens with severe ocular inflammation may develop symblepharon, in which the eyelids and conjunctiva adhere to each other or to the cornea.

With chronic FHV infection, mild, persistent conjunctivitis; linear or nonhealing corneal ulcers; corneal inflammation; and dry eye may occur. (See also the handouts on **Feline Corneal Sequestration**, **Keratoconjunctivitis Sicca [Dry Eye]**, and **Feline Eosinophilic Keratitis**.) Symptoms may persist for a prolonged time or recur sporadically over the life the cat.

Diagnostic Tests

In severe cases and in cases with upper respiratory signs, the signs often allow a presumptive diagnosis to be made. Signs are less specific in chronic cases, although FHV is suspected to play a role in many cases of chronic conjunctivitis of cats. Scrapings may be taken from the conjunctiva to assess the type of cells present and to look for evidence of the virus and other agents. Specialized tests for FHV are available that utilize samples from the eye, nose, windpipe, or blood. If a secondary bacterial infection is suspected, bacterial cultures may be performed.

TREATMENT AND FOLLOW-UP

Rx Treatment Options

Treatment is directed at active FHV infection; there is no effective treatment for latent infection. It is difficult to cure FHV, but the infection may go into remission. Antiviral therapy involves the following:

- Topical antiviral medications, such as idoxuridine, trifluridine, or cidofovir, can be tried. These medications are expensive and are often obtained from compounding pharmacies. They require frequent application and can be irritating.
- Oral antiviral medications, such as famciclovir, may also be used.
- Oral lysine is an inexpensive supplement that can be used long term to try and keep the virus in remission.
- Oral or topical interferon-α may be tried in some cats.

Additional supportive measures may also be helpful:

- Concurrent bacterial (especially chlamydial) infections may require treatment with topical and systemic antibiotics.
- Protective lubricants and topical pain medications are useful in cases of conjunctival swelling and corneal ulceration.
- Application of most, warm compresses helps keep the eyes clean and free of discharge.
- The development of a corneal bulla or bubble or rupture of corneal ulcers may require surgery to repair the lesions or to remove the eye.

FHV infection may be part of an upper respiratory complex in cats (See the handout on **Feline Upper Respiratory Infection**.)

Follow-up Care

Recheck visits are often needed to monitor response to treatment and the healing of corneal ulcers. Medications may be changed or adjusted if signs do not improve. Fluorescein staining of the cornea and tear tests may be performed repeatedly.

Prognosis

Early and adequate vaccination of cats helps prevent FHV, especially the most severe infections. Severe infections do not often recur if the cat has a good immune system, but low-grade signs of FHV may recur sporadically throughout the cat's life. FVH is most likely to reactivate during times of stress, when other illnesses occur, or with prolonged use of anti-inflammatory or immunosuppressive medications (such as steroids). Chronic ocular inflammation can be difficult to treat, and prolonged, diligent therapy is often needed.

SPECIAL INSTRUCTIONS:

Glaucoma in Cats

Rhea V. Morgan, DVM, DACVIM (Small Animal), DACVO

BASIC INFORMATION

Description

Glaucoma is an increase in pressure within the eye. In contrast to dogs, primary or inherited glaucoma is rare in the cat. Both eyes are predisposed with primary glaucoma. Secondary or acquired glaucoma is the most common type of glaucoma in the cat and may affect only one eye, depending on the underlying cause.

Causes

Chronic uveitis (inflammation of the iris and surrounding tissues) is the most common cause of glaucoma in the cat. Other causes of secondary glaucoma include dislocation (luxation) of the lens, bleeding in the eye (hyphema), tumors, trauma, and other conditions. In rare cases, fluid in the front part of the eye may be directed backward, and pressure may become elevated (aqueous misdirection syndrome).

Primary glaucoma is rare but has been seen in Siamese and domestic shorthair cats. Glaucoma most often affects middle-aged to older cats, although it can occur in kittens. Congenital glaucoma is very rare.

Clinical Signs

Acute glaucoma can cause redness, watery discharge, pain (squinting, rubbing the eye), cloudiness, and blindness in the affected eye. Because many cats are quite stoic and can function normally with vision in just one eye, glaucoma may not be discovered until it becomes chronic and the eye enlarges. Signs of glaucoma are also similar to those of many other eye diseases. In some cases, glaucoma is discovered when the eye is examined for other problems, such as uveitis. Acute glaucoma usually affects one eye initially, unless uveitis is present in both eyes.

Diagnostic Tests

Glaucoma is diagnosed by measuring the pressure in the eye using a tonometer. A thorough eye examination is done to search for an underlying cause. If uveitis is present, laboratory testing is often needed to search for the cause of the uveitis. (See the handout on **Anterior Uveitis**.)

Primary glaucoma is diagnosed when none of the causes of secondary glaucoma are found. If the diagnosis, type, and cause of glaucoma are uncertain or if specialized treatment is needed, your veterinarian may refer your cat to a veterinary ophthalmologist for further evaluation.

TREATMENT AND FOLLOW-UP

Treatment Options

The goals of therapy are to lower the pressure, save or maintain vision, and relieve pain. Because primary glaucoma is rare and acute glaucoma is uncommonly recognized, most cats are treated for chronic, secondary glaucoma. Treatment of secondary glaucoma involves administration of anti-glaucoma drugs and therapy for the underlying cause. For example, surgery may be done to remove a dislocated lens, the eye may be removed if a tumor is suspected, or treatment may be started for uveitis.

Topical glaucoma medications are commonly used in both primary and secondary, acute and chronic glaucoma. Many different types of glaucoma medications may be used in cats, and the following are safe to use in the presence of uveitis:
- Beta-blockers: timolol (*Timoptic*), levobunolol (*Betagen*), betaxolol (*Betoptic*)
- Carbonic anhydrase inhibitors: dorzolamide (Trusopt), brinzolamide (*Azopt*)
- Combination products: timolol/dorzolamide (*Cosopt*)

If the glaucoma or underlying cause cannot be successfully controlled and the eye is blind, then an enucleation (removal of the eye) may be considered. In the rare cases of primary glaucoma, topical glaucoma medications are started in the normal eye to prevent or delay the onset of glaucoma in that eye.

Follow-up Care

Eyes with glaucoma require frequent monitoring and adjustment of medications. Over time, affected eyes may become less responsive to topical medications. Changes in medications or an enucleation may be needed, especially if the eye is blind and becoming larger. If the glaucoma can be controlled with medications, therapy may be lifelong.

Mild to moderate alterations in pressure within the eye may not cause a visible change and may be detected only with repeated pressure measurements (tonometry). Notify your veterinarian immediately if any increase in redness, cloudiness, or decreased vision occurs, because these signs may indicate worsening of the glaucoma.

Prognosis

Glaucoma does not always respond to medications; the medications must be administered painstakingly, and some are expensive. Prognosis for secondary glaucoma varies, depending on the cause. Many cats with mild glaucoma associated with uveitis respond well to medications, and vision can be saved. Primary glaucoma is often difficult to treat, and most affected eyes eventually go blind.

SPECIAL INSTRUCTIONS:

Glaucoma in Dogs

Rhea V. Morgan, DVM, DACVIM (Small Animal), DACVO

BASIC INFORMATION

Description

Glaucoma is an increase in pressure within the eye. It is a common eye disease of dogs. Primary or inherited glaucoma occurs in more than 40 different breeds, and both eyes are predisposed. Secondary or acquired glaucoma is also common and may affect only one eye, depending on the underlying cause.

Causes

With primary glaucoma, fluid in the front chamber of the eye backs up because of a malfunction in the drainage area, which causes an increase in pressure. The exact mechanism of the malfunction and the inheritance pattern of glaucoma are not clearly defined in many breeds. Primary glaucoma usually arises in adult dogs. Congenital glaucoma is very rare.

With secondary glaucoma, the movement of the fluid is obstructed somewhere along its usual route, so pressure increases. Causes of secondary glaucoma include uveitis, dislocation (luxation) of the lens, bleeding in the eye (hyphema), tumors, prior intraocular surgery, and other conditions.

Clinical Signs

Acute glaucoma can cause redness, watery discharge, pain (squinting, rubbing the eye), cloudiness, and blindness. Because many dogs are quite stoic and can function normally with vision in just one eye, glaucoma may not be discovered until it becomes chronic and the eye enlarges. Signs of glaucoma are also similar to those of many other eye diseases. Acute glaucoma usually affects one eye initially, unless uveitis (inflammation) is present in both eyes.

Diagnostic Tests

Glaucoma is diagnosed by measuring the pressure in the eye using a tonometer. A thorough eye examination is done to search for an underlying cause. Primary glaucoma is diagnosed when none of the causes of secondary glaucoma are found and the dog is of a predisposed breed. If the diagnosis and cause are uncertain or specialized treatment is needed, your veterinarian may refer your pet to a veterinary ophthalmologist for further evaluation.

TREATMENT AND FOLLOW-UP

Treatment Options

Acute glaucoma can be devastating to the eye and can result in blindness within a few hours. Aggressive therapy must be instituted quickly to try and save vision and relieve pain. Such therapy can involve the administration of intravenous mannitol and/or topical anti-glaucoma medications to bring the pressure down. Sometimes oral medications (glycerin, methazolamide) are also used. If the eye is inflamed, topical steroids may be given. Once

the pressure improves, several choices of therapy exist, depending on whether the eye still has visual function and whether the glaucoma is primary or secondary.

Most cases of primary glaucoma require surgery, because medications do not control the pressure well over the long term. Surgical options for sighted eyes include laser therapy, cryotherapy (freezing), and insertion of valves. Surgical options for blind eyes with glaucoma that cannot be controlled with medication alone include enucleation (removal of the eye), evisceration (removal of the internal contents of the eye) and prosthesis insertion, and sometimes a vitreal injection.

Treatment of secondary glaucoma involves administration of anti-glaucoma drugs and therapy for the underlying cause. For example, surgery may be done to remove a dislocated lens, the eye may be removed if a tumor is suspected, or treatment may be started for uveitis.

Topical glaucoma medications are commonly used for primary and secondary, acute and chronic glaucoma. Many different types of glaucoma medications can be used in dogs, and the choices depend on the type and severity of the glaucoma.

- Beta-blockers: timolol (*Timoptic*), levobunolol (*Betagen*), betaxolol (*Betoptic*)
- Carbonic anhydrase inhibitors: dorzolamide (*Trusopt*), brinzolamide (*Azopt*)
- Prostaglandin agents: latanoprost (*Xalatan*), bimatoprost (*Lumigan*), travoprost (*Travatan*)
- Combination products: timolol/dorzolamide (*Cosopt*), timolol/latanoprost (*Xalacom*), timolol/brimonidine (*Combigan*)
- Pupil constrictors: pilocarpine

Follow-up Care

Eyes with glaucoma require frequent monitoring and adjustment of medications. Over time, affected eyes may become less responsive to topical medications, so changes in medications or consideration of surgical options may be needed. If the glaucoma can be controlled with medications, therapy is lifelong in many cases.

In cases of primary glaucoma, topical medications are usually started to prevent glaucoma in the normal eye, and the pressure in that eye is periodically monitored. Any sign of redness, cloudiness, or decreased vision in the normal eye may indicate the onset of glaucoma, and the animal should be examined *immediately*!

Prognosis

Glaucoma is one of the most frustrating eye diseases to treat. Glaucoma does not always respond to medications; the medications must be administered painstakingly, and some are expensive. Primary glaucoma is extremely difficult to treat, and most affected eyes eventually go blind. The prognosis for secondary glaucoma varies, depending on the cause.

SPECIAL INSTRUCTIONS:

Horner's Syndrome

Rhea V. Morgan, DVM, DACVIM (Small Animal), DACVO

BASIC INFORMATION
Description

Horner's syndrome arises when certain neurologic information (sympathetic innervation or tone) to the eye is lost. Unlike sensory (feeling) or motor (movement) innervation, sympathetic innervation to eye does several unique things. It keeps the eye in the front part of the socket (orbit), the third eyelid recessed down in the corner near the nose, the pupil partially open, and the upper eyelid fully raised.

Sympathetic information begins in the brain, travels down the spinal cord in the neck, and leaves the spinal cord on nerves near the front of the chest. The nerve carrying the information crosses the chest near the first rib, turns back toward the head, and runs up the neck with the vagus nerve in the groove near the jugular vein. The nerve then travels through the middle ear, back into the floor of the brain cavity, and joins with the fifth cranial nerve. This last nerve then travels to the ocular structures, carrying sympathetic innervation with it.

Causes

Horner's syndrome can arise anywhere along the route that the nervous information travels. Common causes include trauma to the neck, such as from bite wounds, automobile accidents, surgery, venipuncture, or insertion of an intravenous catheter. Problems in the front of the chest, such as tumors, bleeding, fractured ribs, or tearing of the nerves from trauma, may cause Horner's syndrome.

Diseases, tumors, and surgery of the middle ear are potential causes. Head trauma, inflammation (meningoencephalitis), tumors, and vascular diseases of the brain are uncommon causes of Horner's syndrome.

Approximately 50% of all cases in dogs arise for unknown reasons and are called *idiopathic*. In cats, it is more common for a cause to be identified. Horner's syndrome typically affects just one eye.

Clinical Signs

The four classic signs of Horner's syndrome are a small pupil (miosis), recession of the eye into the orbit (enophthalmos), protrusion of the third eyelid, and drooping of the upper eyelid (ptosis). Ptosis can be subtle and may not be noticeable in all cases. Depending on the cause, other signs may also be present.

Diagnostic Tests

A tentative diagnosis is made by the presence of the four classic signs. Other causes of these signs must be ruled out by a thorough examination of the eye. Your pet may be referred to a veterinary ophthalmologist if further evaluation of the eye is needed.

Once Horner's syndrome is diagnosed, a search is undertaken for the cause. A complete physical examination is done, with close scrutiny of the ears, neck, and chest. Neurologic evaluations are performed. Routine laboratory tests and chest x-rays may be recommended. If other neurologic abnormalities are present, computed tomography (CT scan) or magnetic resonance imaging (MRI) may be considered. In some cases, pharmacologic testing (application of certain dilating drops on the eye) may be performed to try and determine where in its course the nerve is affected.

If all tests are negative, then the condition is considered idiopathic.

TREATMENT AND FOLLOW-UP

Treatment Options

No specific treatment exists for Horner's syndrome. Instead, treatment is directed at the underlying cause, if one can be found. There is no evidence that topical eye or ear medications affect the outcome.

Follow-up Care

Animals with Horner's syndrome are usually monitored for several weeks to months. The frequency of recheck visits and whether certain tests are repeated depends on the underlying cause. If any other neurological signs develop, notify your veterinarian immediately, as they may indicate the presence of brain disease.

Prognosis

Prognosis for Horner's syndrome varies, depending on the underlying cause. Horner's syndrome associated with chest trauma and tearing of the nerve, tumors of the chest, or brain diseases is often permanent. Horner's syndrome that accompanies trauma, surgery, or irritation to the tissues in the neck may resolve with time. Most cases that arise with inflammation or surgery of the middle ear also improve or resolve.

Approximately 50% of idiopathic cases improve or resolve. In some instances, the signs improve but do not completely disappear. Improvement usually starts within 6-8 weeks. Horner's syndrome is not painful, and most animals are oblivious to it. If it persists, it does permanently change the appearance of the animal.

SPECIAL INSTRUCTIONS:

Hypertensive Retinopathy

Rhea V. Morgan, DVM, DACVIM (Small Animal), DACVO

BASIC INFORMATION

Description

Hypertensive retinopathy includes a number of ocular changes that are produced by high blood pressure (systemic hypertension). Systemic hypertension is defined as a systolic pressure greater than 180 mm Hg or a diastolic pressure greater than 95 mm Hg. Most ocular abnormalities are associated with systolic blood pressures greater than 200 mm Hg. (See also the handout on **Systemic Hypertension**.)

Ocular changes associated with hypertension include retinal hemorrhages, abnormalities in retinal vessels, retinal detachment, and bleeding into the front chamber of the eye (hyphema). Multiple retinal hemorrhages are usually present and range in size from pinpoint to very large. The retina may detach in small, focal areas or completely. In most cases, several of these changes are present in the same eye. Both eyes are typically affected, but the abnormalities can be asymmetrical.

Causes

Chronic kidney disease is a common cause of hypertension in both dogs and cats. In cats, other causes include hyperthyroidism (elevated thyroid hormone), high-salt diets, and certain medications. In dogs, other causes include hyperadrenocorticism (elevated cortisone hormone), tumors of the adrenal gland and kidneys, diabetes mellitus (sugar diabetes), hypothyroidism (low thyroid hormone), and elevated red blood cell counts (polycythemia). Although it is rare, spontaneous (primary, essential) hypertension may occur in dogs and cats.

Clinical Signs

Mild hypertensive retinopathy may cause no vision abnormalities or clinical signs and may only be discovered when the animal is examined for other reasons. Severe retinal hemorrhages and complete retinal detachments lead to blindness. The blindness is often sudden in onset (within hours to days) and may be accompanied by dilated pupils. With hyphema, fresh red blood is seen in the front of the eye. Other clinical signs of the underlying disease are usually present.

Diagnostic Tests

Diagnosis of hypertensive retinopathy depends on finding one or more of the ocular lesions in an animal with hypertension. Hypertension is confirmed by repeated blood pressure measurements. Blood pressure is measured in dogs and cats with a blood pressure cuff in a manner similar to that in people, but special equipment must be used to detect blood flow in their tiny arteries. (See also the handout on **Indirect Blood Pressure Measurement**.)

Once the diagnosis is established, further tests are needed to find the underlying cause of the hypertension, and these may include routine laboratory tests, thyroid tests (cats), chest x-rays, and cortisol tests (dogs). Abdominal x-rays and an ultrasound may also be recommended. An echocardiogram (heart ultrasound) is often done in animals with signs of heart failure or heart murmurs detected on the physical examination. Additional tests, such as blood clotting tests, may be recommended to rule out other causes of ocular bleeding.

TREATMENT AND FOLLOW-UP

Treatment Options

Goals of therapy include control of the hypertension, successful treatment of the underlying cause, and improvement in the ocular changes. Antihypertensive drugs are started, such as amlodipine in cats and angiotensin-converting enzyme (ACE) inhibitors in dogs. If possible, systolic blood pressure is reduced to less than 160 mm Hg and diastolic pressure to less than 100 mm Hg. Appropriate treatments for the underlying cause are also instituted.

Hyphema usually causes inflammation in the eye, so topical steroid (anti-inflammatory) drugs are often used. The pupil may be dilated with atropine so that it does not stick to the lens. If the retinas are detached, oral steroids may be considered, because topical medications applied to the eye do not reach the retina. Oral steroids must be used with caution, however, because they may aggravate uncontrolled hypertension and are contraindicated with some of the underlying diseases that cause hypertension.

Follow-up Care

Eye and physical examinations and blood pressure measurements are commonly repeated every 7-14 days until blood pressures are normal and the ocular signs improve. The frequency of follow-up visits depends on how well the ocular changes respond to therapy and what is required to treat the underlying disease. Periodic monitoring is usually required for the life of the animal.

Prognosis

If the hypertension can be controlled, most ocular abnormalities improve and slowly resolve. It may take several weeks to months for hyphema to dissipate and retinal hemorrhages to fade. Abnormalities of the pupil may persist after hyphema, and retinal scarring is common in areas where hemorrhages occurred. If retinal detachments are diagnosed early and the hypertension is treated aggressively, reattachment of the retina can occur. In these cases, it is possible for some dogs to regain vision, but most cats remain blind.

SPECIAL INSTRUCTIONS:

Hyphema

Rhea V. Morgan, DVM, DACVIM (Small Animal), DACVO

BASIC INFORMATION

Description

Hyphema is blood in the front chamber of the eye. The blood may be clotted, or it may move freely. Free blood often settles when the animal is quiet, then disperses and becomes more noticeable when the animal is active.

Causes

Numerous causes of hyphema exist, including the following:

- Trauma—blunt or penetrating
- Abnormalities of blood clotting
- Hypertension (high blood pressure)
- Excessively high circulating protein levels (hyperviscosity) or number of red blood cells (polycythemia)
- Inflammation of the eye (uveitis), especially uveitis associated with certain tick-borne infections (ehrlichiosis, Lyme disease, and others)
- Movement of the lens within the eye and following retinal detachment
- Tumors of the eye
- Congenital birth defects of the eye, such as persistence of certain blood vessels and structures that should disappear soon after birth or the collie eye anomaly
- As a complication of eye procedures or surgery

Clinical Signs

Hyphema is usually diagnosed by a thorough eye examination. The eye examination often involves tear testing, fluorescein staining of the cornea, glaucoma testing, and evaluation of the deeper structures of the eye.

Diagnostic Tests

Once the presence of hyphema is confirmed, a search is instituted for the cause. A complete physical examination is conducted to look for other evidence of bleeding or an underlying cause. Routine laboratory tests, blood pressure measurement, blood clotting tests, and assays for tick-borne diseases may be recommended.

If there is too much blood in the eye to allow examination of the deeper structures, an ocular ultrasound may be helpful. X-rays of the skull may be done to look for metallic foreign bodies and evidence of trauma. Further testing may be needed if a systemic cause is found, to better define its effects on other organs of the body.

TREATMENT AND FOLLOW-UP

Treatment Options

Therapy for hyphema involves treating both the eye and the underlying cause. Appropriate treatment of the cause often helps prevent further hyphema. Affected animals are kept quiet to decrease the chance of further bleeding.

If the cornea is not ulcerated, topical steroids are started, because the hyphema commonly causes inflammation within the eye. Topical atropine is often used to dilate the pupil, unless secondary glaucoma is present. If glaucoma is detected, then anti-glaucoma drugs are started. Injection into the eye of drugs that dissolve clots may be tried when hyphema occurs after surgery on the eye.

Follow-up Care

Close monitoring of the eye is needed until the hyphema resolves, which can range from days to months. Repeated staining of the cornea and glaucoma testing are performed. Laboratory tests and blood pressure measurements may be repeated periodically, depending on the underlying cause.

Prognosis

Prognosis is highly variable. If the hyphema is mild and associated with trauma or a disease that can be effectively treated, the prognosis is good. Mild hyphema may resolve within days and may have no effect on vision.

If hyphema is severe, or if it is accompanied by bleeding into the back of the eye or by a retinal detachment, then the eye will be permanently blind. Severe hyphema may also lead to either shrinkage of the eye (over several weeks to months) or secondary glaucoma. If severe, unresponsive secondary glaucoma develops, then removal of the eye may be considered.

Hyphema that does not respond to topical therapy or is caused by diseases that are difficult to treat has a poor to guarded (uncertain) prognosis. In these cases, the hyphema can persist for long periods of time and can recur. Long-standing hyphema can disrupt the nutrition of the lens, which leads to cataract formation.

SPECIAL INSTRUCTIONS:

Intraocular Tumors

Rhea V. Morgan, DVM, DACVIM (Small Animal), DACVO

BASIC INFORMATION
Description
Intraocular tumors are masses that develop from structures within the eye (primary) or spread to the eye from other areas of the body (metastatic or secondary). These tumors may arise in the front or the back part of the eye.
Causes
The intraocular sarcoma of cats is the only tumor for which the cause is known. These tumors tend to arise from prior penetrating trauma and rupture of the lens. They can also be induced by substances injected into the eye.

Primary tumors of the eye may arise from the brown, pigmented layer (uvea) of the eye. Melanomas and ciliary body tumors may develop in the uvea. Tumors of retinal and neurologic tissues may develop in the back of the eye and include the medulloepithelioma, glioma, and astrocytoma.

Metastatic tumors occur most often in the back of the eye. Examples include adenocarcinomas originating from the kidneys, mammary glands, pancreas, or thyroid gland. Almost any tumor that metastasizes may eventually spread to the eye.

Lymphoma may develop as a primary or secondary intraocular tumor. It can arise in either the front or the back of the eye and is one of the few tumors that commonly affects both eyes.

Clinical Signs
When the tumor is in the front of the eye, it may be clearly visible as a brown or pink mass. The mass may involve the iris or the area immediately behind the iris, or it may occasionally be visible as a mass under the conjunctiva. The mass may distort the size and shape of the pupil, cause bleeding into the eye, or cause inflammation within the eye (uveitis).

Masses in the back of the eye may cause no outward clinical signs. As they enlarge, however, they may cause bleeding and inflammation. The retina may detach, resulting in blindness and a dilated pupil. The lens may dislocate, or glaucoma may develop.

The affected eye may eventually become red and painful. Other clinical signs may be present in cases of lymphoma and other metastatic tumors.

The age at onset of these tumors varies. Medulloepitheliomas occur most often in younger adult dogs. Lymphoma can occur at any age. Feline intraocular sarcoma may develop 1-10 years after the traumatic event. Other tumors are more likely in older animals.

Diagnostic Tests
A tentative diagnosis may be made from an eye examination, but many tumors appear similar to various forms of uveitis. Your pet may be referred to a veterinary ophthalmologist if further evaluation of the eye is needed. A thorough physical examination, routine laboratory tests, and chest and abdominal x-rays are often done to search for evidence of tumors elsewhere.

An ocular ultrasound may be recommended to better examine the eye, especially if bleeding makes it difficult to see intraocular structures. An abdominal ultrasound may be indicated if metastatic tumor is suspected. Tests may be conducted to rule out causes of uveitis that can result in similar signs and ocular findings. If the tumor is growing in the front of the eye, fluid may occasionally be aspirated from the front chamber (with the animal under anesthesia) and sent for microscopic analysis.

Definitive diagnosis requires biopsy. For secondary tumors, this may mean biopsying the main tumor in another organ. For primary tumors, biopsy often involves removing the eye and submitting the whole eye for evaluation.

TREATMENT AND FOLLOW-UP
Treatment Options
Removal of the eye (enucleation) is the most common treatment used for primary tumors. In rare instances, small, benign primary tumors may be treated with laser therapy or surgical removal, but most tumors are discovered too late (and are too large) for these therapies.

Because metastatic tumors originated elsewhere in the body, enucleation does not solve the problem. It may be done, however, to improve the quality of the animal's life if the eye is painful. Treatment of lymphoma and other secondary tumors often involves chemotherapy.

Follow-up Care
Little follow-up is needed after removal of eyes with benign tumors. Continuous monitoring and periodic testing are needed for the life of the animal when a malignant tumor is diagnosed.
Prognosis
Prognosis is good for benign tumors, because enucleation is curative. Prognosis is fair for primary malignant tumors that are diagnosed and removed early, before they have spread elsewhere. Prognosis is poor to grave for most other tumors. Not only is the eye usually lost, but the animal often succumbs to the cancer within several months. Chemotherapy may induce prolonged remission in animals with lymphoma.

SPECIAL INSTRUCTIONS:

Iridociliary Cysts

Rhea V. Morgan, DVM, DACVIM (Small Animal), DACVO

BASIC INFORMATION
Description

Iridociliary cysts are small, pigmented, fluid-filled structures that arise from the posterior surface of the iris or the ciliary body. The back of the iris is covered by a thin layer of cells that may become separated and filled with aqueous humor (fluid that is made by the ciliary body of the eye). The ciliary body is located behind the base of the iris. These cysts may also be called *anterior uveal cysts,* because the anterior uvea is composed of the iris and ciliary body.

Iridociliary cysts occur more often in dogs than in cats. Commonly affected breeds include the beagle, golden retriever, Labrador retriever, Great Dane, and Boston terrier. In most cases the cysts do not adversely affect the eye unless they are large and located directly in the center of the pupil. In the golden retriever breed, however, iris cysts may be associated with chronic pigmentary uveitis (inflammation of the iris and ciliary body) and glaucoma. Glaucoma has also been sporadically diagnosed in association with iridociliary cysts in Great Danes.

Causes

These cysts can be either congenital (present at birth) or acquired. Congenital cysts result from minor developmental abnormalities and may not become visible for several years. Acquired cysts may arise spontaneously, or they may develop after inflammation, degeneration, or trauma involving the iris or ciliary body. The tendency to form cysts may be inherited in the golden retriever. Usually the underlying cause is not known.

Clinical Signs

Most animals have no clinical signs associated with the cysts. Sometimes the cysts are discovered by the owner and appear as small, dark brown or black spots in the front aspect of the eye. Cysts can vary in size, shape, and color (from dark to almost transparent). One or more cysts may be noted. Cysts may be attached to the edge of the pupil, or they may float freely in the front chamber of the eye.

In some animals, the cysts are discovered only when a thorough eye examination is performed. Cysts that are still attached to the back of the iris or ciliary body may be seen only when the pupil is dilated. Eyes that are also inflamed or have glaucoma may be red, cloudy, and, occasionally, painful.

Diagnostic Tests

Diagnosis can usually be made by examination of the eye using magnification, especially when a slit-lamp biomicroscope is used. Occasionally, an ocular ultrasound is needed to document that the center of the cyst is fluid-filled and not solid. Testing for glaucoma and close scrutiny of the eye for inflammation are commonly done. Your pet may be referred to a veterinary ophthalmologist for further evaluation to confirm that the lesion is a cyst and not a solid tumor such as a melanoma.

TREATMENT AND FOLLOW-UP
Treatment Options

Most cysts require no treatment. If the cyst is large, is located within the front chamber or pupil, and interferes with vision, it may be deflated by the use of a laser or by aspiration of its fluid with a needle. Aspiration is commonly done with the animal under general anesthesia. Laser therapy may be done with either sedation or anesthesia. Both techniques cause inflammation within the eye, can result in damage to other nearby structures, and are rarely indicated.

Follow-up Care

Periodic eye examinations may be recommended to monitor for progressive enlargement, the development of more cysts, and the onset of complicating factors (uveitis, glaucoma).

Prognosis

Prognosis is good in almost all cases. Iridociliary cysts are usually incidental lesions that cause few problems within the eye. Monitoring for glaucoma and uveitis is warranted in affected golden retrievers, and occasionally in Great Danes.

SPECIAL INSTRUCTIONS:

Iris Melanosis of Cats

Rhea V. Morgan, DVM, DACVIM (Small Animal), DACVO

BASIC INFORMATION

Description

Iris melanosis is darkening of the iris of cats that occurs from proliferation of cells that produce a brown pigment called *melanin*. Iris melanosis may begin as a focal, dark spot or as several spots. A single spot of flat, irregular pigmentation may be called a *freckle*. If the spot becomes darker and more defined, it may be called a *nevus*. Neither freckles nor nevi alter the surface contours of the iris or adversely affect the eye.

If multiple spots develop and coalesce (run together), the condition is called *diffuse iris melanosis*. Early in its course, iris melanosis is a benign condition. If the pigmentation steadily progresses, however, it may become a form of malignant melanoma. Although freckles and nevi may occur in one or both eyes, the diffuse form of the disease typically affects only one eye.

The condition may occur in cats with any color of eye and at any age. In many cats, the progression of the melanosis is very slow (several years). Melanosis in young cats tends to change more quickly. With progressive melanosis, raised masses may develop on the surface of the iris or spread toward the back of the eye. The size and shape of the pupil may become abnormal. Secondary glaucoma may occur.

Causes

The cause is unknown.

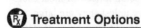 Clinical Signs

The most obvious sign is the development of brownish spots in areas of the iris that were previously golden yellow or green. Initially, the spots may be very light brown in color, but over time they usually turn very dark brown. The spots may be round, irregular, or streaky in shape. A single spot or many spots may be seen in the same iris.

If the melanosis is affecting the iris muscle, the pupil may be irregular in shape and a different size from the pupil of the other eye. If glaucoma is present, the eye may appear red and cloudy. Most cats are oblivious to the condition unless glaucoma is present and causes pain.

Diagnostic Tests

Diagnosis of iris melanosis can be made from an eye examination, but it is difficult to distinguish benign melanosis from malignant disease. Examination of the eye under magnification with a slit-lamp biomicroscope is very helpful in detecting evidence that the melanosis may be serious. Your cat may be referred to a veterinary ophthalmologist for slit-lamp examination and further evaluation of the eye.

Routine laboratory tests and chest x-rays may be recommended to ensure that there is no evidence of tumor elsewhere. Although aspiration and microscopic analysis of cells from the surface of the iris has been tried as a method to detect the malignant form, this procedure has had disappointing results. Currently, the only way to determine whether the melanosis is benign or malignant is to remove the eye and submit it for biopsy.

TREATMENT AND FOLLOW-UP

Treatment Options

No treatment is needed for freckles and nevi that are not changing. Some nevi may be destroyed by a laser, but this therapy in cats is somewhat controversial.

Currently, the only treatment for diffuse iris melanosis and the best way to prevent melanosis from converting to a malignant form and spreading elsewhere in the body is to remove (enucleate) the eye. Because the rest of the eye is normal in most case of diffuse iris melanosis, your veterinarian may recommend that enucleation be delayed and the eye closely monitored for a period of time. If the condition changes very slowly, the eye may not have to be removed for years. If enucleation is done, the eye should always be submitted for histopathologic analysis.

Follow-up Care

If monitoring is chosen, then repeated examinations by a veterinary ophthalmologist are usually needed. The frequency of recheck visits depends on the appearance of the melanosis. If any evidence of possible transformation is detected on subsequent eye examinations, enucleation is usually recommended. Changes compatible with a more serious form of the condition include widespread involvement of the iris, development of raised masses on the surface of the iris, spread of the melanosis to the back of the eye, distortion of the pupil, and secondary glaucoma.

Prognosis

Prognosis for all benign forms of diffuse iris melanosis is good. Some eyes may never need to be enucleated, and enucleation is curative. If a biopsy shows a malignant melanoma, the long-term prognosis is fair to guarded (uncertain). This type of melanoma is usually slow to metastasize (12-24 months), and enucleation may prevent metastasis in some cats.

SPECIAL INSTRUCTIONS:

Keratoconjunctivitis Sicca (Dry Eye)

Rhea V. Morgan, DVM, DACVIM (Small Animal), DACVO

BASIC INFORMATION

Description

Keratoconjunctivitis sicca (KCS) is the Latin term for *dry eye*. KCS usually arises from inadequate production of watery tears. Blockage of the tear ducts is not often involved. There are two major tear glands in animals, one beneath the upper eyelid and one that resides on the back side of the third eyelid.

Causes

Potential causes in dogs include the following:

- Dry eye often arises from an immune-mediated inflammation of the tear glands and is common in the American cocker spaniel, English bulldog, Lhasa apso, shih tzu, West Highland white terrier, Cavalier King Charles spaniel, and others.
- Removal of a prolapsed gland of the third eyelid can cause KCS, often years later.
- Certain drugs are toxic to the tear glands, including sulfa drugs, etodolac, 5-aminosalicylic acid, and others.
- Canine distemper virus infection can cause KCS.
- Neurogenic KCS is a rare disease in dogs in which the tear gland and membranes of the nostril on the same side are affected.
- Congenital underdevelopment of the tear glands can lead to KCS very early in life; this occurs most often in the Yorkshire terrier.

Potential causes in cats include the following:

- Feline herpesvirus infection may be the most common cause of dry eye in cats. Whether the tear glands are affected by the virus or the tear ducts become scarred and blocked by chronic conjunctivitis is unclear.
- Removal of a prolapsed gland of the third eyelid can also result in dry eye, but prolapsed glands are uncommon except in the Burmese.

Potential causes in both dogs and cats include the following:

- General anesthesia and use of topical atropine may cause decreased tear production, which is often temporary.
- Trauma, radiation therapy to the head, corneal ulceration, and proptosis of the globe may result in dry eye, usually on one side.
- Damage to the facial nerve, which activates the tear glands, can cause KCS and usually arises from chronic ear disease.

📋 Clinical Signs

Drying and inflammation of the surface tissues of the eye occur. The conjunctiva and cornea become red and inflamed. The cornea may become pigmented and scarred, with decreased vision. Corneal ulceration may occur. Mucus and oily secretions produced by glands of the eyelid and conjunctiva may build up and become infected (yellow-green in color). A classic sign of dry eye is thick ocular discharge.

If the onset of KCS is sudden, the eye is often painful (squinty). The nostril on the same side may be dry and filled with thick material, particularly in dogs with neurogenic KCS. The eyelids may be crusted over with discharge.

🔬 Diagnostic Tests

KCS may be tentatively diagnosed based on clinical signs and confirmed by measurement of tear production using the Schirmer tear test. The tear test may be performed on more than one occasion, because the results can vary somewhat, especially in cats. Other causes of conjunctivitis, keratitis, and thick discharge are ruled out with a thorough eye examination.

TREATMENT AND FOLLOW-UP

℞ Treatment Options

The main goal is to increase tear production. Cyclosporine is commercially available as an ointment and can be obtained as a solution from compounding pharmacies. Ocular tacrolimus is not yet approved for use in the United States but is available from compounding pharmacies. Either of these drugs is administered 1-3 times daily, often indefinitely. Pilocarpine applied to the food is usually tried in cases of neurogenic KCS. Tear production may increase within 3-4 weeks, but it can take as long as 12 weeks to see a response. Not all patients respond to these agents.

Another goal is to keep the eye well lubricated, and a variety of products manufactured for people and animals are available for this purpose. They include artificial tear solutions, gels, and ointments.

Topical anti-inflammatory agents and antibiotics may also be administered. For patients that do not respond to the tear stimulants and do poorly on lubricants alone, surgery to transplant a salivary duct up to the eye (parotid duct transposition) may be considered.

🐾 Follow-up Care

Periodic rechecks, with repeated tear tests, are required for the life of the animal. Medications often need adjustment to maintain good surface health of the eye. Continuous and diligent treatment by the owner is key to managing this disease.

Prognosis

KCS is usually a lifelong, chronic disease that may be controllable but is not often curable. Eyes that respond to tear stimulants have a good prognosis.

SPECIAL INSTRUCTIONS:

Lens Luxation and Subluxation

Rhea V. Morgan, DVM, DACVIM (Small Animal), DACVO

BASIC INFORMATION

Description

Luxation is complete dislocation and *subluxation* is partial dislocation of the lens from its normal position within the eye. The lens is suspended and centered behind the pupil by a ring of tiny fibers. When these fibers degenerate or break, the lens becomes unstable and may move.

Causes

The terrier breeds, border collie, German shepherd dog, and Chinese shar-pei are predisposed to *primary lens luxations,* because they have an inherited tendency for the suspensory fibers to break. Although lens movement may occur in only one eye initially, the other lens is also prone to luxation. Most affected dogs are 3-7 years of age.

Secondary luxations or subluxations can occur when the eye stretches as a result of glaucoma or the suspensory fibers are destroyed by inflammation (uveitis). Secondary luxations are the most common type in the cat. Rarely, subluxations may occur from tumor growth or serious infection behind the lens. In some instances, the cause of the lens movement is not identified and is termed *idiopathic.*

Clinical Signs

No specific clinical signs may occur with posterior subluxations and luxations (those in which the lens remains behind the pupil). In these cases, the lens movement may be discovered only when the eye is examined.

Forward (anterior) movement of the lens can disrupt the normal flow of fluid in the eye and cause acute, serious glaucoma. Glaucoma is most likely when the lens becomes trapped within or in front of the pupil. Signs of acute glaucoma include pain (squinting, blinking, and lethargy), bluish-white discoloration of the cornea, redness, and blindness in the eye. If the lens is opaque from a cataract, then the front of the eye may suddenly become very white. Because the lens is most likely to move when the pupil is dilated (at night, in darkness), it is common for signs of lens luxation to first be present in the morning.

If the lens luxation is secondary to another eye condition, then signs of that condition may also be noted.

Diagnostic Tests

Diagnosis is confirmed by a thorough eye examination, which includes glaucoma testing. If the eye is opaque and an adequate examination cannot be performed, your pet may be referred for slit-lamp examination or an ocular ultrasound or both. A search for an underlying cause is also indicated if lens movement is thought to be secondary.

TREATMENT AND FOLLOW-UP

Treatment Options

Posterior luxation and many subluxations of the lens require no treatment other than that indicated for the underlying cause. In contrast, acute anterior subluxations and luxations are usually considered emergencies because of the extremely high pressures that can develop in the eye within a few hours.

Initially, the animal may be given medications to decrease the pressure in the eye. If there is a chance that vision can be saved in the eye, your pet may be referred to a veterinary ophthalmologist for surgical removal of the lens (lensectomy). This type of surgery is very similar to that performed for cataracts and requires hospitalization and general anesthesia.

If the affected eye is blind, then an attempt to control the glaucoma may be made with medications. If the pressures cannot be controlled, removal of the eye may be recommended. Treatment of underlying conditions is also instituted.

Follow-up Care

Lensectomy surgery requires a major financial and time commitment on the part of the owner. Postoperatively, medications must be administered several times daily for weeks to months, and numerous recheck visits are needed. Close monitoring for complications, such as postoperative uveitis, glaucoma, and retinal detachments, is important. Often the animal must wear an Elizabethan collar for 3-4 weeks while the incision is healing.

Eyes that are treated with medications alone also require long-term monitoring, because the medications can become less effective over time. In dogs with primary lens luxation, the opposite eye must be monitored periodically for evidence that the lens is becoming loose. If any lens movement is detected, then lensectomy may be recommended in that eye.

Prognosis

Prognosis is highly variable, depending on which direction the lens moves, whether the eye was blind before the movement, and whether the luxation is primary or secondary. In dogs with primary, acute, anterior lens luxation, time is of the essence. Permanent blindness can occur within a few hours due to the extremely high intraocular pressures that occur. If these pressures are alleviated and the lens is removed, then the short-term prognosis can be good. Postoperatively, many of these dogs are still prone to glaucoma and may require lifelong therapy.

SPECIAL INSTRUCTIONS:

Lipid Keratopathy

Rhea V. Morgan, DVM, DACVIM (Small Animal), DACVO

BASIC INFORMATION

Description

Lipid keratopathy is the accumulation of fatty substances (often cholesterol crystals) in the cornea. The cornea is the clear outer part of the front of the eye. Lipid keratopathy occurs most often in dogs but can be seen sporadically in cats.

Causes

In the dog, there are three main causes:

* Spontaneous, inherited forms occur in many breeds of dogs, including the Afghan hound, cocker and Cavalier King Charles spaniels, Siberian husky, Boston terrier, collie, Shetland sheepdog, German shepherd dog, beagle, Airedale terrier, and many others. The reason why lipid deposition occurs in the corneas of these breeds is unknown. Both eyes are usually affected.
* Lipid may also be deposited in corneas after episodes of ocular inflammation, such as dry eye, corneal ulceration, corneal or scleral inflammation (keratitis, scleritis), or inflammation within the eye (uveitis), or following ocular surgery. This form of lipid keratopathy may occur in one or both eyes.
* Occasionally, lipid deposition occurs in the cornea when cholesterol levels in the blood are too high. Causes include high dietary fat intake and hypothyroidism (low thyroid hormone levels). Both eyes are often affected.

In the cat, lipid deposition is uncommon and usually occurs subsequent to inflammation or ulceration of the cornea. It may occur in one or both eyes.

Clinical Signs

Lipid appears as a shiny, crystalline material in the front third of the cornea. The surface of the cornea often remains smooth and rounded. With the exception of lipid punctate keratopathy in Shetland sheepdogs, the condition is not painful. The location and shape of the lipid varies, depending on the cause:

* Many inherited forms are oval or circular lesions located near the center of the cornea. The Siberian husky and Samoyed have a donut-shaped lesion, with a clear center. In shelties, circular, pitted (punctate) lesions may be scattered around the cornea. The unaffected portions of the cornea are usually normal in appearance.
* Postinflammatory lesions may also be circular, but they vary widely in shape and location. Deposition of lipid that arises with scleritis often forms a white arc at the limbus (where the cornea and sclera meet). These lesions may be accompanied by blood vessels and scarring in the cornea, and the cornea may have an irregular surface.
* Lipid keratopathy associated with high cholesterol often forms near the limbus and appears as a white arc, similar to that associated with scleritis.

Diagnostic Tests

A thorough eye examination is performed to look for any evidence of active or prior inflammation. This can include fluorescein staining of the cornea, tear testing, glaucoma testing, and examination of the interior structures of the eye. A 12-hour fasting cholesterol level may be measured to rule out high cholesterol. If the cholesterol is elevated, then thyroid tests may be done. A diagnosis of the inherited forms is made when all other causes of lipid keratopathy are ruled out.

TREATMENT AND FOLLOW-UP

Treatment Options

No specific therapy exists for this condition. No topical or systemic drugs are available that remove the lipid, and the lipid invariably returns, even if it is surgically removed. Fortunately, lipid keratopathy does not usually affect vision to any significant degree. Most inherited forms progress to a certain point and then remain static for the life of the dog. The lipid does not cause any secondary changes within the eye.

For dogs with high cholesterol, low-fat diets are indicated. Human oral cholesterol-lowering agents are not routinely used in animals because of their side effects. Thyroid supplementation is started in dogs with hypothyroidism. Correction of the high cholesterol may prevent the lipid keratopathy from getting worse, and occasionally the lipid infiltrate may improve.

Control of any ocular inflammation and dry eye is also important. Blood vessels and active inflammation may be treated with topical steroids. Shetland sheepdogs can be treated with topical antibiotics and pain medications when they have episodes of discomfort. Topical cyclosporine may also be used in these dogs to decrease progression of the lesions.

Follow-up Care

Most monitoring is related to the presence of underlying inflammation or metabolic or hormonal problems. Cholesterol and thyroid tests may be repeatedly periodically. Cases of inherited lipid keratopathy do not often require follow-up visits. Notify your veterinarian if the lesions change appearance or if the animal develops ocular symptoms.

Prognosis

Although lipid keratopathy cannot be cured, long-term prognosis is good, because it does not usually affect vision or cause pain. Most animals are not bothered by this condition.

SPECIAL INSTRUCTIONS:

Orbital Cellulitis and Abscessation

Rhea V. Morgan, DVM, DACVIM (Small Animal), DACVO

BASIC INFORMATION

Description

The orbit is the bony socket that surrounds most of the eyeball. Cellulitis is inflammation and infection in the orbit, behind the eye. Abscessation is collection of infected material in one area behind the eye. The area behind the eye is called the *retrobulbar space*.

Causes

In many cases, the cause of the inflammation and infection is migration of foreign material from the mouth into the retrobulbar area. Although the exact material may never be found, plant material is a common cause, including grass fragments, awns, seed hulls, and wood splinters. It is thought that the plant material enters the mouth when the animal chews or carries it, or when it licks the material from its fur. Small pieces of the material may become stuck behind the last upper molar tooth, work their way through the roof of the mouth into the retrobulbar space, and begin to deteriorate.

Extension of infection from nearby structures, such as the sinuses, tooth roots, or salivary glands, may also affect the orbit. Rarely, an infection may spread to the orbit through the blood, or a parasite larva may migrate to the orbit from elsewhere in the body.

Clinical Signs

Cellulitis usually develops suddenly (within 24-48 hours) and results in swelling and pain. The swelling pushes the eye forward and the third eyelid upward, so that the eye protrudes and becomes red and inflamed. If the eye dries out and the cornea ulcerates, the animal may squint or paw at the eye. Occasionally, the external eyelids and the side of the face also become swollen and inflamed. Usually, only one eye is involved.

The animal may be reluctant to open its mouth or to chew on hard food, treats, or toys. Some affected animals act systemically ill, with signs of lethargy, fever, and inappetence. If the cellulitis has spread from an infection elsewhere in the body, other clinical signs may be present.

Diagnostic Tests

A preliminary diagnosis can often be made from the following history, signs, and physical findings:
- Sudden onset of protrusion of one eye
- Pain on opening the mouth and with pressure on the eyeball

- Localized swelling in the roof of the mouth behind the last upper molar tooth on the same side

Laboratory tests may be recommended to look for evidence of infection and to assess the health status of the animal prior to surgery. An ultrasound of the retrobulbar space may show widespread changes suggestive of cellulitis or a focal abnormality compatible with an abscess. X-rays of the skull may be recommended to look for metallic foreign bodies, such as sewing needles in cats. Other tests may be needed to rule out diseases of the muscles around the orbit, as well as tumors or hemorrhage within the orbit.

TREATMENT AND FOLLOW-UP

Treatment Options

Some animals respond to antibiotics alone, but most require surgery to provide drainage of the retrobulbar space. With the animal under general anesthesia, a small incision is made through the roof of the mouth, behind the last upper tooth on the affected side. A surgical hemostat is gently inserted into the retrobulbar space, so that an open tract is created to the mouth. A swab of the retrobulbar space may be taken for culture; if abnormal tissue is seen, it may be submitted for biopsy.

Frank pus may be encountered if an abscess if present, but this is uncommon. Typically, little drainage occurs during surgery, but when the animal awakens and resumes a normal, upright position, gravity helps any infected material drain back down into the mouth.

After surgery, antibiotics are administered and may be given by injection initially. Nonsteroidal anti-inflammatory drugs or pain-relieving medications may be given for a few days. Topical antibiotics may be applied to the eye if it is ulcerated or inflamed. Warm compresses may be applied to the eyelids and the side of the face, if they are swollen. Soft foods may be recommended until the pain subsides.

Follow-up Care

The animal may be rechecked 24-72 hours after surgery to ensure that signs are resolving. Antibiotics are often continued for 14 days or longer.

Prognosis

Most signs improve within 2-3 days and resolve within 2 weeks. If signs do not improve, then further diagnostic testing is indicated. If orbital cellulitis is diagnosed early and treated aggressively, prognosis is good. Failure to act swiftly can result in severe damage to the eye and blindness.

SPECIAL INSTRUCTIONS:

Orbital Tumors

Rhea V. Morgan, DVM, DACVIM (Small Animal), DACVO

BASIC INFORMATION

Description

The orbit is the bony socket that surrounds most of the eyeball. Within the orbit are the eyeball, the muscles of the eye, fat, nerves, blood vessels, and tear glands. *Primary tumors* of the orbit arise from one of these tissues. Secondary tumors arise from nearby structures, such as the nose, a salivary gland, or the roof of the mouth, and extend into the orbit as they enlarge. Tumors that spread (metastasize) from other sites in the body are called *secondary tumors*.

Causes

The cause of most orbital tumors is unknown. Most orbital tumors in dogs and cats are malignant. Examples of primary cancers include the osteosarcoma (from bone), fibrosarcoma, chondrosarcoma (from cartilage), meningioma of the optic nerve, rhabdomyosarcoma (from muscle), mast cell tumor, neurofibrosarcoma (from nerves), and hemangiosarcoma (from blood vessels). Lymphoma can also develop in the orbit, as either a primary or a secondary tumor.

Secondary tumors that arise in nearby tissues include nasal and salivary gland adenocarcinomas, squamous cell carcinoma, melanoma, and myxoma/myxosarcoma. Examples of metastatic tumors are adenocarcinomas from the uterus, mammary glands, or kidneys, and transitional cell carcinoma from the bladder.

Clinical Signs

With the exception of lymphoma (which can occur at any age), most tumors arise in older animals. Average age in dogs is 8-9 years, and in cats it is 12.5 years. Most tumors grow slowly and are not painful. When the tumor is behind the eye, the eye is pushed forward and the third eyelid protrudes as the tumor enlarges. The eye may also be deviated out to the side or upward. If the tumor arises beneath the eye and grows towards the front of the orbit, then the eye may be pushed back into the socket (uncommon).

Eyes that protrude often become red and inflamed, and the cornea may ulcerate, which leads to tearing, squinting, and sometimes infection. If the tumor affects the optic nerve, then blindness can occur and the pupil will dilate. Tumors usually affect only one orbit early in the course, but they can eventually break through the bones between the eyes and affect the other side. Other signs may be present if the tumor is secondary and depend on the tissue of origin.

Diagnostic Tests

An orbital tumor may be suspected in an older animal with slowly developing, nonpainful protuberance of the eye. On physical examination, the eye cannot be pushed back into the socket, as the other (nonaffected) eye can, and sometimes the edge of the tumor can be felt beneath the eye. If the tumor is expanding toward the roof of the mouth, a small bulge may be seen behind the last upper molar tooth on the same side. Routine laboratory tests and chest and abdominal x-rays may be recommended to search for evidence of infection or tumors elsewhere.

An ocular ultrasound may show a mass behind the eye that is compatible with tumor, but it does not provide information as to tumor type. X-rays of the skull may reveal bony or nasal cavity changes with some tumors. Advanced imaging with computed tomography (CT scan) or magnetic resonance imaging (MRI) may be recommended to better define the extent of the mass and provide information as to the best approach to treatment.

Definitive diagnosis requires a biopsy. Biopsy samples can sometimes be acquired with a small, cutting needle instrument passed through the roof of the mouth into the retrobulbar space. Biopsy samples may also be taken when the orbit is opened surgically.

TREATMENT AND FOLLOW-UP

Treatment Options

For primary tumors, it is often necessary to sacrifice the eye (enucleate it) in order to surgically remove the tumor. Occasionally, localized tumors in the outer aspect of the orbit can be approached by temporarily removing the bone on the side of the face.

Several options may be considered for secondary tumors, depending on the tissue of origin and tumor type. Chemotherapy, radiation therapy, surgery, or combinations of these therapies are all possibilities.

Follow-up Care

Follow-up visits are needed for the rest of the life of the animal to monitor progression of the disease, to administer chemotherapy, and to watch for side effects of therapy. Laboratory tests and x-rays are periodically repeated.

Prognosis

Prognosis for most orbital tumors is grave. Surgical removal often provides temporary relief, but recurrence is common within 6-12 months for most tumors. Chemotherapy may provide longer remission times. Euthanasia may be considered if the tumor has already invaded multiple tissues of the face and brain at the time of diagnosis.

SPECIAL INSTRUCTIONS:

Pannus

Rhea V. Morgan, DVM, DACVIM (Small Animal), DACVO

BASIC INFORMATION

Description

Pannus is an infiltration of the corneas and/or third eyelids with certain white blood cells, blood vessels, and brown pigment. It is also called *chronic superficial keratitis*. The German shepherd dog is predisposed to the condition. It may occur sporadically in other breeds, such as the greyhound, Rottweiler, golden retriever, Belgian tervuren, border collie, and others.

Causes

The disease is probably an immune-mediated condition, which is an inflammation that is induced by an abnormal immune response. Pannus is aggravated by ultraviolet radiation and pollution. Clinical signs are most severe in dogs residing at high altitudes or in environments with high levels of pollution.

Clinical Signs

Both eyes are typically affected. A red-gray film starts at the 4 and 8 o'clock positions and spreads across the cornea to meet in the middle. If untreated, the entire cornea may become covered, with loss of vision. With time brown (melanin) pigment invades the cornea and may persist despite treatment.

With the third eyelid form of the disease (also known as *plasmoma*), the leading edge and front surface of the third eyelids become thickened, red, depigmented, and irregular. Plasmoma may occur alone or with the corneal disease.

Diagnostic Tests

Diagnosis is usually made by close examination of the corneas and third eyelids. Additional testing for dry eye and corneal ulcers is usually done. Scrapings may be submitted for microscopic analysis (cytology) to identify the type of white blood cells present, which are usually lymphocytes and plasma cells. Other causes of corneal cloudiness must also be ruled out.

TREATMENT AND FOLLOW-UP

Treatment Options

Topical steroid and cyclosporine medications are the most common therapies used for pannus. In mild to moderate cases, topical steroids may be used alone. In severe cases, topical steroids may be combined with a steroid injection into the adjacent conjunctiva or with topical cyclosporine. For severe, refractory cases of pannus with significant loss of vision, beta radiation or cryotherapy (freezing of the cornea) may be considered.

Although corneal ulcers are uncommon with pannus, topical antibiotics are usually administered if they are identified.

Follow-up Care

Periodic recheck visits are used to assess response to treatment and to make adjustments in the frequency and type of medications administered. If the disease does not respond to one type of steroid, it may respond to another or to a combination of steroids and cyclosporine. Because topical steroids are usually needed long term, the cornea is also monitored for ulcers with fluorescein staining.

The goal of therapy is to clear the cornea of the pink-gray film and then attempt to improve any pigmentation. Once the active pannus has receded, the frequency of medications is decreased to the lowest amount that keeps the condition in remission. Notify your veterinarian immediately if you see any worsening of the film in the cornea or any onset of pain (squinting or increased tearing). If the eye becomes painful while a topical steroid is being given, stop the drug until the eye can be re-examined.

Prognosis

Pannus and plasmoma can often be controlled but are rarely cured, especially in German shepherd dogs. Treatment is usually needed for the life of the dog. Active pannus may respond quickly or slowly, but it usually does recede with appropriate therapy.

Corneal pigmentation can be very difficult to treat and may persist. It is much easier to prevent corneal pigmentation by early intervention and treatment than it is to get rid of the pigment once it is in the cornea. After the pannus has receded, the cornea may be left with mild, cloudy scarring or spots of lipid deposits. These latter conditions do not usually affect vision, but vision can be severely affected by pigmentation.

Vigilant monitoring is required to detect recurrences. Many cases of pannus flare up, sometimes at the same time each year. In some geographic areas, flare-ups are more common during the summer; in others, recurrences are more likely during the winter. Pannus almost always recurs if medications are stopped for any length of time, and the recurrence can be more difficult to treat than the original condition.

SPECIAL INSTRUCTIONS:

Persistent Corneal Erosions

Rhea V. Morgan, DVM, DACVIM (Small Animal), DACVO

BASIC INFORMATION
Description

Persistent corneal erosions are superficial ulcers that do not heal and persist for at least 2 weeks beyond the expected healing time. Although the cornea successfully creates a new surface layer to cover the defect, it does not stick to the underlying layer. The new layer slides around, preventing the ulcer from healing. This condition is also known as a *nonhealing ulcer, indolent ulcer, boxer ulcer,* or *spontaneous chronic corneal epithelial defect.*

This type of ulcer occurs more often in dogs than in cats. The boxer, golden retriever, and Pembroke Welsh corgi are predisposed, but a wide variety of purebred and mixed-breed dogs may be affected. Middle-aged to older dogs (average age, 9 years) are affected most often. Usually only one eye is ulcerated, although the other eye may develop a similar ulcer at some time in the future.

Causes

In dogs, several different microscopic structural or neurologic defects can occur in the cornea that delay healing. Corneas that are edematous (fluid is retained in the middle layer of the cornea) are prone to these ulcers, because the surface layer becomes waterlogged and soft. Feline herpesvirus infection has been incriminated in the development of these ulcers in cats.

Clinical Signs

In some animals, tearing is the only symptom. Other animals show evidence of pain, with squinting and pawing or rubbing at the eye. The eye may be red, and the third eyelid may be elevated. The cornea may be cloudy if edema is present, it may be red if vessels have grown into the ulcer, or it may remain clear.

Diagnostic Tests

Diagnosis is made by close examination of the eye. These ulcers are only one layer deep and have loose surface tissue at their edge. Fluorescein staining highlights the ulcer and often demonstrates the loose edges of the ulcer. Other causes must be excluded, including trauma, eyelid abnormalities, dry eye, and bacterial infection. If both eyes are affected, further testing for underlying medical problems may be considered.

TREATMENT AND FOLLOW-UP

Treatment Options
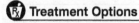

These ulcers can be very difficult to get to heal, and healing may not occur for several weeks to months. No single therapy achieves healing in all ulcers, so many different types of treatments may be tried. Some treatments are minor procedures that are done on an outpatient basis, whereas others require hospitalization and general anesthesia.

- Removal of the loose surface tissue (débridement) is done on most of these ulcers, using a sterile cotton swab or other device. In some cases, the animal may be taken to surgery so that the all abnormal layers of the cornea can be removed (superficial keratectomy).
- Topical antibiotics are used to prevent infection, and topical pain medications are often administered. Use of an Elizabethan collar prevents rubbing of the eye.
- In addition to débridement, the second layer of the cornea may be roughened to improve bonding with the surface layer via procedures such as a punctate or grid keratotomy. Keratotomies are most often performed in dogs and can be repeated.
- Bandage contact lenses or collagen shields (dissolvable lens) may be applied to the cornea, or a third eyelid flap may be sutured over the eye. Lenses and flaps protect the ulcer and prevent the eyelids from rubbing the ulcerated area during blinking.
- A variety of other topical therapies (such as an *Adequan*-tear solution in dogs or interferon-tear solution in cats) can be tried for these ulcers but have had mixed success.
- Ulcers that fail to heal with all other techniques may require surgical grafting.

Ulcers that arise in edematous corneas can be particularly stubborn. The application of topical 5% sodium chloride may be considered, and a specialized cautery procedure (thermokeratoplasty or TKP) may be tried for unresponsive ulcers.

When these ulcers occur in cats, additional treatments for feline herpesvirus infection may be helpful. (See the handout on **Feline Herpesvirus Keratoconjunctivitis**.)

Follow-up Care

Recheck visits are often scheduled every 7-14 days. If the ulcer persists beyond 14-21 days following initial treatment, then treatment is often modified or a different therapy is tried. Notify your veterinarian if any signs worsen or if additional signs occur (more pain occurs, discharge turns from watery to thick or from clear to yellow-green, cornea becomes cloudier, and so on).

Prognosis

Although these ulcers are hard to heal, many do improve within 4 weeks. With persistence and diligent treatment, they eventually heal. Some corneas may be left with cloudy scarring, but vision is usually unaffected unless the cornea is edematous.

SPECIAL INSTRUCTIONS:

Pigmentary Keratitis

Rhea V. Morgan, DVM, DACVIM (Small Animal), DACVO

BASIC INFORMATION

Description

Pigmentary keratitis is the migration of brown (melanin) pigment into the cornea. The pigment usually affects the surface of the cornea, and one or both eyes may be involved. The pigment may or may not be accompanied by inflammation. Pigmentary keratitis occurs most often in the dog; it is rare in cats.

Causes

Pigment usually invades the cornea as a result of chronic irritation. Causes of irritation include the following:

* Extra or abnormal eyelashes or hair rubbing on the cornea
* Exposure of the cornea in dogs with prominent eyes and large eyelid openings, especially in the flat-faced breeds of dogs
* Dry eye (keratoconjunctivitis sicca) from lack of tear production
* Inability of the eyelids to protect the eye because of decreased blinking or enlargement of the eye from glaucoma
* Corneal ulceration
* Chronic corneal inflammation (keratitis), such as pannus in the dog

🗒 Clinical Signs

Depending on the underlying cause, the dog may show no clinical signs except for the development of a dark brown film on the eye. This film may cover only a small portion of the cornea and only be detected by your veterinarian during an examination. If the pigment progresses to cover most of the cornea, then decreased vision may be noted. Other signs usually pertain to the underlying cause and can include pain; tearing; increased thick, ropey discharge; enlargement of the eye; redness; and other ocular symptoms.

🔬 Diagnostic Tests

The presence of corneal pigment is confirmed by examination of the eye, often with the use of magnification. Other diagnostic tests, such as tear testing, fluorescein staining, and glaucoma testing, are used to determine the underlying cause. The eyelids, blink responses, and position and shape of the eye are also thoroughly examined.

TREATMENT AND FOLLOW-UP

℞ Treatment Options

The first priority of treatment is to correct any underlying causes. Eyelid abnormalities and extra eyelashes may require surgery. Medications for dry eye, pannus, and glaucoma are started when indicated.

If the pigment is present in one of the flat-faced breeds of dog and is secondary to the typical anatomy of these breeds (large, prominent eye; lashes or hair growing near the eye; large eyelid opening), then conservative therapy with topical lubricants may be started.

* If the pigment affects the central cornea or progressively worsens, then prolonged therapy with cyclosporine or tacrolimus may be helpful. These drugs increase tear production and encourage the pigment to thin and disperse over time.
* If the pigment threatens vision or does not respond to medications in these breeds, then surgery (canthoplasty) may be considered to remove hair from near the cornea and to make the opening of the eyelids smaller.
* Surgery to remove the pigment from the cornea is no longer performed in most cases, because the pigment is likely to return and may be accompanied by postoperative scarring of the cornea.

🐾 Follow-up Care

Periodic recheck visits are used to monitor both the pigmentation and the underlying cause. If the pigmentation visibly worsens despite therapy or any new signs develop, notify your veterinarian. Following re-examination, the frequency or types of medications may be changed.

Prognosis

It is easier to prevent pigment from spreading than it is to make it recede. When pigment does recede, the process can be slow and take many months. Stopping the progression of the pigment often depends on whether the underlying condition can be successfully treated. If the pigment does not cover the pupil or is not very thick, it may have minimal effects on vision. Thick, widespread pigmentation can result in blindness. Prolonged treatment and diligent monitoring may be required for the life of the dog.

SPECIAL INSTRUCTIONS:

Progressive Retinal Atrophy

Rhea V. Morgan, DVM, DACVIM (Small Animal), DACVO

BASIC INFORMATION
Description

Progressive retinal atrophy (PRA), or generalized retinal degeneration, is a group of inherited diseases of the retina that lead to blindness. Two forms of PRA exist. In the early form, the cells in the retina that detect light (photoreceptors) do not develop normally. In the late form, the photoreceptors develop properly, work well for several years, and then degenerate. PRA affects more than 40 different breeds of dogs. It can also occur in Persian, Abyssinian, and, rarely, mixed-breed cats.

Causes

Most forms of PRA arise from genetic mutations that adversely affect specific enzymes in the photoreceptors, especially the rods. Rods are responsible for dim-light vision and are much more numerous than cones (which are responsible for bright-light and color vision) in the retinas of dogs and cats. Most forms of PRA are inherited as an autosomal recessive trait, which means that the affected dog has inherited one abnormal gene from each parent.

Based on the enzyme affected, different subtypes of the disease exist:

- Rod-cone dysplasia (RCD) 1 of Irish setters
- RCD 2 of collies
- Rod-cone early retinal degeneration (ERD) of Persian cats
- X-linked PRA of Siberian huskies (in which females are carriers and males are affected)
- ERD of Norwegian elkhounds
- Progressive rod-cone degeneration (PRCD) 1, a late-onset form of many different breeds, including poodles, cocker spaniels, Labrador retrievers, and Portuguese water dogs
- PRCD 2, an early-onset disease of Tibetan terriers
- Dominant PRA of mastiffs and Abyssinian cats (in which only one abnormal gene is needed to produce the disease)
- Early-onset cone degeneration of German shorthaired pointers

Clinical Signs

PRA affects both eyes. Because rods are involved initially in most cases, nighttime vision is lost first. Eventually, cones are affected and the animal goes completely blind. The age at onset and rate of progression depend on the type of PRA present. Most early-onset forms begin when the animal is several weeks old; signs are noticeable by 4-6 months of age, and the animal is often blind by 6-12 months of age. With late-onset forms, the disease begins at 2-6 years of age in some breeds and is delayed until 8-10 years in others.

Signs that may initially be noticed at home include reluctance to go down stairs in dim light, into darkened rooms, or outside at night. At the disease progresses, the animal may bump into objects in dim light, may not be able to catch tossed objects, or may act lost or confused. Eventually, the animal bumps into objects in bright light, the pupils become dilated, and the eye shine (tapetal reflex) from the back of the eye may become more visible.

Because vision is not the most important sense for dogs and cats, and their senses of smell and hearing are much better than ours, many affected animals behave normally early in the disease. The disease can be quite advanced before any symptoms are detected, and the actual onset of complete blindness can be hard to determine.

Diagnostic Tests

Early in the course of the disease, few changes may be detected in the eye examination of affected animals. If PRA is suspected, an electroretinogram (ERG) may be recommended, and your pet may be referred to a veterinary ophthalmologist for the procedure. The animal is often sedated for the ERG and wears a contact lens (containing a gold electrode) that is attached to a recording device. Different-colored lights are shone into the eye, and the reaction of the retina is evaluated by a computer program. ERG abnormalities compatible with PRA (such as a decreased response to blue and white light) can be detected prior to physical changes in the retina.

Later in the disease, evidence of retinal degeneration can be seen on the eye examination. A genetic test has been developed for several dog breeds that can detect affected, normal, and carrier animals. The test is available from OptiGen (*www.optigen.com*).

TREATMENT AND FOLLOW-UP

Treatment Options

No treatment is available for this genetic disease. Ongoing research is being performed on gene therapy for PRA. Secondary cataracts may develop from PRA, but removal of the cataract provides no benefit to the animal.

Follow-up Care

Little follow-up is needed unless secondary cataracts develop in the future. The disease is not painful and does not affect the rest of the body.

Prognosis

All affected animals eventually go blind. Animals with late-onset disease often go blind over a period of about 2 years.

SPECIAL INSTRUCTIONS:

Prolapse of the Gland of the Third Eyelid

Rhea V. Morgan, DVM, DACVIM (Small Animal), DACVO

BASIC INFORMATION

Description

A small gland is present on the back side of the third eyelid, the side that lies against the eye. Normally this gland is not seen. In some breeds of dogs and cats, the gland enlarges and moves upward until it becomes visible. This protrusion of the gland usually occurs in animals younger than 1 year of age and may affect one or both eyes. Commonly affected breeds of dogs include the American cocker spaniel, basset hound, beagle, English bulldog, Lhasa apso, Chinese shar-pei, and Newfoundland. The Burmese cat is also predisposed to this condition.

Causes

A small ligament that holds the gland in place apparently stretches or breaks for unknown reasons. Some glands appear to enlarge prior to breaking of the ligament, but most swelling develops after the gland is exposed.

This gland produces about 35% of the watery tears, and the longer it stays out and is exposed, the less functional it becomes. Eyes that have had a prolapsed gland are prone to dry eye, which may develop years after the event.

🔲 Clinical Signs

A smooth, round, pink or red mass is visible in the corner of the eye nearest the nose. The mass looks like a cherry pit, which gives rise to the common name of *cherry eye* for this condition. Thick ocular discharge may be present, and sometimes the dog will try to paw at the eye. The condition is not usually painful.

🔲 Diagnostic Tests

Diagnosis is based on the classic clinical appearance, especially in a young animal of a susceptible breed. A thorough ocular examination is often performed and may include a Schirmer tear test to measure tear production and fluorescein staining of the cornea.

TREATMENT AND FOLLOW-UP

💊 Treatment Options

Because this gland is responsible for about one third of the eye's watery tear production, the preferred treatment is to surgically replace the gland. One of the following techniques may be recommended:

- With the *pocket technique,* two incisions are made on the back side of the third eyelid, one on each side of the gland. The outer edges of the two incisions are sewn together, creating a pocket that covers the gland.
- The *orbital rim tacking procedure* uses suture to anchor the gland to the bony orbit, deep to the lower eyelid.
- With *pursestring* and *modified pursestring* techniques, suture is placed in the conjunctiva around the gland on the posterior surface, then pulled tight to pull the conjunctiva over the gland or to pull the gland downward and backward.
- Combinations of these techniques may also be performed.

Surgical removal of the gland may be considered as a last resort if the replacement techniques fail or if the gland has been prolapsed for so long that it is no longer functional.

🐾 Follow-up Care

Postoperative recheck visits are usually scheduled to check for healing of the incisions. Tear production may also be monitored long term by periodic Schirmer tear tests.

Prognosis

Although no surgical technique guarantees success, many glands remain in place following surgery. Success is highest when the surgery is done soon after the prolapse has occurred and when the gland is not terribly inflamed or enlarged.

Many breeds of dogs that are affected by this condition have an inherent incidence of dry eye (5-6%) in eyes that never develop a prolapsed gland. The incidence of dry eye increases to 42-44% for eyes that develop a prolapse of the gland that is either removed or left untreated. With surgical replacement of a reasonably healthy gland, the incidence of dry eye is lowered to about 14%.

SPECIAL INSTRUCTIONS:

Proptosis of the Eye

Rhea V. Morgan, DVM, DACVIM (Small Animal), DACVO

BASIC INFORMATION

Description

Proptosis is the movement of the eyeball beyond the bony socket and eyelids. As the eye moves forward, the eyelids become folded behind it, which prevents the eye from returning to its normal location. The eye quickly becomes inflamed and dry, and the surface may ulcerate. Typically, only one eye is involved.

Causes

Proptosis is usually caused by trauma. In dogs, it is most likely to occur in the small, flat-faced breeds, because their eyes are so prominent naturally. A common cause in these breeds is a dog fight, especially when a large dog grabs the small one by the scruff of the neck. Choking injuries can also cause a proptosis.

In cats and in other types of dogs, blunt trauma, as from an automobile accident or being kicked by a horse, is a more common cause. Occasionally, restraining the dog by the scruff of the neck can cause a mild or temporary proptosis.

Clinical Signs

Extreme protrusion of the eye is present. The conjunctiva is often bruised, bloody, and swollen. The eye may be deviated to the outside; the cornea is often cloudy or discolored; and blood may be seen in the front of the eye. Wounds and other signs of trauma may be noted on the head and elsewhere on the body. The animal is often painful around the head, and the eye is usually blind (at least temporarily). In some cases, the attachments of the eye are partially severed.

Diagnostic Tests

Diagnosis is based on the clinical appearance of the eye. A thorough physical examination is indicated to search for injuries elsewhere and to ensure that the opposite eye is unharmed. Routine laboratory tests and chest x-rays may be recommended prior to surgery. Skull x-rays may be considered during surgery if deep bite wounds or fractures of the head are suspected.

TREATMENT AND FOLLOW-UP

Treatment Options

In most cases, proptosis is an emergency and must be treated immediately with surgery. Animals that have other serious head or internal injuries must often be stabilized for a few days before they can be safely anesthetized. In all other cases, treatment is instituted as soon as possible.

If the eye is not severely damaged, then surgical replacement is usually recommended. With the animal under anesthesia, the eye and surrounding tissues are cleaned, the lids are unrolled, the eye is replaced in the socket, and the external eyelids are temporarily closed with sutures (temporary tarsorrhaphy). Following replacement, topical antibiotics and pain medications are commonly applied to the eye.

If the eye is severely damaged or surgery must be delayed for several days, then removal of the eye (enucleation) may be recommended. The damaged eye and orbital tissues are removed, the edges of the external eyelids are removed, and the eyelids are permanently sewn together.

Following either surgery, oral antibiotics are commonly started. An Elizabethan collar is used, and warm or cold compresses (depending on the circumstances) may be applied to the area if the animal allows it. Oral nonsteroidal anti-inflammatory drugs or pain-relieving medications may also be administered.

Follow-up Care

Following surgical replacement, the eyelids and suture line are monitored for excessive swelling; thick, yellow-green discharge; and pain. Notify your veterinarian if any of these signs occur or if the animal acts lethargic or ill or begins to run a fever. Sutures are usually removed in 10-14 days but may be removed sooner if an infection is suspected. After the sutures are removed, the position of the eye, the health of the cornea, and the presence of vision are assessed. If the eye is blind and the results are unacceptable, then an enucleation may be considered. If the eye remains deviated to the outside, further surgery may be recommended. Prolonged medical therapy may be needed in some cases to protect the cornea.

Following enucleation, the sutures are removed in 10-14 days, and no further treatment is usually needed.

Prognosis

Prognosis for vision is always poor. The best chance to save vision occurs in those eyes that are not severely proptosed, when the animal is brought to the veterinary facility immediately and surgery is performed within a couple of hours after the injury.

SPECIAL INSTRUCTIONS:

Retinal Detachment

Rhea V. Morgan, DVM, DACVIM (Small Animal), DACVO

BASIC INFORMATION

Description

Retinal detachment is separation of the retina from the back of the eye. The retina is the portion of the eye that detects light and sends information to the brain so that an image can be created. Detachment of the retina decreases vision. Retinal detachment can affect one or both eyes, and it can involve a part of the retina or the entire retina.

Causes

In animals, the most common cause of retinal detachments is the accumulation of fluid, cells, or blood beneath the retina. This type of detachment usually arises in association with some other disease, and it represents an ocular manifestation of a systemic problem. Examples of systemic diseases that can cause retinal detachment include infections, high blood pressure (hypertension), immune diseases, excessively high circulating proteins (hyperviscosity), and cancer.

Some retinal detachments occur from abnormal development of the retina or the rest of the eye. Most these problems are inherited, such as collie eye anomaly, severe retinal dysplasia, and abnormalities of the vitreous (gel in front of the retina).

Occasionally the retina may tear or break, become loose, and eventually detach. This type of detachment (rhegmatogenous) can occur after injury or cataract surgery or in association with long-standing cataracts and vitreal degeneration. Spontaneous retinal detachments occur for unknown reasons in the shih tzu.

Clinical Signs

Animals with partial detachments or a complete detachment in only one eye may show no clinical signs. If both retinas detach completely, the animal is blind and the pupils are often widely dilated. In most animals, the main clinical signs are those of the underlying disease. It is not uncommon for retinal detachments to be discovered only when the animal is examined for some reason other than blindness or eye problems.

Diagnostic Tests

Retinal detachments can often be seen on an eye examination. Sometimes specialized equipment is needed to see the detachment, so your pet may be referred to a veterinary ophthalmologist for evaluation. If the front of the eye is cloudy or a cataract (opaque lens) is present, an ultrasound of the eye may be needed to detect the detachment.

Once a retinal detachment is diagnosed, a thorough search must be conducted for the underlying cause. If there is no obvious evidence of other eye problems, then laboratory (blood and urine) tests, chest and abdominal x-rays, blood pressure measurement, an abdominal ultrasound, and possibly other studies are often needed to find the cause.

TREATMENT AND FOLLOW-UP

Treatment Options

No treatment is available for complete retinal detachments caused by serious inherited eye defects. Several different treatments may be tried for partial detachments that arise from vitreal degeneration, after cataract surgery, or spontaneously. Potential therapies include laser therapy, cryotherapy (freezing), and various surgical procedures. Because partial detachments are uncommonly detected (since they produce few clinical signs), these treatments are not often performed in dogs and cats.

The primary treatment for retinal detachments caused by the accumulation of fluid, cells, or blood is to treat the underlying disease. For example, if hypertension is the cause, then therapy is instituted to lower the blood pressure. If fungal infection is the cause, then antifungal drugs are started. If an immune-mediated disease is present, steroid medications are administered. Treatment is also started for any other eye problems, such as inflammation and glaucoma, that may accompany retinal detachments.

Follow-up Care

Follow-up examinations are important to monitor the response of the systemic illness, as well as the retinal detachment, to treatment. The frequency of visits and repeated testing depends on the underlying cause of the detachment.

Prognosis

Prognosis for partial detachments that are treated with laser therapy or surgery ranges from poor to good. Although the portion of the retina that is detached may remain separated, therapy may prevent the detachment from progressing to a complete one.

Prognosis for detachments associated with the accumulation of fluid, cells, or blood is poor to guarded (uncertain). Detachments associated with cancer, fungal infections, or severe ocular bleeding rarely improve. Even if the underlying problem resolves, the retina is usually so scarred that the animal remains blind. Detachments associated with hypertension may resolve when blood pressure is controlled. If they are diagnosed and treated early, reattachment of the retina can occur. In these cases, it is possible for dogs to regain vision, but most cats remain blind.

Detachments associated with immune-mediated diseases (primarily in dogs) may respond to steroids and other immune-suppressive drugs. With early and aggressive treatment, it is possible for the retinas to reattach and vision to return in some dogs.

SPECIAL INSTRUCTIONS:

Retinal Dysplasia

Rhea V. Morgan, DVM, DACVIM (Small Animal), DACVO

BASIC INFORMATION

Description

Retinal dysplasia is abnormal development of the retina that results in retinal folds or round, medallion-shaped lesions in the retina. If the retina is severely affected, it may detach, which results in blindness. Retinal dysplasia is present at birth, and, with the exception of retinal detachment, the lesions do not change or worsen with time. Usually, both eyes are affected.

Causes

In purebred dogs, the condition is often inherited. It occurs in numerous breeds, such as the American cocker spaniel, Labrador retriever, golden retriever, Pembroke Welsh corgi, English springer spaniel, Akita, Rottweiler, Samoyed, Bedlington terrier, and others. Retinal dysplasia may occur alone, or it may be accompanied by other inherited ocular defects.

Retinal dysplasia can also be caused by certain neonatal infections and events. The retina continues to develop for several weeks after birth, so is highly sensitive to agents that disrupt retinal development in the neonatal period. Infections that can cause retinal dysplasia include canine adenovirus, herpesvirus, and parvovirus in the dog and feline panleukopenia and leukemia virus in the cat. Exposure to toxins or radiation and a dietary deficiency of vitamin A are also potential causes.

Clinical Signs

Retinal dysplasia can be classified into three forms:

- The mildest form is single to multiple retinal folds. No clinical signs or alteration in vision are caused by these folds.
- Geographic, medallion-shaped lesions are a moderate form of the disease. These lesions involve more of the retina but do not often cause clinical signs or detectable vision abnormalities. On retinal examination, it may be difficult to tell these lesions from retinal scars secondary to inflammation, especially when the animal is an adult.
- The most severe form is widespread retinal folding that may lead to retinal detachment or be accompanied by that ocular defects such as cataracts, abnormally small eyes, and vitreal problems. In the Samoyed, the German shepherd dog, and some Labrador retrievers, severe retinal dysplasia is accompanied by skeletal dwarfism. Retinal detachment from severe dysplasia usually occurs within the first 6-9 months of life

and leads to complete blindness. Occasionally, bleeding in the back of the eye or secondary glaucoma may occur with retinal detachment.

Diagnostic Tests

Retinal dysplasia is diagnosed in most animals by examination of the retina with an ophthalmoscope. Since the condition is present at birth or develops soon after birth, it can be seen as early as 6 weeks of age in most animals. Retinal examination is facilitated by application of drops to dilate the pupils. It is common for entire litters of puppies to be examined by a veterinary ophthalmologist at 6-7 weeks for retinal dysplasia and other inherited eye defects. Examination at an early age helps to differentiate retinal dysplasia from retinal scars that may show up later in life.

Retinal dysplasia must be differentiated from normal folds in the retinas of growing animals. Normal folds tend to appear as white, worm-like (vermiform) streaks in the dark part of the retina. Vermiform streaks occur in both purebred and mixed-breed animals, and more than 80% disappear as the retina reaches its adult size.

TREATMENT AND FOLLOW-UP

Treatment Options

No treatment exists for retinal dysplasia. To date, no effective treatment is available to prevent the retinal detachments associated with this condition. Most affected animals should not be used for breeding.

Follow-up Care

Animals with severe retinal dysplasia may be rechecked for several months to monitor for retinal detachment. Notify your veterinarian if any decrease in vision occurs. If retinal folds are believed to be vermiform streaks, the animal may be re-examined periodically to check for their disappearance.

Prognosis

Prognosis is excellent for animals with mild or moderate folds. Because the offspring of affected dogs may develop more severe forms of retinal dysplasia, breeding of even mildly affected dogs is discouraged for most breeds. Prognosis is poor for animals with severe retinal dysplasia, because many go blind before 1 year of age.

SPECIAL INSTRUCTIONS:

Sudden Acquired Retinal Degeneration

Rhea V. Morgan, DVM, DACVIM (Small Animal), DACVO

BASIC INFORMATION
Description
Sudden acquired retinal degeneration (SARD) is an acute loss of function of the entire retina of both eyes that results in blindness. SARD occurs only in dogs and affects primarily adult, large-breed dogs. Dachshunds and miniature schnauzers are small breeds that are predisposed to SARD.

Causes
Although several theories have been proposed, the cause of SARD is unknown. For some reason, the cells that detect light in the retina (photoreceptors) stop functioning. Both types of photoreceptors (rods and cones) are affected. After the photoreceptors stop functioning, the retina slowly degenerates.

Clinical Signs
The deterioration in vision caused by SARD occurs quickly. Dogs often go blind within 30 days and sometimes within a few days. Affected dogs start bumping into objects (in both bright and dim light) and often act very disoriented. Some dogs become afraid and are easily startled. Both pupils are usually dilated and do not respond well to light. Affected dogs may blink their eyes less often, stare into space, and have mild eye redness and tearing.

At about the time that vision begins to deteriorate, many dogs develop increased thirst and appetite, subsequently urinating more often and gaining weight.

Diagnostic Tests
SARD may be suspected with a history of rapidly developing blindness and signs of increased thirst, urination, and appetite. The eye examination is often normal and helps to rule out glaucoma, retinal detachments, and intraocular inflammation as the cause of blindness. Early in the course of the disease, the retina usually appears normal or may show subtle changes in the blood vessels. Routine laboratory tests sometimes reveal mild changes in blood protein levels and in several liver-related tests.

Definitive diagnosis of SARD requires an electroretinogram (ERG), which can usually be performed by a veterinary ophthalmologist. For an ERG, the animal is sedated and wears a contact lens (containing a gold electrode) that is hooked to a computer. Different-colored lights are shone into the eye, and the reaction of the retina is evaluated by a computer program. Typically with SARD, retinal response is absent regardless of the type of light used, which indicates that the photoreceptors are not functioning.

The ERG is important, because it distinguishes SARD from inherited retinal degenerations and neurologic disorders (such as inflammation or malfunction of the optic nerve and certain diseases of the brain) that can cause blindness. Several weeks to months after the dog becomes blind, evidence of retinal degeneration can be seen on the eye examination, but this degeneration can appear exactly like that produced by inherited retinal degenerations.

Laboratory tests may also be performed for Cushing's disease (hyperadrenocorticism), which is a more common cause of increased thirst, urination, and appetite. Several different laboratory tests may be used to search for the presence of Cushing's disease, and an abdominal ultrasound may be used to evaluate the adrenal glands (which are responsible for Cushing's disease). Early in the course of the disease, some of these tests may be abnormal, indicating that the body is producing too much cortisone hormone. However, it is believed that most dogs with SARD do not have true Cushing's disease, because the laboratory abnormalities usually return to normal within 2-4 months without treatment.

TREATMENT AND FOLLOW-UP
Treatment Options
There is no scientifically proven treatment for SARD, and most dogs are irreversibly blind. A few dogs have responded to an experimental treatment with intravenous human immunoglobulin. This treatment is offered at very few veterinary facilities and is quite expensive. Of the dogs that responded, some retained a little vision, and others seemed to improve. However, the ERG remained abnormal in all treated dogs, so the effectiveness of the treatment is still in question. No medications, hormones, or supplements have been shown to have any beneficial effect.

Follow-up Care
Little follow-up is needed unless increased thirst and appetite do not slowly resolve. If these signs persist, then laboratory tests for Cushing's disease may be repeated in a few months; if they are abnormal, treatment may be considered for that condition. SARD is not painful and does not affect the rest of the eye.

Prognosis
After an initial adjustment period of about 6 weeks, most dogs do very well. They learn to rely on their senses of smell and hearing, which are much better than ours. Although many dogs are initially lethargic and quiet, with encouragement, their activity levels and interactions with other animals and family members often return to almost normal.

SPECIAL INSTRUCTIONS:

Taurine Retinopathy

Rhea V. Morgan, DVM, DACVIM (Small Animal), DACVO

BASIC INFORMATION
Description

Taurine retinopathy, also called *feline central retinal degeneration*, is deterioration and death of the retina that is caused by a deficiency of taurine in the diet of cats. Taurine is an essential amino acid (a building block of proteins) that must be supplied in their diet because cats cannot manufacture it themselves.

Within 10 weeks of eating a diet low in taurine, the cone photoreceptors of the retina begin to deteriorate. The cones are responsible for bright-light and color vision. Within 20 weeks, many of the cones are dead. If taurine remains deficient, eventually the rod photoreceptors (responsible for dim-light vision) are also affected. Taurine affects both eyes in a symmetrical fashion, and the end result is complete blindness.

Taurine deficiency also causes dilated cardiomyopathy in cats, a disease of heart muscle. The two conditions can occur alone or together in any individual cat.

Cause

Since the discovery in 1987 that taurine deficiency can cause dilated cardiomyopathy, commercial cat foods have been manufactured with a higher content of taurine. For the past 2 decades, the incidence of taurine retinopathy has steadily declined. Cats that consistently eat a well-balanced commercial food rarely develop the disease.

Taurine retinopathy may occur in cats that eat predominantly dog food, because taurine is not supplemented in canine diets. Dogs can make taurine themselves from other dietary components. Taurine retinopathy is also sometimes found in cats that have been strays and in those exposed to poor-quality food. Rarely, the retinopathy occurs in cats that are fed good-quality commercial foods containing adequate taurine levels (500-750 parts per million), for reasons unknown.

Clinical Signs

Initially, vision is not substantially altered, and affected cats have no clinical signs. As the disease progresses, the cat may bump into objects, stop playing with toys or chasing objects, be reluctant to go outside, or act lost and confused. Eventually, the pupils become dilated, and the eye shine (tapetal reflex) from the back of the eye may become more visible.

Diagnostic Tests

Taurine retinopathy can often be diagnosed from an eye examination, because certain changes characteristic of taurine deficiency can be seen in the retina. As the disease worsens and creates widespread changes in the retina, the condition becomes similar in appearance to inherited progressive retinal atrophy (another slowly developing retinal degeneration of cats; see the handout on **Progressive Retinal Atrophy**). If the diagnosis is uncertain, your cat may be referred to a veterinary ophthalmologist for evaluation of the retinas.

If taurine retinopathy is discovered or suspected, a blood taurine test is frequently recommended. If the blood taurine level is low, the diagnosis of taurine retinopathy is confirmed, and further evaluation of the heart is indicated.

TREATMENT AND FOLLOW-UP

Treatment Options

If the cat is on a poor or unbalanced diet, then a good-quality commercial cat food is provided. Treatment also involves supplementing the cat with extra taurine, usually once or twice daily in pill or powder form. Supplementation is often continued indefinitely. Additional treatments are needed if dilated cardiomyopathy is present. (See the handout on **Dilated Cardiomyopathy in Cats**.)

Follow-up Care

Periodic examinations are performed to monitor for progression of the retinopathy. If the retinal lesions continue to worsen, taurine supplementation may be inadequate. Blood taurine levels may be measured periodically until they become normal. Additional monitoring is needed if dilated cardiomyopathy is present.

Prognosis

Taurine retinopathy can be stopped but not reversed. The areas in the retina that have degenerated by the time of diagnosis will never function again. With adequate taurine supplementation, the remaining healthy part of the retina is protected and the disease does not progress (worsen). If the cat is already blind, the blindness is irreversible. Even in blind cats, however, taurine supplementation is worthwhile, because it will prevent dilated cardiomyopathy.

SPECIAL INSTRUCTIONS:

SECTION 14

Diseases of the Ear

Section Editor: Lynette K. Cole, DVM, MS, DACVD

Aural Hematoma
Deafness
Otitis Externa

Otitis Interna
Otitis Media

Aural Hematoma

Lynette K. Cole, DVM, MS, DACVD

BASIC INFORMATION
Description
An aural hematoma is the accumulation of fluid or blood within the ear flap (pinna).
Causes
An aural hematoma occurs when scratching the ear or shaking the head causes a blood vessel in the ear to rupture and blood leaks into the tissues of the pinna. Occasionally, hematomas also arise from trauma and bite wounds.

Clinical Signs

A noticeable swelling is present in the pinna that may be either firm or soft. The swelling may be small, or it may involve the entire pinna and extend into the ear canal. Aural hematomas occur most often in dogs but can also occur in cats.

Diagnostic Tests

An aural hematoma can often be diagnosed from the typical clinical appearance. In some instances, the swelling may be aspirated with a needle to obtain cells that can be examined under the microscope. Your veterinarian may recommend other tests to investigate an underlying cause of the hematoma, such as an external ear infection.

TREATMENT AND FOLLOW-UP

Treatment Options

Aspiration of the fluid can be attempted. This is the simplest and most conservative method of treatment. It is effective in relieving any associated pain, but recurrence of the aural hematoma is common following aspiration.

Surgical drainage of the fluid also decreases pain, and there is less likelihood of a recurrence. Several surgical methods are available, including the following:

- Silastic drain placement: A drain is inserted into the top and the bottom of the hematoma to allow blood to drain from the hematoma.
- Teat cannula placement: A teat cannula is a small tube with holes at both ends that can be inserted into the opening of the nipple on the udder of a cow. In this instance, the tube is inserted into the bottom part of the hematoma to allow drainage.
- Closed suction catheter system: A catheter is inserted into the bottom of the hematoma. One end of the catheter is attached to a container that collects drainage from the hematoma.
- Incisional drainage: An incision is made from the top to the bottom of the hematoma, and stitches are placed on either side of the incision, all the way through both sides of the pinna.
- Laser procedure: A laser is used to make multiple circular skin incisions that allow the hematoma to drain.

Any ear infection that is present is treated with appropriate topical medications. If underlying allergic disease is present, such as atopic dermatitis or adverse food reactions (food allergy), these diseases also must be controlled to prevent head shaking and scratching.

Follow-up Care

Sutures are removed in 10-14 days, whereas drains are usually removed in 3 weeks. An Elizabethan collar may be used to prevent premature removal of the sutures or drains.
Prognosis
Most hematomas resolve without complications after surgical drainage. Some hematomas recur; however, even with surgical drainage. Although it is uncommon, disfigurement of the pinna can occur after surgical drainage, and it is more noticeable in animals with erect ears. Pinnal scarring and disfigurement are more common with untreated and recurrent hematomas.

SPECIAL INSTRUCTIONS:

Deafness

Lynette K. Cole, DVM, MS, DACVD

BASIC INFORMATION
Description
Deafness can be divided in to several classes based on the specific problem, as follows:

- *Conductive hearing loss* results from failure of sound energy to be translated into mechanical energy in the outer and middle ear structures.
- *Sensorineural hearing loss* is caused by loss of electrical energy transfer from the cochlear sensory receptors or cochlear nerve.
- *Central-mediated hearing loss* is failure to process auditory information at the level of the brain.
- *Presbycusis* is old age–related hearing loss that is not associated with a specific pathologic process but arises from degeneration of the inner ear structures.

Causes
Conductive hearing loss may be caused by outer ear diseases such as otitis externa, ear wax impaction, foreign bodies, cancerous tumors, benign inflammatory polyps, and trauma. Middle ear diseases such as infectious otitis media, primary secretory otitis media (PSOM), foreign bodies, and tumors are also causes.

Congenital, hereditary sensorineural deafness occurs in some dogs and cats with white coat color and blue eyes. It also affects numerous purebred dogs, such as the Dalmatian, Australian blue heeler, English setter, Argentine dogo, bull terrier, Australian shepherd, Jack Russell terrier, and Cavalier King Charles spaniel.

Acquired sensorineural deafness may develop from certain systemic drugs (aminoglycoside antibiotics) and topical otic medications (ceruminolytic agents), trauma, tumors, or presbycusis.

Clinical Signs
Conductive hearing loss can occur at any age, depending on the underlying cause. It rarely results in complete hearing loss. Congenital, hereditary deafness is present soon after birth. With acquired deafness, hearing loss may be sudden or slow in onset; in some cases, balance (vestibular) problems may be detected.

Diagnostic Tests
Physical examination findings are usually normal. Specialized hearing tests are used to confirm deafness, to pinpoint where the hearing loss is occurring in the hearing pathway, and to determine whether the hearing loss is conductive or sensorineural in nature. For the best results, these tests are often performed with the animal sedated or anesthetized, and they are usually available only at veterinary specialty or university hospitals. Examples include the following:

- Impedance audiometry is performed by inserting ear plugs into the ear canal and measuring the change in mobility of the eardrum (tympanic membrane) and the involuntary contraction of the muscles in the middle ear. This test helps to assess the integrity of the middle ear.
- The brainstem evoked auditory response (BAER) test measures specific components of the hearing pathway and can be used to characterize conductive and sensorineural hearing loss.

TREATMENT AND FOLLOW-UP
Treatment Options
Conductive hearing loss is usually reversible and requires removal of any obstruction, such as wax from the external ear canal or mucus from the middle ear (especially in dogs with PSOM). Congenital hereditary sensorineural hearing loss and presbycusis are not treatable and are irreversible. Drug-induced hearing loss is usually permanent but may improve once the drug has been discontinued.

Follow-up Care
Animals with conductive hearing loss from otitis externa and/or media are periodically rechecked to prevent a recurrence of the otitis and hearing loss. Animals with congenital, inherited hearing loss should not be bred.

Prognosis
Prognosis is good for conductive hearing loss. Prognosis is poor for sensorineural hearing loss; however, behavioral modification techniques (such as hand signals) may be used to train the dog.

SPECIAL INSTRUCTIONS:

Otitis Externa

Lynette K. Cole, DVM, MS, DACVD

BASIC INFORMATION

Description

Otitis externa is inflammation of the external ear canal. In many cases, the ear pinna (flap), middle ear, or both are also involved.

Causes

Many different factors are involved in the development of otitis externa, including predisposing factors, primary causes, and perpetuating factors. Predisposing factors alter the environment of the external ear canal, thereby allowing secondary bacterial and yeast infections to develop. Some examples are:

- Pendulous (floppy) ears
- Ear canals with a small or narrow diameter (stenotic)
- Numerous glands in the ear canals that overproduce wax
- Excess hair in the canal
- Frequent swimming ("swimmer's ear")
- Mechanical trauma to the ear canal from overzealous cleaning with potent drying agents, use of cotton-tipped applicators for cleaning, or vigorous plucking of hair from the canal

Primary causes include conditions that directly induce ear inflammation, such as the following:

- Parasites, such as mites or ticks
- Plant material, such as grass awns
- Allergic skin disease, such as atopic dermatitis or food allergy
- Autoimmune skin diseases, in which the immune system attacks components of the skin
- Keratinization disorders, such as idiopathic seborrhea, that result in excessive wax production in the ear canal
- Hormonal disorders, such as low thyroid levels (hypothyroidism)
- Masses in the ear canal, such as benign inflammatory polyps and tumors
- Foreign bodies

Perpetuating factors prevent resolution of the ear inflammation or worsen an existing ear disease and may include the following:

- Bacterial and yeast infections
- Inflammation of the middle ear (otitis media)
- Progressive or persistent changes in the ear canal, such as swelling, scarring, and mineralization (calcification)

Clinical Signs

Otitis externa occurs in dogs more frequently than in cats, and in animals of any age or gender. The most common breeds of dog affected include the cocker spaniel, golden retriever, Labrador retriever, and miniature poodle; however, otitis externa may affect any dog.

The most common signs of otitis externa are discharge and odor from the ear, redness and swelling of the ear, rubbing or pawing at the ear, shaking of the head, and decreased hearing.

Diagnostic Tests

Physical and dermatologic examinations are performed to identify predisposing factors and primary causes of the otitis. An ear examination with an otoscope is done to evaluate the amount of debris and exudate in the ear, to look for changes in the ear canal, and to evaluate the eardrum (tympanic membrane). The ear canal is swabbed, and the material collected is examined under the microscope to look for bacteria, yeast, and ear mites. In certain cases (especially in chronic otitis), an ear swab may be submitted for bacterial culture.

Diagnosis of underlying diseases often requires further testing, such as laboratory and hormonal tests, allergy testing, skin scrapings, and biopsies.

TREATMENT AND FOLLOW-UP

Treatment Options

The goals for treatment of otitis externa are to remove debris from the ears, relieve inflammation, resolve infections, control predisposing and perpetuating factors, and treat the primary cause. Common medications applied to the ear include cleaning and drying agents, antibiotics and antifungals to treat the infection, and steroids to relieve itching and swelling. In severe cases, oral medications (steroid, antibiotic, antifungal) may also be prescribed.

Specific treatment for any underlying conditions is also started. Treatment of ear mites requires that all animals in the household be treated, because ear mites are contagious to other animals.

In some cases of otitis externa, the changes in the ear canal cannot be managed with medications, and surgery is needed. The most common surgery performed is a total ear canal removal (ablation) and bulla osteotomy. Surgery relieves pain, helps resolve infection, and can be used to remove masses in the external and middle ear.

Follow-up Care

Follow-up visits are critical to the management of otitis externa. It is important to continue all prescribed medications until the recheck examination, because, although the clinical signs may resolve soon after starting the medications, infection may still be present. Contact your veterinarian if the signs worsen or recur.

Prognosis

Some cases of otitis externa (such as ear mites) are easy to resolve, but others are not easily cured and may only be controllable. Prognosis is good if early treatment and resolution of the primary causes and predisposing and perpetuating factors are achieved. Chronic, recurrent otitis externa, especially those cases complicated by severe bacterial infections, may be difficult to control and may require surgery.

SPECIAL INSTRUCTIONS:

Otitis Interna

Lynette K. Cole, DVM, MS, DACVD

BASIC INFORMATION
Description
Otitis interna is an inflammatory condition of the structures of the inner ear.
Causes
Otitis interna may be caused by bacterial, fungal, and rickettsial (tick-borne) infections. Noninfectious causes include the following:

- Idiopathic (cause unknown) congenital disease, in which signs occur at birth, can cause otitis interna. It is more common in purebred dogs, such as the Doberman pinscher, German shepherd dog, English cocker spaniel, and beagle. It also occurs in Burmese and Siamese cats.
- Idiopathic acquired diseases, such as old dog and feline vestibulitis, affect the vestibular apparatus (partially responsible for balance) in the ear.
- Metabolic diseases, such as hypothyroidism (low thyroid hormone levels) and hyperadrenocorticism (elevated cortisol hormone levels), may be involved.
- Traumatic and compressive events, such as foreign bodies in the ear, trauma, cancerous tumors, and benign inflammatory polyps, may cause otitis interna.

Clinical Signs

Signs include head tilt, falling, circling, nausea and vomiting, and abnormal eye position or abnormal movements of the eye.

Diagnostic Tests

A complete neurologic examination is usually performed to determine which part of the nervous system is involved.

For infectious diseases, there is usually a prior history of chronic otitis externa and/or otitis media. Initial diagnostic tests are similar to those used in animals with otitis externa or otitis media. They include otoscopy as well as cytologic examination and culture of exudate from the external and middle ear. In addition, laboratory tests for rickettsial or fungal diseases and advanced imaging may be recommended; magnetic resonance imaging is the preferred test. A deep ear flush may be needed. A spinal tap and analysis of cerebral spinal fluid (CSF) is indicated in certain circumstances.

For noninfectious diseases, radiographic imaging is needed to determine whether a benign inflammatory polyp or tumor is present and to look for signs of trauma. For idiopathic acquired vestibular disease, it is important to rule out underlying causes and other diseases with similar signs.

TREATMENT AND FOLLOW-UP

Treatment Options

Treatment of infections includes long-term systemic (oral) antimicrobial medications. For noninfectious diseases, supportive care in the hospital (adequate fluid therapy, nutrition, nursing care) is often required during the early stages, since the animal may have trouble eating, drinking, and walking. Antivertigo drugs may be prescribed for dizziness. Surgery is often needed if a benign inflammatory polyp or tumor of the ear is present.

Follow-up Care

Animals with infectious otitis interna are usually rechecked in 2-4 weeks. If the condition worsens, notify your veterinarian so that the animal can be seen sooner. In most cases, improvement occurs during the first week of treatment. Recurrent episodes of infectious otitis interna are most common when chronic bacterial otitis media is also present.

Animals with idiopathic, acquired vestibular disease usually improve within 2 weeks after the onset of the signs, but it may take several weeks for the signs to stabilize. The need for recheck examinations varies, depending on whether the signs steadily improve. Recurrent episodes of idiopathic, acquired vestibular disease are uncommon.

Prognosis
Prognosis for infectious otitis interna is fair to excellent with appropriate antimicrobial therapy but is worse for fungal infections. Prognosis for noninfectious otitis interna is variable, depending on the cause. It is excellent for idiopathic, acquired vestibular disease; fair for idiopathic, congenital vestibular disease; and excellent for benign inflammatory polyps that can be surgically removed.

SPECIAL INSTRUCTIONS:

Otitis Media

Lynette K. Cole, DVM, MS, DACVD

BASIC INFORMATION

Description

Otitis media is inflammation of the middle ear. Otitis media is an important cause of recurrent otitis externa (external ear inflammation and infection). In addition to diagnosing and treating the otitis media, the underlying cause of otitis externa must also be addressed. (See handout on **Otitis Externa.**)

Causes

Causes may include infections (bacterial, fungal) and noninfectious problems such as trauma, tumors (cancer, benign polyps), and foreign bodies (grass awns). A primary secretory otitis media (PSOM) occurs mainly in the Cavalier King Charles spaniel.

Clinical Signs

The most common sign of otitis media is recurrent otitis externa, with discharge from the ear, pawing and rubbing of the ear, head shaking, and pain around the ear. Additional signs in some dogs include facial drooping and balance problems (incoordination, stumbling). Cavalier King Charles spaniels with PSOM may have head and neck scratching and pain, facial drooping, balance problems, and/or hearing loss.

Diagnostic Tests

Initially, general, dermatologic, and neurologic examinations are performed. An ear examination with an otoscope is done to evaluate the amount of debris and exudate in the ear, to look for changes in the ear canal (narrowing or thickening), and to evaluate the eardrum (tympanic membrane). The ear canal is swabbed, and the material collected is examined under the microscope to look for bacteria, yeast, and ear mites. In certain cases (especially in chronic otitis), an ear swab may be submitted for bacterial culture.

Diagnosis of underlying diseases requires further testing, which may include laboratory and hormonal tests, allergy testing, skin scrapings, biopsies, and so on. Additional tests performed with the animal under sedation or anesthesia are needed to evaluate the middle ear. These tests may include x-rays, computed tomography (CT scan), or magnetic resonance imaging (MRI), and they are often followed by a deep flushing of the external ear canal and middle ear. A myringotomy (incision into the tympanic membrane) is performed to remove any material from the middle ear and to flush the middle ear and allow it to drain. Cytology and bacterial cultures are obtained from the external ear canal and middle ear to identify any bacterial or yeast infections.

TREATMENT AND FOLLOW-UP

Treatment Options

Bacterial and yeast infections of the middle ear are treated with systemic (oral) and topical otic (ear) antimicrobial medications. If the ear canals are swollen, then systemic or topical steroids (or both) may be prescribed. An ear cleaning and drying agent may also be recommended. Cavalier King Charles spaniels with PSOM usually do not have secondary infections in their middle ears and are treated with a short course of oral steroids and agents that break up mucus (mucolytic).

Follow-up Care

A recheck appointment is usually scheduled 2-4 weeks after flushing. Follow-up visits are critical to the management of otitis media. At the recheck appointment, an otoscopic examination, along with repeat cytologic evaluation and culture, may be performed to monitor response to therapy. It is important to continue all prescribed medications until the recheck examination, because although the clinical signs may resolve soon after starting the medications, infection may still be present. In some cases, it takes months before the infection is under control. Contact your veterinarian if the clinical signs worsen or recur.

Complications are possible from deep ear flushing procedures and include facial drooping, head tilt, balance problems, and hearing loss. In the dog, these complications are very rare. In the cat, they occur more commonly but are usually reversible over a period of 3-6 weeks.

Topical otic medications are important in the treatment of otitis media, but none of these medications has been tested for safety in the middle ear, and their use could result in ototoxicity (deafness, balance problems). However, these problems rarely occur. If any of these signs are noted after the flushing or while the animal is on topical otic medications, the medications should be discontinued and a recheck appointment scheduled immediately.

Prognosis

In most cases, the prognosis for control of otitis media is good with appropriate treatment of the infection (both external ear and middle ear) and control of the primary cause. In some cases, the middle ear infection does not completely resolve and becomes a recurrent otitis media requiring surgery (total ear canal ablation and/or bulla osteotomy). In Cavalier King Charles spaniels with PSOM, removal of the mucus plug and flushing of the middle ear may need to be repeated multiple times for the condition to resolve.

SPECIAL INSTRUCTIONS:

SECTION 15

Infectious Diseases

Section Editor: Lynn F. Guptill, DVM, PhD, DACVIM (Small Animal)

Bartonellosis
Blastomycosis
Borreliosis (Lyme Disease)
Brucellosis in Dogs
Campylobacteriosis
Canine Distemper Virus
Canine Infectious Tracheobronchitis (Kennel Cough)
Canine Influenza
Coccidioidomycosis
Coccidiosis, Enteric
Cryptococcosis
Cryptosporidiosis
Cytauxzoonosis
Ehrlichiosis and Anaplasmosis in Dogs
Feline Coronavirus
Feline Immunodeficiency Virus
Feline Leukemia Virus
Feline Upper Respiratory Infection

Giardiasis
Helicobacteriosis
Hepatozoonosis in Dogs
Histoplasmosis
Leishmaniasis
Leptospirosis
Methicillin-Resistant *Staphylococcus* Infections
Neosporosis in Dogs
Parvovirus in Cats
Parvovirus in Dogs
Prototheocosis in Dogs
Pythiosis
Rabies
Rocky Mountain Spotted Fever
Tetanus
Toxoplasmosis
Tritrichomoniasis in Cats

Bartonellosis

Lynn F. Guptill, DVM, PhD, DACVIM (Small Animal)

BASIC INFORMATION

Description

Bartonellosis is a bacterial infection with variable manifestations that affects dogs, cats, and many other species, including humans.

Causes

Bartonellosis is found worldwide and is caused by gram-negative bacteria of the genus *Bartonella*. These bacteria are transmitted in the feces of fleas and probably by tick saliva. Direct transmission among animals has not been demonstrated. *Bartonella henselae, Bartonella vinsonii* subspecies *berkhoffii,* and *Bartonella clarridgeiae* are among the most common *Bartonella* species infecting dogs and cats.

Cats are considered the primary reservoir for *B. henselae,* and dogs are the probable reservoir for *B. vinsonii* subsp. *berkhoffii.* Animals may be infected with more than one *Bartonella* species. Many cats (50-90% in some areas) are infected with *Bartonella,* so it can be difficult to know whether a clinical condition is truly related to *Bartonella* infection or to some other process.

Clinical Signs

Most cats infected with *B. henselae* or *B. clarridgeiae* seem to have no clinical illness as a result of the infection. The clinical syndromes associated with bartonellosis are poorly understood; the most information is known about *B. henselae* infection of cats. The following is a list of potential clinical signs in cats:

- Most infected cats have no apparent signs.
- Fever, lethargy, decreased appetite, and enlarged lymph nodes (glands) are possible, particularly within a few weeks of the initial infection.
- Inflammation of the eye (uveitis) is possible.
- Muscle pain and some nervous system problems have been reported, but a definite association with *Bartonella* has been hard to establish.
- Infection of the heart valves is reported in some infected cats.
- Occasionally, central nervous system signs such as tremors, altered behavior, and decreased responsiveness to stimuli are attributable to *Bartonella* infection.

Clinical syndromes reported in dogs include the following:

- Infection of the heart valves (endocarditis), especially the aortic valve
- Granulomas (masses of inflammatory cells) in various tissues
- Neurologic abnormalities

Diagnostic Tests

Diagnosis is challenging. In cats, the infection may be diagnosed by blood culture or polymerase chain reaction (PCR) testing for bacterial DNA in blood or other tissues. Finding infection, however, does not prove that it is the cause of a particular clinical condition. Positive blood antibody tests indicate past exposure to the bacteria but do not prove that an active infection is present. If no other disease or problem is found to explain the clinical signs, then bartonellosis may be considered a potential cause.

Tests that may be recommended include routine laboratory tests; fine needle aspiration or biopsy of enlarged lymph nodes for microscopic analysis; special imaging of the central nervous system, such as computed tomography (CT scan) or magnetic resonance imaging (MRI); and a spinal tap to retrieve cerebrospinal fluid for analysis. Blood cultures have a poor yield in dogs, but in cats *Bartonella* bacteria can persist in the blood in variable numbers for several years.

TREATMENT AND FOLLOW-UP

Treatment Options

No antibiotics have been proven effective for clearing *Bartonella* infections. Antibiotics that are commonly used include doxycycline and azithromycin. Treatment is recommended when an animal has clinical signs consistent with bartonellosis and no other cause is found for those signs. Treatment is often continued for at least 4-6 weeks. Treatment of asymptomatic animals is not recommended.

Follow-up Care

So little is known about treatment of *Bartonella* infections that follow-up testing is difficult to define. Sometimes a repeated blood culture is recommended in cats and tests for antibodies are repeated in dogs and cats. Because the length of time that antibodies persist after treatment is unknown, it is difficult to know the best time at which to do follow-up testing.

Bartonella infections do not result in immunity to bartonellosis. Control of fleas and ticks is the most effective means of preventing infection. A thorough flea and tick control program should be instituted for any animal with suspected bartonellosis. No vaccines are available for the disease.

Prognosis

Prognosis has not been established in animals. *B. henselae* causes cat scratch disease in people, as well as numerous other illnesses. Other *Bartonella* species are also associated with clinical illnesses in humans, some of which are serious. Immunocompromised people are especially susceptible to *Bartonella* infections, and clinical infections can be life-threatening. Precautions should be taken to minimize any bites or scratches from animals infected with *Bartonella.*

SPECIAL INSTRUCTIONS:

Blastomycosis

Anisa D. Dunham, AS, RVT
Lynn F. Guptill, DVM, PhD, DACVIM (Small Animal)

BASIC INFORMATION

Description

Blastomycosis is a fungal infection that usually starts in the lungs and then spreads to other parts of the body. Dogs and cats are both susceptible, but the disease occurs most often in dogs.

Cause

Blastomycosis is caused by the fungus *Blastomyces dermatitidis*. It is an organism that grows in and receives its nourishment from dead or decaying organic matter in the soil. It can survive in a wide range of moistures and temperatures. In the United States, it occurs most commonly in the Ohio, Mississippi, Missouri, Tennessee, and St. Lawrence River valleys. It can also be found in the southern Great Lakes region and in the mid-Atlantic states.

Infection occurs most commonly via inhalation or ingestion of the fungus from the environment. Infection may be limited to the lungs or may spread to multiple sites in the body.

Clinical Signs

Signs may initially be nonspecific and include lethargy, decreased appetite, and weight loss. Increased respiratory rate, difficulty breathing, and coughing may occur. Inflammation of the eyes, vision changes, enlarged lymph nodes (glands), and lameness from bony involvement are other possible signs.

Skin lesions occur in about half of the cases and are usually crusty bumps that drain a thick liquid. Organisms present in this liquid may spread the infection if it contaminates an open wound. Feet and nail beds are sometimes affected.

Altered mental attitude and difficulty walking are signs of central nervous system (primarily brain) disease. Other organs that may be affected include the testicles, prostate, and mammary glands (breast tissue). Gastrointestinal signs are uncommon.

Diagnostic Tests

Routine laboratory tests and chest x-rays are commonly recommended to investigate the clinical signs. X-rays of the legs may be done if lameness and bone pain are present. Blood tests are available for blastomycosis at certain outside laboratories. Although these tests are sensitive, false-negative and false-positive results can occur.

Finding the organism in affected tissues is the best diagnostic test. Needle aspiration or biopsy of an enlarged lymph node, skin lesion, blind eye, or other affected tissue may be done. A tracheal wash (collecting fluid from the airway through a catheter inserted into the windpipe) or bronchoscopy (examination of the airway through a fiberoptic viewing scope) may be considered if the lungs are involved. In cases of central nervous system involvement, a spinal tap may be considered to collect cerebrospinal fluid. The fluid is then submitted for analysis and culture. In some cases, the fungal agent can be cultured from infected tissues.

TREATMENT AND FOLLOW-UP

Treatment Options

The oral antifungal drugs, itraconazole and fluconazole, are generally considered effective but must be given for a prolonged period (months). Ketoconazole may be less expensive, but it is also less effective and has more side effects. Intravenous amphotericin B may be needed in animals with severe disease, especially if they do not respond to or do not tolerate oral medications. Amphotericin B is used cautiously, because it is toxic to the kidneys. Some forms are less toxic than others.

Seriously ill animals often require hospitalization, with intensive treatment and monitoring for the first several days of treatment. Dogs with severe lung disease may need supplemental oxygen. Death of the fungal organisms that occurs within the first few days of therapy may make the lung changes temporarily worse. Eyes that are blind and have persistent inflammation or glaucoma may be surgically removed.

Follow-up Care

Periodic recheck visits and repeated laboratory testing are required for several months to monitor the response to treatment and for side effects of the medications. Treatment is continued for at least 2-3 months, and for 1 month beyond the disappearance of all clinical signs.

After therapy is completed, the animal is commonly re-evaluated for up to 6 months to assess for relapses, which can occur in as many as 20-25% of treated animals. Strict adherence to treatment protocols is needed for the best response.

Prognosis

Prognosis is variable and depends on the extent and severity of the disease, as well as the initial response to treatment. Prognosis is better in animals with mild clinical signs or signs limited to one organ system. Prognosis is guarded (uncertain) in animals with widespread disease, central nervous system involvement, or severe involvement of any organ system.

SPECIAL INSTRUCTIONS:

Borreliosis (Lyme Disease)

Lynn F. Guptill, DVM, PhD, DACVIM (Small Animal)

BASIC INFORMATION

Description

Borreliosis (Lyme disease) is a tick-borne disease that affects animals and people worldwide.

Causes

Borreliosis is one of a large group of tick-transmitted diseases caused by spirochete bacteria. This handout focuses on Lyme disease. The causative agent of Lyme disease in the United States is *Borrelia burgdorferi,* which is transmitted most commonly by deer ticks. Most cases of Lyme disease in the United States occur in the eastern coastal states and upper midwestern states. Lyme disease primarily affects dogs; cats are much more resistant to the disease.

Clinical Signs

Approximately 5-10% of dogs exposed to *B. burgdorferi* develop signs of Lyme disease, which is a low number. Initially, fever, lethargy, decreased appetite, and lameness are the most common signs. Lameness tends to shift from one leg to another over several weeks. Joint swelling and enlarged lymph nodes may occur. Multiple joints may be affected. Inflammation of the eyes (uveitis) may develop.

Rarely, and possibly more frequently in Labrador and golden retrievers, severe kidney disease occurs. Dogs with kidney disease often have sudden onset of lethargy, decreased appetite, vomiting, and weight loss. This manifestation of Lyme disease may progress rapidly to kidney failure.

Diagnostic Tests

Routine laboratory (blood and urine) tests, abdominal and joint x-rays, and an abdominal ultrasound may initially be recommended to investigate the source of the clinical signs. Biochemistry panels may show low blood protein levels and evidence of kidney malfunction or failure. Urine analysis may show increased protein in the urine, poor ability of the kidneys to concentrate the urine, or both. A joint tap and analysis of joint fluid may also be recommended.

Tests for antibodies to *B. burgdorferi* may be done on blood samples. Two tests may be run 2-3 weeks apart to determine whether the antibody levels are increasing. In dogs that have been vaccinated for Lyme disease, special tests may be needed to differentiate whether the antibodies are from the vaccination or from natural exposure to the bacteria. Dogs with positive antibody tests may not have clinical disease; they may only have been exposed to the bacteria.

Bacterial culture is not often practical but may be attempted. Skin biopsies from near the site of attachment of a tick may provide the best tissue to culture. Polymerase chain reaction (PCR) tests for bacterial DNA may be done in some cases (when available) on biopsies of skin or joint tissue.

TREATMENT AND FOLLOW-UP

Treatment Options

Treatment is recommended when the history, clinical signs, and laboratory test results are consistent with possible Lyme disease. Doxycycline is the most commonly recommended antibiotic and is usually administered for 3-6 weeks. Doxycycline has antiinflammatory properties that may also be helpful. Amoxicillin, given for 1 month, is also considered an effective treatment. Side effects of doxycycline and amoxicillin in dogs are usually limited to mild vomiting or diarrhea. These drugs are often given with food to decrease these side effects.

Nonsteroidal antiinflammatory drugs (NSAIDs) may be recommended to relieve joint pain. (See also the handout on **Immune-Mediated Arthritis.**) Side effects of NSAIDs include vomiting, diarrhea, and sometimes stomach or intestinal ulceration. Stop the medication and notify your veterinarian immediately if any of these problems occur.

Antibiotic treatment of dogs that are clinically healthy but have a positive screening test for *B. burgdorferi* is considered controversial. Dogs with kidney disease require specific treatment for that disorder in addition to antibiotic treatment. (See also the handouts on **Protein-Losing Nephropathy in Dogs** and **Acute Kidney Failure.**) NSAIDs must be used with caution in animals with kidney disease.

Follow-up Care

B. burgdorferi may be difficult to completely clear from an infected dog, and clinical signs may recur weeks to months after treatment. Treatment also does not protect the animal against reinfection. Vaccination may be recommended in some areas where Lyme disease is common.

Ticks should be removed from dogs each day during the tick season. Strict tick control is an important means of preventing exposure to Lyme disease. Sometimes it is recommended that dogs exposed to *B. burgdorferi* be periodically tested for protein in their urine.

Prognosis

Most dogs treated for Lyme disease have a good prognosis, although relapse, re-exposure, and reinfection are possible. Dogs with severe kidney disease attributed to Lyme disease have a poor prognosis.

SPECIAL INSTRUCTIONS:

Brucellosis in Dogs

Anisa D. Dunham, AS, RVT
Lynn F. Guptill, DVM, PhD, DACVIM (Small Animal)

BASIC INFORMATION

Description

Brucellosis is a zoonotic disease (a disease that can be transmitted from animals to humans) that affects primarily reproductive organs. It can also infect other tissues of the body, such as intervertebral discs of the spine, eyes, and kidneys.

Cause

Brucellosis in dogs is caused by the bacterial organism *Brucella canis*. Transmission usually occurs during breeding, at birth, or from intimate contact with infected animals, possibly via inhalation of aerosols associated with abortion or vaginal discharges. The organisms reside within cells, making them difficult to eliminate.

Clinical Signs

Reproductive problems include failure to conceive after breeding, abortion of dead puppies, production of stillborn or weak puppies, and testicular abnormalities. Nonreproductive problems may include back pain, lameness, weakness, and partial paralysis. Uveitis, an inflammation of the eye, may also be seen.

Diagnostic Tests

Initially, routine laboratory tests or x-rays may be recommended, depending on the clinical signs. Diagnosis of brucellosis can be made based on several tests, such as the following:

- Blood tests are the primary method of diagnosis. Some rapid, in-clinic tests are very sensitive and can have false-positive results. Positive tests must be confirmed by specialized assays done at outside reference laboratories, such as state diagnostic laboratories.
- Bacterial culture of the blood may be done, but false-negative results may occur, because the bacteria are not always present in the blood. Urine, semen, and intervertebral disc material may also be cultured.

Semen analysis may be done in infertile male dogs. Abnormalities seen may include immature or deformed sperm. Biopsy and microscopic evaluation of reproductive tissues can support the diagnosis. Other tests may be indicated to rule out other diseases that cause similar clinical signs.

TREATMENT AND FOLLOW-UP

Treatment Options

Treatment for brucellosis may not be advisable, since the infection can be zoonotic, and eradication from tissues is uncertain and difficult to prove. If infected dogs are treated, they *must* be removed from breeding programs and neutered. Combinations of antibiotics are needed to treat the disease. The combination of a tetracycline (such as doxycycline, minocycline) and an aminoglycoside (such as gentamicin) antibiotic is most likely to be effective. Resolving the infection is difficult, and relapses are common. Multiple courses of therapy separated by 1-2 months may be needed. (See the handouts on **Discospondylitis** and **Anterior Uveitis** for more details on the treatment of these two conditions.)

Follow-up Care

Periodic recheck visits and repeated testing (x-rays, laboratory tests) are usually needed to monitor response to treatment. Blood tests for brucellosis may be repeated every 3-6 months to monitor for relapse.

Kennels containing animals that are positive for brucellosis are usually quarantined and infected animals removed. All dogs in the kennel are then tested monthly, and the kennel is released from quarantine only after all dogs have had two consecutive negative tests. Cleaning and disinfection procedures must be carefully followed. People working with infected animals should wear gloves and other appropriate personal protective equipment.

Prevention

Preventive measures are very important in breeding kennels and in any facility that houses a large number of dogs. New animals should be quarantined until two negative test results are obtained, 1 month apart. Dogs that leave the facility should be tested again before being allowed to return.

Prognosis

Although adult dogs are not often seriously ill, relapses are common. Since brucellosis can be transmitted to people and there is no known cure for brucellosis, euthanasia of infected dogs should be considered. All breeding animals should be tested for brucellosis 3-4 weeks before each breeding. Dogs used as blood donors are also commonly tested.

SPECIAL INSTRUCTIONS:

Campylobacteriosis

Lynn F. Guptill, DVM, PhD, DACVIM (Small Animal)

BASIC INFORMATION

Description

Campylobacteriosis is an infection associated with diarrhea. It affects many species of animals, including dogs, cats, and cattle, as well as humans.

Causes

Campylobacteriosis is caused by several species of gram-negative bacteria in the genus *Campylobacter*. Transmission occurs when the organism is swallowed, often in water or food contaminated with feces. The organism can persist in the environment for several days, and possibly longer at cooler temperatures and when contained in organic material.

 ### Clinical Signs

Dogs and cats are often asymptomatic carriers. Clinical signs are believed to develop more often (and are more severe) in animals that are young, are immune suppressed, or have another infection. Animals with campylobacteriosis are likely to be at risk for other intestinal infections, such as coccidiosis, giardiasis, or *Salmonella* infection. Diarrhea may contain mucus or blood and is often watery. A more widespread (systemic) disease has been reported in a few dogs, with signs of fever, decreased appetite, or jaundice (yellow color to the skin and mucous membranes of the eyes and mouth).

 ### Diagnostic Tests

Diagnosis of campylobacteriosis may be suspected based on the clinical presentation and can be confirmed through several laboratory tests. Testing can involve the following:

- Microscopic examinations of fecal samples using specialized methods may identify the curved ("gull-wing" shaped) *Campylobacter* bacteria. *Helicobacter* bacteria may look similar; however, so other tests are needed to confirm campylobacteriosis.
- Culture of fresh feces or a rectal swab is often recommended, and specialized culture conditions are required. The best culture results are achieved when feces are transported to the laboratory quickly.
- Additional testing on the cultured bacteria may be recommended to determine which *Campylobacter* species is present.

- Identification of the species can be important in locating the source of the infection and whether it is likely to be transmissible to humans.

Laboratory tests, other fecal assays, x-rays, and other tests may be recommended if affected animals are systemically ill and to rule out other diseases that cause similar clinical signs.

TREATMENT AND FOLLOW-UP

 ### Treatment Options

The effectiveness of antibiotic therapy for campylobacteriosis in dogs and cats is unknown. It is possible that the diarrhea may stop without treatment in some animals. It is also not known whether antibiotics will stop the shedding of the bacteria in the feces. Antibiotics that are commonly prescribed include erythromycin and second-generation cephalosporins. Fluoroquinolone antibiotics, metronidazole, and sulfadimethoxine are not often used, because *Campylobacter* species can become resistant to these drugs.

Follow-up Care

Strict sanitation and hygiene practices are needed to limit the spread of *Campylobacter* organisms and prevent reinfection. Crowding and close confinement of multiple animals should be avoided. Fecal material must be removed daily. Clean all organic material (feces, dirt) from all surfaces (cages, kennels, food bowls) prior to disinfecting them. Bathing the animals during treatment may be helpful, because it removes fecal material and decreases bacterial contamination.

Some animals continue to shed *Campylobacter* even when treated with antibiotics.

Campylobacter species are transmissible to humans and can cause severe gastrointestinal disease, particularly in immune-compromised individuals. Caution should be exercised (wear gloves, wash hands thoroughly) when handling and treating animals with campylobacteriosis.

Prognosis

Prognosis is good for most animals with campylobacteriosis.

SPECIAL INSTRUCTIONS:

Canine Distemper Virus

Lynn F. Guptill, DVM, PhD, DACVIM (Small Animal)

BASIC INFORMATION

Description

Canine distemper virus (CDV) is very contagious and infects the respiratory tract, the gastrointestinal (GI) tract, and the central nervous system (CNS, including brain and spinal cord). The disease can be prevented by vaccination.

Cause

CDV is an enveloped virus closely related to measles virus. It is highly concentrated in respiratory tract secretions and is also found in other body fluids, such as urine. CDV is commonly spread through the air and survives in cold, freezing environments. The virus can be destroyed by sunlight, high heat, drying, and many common disinfectants.

Clinical Signs

Clinical signs vary widely in severity. Signs may be very mild, with only fever, lethargy, and slight nasal or eye discharge. Severe systemic infection occurs most often in young puppies and unvaccinated adult dogs. Clinical signs in severe cases may include fever, watery or cloudy nasal and eye discharge, and coughing that may be accompanied by difficulty breathing. Decreased appetite, vomiting, and diarrhea may also occur. Examination of the eyes with an ophthalmoscope may reveal inflammation in the retina.

CNS signs include seizures, behavioral changes, weakness, and difficulty walking. Involuntary repetitive contractions (tic, myoclonus) of certain muscles, often in one limb, and twitching of facial muscles may be seen. Neurologic signs may occur at the same time as respiratory and GI signs, or they may occur several weeks after recovery from those signs.

Other findings may include thickened foot pads (known as *hard pad disease*); abnormal tooth enamel (pits, discoloration); and dry, painful eyes from decreased tear production. In some cases, infected dogs have minimal clinical signs initially, then months to years later develop CNS signs. This variant of CDV disease is called *old dog distemper*.

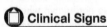 Diagnostic Tests

No single test is available to make the diagnosis of CDV infection, so a number of tests are usually recommended to search for evidence of the disease, such as the following:

- A complete blood count may show low numbers of lymphocytes (a form of white blood cell affected by the virus).
- A biochemistry panel may show blood protein abnormalities.
- Analysis of cerebrospinal fluid (CSF) taken by a spinal tap may be recommended and may show increased numbers of lymphocytes and high protein concentrations.

- X-rays of the chest and abdomen may be recommended if respiratory or GI tract signs are present.
- Tests for antibodies to CDV in the blood and/or CSF may help identify an active infection.
- Special stains on scrapings or swabs taken from the conjunctiva, skin, or other samples can sometimes reveal viral components in the cells, but false-negative results are common.

Other tests may be recommended to rule out other diseases that cause similar clinical signs.

TREATMENT AND FOLLOW-UP

Treatment Options

Dogs with suspected CDV infection should be isolated from other dogs because of the highly contagious nature of the virus. No drug is available that will destroy the virus or rid it from the body, so supportive care is usually instituted.

Supportive care for respiratory and GI infection may include intravenous fluids and antivomiting medications. Nebulization and physical therapy (coupage) of the chest may be done to loosen and remove thickened respiratory secretions. Secretions are also cleaned from the nose and eyes. Antibiotics may be needed to treat secondary bacterial infections.

Animals with CNS disease may require anticonvulsant medications to control seizures, and steroids (prednisone) may be used in some animals to treat CNS inflammation.

Follow-up Care

Animals that appear to recover from respiratory and/or GI illness may develop CNS signs a few weeks to months later. Close monitoring is needed to watch for neurologic abnormalities. Recovering dogs may shed virus for several weeks, and care must be exercised to minimize or prevent interaction with other dogs, particularly dogs that are not vaccinated.

Prior to disinfection of cages and floors, all organic material must be removed. Disinfectants must contact treated surfaces for prolonged periods, depending on label directions. Immunity to CDV persists for many years following recovery from infection.

Prognosis

Animals with mild respiratory or GI tract signs may recover; however, many infected dogs will develop CNS disease. Prognosis for dogs with CNS disease is guarded (uncertain) to poor. Some dogs may recover but have permanent problems, such as seizures (that can be controlled with medication), vision abnormalities, and/or involuntary muscle tics. Euthanasia may be considered for severely ill animals that do not respond to supportive therapy.

SPECIAL INSTRUCTIONS:

Canine Infectious Tracheobronchitis (Kennel Cough)

Lynn F. Guptill, DVM, PhD, DACVIM (Small Animal)

BASIC INFORMATION

Description

Canine infectious tracheobronchitis (ITB), also known as *kennel cough*, results from infection of the respiratory tract with one or more viruses and bacteria. It is highly contagious.

Causes

The most common causes include canine parainfluenza virus, canine adenovirus 2, canine influenza virus, and bacteria such as *Bordetella bronchiseptica* and *Mycoplasma* species. ITB may develop from a single agent, or it may be a mixed infection. Common mixed infections involve *B. bronchiseptica,* canine parainfluenza virus, and/or canine adenovirus 2.

Viruses and *B. bronchiseptica* are spread through the air via close contact or by fomites (contaminated inanimate objects). Direct contact with infected secretions is the most common way that ITB spreads from dog to dog. Clinical disease often follows exposure to other infected dogs at kennels, dog parks, and dog shows.

Clinical Signs

The most common sign is coughing that often comes in spasms. The cough may be dry and hacking ("goose honk") or productive (gagging or coughing up secretions). These signs are sometimes mistaken for something caught in the dog's throat. Coughing episodes may be triggered by excitement, activity, or pressure on the neck (such as pulling against a collar).

Pneumonia and other generalized signs (nasal discharge, fever, decreased appetite, respiratory difficulty) may occur with complicated or serious infections. Unvaccinated and young dogs are most susceptible to complicated ITB. Secondary bacterial infections may also lead to bronchopneumonia.

Diagnostic Tests

Classic clinical signs and a history of recent exposure to other dogs are suggestive of ITB. Routine laboratory tests, such as a complete blood cell count and biochemistry profile, are often normal unless pneumonia or other complications are present. Chest x-rays may be recommended if pneumonia is suspected.

Special procedures, such as a tracheal wash (collecting fluid from the airway through a catheter inserted into the windpipe) or bronchoscopy (examination of the airway through a fiberoptic viewing scope), may be needed in complicated ITB cases or in dogs with pneumonia. Collected fluids are usually analyzed microscopically and submitted for bacterial culture and antibiotic susceptibility testing. Tests for antibodies in the blood and cultures for viruses may be done in some cases but are not often needed.

TREATMENT AND FOLLOW-UP

Treatment Options

Treatment for uncomplicated ITB is mainly supportive and involves administration of cough-suppressant medications. Cough suppressants are not recommended if the cough is productive or if pneumonia is present. Increasing the humidity in the environment can ease breathing and loosen respiratory secretions. Most uncomplicated infections resolve with time and do not require antibiotics. Antibiotics may be given to treat complicated ITB or secondary bacterial infections.

Dogs with pneumonia may require intensive care in an isolation ward, with intravenous fluids, supplemental oxygen, and antibiotics. Inhalation therapy with saline, a bronchodilator drug, and/or antibiotics may also be recommended.

Follow-up Care

It is important to prevent the spread of this disease to other dogs by taking the following steps:

- Isolate dogs with ITB from other dogs until all clinical signs have resolved.
- Keep recovered dogs away from unvaccinated or immune-compromised dogs and puppies.
- Most of the infectious agents that cause ITB are inactivated by bleach. Disinfect all items (cages, bowls, brushes) that have come in contact with the infected dog with a solution of bleach diluted (1:32) in water.
- ITB may be transmitted by fomites and by a person who has been exposed to an infected dog. To prevent this type of transmission, isolation of infected dogs and strict disinfection of facilities and equipment is essential. It is sometimes necessary to close facilities that house dogs for awhile when outbreaks of ITB occur.

Vaccines are available for *B. bronchiseptica*, parainfluenza virus, and adenovirus 2. Puppies are initially given two or three vaccinations 2-3 weeks apart. The vaccines are repeated at 1 year of age and then every 3 years. *Bordetella* vaccines may be required more often for dogs that are frequently kenneled. Vaccines do not prevent all infections, but they usually decrease the severity of disease.

It is possible for *B. bronchiseptica* to be transmitted from dogs to immune-compromised people, so preventive measures should be taken when caring for an infected animal.

Prognosis

For most dogs, prognosis is very good. The disease can be life-threatening in young puppies and in dogs compromised by other illnesses. For dogs with pneumonia, prognosis depends on the severity of the pneumonia and any other complicating conditions.

SPECIAL INSTRUCTIONS:

Canine Influenza

Anisa D. Dunham, AS, RVT
Lynn F. Guptill, DVM, PhD, DACVIM (Small Animal)

BASIC INFORMATION

Description

Canine influenza (CI) is a newer influenza strain that was first reported in 2004 at a Florida greyhound track. The virus first affected pet dogs in 2005. Dogs are the only known susceptible species. This strain (H3N8) is not known to infect humans.

Cause

Canine influenza is caused by an H3N8 strain of the influenza A virus family. It is a mutated strain of an equine influenza virus. Healthy dogs of all ages are susceptible. The influenza is thought to be transmitted by an infected dog sneezing or coughing on another dog, much the same way as influenza is spread among humans. It can also be transmitted via contaminated inanimate objects (fomites) and by people who touch both infected and uninfected dogs.

The incubation period is usually 2-5 days. Infected dogs shed the virus for 7-10 days after clinical signs appear. Since the virus is new, all dogs are considered susceptible to infection, and most dogs exposed to CI become infected. Approximately 80% of infected dogs develop clinical signs. Infected dogs that do not exhibit clinical signs can still shed the virus and spread the infection.

Clinical Signs

The disease may be mild or severe. Most dogs exhibit the mild form of the disease. The most common clinical sign is a cough that lasts 10-30 days despite treatment with antibiotics and cough suppressants. Most dogs have a soft, productive (moist) cough, but others have a dry cough that is similar to kennel cough. Many dogs have a nasal discharge that is purulent (contains pus) and a low-grade fever. Some dogs are more severely affected and may develop pneumonia with a high fever (104-106° F) and difficulty breathing.

Diagnostic Tests

Serologic tests that measure antibodies in the blood are commonly used to confirm a CI infection. Antibodies can be detected as early as 7 days after the onset of clinical signs. The first sample is tested within these 7 days, and a second sample is taken 2-3 weeks later. A fourfold increase in antibody levels from the first (acute) sample to the second (convalescent) sample indicates a positive diagnosis of CI. If no early sample was obtained, a positive convalescent sample confirms that the dog was exposed but does not indicate whether an infection was present.

A disadvantage of serology is that it cannot be used to confirm the presence of an acute, active infection. A rapid test is available that can be used to tentatively diagnose an active infection. The test can be run on a nasal swab and is most sensitive during the first 2-3 days of illness. Polymerase chain reaction tests done at outside laboratories are more accurate.

TREATMENT AND FOLLOW-UP

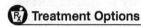 Treatment Options

Treatment is mostly supportive. In the mild form of the disease, nasal discharge may indicate a secondary bacterial infection, so treatment with a broad-spectrum antibiotic may be recommended. Pneumonia associated with the severe form of the disease can also be complicated by a bacterial infection, so broad-spectrum antibiotics are also commonly recommended in those cases. Intravenous fluids may be needed for dehydrated dogs. Cough suppressants are not very helpful in most cases.

Antiviral drugs developed for treatment of influenza in humans, such as *Tamiflu*, are not used to treat CI, because the appropriate dose and duration of treatment in dogs are unknown. In addition, when used in humans, the drug needs to be started within 48 hours of infection, and canine influenza is rarely diagnosed that early.

Follow-up Care

Dogs showing signs of CI should be isolated as soon as possible, to prevent spread of the disease to other dogs. Do not take these dogs to dog parks, boarding facilities, or other places where other dogs can be exposed to the virus. Recovering animals are also isolated for a couple of weeks to prevent transmission or possible reinfection before the dog has time to build up an adequate immune response to the virus. Wash your hands thoroughly after handling each dog. Thoroughly disinfect areas where the dog is housed with dilute bleach or another suitable disinfectant. All surfaces, equipment, and cages that have come in contact with an infected dog should be thoroughly cleaned and disinfected.

Prognosis

Prognosis is good in most cases. Good nursing care and nutrition are essential for a full recovery. Approximately 5-8% of clinically ill dogs die of this disease.

SPECIAL INSTRUCTIONS:

Coccidioidomycosis

Anisa D. Dunham, AS, RVT
Lynn F. Guptill, DVM, PhD, DACVIM (Small Animal)

BASIC INFORMATION
Description
Coccidioidomycosis is a systemic (affecting the whole body) fungal infection that typically originates in the lungs and may spread to the lymph glands, bones, and other organs. It has also been called *valley fever* and *San Joaquin Valley fever*.

Cause
Coccidioidomycosis is acquired from the environment. The fungus *Coccidioides immitis* is found most commonly in sandy, alkaline soil. Distribution in the United States is considered to be limited to the southwest desert regions. Coccidioidomycosis also occurs in Mexico, Central America, and some areas of South America. Outbreaks of disease can occur when drought is followed by conditions that allow the release and spread of fungal elements into the air.

Infection occurs via inhalation of the organism from the environment into the lungs or, rarely, from direct inoculation of the organism into the skin. Infection can spread from the lungs to other tissues.

Clinical Signs
Any tissue may be affected. In dogs, sites commonly affected include the lungs, bones, liver, spleen, kidneys, heart, reproductive tract, eyes, and central nervous system (especially brain). In cats, the skin is affected more commonly. Skin lesions may appear as draining tracts and abscesses.

Systemic (widespread) infection probably occurs more commonly in dogs than in cats. Infected cats and dogs may cough. Nonspecific signs, such as decreased appetite, lethargy, and weight loss, are also common. Other signs depend on the tissue affected. Lameness occurs in animals with bone or joint involvement, and seizures or behavioral changes may occur in animals with brain infection.

Diagnostic Tests
Finding the organism in infected tissues is the best diagnostic test. Procedures such as needle aspiration or biopsy of lymph nodes or other affected tissue may be done. Tracheal wash or bronchoscopy (examination of the airways through a small fiberoptic viewing scope) for collection of fluid from the lungs may be needed. Potential additional tests include the following:
- X-rays of the lungs may reveal abnormalities compatible with fungal infection. If lameness is present, x-rays of affected limbs are also indicated.

- Routine blood and urine tests help determine how the infection is affecting various organ systems.
- If neurologic signs are present, cerebrospinal fluid collection (spinal tap) and analysis may be recommended.
- Blood tests for serum antibodies to *Coccidioides* may be useful.

TREATMENT AND FOLLOW-UP
Treatment Options
The antifungal drugs, itraconazole and fluconazole, are generally effective. These drugs must be given for prolonged periods (months), and the response to treatment should be regularly evaluated by a veterinarian. Severely affected animals often initially require hospitalization and intensive care, sometimes for 1-2 weeks. Treatment is continued for at least 1 month beyond resolution of all clinical signs. Another drug, amphotericin B, may be given to animals with severe disease. It is not used in many cases because it is potentially toxic to the kidneys and must be given by injection. Some forms are less toxic than others.

Follow-up Care
Blood tests are commonly done before and 2 weeks after beginning treatment, and then monthly during treatment to monitor for possible adverse effects. Other monitoring tests (x-rays, eye examinations, others) are also performed at regular intervals to assess response to treatment. Animals are often re-evaluated at 1, 3, and 6 months after treatment is discontinued to look for evidence of relapse. Notify your veterinarian if any signs return after treatment is stopped.

Prognosis
Prognosis is variable, depending on the extent of disease, severity of clinical signs, and initial response to treatment. Prognosis is best in animals with less severe involvement and clinical signs limited to one organ system. Prognosis is guarded (uncertain) to poor in animals with widespread disease, central nervous system infection, or very severe involvement of any organ system.

Strict adherence to treatment protocols is needed for the best response. Treatment of systemic fungal infections requires a commitment to months of medication and follow-up evaluations with your veterinarian. Relapses occur, and follow-up visits (after treatment is completed) are important to help recognize signs of possible relapse.

SPECIAL INSTRUCTIONS:

Coccidiosis, Enteric

Lynn F. Guptill, DVM, PhD, DACVIM (Small Animal)

BASIC INFORMATION

Description

Enteric coccidiosis is a worldwide intestinal disease that causes diarrhea in dogs and cats.

Causes

Several species of microscopic, single-celled, protozoan parasites cause enteric coccidiosis. The most common one to infect dogs and cats is *Isospora* (*Cystoisospora*). All enteric coccidia are spread by the fecal-oral route, which means that the organisms are commonly swallowed in water or food contaminated with feces. Some infections may occur by eating tissues from infected animals. Most coccidial organisms are hardy and can persist in the environment.

Clinical Signs

Some infections cause no clinical signs, and the animal may be a silent carrier. In other animals, diarrhea (sometimes bloody), weight loss, and dehydration occur. Diarrhea is more likely in young and immune-suppressed animals.

Diagnostic Tests

Microscopic examination of feces usually reveals the organism in infected animals. Because the organisms may be shed intermittently, examination of more than one fecal sample may be necessary.

TREATMENT AND FOLLOW-UP

Treatment Options

Treatment with sulfadimethoxine is the most common therapy used in dogs and cats. Other sulfa drugs may also be effective. Supportive care, such as fluid therapy for dehydration, may also be necessary.

Follow-up Care

To prevent and control the spread of intestinal coccidiosis, overcrowding of animals must be avoided, and good hygiene should be maintained. Organisms are resistant to most disinfectants but can be killed by steam. Some commercial formulations of ammonia are effective, but they should be used only by trained, experienced people using appropriate personal protective equipment.

Removal of all organic material (dirt, feces) is important in preventing infection. Bathing affected animals during treatment helps remove fecal material containing infectious organisms. In certain kennel and cattery situations, treatment may be recommended for all animals in contact with the infected animal.

Prognosis

Prognosis for infected dogs and cats is generally good, because most respond well to therapy and recover quickly from the disease.

SPECIAL INSTRUCTIONS:

Cryptococcosis

Anisa D. Dunham, AS, RVT
Lynn F. Guptill, DVM, PhD, DACVIM (Small Animal)

BASIC INFORMATION

Description

Cryptococcosis is a systemic (present throughout the body) fungal infection that occurs worldwide. It usually originates in the nasal cavity, in tissues alongside the nose, or in the lungs. It may spread to the skin, eyes, or central nervous system (CNS) (brain and spinal cord). Cats are affected most often.

Causes

The most common causes are *Cryptococcus neoformans* and *Cryptococcus gattii*. *C. neoformans* is often associated with pigeon droppings, bird habitats, or roosts, such as barn lofts, hay mows, statues, and certain buildings.

Pigeons are considered to be an important vector (agent that spreads the disease from one host to another) of *C. neoformans*. Unlike other systemic fungal infections, it is not confined by any geographic boundaries. The organism may survive in the environment for years. *C. neoformans* may be found in nasal washes of dogs and cats as an incidental finding; it may or may not progress to clinical disease.

C. gattii is a more geographically restricted organism. It is associated most commonly with the bark and leaf litter of certain eucalyptus trees found in tropical and subtropical environments, and in the Pacific Northwest. It is inactivated by direct exposure to sunlight.

Cryptococcosis is not spread from animal to animal; rather, the infection usually occurs via inhalation of the organisms from the environment. Most of the yeast organisms are too large to be inhaled directly into the lungs, so they often stop in the nasal passages. The small dried forms of the organism can be inhaled directly into the lungs. After the organism is inhaled, it may spread to nearby tissues by direct extension or to other locations via the blood.

Clinical Signs

Lethargy and loss of appetite are common. Fever is uncommon. Upper respiratory signs (sneezing and nasal discharge) are seen in most affected cats. Soft tissue masses or ulcerated lesions may occur in the nasal passage, the bridge of the nose, or in the mouth. Nodules may be seen if the skin or underlying tissues are affected, including the footpad and nail beds.

Behavioral changes, mental dullness, seizures, circling, neck pain, paresis (partial paralysis or impaired movement), and ataxia (lack of coordinated muscle movements) are seen if the CNS is involved. Lameness, blindness, kidney failure, and enlarged lymph nodes may also occur. Most animals with CNS involvement also have the disease in other organs.

Diagnostic Tests

Diagnosis of cryptococcosis can be made on the basis of several laboratory tests:

- A complete blood cell count is often normal, but a mild anemia may be seen. The serum biochemistry profile is usually normal.
- Chest x-rays are usually normal but may show abnormal lung patterns or fluid in the chest.
- The organism can often be identified microscopically in nasal swabs, discharge from skin lesions, or samples taken from soft tissue masses.
- Bronchoscopy (examination of the airways of the lungs using a fiberoptic viewing scope) or rhinoscopy (examination of the nasal passages) may be needed to confirm the diagnosis.
- Fungal culture can also be done.
- Special imaging, such as computed tomography (CT scan) or magnetic resonance imaging (MRI) of the skull or CNS and collection of cerebrospinal fluid (spinal tap) may be recommended.
- A test for cryptococcal antigens (proteins of the organism) in the blood or cerebrospinal fluid is very reliable and is used for diagnosis and to monitor response to treatment.

TREATMENT AND FOLLOW-UP

Treatment Options

Antifungal drugs, such as fluconazole, itraconazole, or amphotericin B, are effective treatments. Fluconazole may be the preferred treatment for CNS disease. Amphotericin B is very effective; however, it is expensive, is usually administered intravenously, and can be toxic to the kidneys. Large lesions may be reduced in size with surgery before medical therapy is started. Treatment is needed for many months and is continued for 1 month after resolution of all clinical signs.

Follow-up Care

Physical and eye examinations are usually performed monthly and include a serum biochemistry profile to check for liver abnormalities that may be caused by the medications. It may be useful to repeat the antigen test to monitor treatment response. Animals are commonly re-examined 3-6 months after treatment is discontinued to check for relapses.

Prognosis

Prognosis depends on the extent of disease. Animals with primarily skin involvement have the best prognosis. Cats with feline leukemia virus or feline immunodeficiency virus infection may require longer therapy. Prognosis is guarded (uncertain) for animals with CNS involvement or severe systemic illness.

SPECIAL INSTRUCTIONS:

Cryptosporidiosis

Lynn F. Guptill, DVM, PhD, DACVIM (Small Animal)

BASIC INFORMATION

Description

Cryptosporidiosis is an intestinal disease that causes diarrhea in many species, including dogs, cats, farm animals, and humans.

Causes

Cryptosporidium species are microscopic, single-celled, protozoan parasites that are found all over the world. Several distinct species exist, and those that infect dogs and cats do not seem to commonly infect humans.

Cryptosporidiosis is spread by the fecal-oral route, which means the organism is often swallowed in food or water contaminated by feces. The organism is very hardy and persists in the environment for prolonged periods.

Clinical Signs

Many infections in dogs and cats cause no clinical signs or only a mild, self-limited (short-lived) diarrhea. Diarrhea, when it occurs, is characterized by a high volume of semiformed to liquid feces and normal frequency of defecation. Weight loss may be seen in animals with persistent diarrhea. Diarrhea is more likely in young and immune-suppressed animals.

Diagnostic Tests

Diagnosis can be made using a number of different methods, such as the following:

- Microscopic examination of fresh feces may reveal the organism. Routine methods of fecal examination are not sensitive enough to detect *Cryptosporidium.* and special techniques are often needed to identify the organisms. It is often recommended that fecal samples be sent to an outside laboratory that is capable of making the diagnosis.
- Tests that detect antigens (proteins of the organism) in the feces of affected animals may be useful.
- Parasite DNA may also be detected in feces by polymerase chain reaction (PCR) testing, but this assay is not always available.
- Organisms may be seen on microscopic examination of intestinal biopsy samples.

TREATMENT AND FOLLOW-UP

Treatment Options

Because the diarrhea often resolves on its own in healthy animals, treatment may not be necessary. Few medications are proven to be effective for cryptosporidiosis in dogs and cats, but drugs, such as azithromycin and nitazoxanide, may be tried. Tylosin has been used for treating infected cats.

Follow-up Care

To prevent and control the spread of *Cryptosporidium,* avoid overcrowding of animals and maintain good hygiene. *Cryptosporidium* is resistant to most disinfectants. It can be killed by steam. Some commercial formulations of ammonia are effective, but they should be used only by trained, experienced people using appropriate personal protective equipment. Removal of all organic material (dirt, feces) is important in preventing infection.

Cryptosporidium can infect humans. Immune-compromised individuals are at a much higher risk for infection. Immune-compromised people should avoid handling infected animals, their feces, or articles contaminated by infected feces.

Prognosis

Prognosis for infected dogs and cats is generally good. Most animals recover from the infection. No vaccination is currently available for this disease.

SPECIAL INSTRUCTIONS:

Cytauxzoonosis

Anisa D. Dunham, AS, RVT
Lynn F. Guptill, DVM, PhD, DACVIM (Small Animal)

BASIC INFORMATION

Description

Cytauxzoonosis is a tick-borne blood disease of cats that occurs in central, south central, and southeastern states in the United States. It is also found in many locations worldwide. Infection of domestic cats often results in a rapidly progressive, fatal disease. Bobcats are believed to be the reservoir host for the parasite. Affected bobcats may have long-term, usually asymptomatic infections.

Causes

Cytauxzoon felis, a protozoan (one-celled) parasite, causes cytauxzoonosis. Ticks transmit the infection in nature. Cats usually become ill 2-3 weeks after exposure to infected ticks. Most infections are seen between March and September.

🗋 Clinical Signs

Affected cats initially have nonspecific signs, such as decreased appetite and lethargy. A rapid course of severe illness and death follows, usually in fewer than 5 days. Difficulty breathing, dark urine, dehydration, anemia, jaundice (yellow color to the skin and membranes of the eyes and mouth), and fever may occur. Low body temperature and coma may develop shortly before death.

🔬 Diagnostic Tests

Diagnosis is complicated by the fact that infected cats deteriorate so rapidly and may die before any testing can be performed. Early in the clinical course, diagnosis can be made by utilizing laboratory tests, such as the following:

- A complete blood cell count usually shows anemia. A very low white blood cell count, a low platelet count, or both occur later in the course of the disease.
- A blood biochemistry profile shows high total bilirubin, and a urinalysis shows bilirubin in the urine, both of which are related to the jaundice produced by the disease.
- Definitive diagnosis can be made by finding the parasite in red blood cells on blood smears.

- Parasites may also be found in aspirates of lymph nodes (glands), spleen, liver, or bone marrow.
- Polymerase chain reaction tests are used to detect parasite DNA in blood or tissues of ill cats and can be performed at some specialized laboratories. However, results may not be reported for several days.

Other tests may be recommended to rule out other diseases that cause similar signs. Such tests include chest and abdominal x-rays, an abdominal ultrasound, and tests for other parasites. A necropsy (similar to an autopsy in people) can confirm the diagnosis after death of the animal.

TREATMENT AND FOLLOW-UP

℞ Treatment Options

Treatment is often unsuccessful. Domestic cats appear to be highly susceptible to this organism. Drugs used for treatment include a combination of atovaquone and azithromycin (currently believed most effective) or imidocarb (alone). Supportive care is of utmost importance. Intravenous fluids, treatment for bleeding disorders, and blood transfusions are often necessary.

🐾 Follow-up Care

If the cat survives, blood smears are usually monitored regularly to check for the parasite. Other tests may also be repeated to monitor response to treatment. A program of strict tick control and keeping cats indoors may help prevent cytauxzoonosis. Most cases of cytauxzoonosis have involved cats that roamed freely in wooded, tick-infested areas. The disease appears to be increasing in incidence in many areas of the southeastern United States where bobcat populations have rebounded in recent years.

Prognosis

Prognosis is poor in most cases. Recently, an increasing number of cats have survived natural infections, perhaps due to early recognition and treatment of the disease. In many cases; however, the death rate is high even with treatment using the most effective drugs.

SPECIAL INSTRUCTIONS:

Ehrlichiosis and Anaplasmosis in Dogs

Lynn F. Guptill, DVM, PhD, DACVIM (Small Animal)

BASIC INFORMATION

Description

Ehrlichiosis and anaplasmosis are systemic diseases caused by rickettsial bacteria that are transmitted by ticks.

Causes

Ehrlichiosis may be caused by *Ehrlichia canis, Ehrlichia chaffeensis,* or *Ehrlichia ewingii.* Anaplasmosis may be caused by *Anaplasma phagocytophilum* or *Anaplasma platys.* The clinical manifestations of infection with these agents have many similarities, so they are discussed here as a group. It is important to consider that any animal bitten by a tick may develop clinical signs as a result of infection with one or more of these rickettsia. Many animals are bitten by more than one tick, and ticks may carry more than one infectious agent.

Clinical Signs

Acute (recent) infection with any of these agents may cause clinical signs. However, some rickettsia cause chronic, asymptomatic infections, with clinical signs developing months to years after the original infection.

Clinical signs vary widely, depending on whether the animal was recently infected or has a chronic infection. Many organ systems may be affected. A list of potential signs follows:

- Fever, lethargy, decreased appetite, and possible weight loss
- Enlarged lymph nodes and spleen, as well as areas of bruising or bleeding under the skin, in the mouth, or from the nose
- Inflammation and hemorrhages within the eye, retinal detachments, vision abnormalities
- Joint and muscle pain, joint swelling, lameness (possibly shifting from leg to leg)
- Central nervous system signs, such as seizures, neck pain, uncoordinated movement (ataxia), head tilt, falling, and others
- Increased thirst and urination that may indicate kidney disease

Diagnostic Tests

Diagnosis often involves comprehensive laboratory testing and other diagnostic procedures:

- A complete blood cell count may show low numbers of platelets, certain white blood cells, and red blood cells (anemia).
- A biochemistry profile may show abnormally high protein levels, elevated liver tests, and evidence of decreased kidney function.
- X-rays of the abdomen and chest, as well as an abdominal ultrasound, may be recommended, depending on the signs.
- Computed tomography (CT scan) or magnetic resonance imaging (MRI) and a spinal tap for collection of cerebrospinal fluid may be considered when neurologic signs are present.

- X-rays of affected joints and joint taps to collect fluid for analysis are commonly done when joints are swollen and inflamed.
- Two blood tests for antibodies to *Ehrlichia* and *Anaplasma* species are commonly done 2-3 weeks apart to determine whether the antibody levels are increasing. Several different tests may be requested for the various species that could be involved.

TREATMENT AND FOLLOW-UP

Treatment Options

Doxycycline antibiotic is often administered for at least 4 weeks. Other tetracycline-type antibiotics (oxytetracycline, tetracycline) may also be considered. Because these drugs can cause gastrointestinal tract upset (decreased appetite, vomiting, diarrhea), they are often given with food.

If doxycycline does not appear to be effective, treatment with imidocarb dipropionate may be recommended. Other appropriate treatments are often needed, depending on the clinical signs. Nonsteroidal anti-inflammatory drugs (NSAIDs) may be given for arthritis. (See also the handout on **Immune-Mediated Arthritis.**) Steroid drugs are sometimes recommended but must be used with caution. Steroids should not be used with NSAIDs, because the combination can cause severe gastrointestinal damage, such as bleeding ulcers and intestinal perforation.

Follow-up Care

Improvement of clinical signs often occurs within 48-72 hours of starting antibiotic therapy. Follow-up examinations and repeated laboratory tests are commonly used to monitor response to treatment and may be continued for 4 weeks after completion of the antibiotics. The frequency of visits depends on the severity and clinical manifestations of the disease. A good tick control program must be instituted for all infected animals.

Prognosis

Prognosis is generally good for animals that do not have severe disease. Prognosis is guarded (uncertain) for animals that are seriously ill, especially those with severe central nervous system signs, anemia, or kidney disease.

Public Health Information

Ehrlichiosis and anaplasmosis are considered zoonotic; that is, they can be transmitted from animals to humans. Transmission does not occur directly from animals to people but takes place through a vector (intermediate host), such as a tick. If an animal is suspected of having ehrlichiosis or anaplasmosis, people in contact with the animal should take precautions to prevent tick bites.

SPECIAL INSTRUCTIONS:

Feline Coronavirus

Anisa D. Dunham, AS, RVT
Lynn F. Guptill, DVM, PhD, DACVIM (Small Animal)

BASIC INFORMATION

Description

Feline coronavirus (FCoV) is a highly contagious intestinal (enteric) infection that causes few problems in most infected cats. In some cats, however, the intestinal form of FCoV mutates and gives rise to feline infectious peritonitis (FIP), a disease that is generally fatal. Two forms of FIP may occur, effusive (wet) and noneffusive (dry).

Causes

Enteric FCoV is highly contagious via fecal-oral transmission, which means that the virus is swallowed in contaminated materials. Most infected cats intermittently shed the virus. Eventually many cats stop shedding the virus, although persistent shedding occurs in some. Interestingly, lifelong shedders do not usually develop FIP, and the FIP virus is rarely shed in feces. Even though FCoV is inactivated by most disinfectants, it may remain in the environment.

Clinical Signs

Enteric FCoV may cause no signs or only mild diarrhea. FIP tends to affect cats younger than 2 years of age and elderly cats. Signs of the wet form of FIP include fever, pale gums (anemia), jaundice (yellow discoloration of the skin and whites of the eyes), difficulty breathing, and a distended abdomen. With the dry form of FIP, signs reflect the organ system that is affected. Neurologic signs (such as seizures), eye inflammation (uveitis), and difficulty breathing may be seen. Fever and weight loss are also common with the dry form.

Diagnostic Tests

Because there is no single, definitive laboratory test for FIP, a number of tests are commonly performed to look for evidence of the disease. Abnormalities may include the following:
- A complete blood cell count may show anemia.
- A blood biochemistry profile may show increased blood proteins, as well as abnormal liver and kidney tests. A protein electrophoresis test may be recommended to determine what blood proteins are elevated.
- X-rays may show fluid in the chest or abdomen, especially with the wet form of FIP. X-rays and an abdominal ultrasound may show other abnormalities in the lungs and abdominal organs.
- Microscopic analysis of fluid removed from the chest or abdomen can support the diagnosis of FIP.
- Further tests (fecal examination, urinalysis, others) may be recommended to rule out other diseases that cause similar signs.

Tests for antibodies in the blood can indicate exposure to FCoV, but they are not diagnostic for FIP because they do not distinguish enteric FCoV from FIP. Antibody titers also do not indicate whether fecal shedding of the virus is present. Newer tests are being developed that evaluate cells from abdominal or chest fluid, but they still may not provide a definitive diagnosis.

Histopathologic evaluation of tissue samples is currently the best method to diagnose FIP. A definitive diagnosis of intestinal FCoV may be accomplished via electron microscopy or polymerase chain reaction (PCR) testing of feces.

TREATMENT AND FOLLOW-UP

Treatment Options

Since enteric FCoV often causes few signs or only mild, short-lived diarrhea, specific therapy is often not necessary. No known treatment reduces the chance that FCoV-infected cats will develop FIP.

Treatment for FIP is often unsuccessful, and the disease is usually fatal. Supportive care with nutritional supplementation, removal of chest and abdominal fluid, intravenous fluid therapy, blood transfusions, and antibiotics for secondary infections may help prolong and improve the quality of the cat's life. Suppressing or altering the immune system with steroids and other drugs may benefit a small number of cats. Although various treatments have been recommended for FIP, little scientific evidence exists regarding their benefit. Cats with FIP should be isolated from other cats.

Follow-up Care

Animals with FIP require periodic monitoring for progression of the disease. When catteries or multicat households are exposed to FIP, exposure to feces must be avoided and all equipment and cages must be disinfected. Isolate any cats that are potential or identified shedders of the virus. Keep all cats indoors, and remove kittens from antibody-positive queens (mothers) at 5-6 weeks of age.

An intranasal vaccine is available that appears to be safe, but its effectiveness is not well documented. Vaccination of low-risk cats, such as adults or cats in single-cat households, is not usually done. Kittens that are at risk (exposed to multiple cats or infected adult cats) may benefit from vaccination. Vaccination is not recommended for routine use and does not prevent mutation of FCoV in an already infected cat.

Prognosis

Prognosis for the intestinal form of FCoV is good. Cats with FIP have a grave long-term prognosis, because the disease is usually fatal.

SPECIAL INSTRUCTIONS:

Feline Immunodeficiency Virus

Lynn F. Guptill, DVM, PhD, DACVIM (Small Animal)

BASIC INFORMATION
Description
Feline immunodeficiency virus (FIV) can cause a permanent infection that eventually leads to diminished function of the immune system and various associated clinical conditions.
Cause
The virus can infect any cat. It is spread by close contact (most often via bite wounds) and from mother to kittens across the placenta. It may also be spread by blood transfusions or by equipment that is contaminated with infected blood or other body fluids. The virus is shed in most body fluids.

The virus is susceptible to drying, sunlight, disinfectants, and detergents, and it does not survive well in the environment. It can sometimes persist long enough in shared food and water bowls, litter boxes, and on other items to be transmitted to other cats.

Clinical Signs
Signs are quite variable. Fever, enlarged lymph nodes (glands), and lethargy may occur soon after infection, but may be so mild that they are not noticed. Cats then enter a prolonged asymptomatic phase of infection that may last from months to years. The final phase of infection occurs when cats are severely immune deficient, and during this phase secondary infections and other conditions may be seen.

Signs that may occur include intermittent fever, lethargy, and infections of the mouth (gingivitis and stomatitis). Neurologic signs, such as a wobbly gait (ataxia), altered mental awareness, and seizures (rare) may be seen. Inflammation in the eyes (uveitis) and various cancers may develop. When a sick cat is diagnosed with FIV infection, it may be difficult to determine whether the presenting problem is caused by FIV or by some other disease.

Diagnostic Tests
Because cats can be asymptomatic shedders of virus and transmit the infection to other cats, it is commonly recommended that cats be tested for FIV at some point in their lives. Testing may occur when cats are acquired as a new pet; when they are exposed to an infected cat; when they are potentially exposed after escaping from the house or being allowed to roam outside; or when they are ill. Testing is also done prior to vaccination against FIV.

Routine laboratory tests and x-rays are often recommended to investigate the clinical signs. Further testing depends on what organ systems are involved. Any results or signs that indicate an abnormal immune system may prompt testing for FIV and feline leukemia virus.

Diagnosis of FIV infection is commonly made from a blood test that is available in most veterinary clinics. Initial FIV test results may be verified in some cases by tests that are done at outside laboratories. For example, your veterinarian may recommend verifying positive test results. Verification is done not only by performing more than one type of test but also by testing the cat at different times.

TREATMENT AND FOLLOW-UP
Treatment Options
No treatment is proven to eliminate FIV infection. Some antiviral drugs and immune-modulating drugs have been tried, but no treatment is curative. Healthy FIV-positive cats do not require any specific treatment. Cats that are FIV-positive and have clinical signs are treated with appropriate medications and supportive care for those signs.

Follow-up Care
Cats with FIV infection should be kept indoors and isolated from noninfected cats. Infected cats should not be bred, because the virus may be transmitted to the unborn kittens. The American Association of Feline Practitioners recommends that healthy FIV-infected cats visit a veterinarian at least twice a year for a complete physical examination and that a complete blood count, biochemistry panel, and urinalysis be done at least once a year.

FIV-positive cats do not benefit from vaccination for FIV; however, they may receive other routine feline vaccinations (for feline rhinotracheitis, calicivirus, and panleukopenia virus, as well as rabies) as long as they remain healthy. Vaccination for FIV is not currently recommended routinely for all cats, because it does not provide 100% protection and may be unnecessary in cats that are not allowed outside.
Prognosis
Cats with FIV infection may have a normal, healthy life for many years. In the later stages of infection (when the cat is immune-compromised and has a variety of secondary conditions), prognosis is guarded (uncertain) to poor. Euthanasia is not usually recommended based on a positive FIV test alone.

SPECIAL INSTRUCTIONS:

Feline Leukemia Virus

Lynn F. Guptill, DVM, PhD, DACVIM (Small Animal)

BASIC INFORMATION

Description

Feline leukemia virus (FeLV) can cause a permanent infection that eventually leads to suppression of the immune system, various bone marrow disorders (such as anemia or leukemia), or cancer.

Cause

The virus can infect any cat. It is spread by close contact and from mother to kittens across the placenta and through the milk. It may also be spread by blood transfusions or equipment that is contaminated with infected blood or other body fluids. It is shed in saliva, tears, urine, feces, and milk.

The virus is susceptible to drying, sunlight, disinfectants, and detergents, and it does not survive well in the environment. However, it may persist long enough in shared food and water bowls, litter boxes, and other items to be transmitted to other cats.

Clinical Signs

Some infected cats have no clinical signs. When a sick cat is diagnosed with FeLV infection, it may be difficult to determine whether the presenting problem is caused by FeLV or some other disease.

Fever, lethargy, enlarged lymph nodes (glands), and weakness from anemia may occur. Some infected cats develop cancer, usually of the lymph nodes or bone marrow. Signs of gastrointestinal disease, such as weight loss or diarrhea, occur in some cats. Infected cats are often more susceptible to infections with other viruses and bacteria, and they may show signs of multiple infections (skin lesions, coughing, vomiting, diarrhea, others). Pregnancy failure and delivery of weak kittens may also occur.

Diagnostic Tests

Because cats can be asymptomatic shedders of FeLV and transmit the infection to other cats, it is commonly recommended that cats be tested for FeLV at some point in their lives. Testing may occur when cats are acquired as a new pet; when they are exposed to an infected cat; when they are potentially exposed after escaping from the house or being allowed to roam outside; or when they are ill. Testing is also done prior to vaccination against FeLV.

Routine laboratory tests and x-rays are often recommended to investigate the clinical signs. Further testing may include aspiration of enlarged lymph nodes and the bone marrow, especially if anemia, leukemia, low white blood cell counts or low platelet counts are found. Any results or signs that indicate an abnormal immune system may prompt testing for FeLV and feline immunodeficiency virus.

Diagnosis of FeLV infection is commonly made from a blood test that is available in most veterinary clinics. Initial FeLV test results may be verified in some cases by tests that are done at outside laboratories. For example, your veterinarian may recommend verifying positive test results. Verification is done not only by performing more than one type of test but also by testing the cat at different times.

TREATMENT AND FOLLOW-UP

Treatment Options

Some cats appear to spontaneously clear the infection or to reduce the number of virus particles to such a low level that many FeLV tests are negative and the cat remains healthy.

No treatment is proven to eliminate FeLV infection. Some antiviral drugs and immune-modulating drugs have been tried, but no treatment is curative. Healthy FeLV-positive cats do not require any specific treatment. Cats that are FeLV-positive and have clinical signs are treated with appropriate medications and supportive care for those signs.

Follow-up Care

Cats with FeLV infection should be kept indoors and isolated from noninfected cats. Infected cats should not be bred, because the virus may be transmitted to the unborn kittens. The American Association of Feline Practitioners recommends that healthy FeLV-infected cats visit a veterinarian at least twice a year for a physical examination and a complete blood count, and that a serum biochemistry panel and urinalysis be done at least once a year.

FeLV-positive cats do not benefit from vaccination for FeLV; however, they may receive other routine feline vaccinations (for feline rhinotracheitis, calicivirus, and panleukopenia virus, as well as rabies) as long as they remain healthy. FeLV vaccinations are not routinely recommended for low-risk cats, such as indoor cats, cats in a single-cat household, and cats in a household where all cats have tested negative. Vaccination may be considered for high-risk cats, so discuss this option with your veterinarian.

Prognosis

Adult cats with FeLV infection may live a normal, healthy life for many years. Cats that are infected as kittens or are ill at the time of diagnosis have a guarded (uncertain) to poor prognosis. Euthanasia is not usually recommended based on a positive FeLV test alone.

SPECIAL INSTRUCTIONS:

Feline Upper Respiratory Infection

Anisa D. Dunham, AS, RVT
Lynn F. Guptill, DVM, PhD, DACVIM (Small Animal)

BASIC INFORMATION

Description

Feline upper respiratory infection (URI) complex is a highly contagious infection with one or more viruses and bacteria.

Causes

The most commonly involved agents are feline herpesvirus 1 (FHV-1 or feline rhinotracheitis), feline calicivirus (FCV), and the bacteria, *Bordetella bronchiseptica, Chlamydophila felis,* and *Mycoplasma* species.

URI may develop from a single agent, or it may be a mixed infection. Mixed infections often begin with FHV-1 or FCV infection. Direct contact with infected secretions is the most common way that URI is spread from cat to cat. FCV is easily transmitted via fomites (inanimate objects). In some cats, acute disease is followed by a period of latency (dormancy). Cats infected with FHV-1, FCV, *B. bronchiseptica,* or *C. felis* often become long-term carriers and intermittently show clinical signs (often after some stressful event).

Clinical Signs

The most common signs are nose and eye discharge, conjunctivitis, lethargy, and decreased appetite. Sneezing and fever may also occur. FHV-1 infection may cause salivation and various eye diseases. FCV infection may cause oral ulcers, but sneezing is usually less common. Severe conjunctivitis may be the only sign with *C. felis* infection. *B. bronchiseptica* and rhinotracheitis may cause coughing.

Pneumonia and other generalized signs can occur with complicated infections. Unvaccinated and young cats are most susceptible to complications, such as secondary bacterial infections. Secondary bacterial infections or *B. bronchiseptica* may lead to bronchopneumonia. Lameness may develop with FCV and mycoplasmal infections.

A particular strain of FCV can cause severe illness, with a high death rate. Although this strain is uncommon, it spreads quickly throughout a facility and affects both vaccinated and unvaccinated cats.

Severe URI, especially in young cats, can cause permanent damage to the nasal passages. Affected cats have lifelong upper respiratory problems, such as nasal congestion, conjunctivitis, and bacterial infections of the nose and sinuses.

Diagnostic Tests

A tentative diagnosis is often made from the clinical signs and history, especially if the cat has recently been exposed to other cats or stressed. In mildly affected cats, no other testing may be pursued.

In cats with more severe disease, routine laboratory tests may be recommended, and chest x-rays may be done if pneumonia is suspected. Conjunctival scrapings, oral swabs, and samples from the trachea may be submitted to identify the organism involved.

Skull x-rays, computed tomography (CT scan), or magnetic resonance imaging (MRI) may be needed in cats with chronic nasal disease. Rhinoscopy (examination of the nose with a fiberoptic viewing scope) may also be considered.

TREATMENT AND FOLLOW-UP

Treatment Options

Treatment of uncomplicated URI is mainly supportive. To encourage eating, warm the food or offer strong-smelling foods, such as tuna. If the cat refuses to eat, force-feeding or insertion of a feeding tube may be considered. Humidifying the environment can loosen respiratory secretions and improve breathing. Fluid therapy may also be helpful. Antibiotics, such as amoxicillin or doxycycline, may be given for bacterial infections. Cleansing of the eyes and application of topical medications is commonly needed. Oral lysine may be given if FHV-1 infection is suspected.

Cats with pneumonia may require hospitalization, intravenous fluids, antibiotics, and supplemental oxygen. Inhalation therapy with saline, a bronchodilator drug, and/or antibiotics may also be recommended.

Follow-up Care

It is important to prevent the spread of this disease to other cats by taking the following steps:
- Isolate clinically ill cats.
- Keep recovered cats away from unvaccinated or immune-compromised cats.
- Most of the agents that cause URI are inactivated by bleach. Disinfect all contaminated cages, bowls, brushes, litter boxes, equipment, and other items with a solution of bleach diluted in water (1:32).
- It is sometimes necessary to close facilities that house cats when outbreaks of feline URI occur, particularly with FCV.

Vaccines are available for FHV-1 and FCV, and they are routinely recommended for all cats. Vaccines do not prevent all infections, but they decrease the severity of the disease. Vaccination for *B. bronchiseptica* may also be recommended for some cats.

It is possible for *C. felis* and *B. bronchiseptica* to be transmitted from cats to immune-compromised people, so preventive measures should be taken when caring for an infected animal.

Prognosis

For most cats, prognosis is very good. URI can be life-threatening, however, in kittens, older cats, nursing mothers and their kittens, and any cat whose immune system is already compromised by other illnesses. For cats with pneumonia, prognosis depends on the severity of the pneumonia and the presence of other diseases and complications.

SPECIAL INSTRUCTIONS:

Giardiasis

Anisa D. Dunham, AS, RVT
Lynn F. Guptill, DVM, PhD, DACVIM (Small Animal)

BASIC INFORMATION

Description

Giardiasis is an acute or chronic gastrointestinal (GI) tract disease. It is characterized by diarrhea and weight loss in both dogs and cats.

Causes

Giardiasis is caused by the one-celled, protozoan parasite *Giardia duodenalis*. At least seven genetic groups (called *assemblages*) of *Giardia* may infect dogs and cats. Some of these genetic groups can also infect humans, whereas others infect only dogs and cats.

Giardia is found throughout the world. Transmission is via the fecal-oral route, which means that the cyst form of the parasite is swallowed in food and water contaminated with feces. Cysts enter the small intestines, where they mature into trophozoites (the active feeding stage of the parasite). Both cysts and trophozoites are passed in the feces.

Clinical Signs

Most animals infected with *Giardia* are asymptomatic. When signs are present, the most common one is an acute, self-limited, small-bowel diarrhea that results in the passage of large volumes of watery feces. Intermittent or chronic diarrhea, weight loss, decreased appetite, and vomiting occur less often. Rarely, acute or chronic large-bowel diarrhea may develop, with increased frequency and straining to defecate and the presence of mucus and red blood in the feces.

Diagnostic Tests

Routine laboratory (blood, fecal) tests are usually recommended to investigate the clinical signs. *Giardia* cysts and trophozoites can be identified in the feces. Samples are commonly collected for 3-5 days, because the parasite is shed intermittently. Special types of fecal tests (such as zinc sulfate flotation with centrifugation) may be done to improve the chance of finding *Giardia* in the feces. A test for *Giardia* antigens (proteins of the parasite) in the feces can also be done. A combination of these tests may be recommended, and additional specialized tests (assays for parasite DNA, intestinal biopsies, and others) may be done in some circumstances.

TREATMENT AND FOLLOW-UP

Treatment Options

Fenbendazole or a combination of febantel and praziquantel (commonly used deworming agents) may be given to dogs and cats once daily for 5 days. Metronidazole (an antibiotic) may also be used in dogs and cats. Although metronidazole is a safe drug, side effects, such as decreased appetite and vomiting, are possible. Neurologic signs may occur with high doses or prolonged use. Animals with *Giardia* are commonly bathed at the beginning and during treatment to remove any parasites from the fur.

The animal's immune response to *Giardia* plays an important role in clearing the infection. Nutritional status of the animal, presence of other GI diseases, coinfection with multiple intestinal protozoans, and virulence (aggressiveness) of the *Giardia* strain also affect the severity of the disease.

Follow-up Care

Treatment failure and reinfections are common because of repeated exposure to the parasite in contaminated environments. The environment should be completely cleared of fecal material. Feces should also be removed from the environment immediately after each defecation. Wash as many areas as possible after removing all organic material, and disinfect the premises with a solution of bleach diluted in water (1:32).

If the environment cannot be completely cleaned (for example, some outdoor kennels), remove the animal from that environment. If the infection does not resolve with appropriate medication, bathing, and environmental control, then your veterinarian may recommend repeating the medication, administering the medication for a longer period of time, or treating the animal with both metronidazole and fenbendazole.

Some drug-resistant strains of *Giardia* exist, but many treatment failures occur because the steps outlined here are not accomplished. Animals should not be allowed to drink from puddles, lakes, streams, or other sources of stagnant water. It may be advisable to treat other animals in the same household while treating the infected, symptomatic pet.

Prognosis

Prognosis is generally good. Sometimes the organism is difficult to completely eliminate, so good husbandry practices are essential for a successful outcome. Older animals, animals with other illnesses, and those with compromised immune systems have an increased risk of complications.

Public Health Information

Some genetic groups of *Giardia* are known to infect humans, so appropriate measures should be taken to avoid contact with feces and other contaminated items. Wear gloves and wash hands thoroughly after handling infected animals or contaminated items.

SPECIAL INSTRUCTIONS:

Helicobacteriosis

Anisa D. Dunham, AS, RVT
Lynn F. Guptill, DVM, PhD, DACVIM (Small Animal)

BASIC INFORMATION

Description

Helicobacteriosis is a bacterial infection that causes inflammation of the lining of the stomach (gastritis) in people and possibly in dogs and cats. Some species of *Helicobacter* may cause inflammation of the intestines and liver.

Causes

Helicobacteriosis is caused by spiral-shaped *Helicobacter* species. Transmission is via direct fecal-oral or oral-oral routes, which means that the bacteria are swallowed in materials contaminated with feces or via oral secretions from infected animals. The bacteria may also be transmitted by fomites (inanimate objects).

Clinical Signs

It difficult to know how important *Helicobacter* organisms are in the production of clinical signs in dogs and cats, because many healthy, asymptomatic animals have the bacteria in their gastrointestinal (GI) tract. Vomiting, diarrhea, and weight loss may be seen with infections in the stomach and intestines. If the liver is infected, signs of hepatitis (decreased appetite, vomiting, diarrhea) may occur. In some species of animals (such as ferrets), *Helicobacter* infection may be associated with cancer of the GI tract. The bacteria are not known to cause cancer in dogs or cats.

Diagnostic Tests

Routine laboratory tests (blood, urine, fecal), abdominal x-rays, and an abdominal ultrasound may be recommended to investigate the clinical signs and rule out other diseases that cause similar signs. Diagnosis of the presence of *Helicobacter* organisms requires culture and/or microscopic examination of biopsies or brushings of the lining of the GI tract. An indirect test can also be done on stomach biopsies to detect an enzyme that is produced by the bacteria. Culture of the bacteria is difficult. Samples for testing are often obtained via endoscopy (passage of a fiberoptic viewing scope into the stomach and upper small intestine).

TREATMENT AND FOLLOW-UP

℞ Treatment Options

No one treatment has been identified that is best for helicobacteriosis, so many treatment protocols have been published. The most commonly used treatment is the administration of three oral drugs for 14-28 days. These drugs include a GI protective agent, such as bismuth subsalicylate (*Pepto-Bismol*, in dogs only) or an antacid, such famotidine or omeprazole (in both dogs and cats), combined with the antibiotics metronidazole and amoxicillin.

🐾 Follow-up Care

Treated animals can become sick again from reinfection or relapse, especially if treatment only decreased the number of bacteria present. Humans may also be infected with *Helicobacter*, but the strains that infect people have not been proven to be transmitted by animals. Because transmission of *Helicobacter* to people may be possible, however, preventive measures (such as wearing gloves when treating or cleaning up after animals) should be taken when caring for an infected animal.

Prognosis

Prognosis is generally very good, because most signs resolve with treatment.

SPECIAL INSTRUCTIONS:

Hepatozoonosis in Dogs

Lynn F. Guptill, DVM, PhD, DACVIM (Small Animal)

BASIC INFORMATION

Description

Hepatozoonosis is a systemic infection that affects dogs and very rarely affects cats.

Causes

The cause of canine hepatozoonosis in North America is primarily *Hepatozoon americanum,* a one-celled, protozoan parasite. *Hepatozoon canis* occurs more commonly in other areas of the world but only rarely in North America. The species of *Hepatozoon* that cause feline hepatozoonosis has not been identified. *Hepatozoon* infections are reported primarily in the southern and southeastern United States.

The parasite is maintained in wildlife, most likely foxes, in North America. It is transmitted to dogs when they eat infected ticks. The parasite penetrates the walls of the intestines, enters certain blood cells, and then may spread to other tissues, such as muscles, bones, spleen, lymph nodes (glands), bone marrow, liver, heart, kidneys, and lungs.

Clinical Signs

Clinical signs are different for *H. canis* and *H. americanum* infections. With *H. canis* infection, a low parasite burden may cause few or mild clinical signs, including lethargy, fever, and weight loss. Higher parasite burdens result in severe clinical signs from tissue inflammation and anemia.

Most dogs infected with *H. americanum* have discharge from the eyes, fever, severe muscle and/or bone pain (including neck and back pain), stiffness, lameness, lethargy, and weight loss. *H. americanum* infections are often fatal.

Dogs with hepatozoonosis may also have signs from coinfection with other tick-transmitted diseases, such as ehrlichiosis, anaplasmosis, Lyme disease, and bartonellosis.

Diagnostic Tests

Diagnosis of *H. canis* infection is based on clinical signs, history of tick exposure, residence or travel in areas where hepatozoonosis is known to occur, and laboratory results.

- Finding *H. canis* organisms on a blood smear is a common method for diagnosis. Organisms may also be found in biopsies of liver, spleen, kidneys, and lungs or in fluid collected from the lungs.
- Anemia is the most common finding on a complete blood count. High white blood cell counts and low platelet counts are possible, especially with high parasite burdens.
- A biochemistry panel may show abnormally high liver and muscle enzyme activities, low blood sugar, and low albumin protein.

- A blood test for antibodies to *H. canis* is available but is not commonly used.

Diagnosis of *H. americanum* infection is based on similar evidence:

- In contrast to *H. canis* infections, it is rare to find *H. americanum* organisms on a blood smear. Many organisms are often seen in muscles biopsies, however.
- A very high white blood cell count is the most common finding on a blood count. Mild anemia is also common. A high platelet count may occur.
- Low blood protein (albumin) levels are common in infected dogs. Elevated enzyme activities are surprisingly uncommon, despite severe muscle inflammation.
- A blood test for antibodies to *H. americanum* is available.
- X-rays of affected bones often show marked changes.

TREATMENT AND FOLLOW-UP

Treatment Options

Treatment for *H. canis* is imidocarb dipropionate, which is given every 14 days until the organisms are no longer seen on blood smears. The antibiotic, doxycycline, may be given with imidocarb. Dogs that are systemically ill may require hospitalization and supportive care.

Treatment for *H. americanum* usually includes a combination of medications. Trimethoprim-sulfa, clindamycin, pyrimethamine, and decoquinate are commonly given together for 14 days. Decoquinate is then given daily for at least 2 years after resolution of all signs, and it may be required indefinitely. Prolonged treatment is considered necessary to control the organisms that are encased in cysts in the tissues.

Follow-up Care

Relapses are common, and periodic follow-up is needed. Relapses can occur with *H. americanum,* even in dogs receiving decoquinate. Good tick control is important. Animals that are infected with *Hepatozoon* may also be exposed to other diseases transmitted by insect hosts (such as heartworm disease, ehrlichiosis, anaplasmosis, and leishmaniasis), so screening for these diseases may be warranted.

Prognosis

Prognosis for dogs with mild *H. canis* infection is good. Prognosis for dogs with *H. americanum* infection depends on their initial condition at time of diagnosis and their response to treatment. When response to the initial treatment is good and treatment with decoquinate is continued for at least 2 years, prognosis is good. Prognosis is guarded (uncertain) to poor for dogs with severe disease attributed to either *H. canis* or *H. americanum.*

SPECIAL INSTRUCTIONS:

Histoplasmosis

Anisa D. Dunham, AS, RVT
Lynn F. Guptill, DVM, PhD, DACVIM (Small Animal)

BASIC INFORMATION

Description

Histoplasmosis is a fungal infection that can affect the whole body. It usually starts in the lungs or gastrointestinal (GI) tract and then spreads to other organs.

Cause

Histoplasmosis is caused by the fungus *Histoplasma capsulatum*. The fungus can survive in a wide range of moistures and temperatures. Nitrogen-rich soil (especially soil containing bird or bat feces) is ideal for its growth. *H. capsulatum* is widespread in most temperate and subtropical regions of the world. In the United States, it occurs mainly along the Mississippi, Ohio, and Missouri River valleys.

Infection usually occurs via inhalation or ingestion. It may be limited to the lungs, or it may spread to multiple sites in the body. Infection may occur with no clinical signs in a few animals. The lungs, GI tract, lymph nodes (glands), liver, spleen, bone marrow, eyes, and adrenal glands are most commonly affected in dogs. In cats, the lungs, liver, lymph nodes, eyes, and bone marrow are most commonly affected. Outbreaks of the disease are often associated with exposure to areas heavily contaminated with the organism, such as chicken coops, bat habitats, and starling roosts.

📷 Clinical Signs

Clinical signs in cats are usually subtle and nonspecific, such as lethargy, decreased appetite, and weight loss. Difficulty breathing and increased respiratory rate can occur, but coughing is uncommon. Eyelid nodules, redness or cloudiness of the eyes, vision changes, enlarged lymph nodes, and lameness are also possible. Occasionally, the central nervous system (brain and spinal cord) may be involved. Internal organs (liver or spleen) may be affected, causing jaundice (yellowing) or pale mucous membranes (such as the gums) from anemia.

Dogs may also have nonspecific symptoms, similar to cats. Diarrhea, weight loss, and decreased appetite are common. Enlarged lymph nodes, eye inflammation (pain, blinking, squinting, or vision changes), difficulty breathing, and increased respiratory rate (with or without coughing) may occur.

🔬 Diagnostic Tests

Finding the organism in affected tissues is the best diagnostic test. This may require fine-needle aspiration or biopsy of various tissues or collection of fluid from the lungs. Other tests that may be recommended include the following:

- Routine laboratory tests, x-rays of the chest, and x-rays or an ultrasound of the abdomen to assess the function of various organs and rule out diseases that cause similar signs

- Bone x-rays for any lameness
- Bone marrow tests

Some blood tests for histoplasmosis are available, but assays for serum antibodies are often not useful, because false-negative and false-positive results are common. Newer tests for *Histoplasma* antigen in blood and urine are being developed but are not yet validated for cats and dogs.

TREATMENT AND FOLLOW-UP

💊 Treatment Options

Oral antifungal drugs, such as itraconazole and fluconazole, are usually effective. These drugs must be given for prolonged periods (months), and your veterinarian must regularly evaluate your pet's response to treatment. Treatment is continued for at least 1 month after resolution of all clinical signs. Numerous tests (x-rays, eye examinations, others) may be repeated during therapy.

Ketoconazole is less effective and may have more severe side effects. Intravenous amphotericin B may be used in severely affected animals. Several forms of this drug are available, some more toxic to the kidneys than others. With severe GI infections, oral drugs may not be absorbed well, and treatment, at least initially, may be more successful with medications given intravenously. Seriously ill animals generally require hospitalization and intensive treatment and monitoring for the first week or two. Strict adherence to treatment protocols is needed for the best response.

🐾 Follow-up Care

Blood tests are commonly done before and 2 weeks after beginning treatment, and approximately every month during treatment, to monitor for possible adverse effects. Treatment of systemic fungal infections requires commitment to months of medication and follow-up evaluations with your veterinarian. Relapses occur in as many as 20-25% of treated animals, and follow-up visits after treatment are important to help recognize signs of relapse. Animals are often re-evaluated at 1, 3, and 6 months after treatment is discontinued.

Prognosis

Prognosis is variable and depends on the extent of organ involvement, severity of clinical signs, and initial response to treatment. Animals with only mild to moderate respiratory signs often have a good prognosis. Prognosis is better in animals with mild clinical signs limited to one organ system. Prognosis is guarded (uncertain) to poor in animals with widespread disease, brain involvement, or very severe signs.

SPECIAL INSTRUCTIONS:

Leishmaniasis

Lynn F. Guptill, DVM, PhD, DACVIM (Small Animal)

BASIC INFORMATION
Description
Leishmaniasis is a group of systemic (generalized) or skin diseases that affect dogs and, less commonly, cats. Leishmaniasis occurs worldwide but is most common in the Mediterranean basin, the Middle East, and South America. The disease occurs in the United States, especially in foxhounds.

Causes
Several species of the one-celled, protozoan parasite *Leishmania* cause leishmaniasis. The organism is transmitted by sandflies. Dogs are considered an important reservoir of some *Leishmania* species. Other modes of transmission may be possible, because animals with no exposure to sandflies may become infected with *Leishmania*. Such methods of transmission may include direct contact, bite wounds, ingestion, blood transfusion, or transmission from mother to offspring (congenital).

Clinical Signs
Not all infected dogs have clinical signs, and signs vary from mild to severe (including death). The most common findings are skin lesions, enlarged lymph nodes, weight loss, lethargy, lameness, decreased activity, diarrhea, and eye lesions. Common skin lesions include hair loss and scaliness, ulcerations on the nose or ears, and sometimes nodules in the skin. The skin lesions are not usually itchy.

Cats are rarely diagnosed with leishmaniasis. Skin lesions in cats are similar to those reported in dogs. Other clinical signs are rare, although eye lesions and bone marrow, liver, spleen, and lymph node (gland) involvement have been described.

Diagnostic Tests
A number of tests are commonly needed to reach a diagnosis. Tests that may be recommended include the following:
* A complete blood count commonly shows anemia, low platelet count, and either a high or a low white blood cell count.
* A biochemistry panel may reveal abnormal protein levels (high globulins, low albumin) and evidence of decreased kidney function and liver disease.
* Urine analysis may show mild to severe loss of protein in the urine.

* Microscopic examination of aspirates or biopsies of skin lesions, lymph nodes, bone marrow, and other tissues may show *Leishmania* organisms. Special stains may be used on the biopsy samples to help identify the organisms.
* Blood, lymph nodes, skin, and bone marrow may be tested by polymerase chain reaction (PCR) assays for DNA of the organisms.
* Blood tests for antibodies to the organism may also be done.
* Other tests, such as x-rays of the chest and abdomen or an abdominal ultrasound, may also be recommended.

Animals that are infected with *Leishmania* may also be exposed to other diseases transmitted by ticks and other insects (such as heartworm disease, ehrlichiosis, anaplasmosis, and hepatozoonosis), so screening for these diseases may be warranted.

TREATMENT AND FOLLOW-UP

Treatment Options
For dogs, combination therapy is commonly done with antimony-based drugs (such as meglumine antimonate or sodium stibogluconate) plus allopurinol for 3-4 weeks. Then allopurinol is continued for 6 months or indefinitely.

The best treatment for cats is not well defined, although antimonial compounds have been used.

Follow-up Care
During therapy, animals are re-evaluated regularly, with repeated laboratory tests. Once treatment is discontinued, recheck examinations and laboratory testing are done at least every 6 months to check for relapses. Insecticidal collars should be worn by dogs in areas where the disease occurs, to discourage biting by sandflies. Dogs may also be kept inside during the times of day (dusk through dawn) that sandflies are most likely to be out.

Prognosis
Treatment is not considered curative, relapses are common, and extended or indefinite treatment is often needed.

Public Health Information
Leishmaniasis is transmitted to humans by sandflies, and infected dogs can serve as a source of infection for the sandflies. This is one reason why infected dogs should be treated and closely monitored.

SPECIAL INSTRUCTIONS:

Leptospirosis

Anisa D. Dunham, AS, RVT
Lynn F. Guptill, DVM, PhD, DACVIM (Small Animal)

BASIC INFORMATION

Description

Leptospirosis is a zoonotic (transmitted from animals to humans), multiorgan disease of dogs, livestock, and many other animals, as well as people. It occurs only rarely in cats. Various animals serve as reservoirs, including the mouse, rat, raccoon, opossum, and deer.

Causes

Leptospirosis is caused by different types of *Leptospira* bacteria (leptospires). Leptospires are shed in the urine of infected animals and are transmitted by direct or indirect contact. Direct transmission occurs through contact with infected urine; during breeding; from mother to offspring through the placenta; via bite wounds; or by eating infected tissues. Crowding of dogs in kennels can enhance direct transmission. Indirect transmission occurs through exposure to contaminated water, soil, food, or bedding. Disease outbreaks often occur during or immediately after periods of heavy rain or flooding.

Leptospires enter the blood and other tissues, where they reproduce and cause inflammation that damages many parts of the body, such as the kidneys, liver, spleen, central nervous system (brain and spinal cord), eyes, and genital tract.

Clinical Signs

Clinical signs in cats are mild or inapparent. Signs in dogs can be variable, depending on the organs most affected. In very acute (sudden) infections, large numbers of organisms may circulate in the blood, leading to shock and death. More often, fever, shivering, and decreased appetite are the first signs. Vomiting and dehydration follow. The animal may be reluctant to move. Coughing, difficulty breathing, and inflammation of the eyes (redness, pain) may occur. Progressive deterioration in kidney function may result in decreased or no urine production. Jaundice (yellowing of the skin and gums) may arise from liver damage.

Diagnostic Tests

Results from several laboratory tests can be used to diagnose leptospirosis, including the following:

- A complete blood cell count is important to evaluate red and white blood cell and platelet numbers.
- A blood chemistry profile helps to evaluate liver and kidney function and electrolyte values.
- Urine tests are also used to evaluate liver and kidney function.
- The microscopic agglutination test (MAT) for antibodies in the blood can be used to confirm the diagnosis. Antibody tests early in illness are often negative, so follow-up tests 2-3 weeks after the onset of illness must often be done.

- Polymerase chain reaction (PCR) tests may be done to detect *Leptospira* DNA, but they are not available from all laboratories.

TREATMENT AND FOLLOW-UP

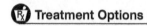 Treatment Options

Severely affected animals need hospitalization and intensive care. Intravenous fluids may be needed to correct dehydration. A urinary catheter may be inserted so that urine output can be accurately measured in animals with decreased or no urine production.

Antibiotics that kill the leptospires are started as soon as possible in order to reduce some of the serious and possibly fatal complications of the disease, such as liver and kidney failure. Penicillin-type antibiotics are often the drugs of choice for initial treatment and are given for 2 weeks. Another antibiotic, doxycycline, may then be started to minimize or eradicate shedding of the bacteria in the urine. It is usually started after penicillin therapy is completed and is usually given for 2-4 weeks. Alternatively, doxycycline may be used for the entire treatment.

During treatment, infected animals should be isolated to prevent accidental contact with other animals. The infection may be transmitted to other pet animals and to humans by contact with infected urine. Gloves are worn when handling bedding and other items that may have been contaminated with urine or when cleaning urine from the environment. Facemasks and goggles may be worn when hosing down contaminated kennels. There is useful information about leptospirosis in pets at the Centers for Disease Control and Prevention website, *www.cdc.gov/ncidod/dbmd/ diseaseinfo/leptospirosis_g_pet.htm*.

Follow-up Care

Intensive monitoring is often needed for hospitalized animals. Following recovery, laboratory tests are usually repeated to evaluate liver and kidney function and, sometimes, antibody levels. It may be necessary to disinfect areas of the animal's environment with diluted bleach. It is very important to remove organic debris (feces, dirt) before disinfecting the area, because the debris can decrease the effectiveness of the disinfectant. Bleach should not be used on grassy areas. Vaccination is available for several *Leptospira* species.

Prognosis

As many as 25% of dogs with very severe leptospirosis do not survive. Most dogs, however, respond well to treatment. Long-term liver or kidney disease may occur, even with appropriate treatment.

SPECIAL INSTRUCTIONS:

Methicillin-Resistant *Staphylococcus* Infections

Lynn F. Guptill, DVM, PhD, DACVIM (Small Animal)

BASIC INFORMATION

Description

Methicillin-resistant *Staphylococcus* (MRS) infections are a growing problem in humans and animals. Methicillin is an antibiotic formerly used to treat staphylococcal infections, and strains resistant to this antibiotic are also commonly resistant to most other antibiotics. A major concern with these infections is the development of strains that will be resistant to all known antibiotics. MRS infections may be localized (wound infections) or become generalized.

Causes

MRS infections are caused by a variety of staphylococcal bacteria. Infections with *Staphylococcus aureus* (MRSA), *Staphylococcus pseudointermedius* (formerly known as *Staphylococcus intermedius*), *Staphylococcus schleiferi* subspecies *coagulans*, and *Staphylococcus epidermidis* are the most common causes in dogs and cats. These organisms may normally live on skin, in the nasal passages, and in the gastrointestinal tract of animals without causing any clinical signs. When a wound occurs, a surgical procedure is performed, or skin is otherwise damaged or inflamed, these bacteria may take advantage of the loss of normal protective barriers and cause an infection.

Most *Staphylococcus* bacteria are susceptible to commonly used disinfectants and hand soaps and are unable to survive for extended periods in the environment in the absence of organic material. Transmission is by direct contact with infected people or animals or via contaminated fomites (inanimate objects).

Clinical Signs

Most MRS infections are associated with wounds, dermatologic conditions (such as pyoderma), ear infections (otitis externa, otitis media), or surgical sites. Infections caused by MRS do not clinically look different from other infections. Most MRS infections produce pus. In humans, MRS infections may resemble spider bites, but this description does not generally apply to infections in animals.

Because animals may carry these bacteria without evidence of infection, it is possible for a wound that is not initially infected with MRS to become infected. Clinical signs may include the following:

- An infected wound with purulent drainage (pus)
- A surgical site that does not heal normally and develops a purulent infection
- Dermatitis or an ear infection that does not improve with standard treatment
- Rarely, coughing or difficulty breathing from pneumonia
- Fever, lethargy, decreased appetite, or other signs of a generalized infection

Diagnostic Tests

Diagnosis of MRS infections may require several tests, such as the following:

- A bacterial culture of the affected area helps prove the presence of staphylococcal bacteria.
- Antibiotic susceptibility testing performed on the culture often shows resistance to multiple or all commonly tested drugs. Further testing may be needed to identify antibiotics to which the bacteria are still sensitive.
- When MRS are detected, special tests may be recommended to type (identify) the bacteria involved. Several well-defined types of MRS exist, and identifying the specific type involved in the infection may help to determine the source of the infection.
- Tests for certain factors or properties that allow MRS bacteria to become more invasive may also be recommended.

TREATMENT AND FOLLOW-UP

Treatment Options

Infected wounds may require only careful local treatment. Topical treatment of infected areas with mupirocin ointment may be recommended.

Most MRS organisms are resistant to all antibiotics in the penicillin and cephalosporin groups, and some are resistant to many other antibiotics. If an antibiotic is needed, the choice is guided by results of culture and antibiotic susceptibility testing.

Follow-up Care

Animals may still harbor these bacteria (remain colonized) after recovering from an MRS infection. Swabbing of the nose or rectum may be done to check for the presence of MRS bacteria. Duration of colonization often depends on the species of MRS. Certain strains of MRSA are believed to subside in approximately 6 weeks without any treatment. Information is not currently available for MRS colonization with *S. pseudointermedius* or other species.

Prognosis

Prognosis is good in most cases when wounds are correctly managed and antibiotic treatment is guided by culture and antibiotic susceptibility testing.

Public Health Information

Most MRSA infections in dogs and cats are believed to be transmitted to animals from humans. All MRS infections may be transmitted between animals and people, so precautions are needed to prevent such transmission. Hand washing and good hygiene practices are the best preventive measures.

SPECIAL INSTRUCTIONS:

Neosporosis in Dogs

Lynn F. Guptill, DVM, PhD, DACVIM (Small Animal)

BASIC INFORMATION

Description

Neosporosis is a worldwide disease of dogs that can cause neurologic signs and muscle inflammation. It also causes reproductive failure in cattle.

Cause

Neosporosis is caused by the microscopic, one-celled, protozoan parasite *Neospora caninum*. It is transmitted via the fecal-oral route by ingestion of (swallowing) contaminated food or water or ingestion of tissue cysts in the muscles of infected animals. Neosporosis can also be transmitted from mother to offspring (congenital transmission), and all puppies in a litter may be affected.

When dogs swallow tissue cysts, the parasites are released and multiply in the gastrointestinal tract. Eggs of the parasites (oocysts) are usually shed in the dog's feces for 1-3 weeks or up to several months. The parasites multiply within intestinal cells and may spread throughout the body. Parasites may enter any tissue and cause illness. Parasitic cysts may form in tissues and remain quiet (dormant) for the life of the animal, or they may become activated and cause illness at a later time.

🔲 Clinical Signs

Signs are believed to develop more often and to be more severe in animals that are young, are immune-suppressed, or have another infection. Weakness, incoordination, and other nervous system problems such as weakness of the neck or difficulty swallowing may be seen. Often the hind legs are severely affected, with loss of muscle mass (atrophy) and limb stiffness. Adult dogs may develop skin lesions or pneumonia.

🔳 Diagnostic Tests

Routine laboratory tests, chest and abdominal x-rays, and an abdominal ultrasound may be recommended to investigate the clinical signs and determine the extent of the disease. Diagnosis may require a combination of several different tests, such as the following:

- Tests for antibodies can be performed on blood samples or on cerebrospinal fluid retrieved by a spinal tap.

- Electromyography (EMG), which is the measurement of electrical activity of muscles, may be recommended and may show numerous abnormalities.
- Microscopic examination of tissue samples, cerebrospinal fluid, and cells obtained from the trachea or lungs can be helpful in identifying the organism and confirming the diagnosis.
- Puppies that have succumbed to the disease may be submitted for necropsy examination (similar to an autopsy in people).

TREATMENT AND FOLLOW-UP

℞ Treatment Options

Clindamycin (an antibiotic) is often the drug of choice for muscle and skin involvement. Trimethoprim-sulfa drugs may also be used, particularly when neurologic disease is present. Additional supportive care in the hospital may be needed. If neosporosis is suspected, treatment is often initiated before results of the diagnostic tests are received.

🐾 Follow-up Care

Signs are often slow to respond to treatment. Complete eradication of tissue cysts is considered unlikely. When possible, treatment of all puppies in a litter should be considered if a diagnosis of neosporosis is made in one littermate.

Transmission of *N. caninum* can be reduced by limiting exposure to oocysts and tissue cysts. Feed dogs only fully cooked foods. Prevent access to livestock when possible. If congenital transmission is suspected, avoid breeding bitches (females) that have had affected litters previously. No treatment is known to prevent transmission from mother to offspring.

Prognosis

Treatment is often unsuccessful or only partially successful. Prognosis depends on how long clinical signs are present and how quickly treatment is instituted. Dogs older than 4 months of age and acutely infected dogs may respond better to treatment than younger puppies or dogs with long-standing clinical signs. Prognosis for animals with widespread systemic disease is guarded (uncertain).

SPECIAL INSTRUCTIONS:

Parvovirus in Cats

Anisa D. Dunham, AS, RVT

BASIC INFORMATION

Description

Feline parvovirus (FPV) causes a disease known as *feline distemper* or *feline panleukopenia*. It is a highly contagious disease of young, unvaccinated cats. A high death rate is associated with the disease.

Cause

FPV is related to the virus that causes canine parvovirus. The virus is shed in all body secretions, but virus present in feces is the primary source of infection. Transmission occurs by contact with infected animals or from contaminated environments or equipment. The virus can also cross the placenta of pregnant animals and infect developing kittens.

The virus infects rapidly growing and dividing cells, such as cells in the lining of the intestines, lymphoid tissues, and bone marrow (especially stems cells that can develop into all blood cell types). FPV occurs most commonly in young kittens between 3 and 6 months of age. Most cats greater than 1 year old are immune because of prior subclinical infection (that produced no clinical signs) or vaccination. Kittens younger than 6-8 weeks of age are often protected by antibodies they received from their mother prior to birth.

Clinical Signs

Adult cats may show no clinical signs. Kittens may die within 12 hours, with few or no signs. More often, fever, depression, lack of appetite, vomiting, and severe dehydration are noted. Diarrhea may occur later and may be bloody.

Infection early in pregnancy may cause fetal resorption (death and dissolution of the embryo) and infertility in apparently healthy queens (mother cats). Infection later in pregnancy may cause abortion of fetuses and stillbirths. A brain abnormality (cerebellar hypoplasia) may occur in kittens exposed to the virus prior to birth. These kittens may have seizures, be uncoordinated, and have poor motor skills.

Diagnostic Tests

Diagnosis of FPV can be made on the basis of several laboratory tests, such as the following:

- Early in the disease, a complete blood cell count shows a severe decrease in the numbers of circulating white blood cells (leukopenia). A decrease in all white blood cell types is called *panleukopenia*; hence, the name for the disease. Anemia and decreased platelets may also be seen.
- A blood biochemistry profile may show evidence of liver inflammation, altered kidney function, and electrolyte imbalances.
- Fecal test kits for canine parvovirus can also detect FPV, but false-positive and false-negative results do occur.
- Dead kittens may be submitted for necropsy examination (similar to an autopsy in people).

Other tests, such as fecal tests, x-rays, and other laboratory assays, may be recommended to rule out other diseases that cause similar signs.

TREATMENT AND FOLLOW-UP

Treatment Options

Treatment consists of supportive care, because no specific antiviral therapy is available for FPV. Fluid therapy is used to correct dehydration. Medications that decrease stomach acid, stop vomiting (antiemetics), and treat secondary bacterial infections (antibiotics) may also be given. Blood transfusions may be needed for severe anemia. Good nursing care is important to prevent urine or fecal scalding on the skin and secondary bacterial infections.

Food is withheld from kittens with vomiting and diarrhea. Once the vomiting has stopped for 12-24 hours, small amounts of water can be offered, and then bland food. After food is well-tolerated, the regular diet can be gradually reintroduced.

Cerebellar hypoplasia is not treatable but usually does not worsen, and uncoordinated kittens may be able to compensate well and lead good-quality lives.

Prevention

The virus is very stable in the environment. It can survive in organic material for months to 1 year at room temperature and for longer periods at lower temperatures. Contaminated surfaces must be washed to remove any organic material and then disinfected. Bleach is a good disinfectant to use for FPV. Materials that may harbor the virus but cannot be washed and disinfected should be discarded.

The virus is highly contagious to all cats. Vaccination is recommended, because clinical disease is rare in vaccinated cats.

Follow-up Care

If the cat recovers, it has lifetime immunity to the disease. The virus can be shed for up to 6 weeks after recovery, so precautions must be taken to protect other cats and the environment.

Prognosis

Infected kittens that survive for longer than 5 days usually recover, but recovery may take several weeks. Older kittens usually have a milder form of the disease and a better prognosis. Kittens with brain involvement often have permanent neurologic abnormalities but may adapt well to living with these disabilities.

SPECIAL INSTRUCTIONS:

Parvovirus in Dogs

Lynn F. Guptill, DVM, PhD, DACVIM (Small Animal)

BASIC INFORMATION
Description
Canine parvovirus (CPV) is very contagious and causes primarily a gastrointestinal (GI) disease. The disease can be prevented by vaccination.
Cause
CPV is highly concentrated in the feces of infected animals. It persists in the environment under a variety of conditions and is resistant to many common disinfectants. CPV is inactivated by sodium hypochlorite (a 1:20 dilution of common household bleach) after 10 minutes of contact time. All organic material must be removed first, so that the bleach can reach the virus. Because parvovirus is so resilient, the virus can be carried on inanimate objects (fomites) such as shoes, clothing, and other materials that touch infected substances. Transmission commonly occurs by swallowing the virus.

Clinical Signs
The primary signs are GI and include diminished appetite, vomiting, lethargy, and diarrhea. Vomiting is often severe, and diarrhea may be profuse and bloody. Fever may be present, and animals can become severely dehydrated very quickly. Affected dogs are often very weak, and shock may develop in some dogs from the dramatic loss of body fluids. Rarely, the heart is affected, which can cause sudden death.

Diagnostic Tests
Because CPV causes many infected dogs to become seriously ill, a number of tests may be recommended to assess its effects on various organs and to confirm the presence of the virus:
* A complete blood count may show low numbers of certain white blood cells and platelets (needed for blood clotting). Anemia may be detected and is sometimes severe.
* A serum biochemistry panel may show low blood protein levels and electrolyte imbalances (such as low potassium) from the vomiting and diarrhea.
* X-rays of the abdomen help rule out other causes of GI signs.
* Specific tests for parvovirus are done on fecal samples. These tests are rapid, may be done in the veterinary clinic, and are very reliable. However, false-positive tests are possible 5-12 days after vaccination for parvovirus, because noninfective virus is shed in the feces after vaccination. False-negative tests are also possible.
* Tests may also be done for antibodies to the virus in the blood but may not be needed.
* Changes typical of CPV may be seen in biopsies of the GI tract. Biopsy is not commonly done to diagnose the disease in

a living animal, but it may be useful to determine the cause of death in dogs that do not survive.

TREATMENT AND FOLLOW-UP
Treatment Options
Dogs with suspected CPV infection should be isolated from other animals because of the highly contagious nature of the virus. Special precautions are needed to prevent transmission to other dogs. Hospitalized animals are commonly quarantined in an isolation ward. To decrease spread of the disease, owners may not be allowed to visit animals that are in isolation.

Treatment of CPV is largely supportive, with intravenous fluids, sometimes plasma transfusions, antivomiting medications, and possibly medications to decrease stomach acid production (to protect the stomach). If anemia is severe, blood transfusions may be administered. Antibiotics may be given for secondary bacterial infections.

Severely ill dogs may develop sepsis, a widespread bacterial infection that occurs when bacteria normally confined to the GI tract are released into the bloodstream as a result of severe damage caused by CPV. When sepsis occurs, it can adversely affect many other organs and usually requires intensive therapy.

Food and water are commonly withheld until no vomiting has occurred for 12-24 hours. Then small amounts of water or ice chips may be offered, and if that is tolerated well, bland food is reintroduced very slowly. Small portions are fed every 2-4 hours initially, after which the amount of food is gradually increased and the time between feedings is gradually lengthened.

Dogs with parvovirus infection may also be treated with deworming medications, because the animals most susceptible to CPV (especially young puppies) are also the ones most susceptible to intestinal parasites. The heart disease caused by CPV often progresses very rapidly, so treatment is not often possible.

Follow-up Care
Dogs that recover from parvovirus disease usually have long-lasting protection from reinfection. Regular vaccination is recommended to maintain good immunity, however.
Prognosis
Dogs that survive the first 2-4 days of treatment are most likely to recover fully. Prognosis is guarded (uncertain) for dogs with prolonged illness. Prognosis is poor for dogs with sepsis. Dogs with CPV-related heart disease often die from the condition.

SPECIAL INSTRUCTIONS:

Prothecosis in Dogs

Anisa D. Dunham, AS, RVT
Lynn F. Guptill, DVM, PhD, DACVIM (Small Animal)

BASIC INFORMATION

Description

Canine protothecosis is an uncommon disease caused by a type of algae. It can cause severe gastrointestinal (GI) disease. It can also affect the skin, the eyes, or the whole body. The organism may infect human beings as well as dogs, cats, and cattle, but it does not spread between animals and people.

Causes

The infectious agents, *Prototheca zopfii* and *Prototheca wickerhamii,* are commonly found in sewage, animal waste, and tree slime. Water and soil may be contaminated by these materials. The disease occurs in North America, Europe, Asia, the Pacific islands, Africa, and Australia. Most cases of protothecosis in the United States occur in the southeastern states. Animals with defective immune systems and those that are very ill with another disease may be more susceptible to protothecosis than healthy animals with normal immune systems. Infection occurs when the organism comes into contact with injured skin or the lining of the GI tract or nose.

There are two forms of the disease, systemic and cutaneous. In the systemic form, the organism is swallowed, infects the GI tract, and then may spread to other areas in the body through the bloodstream or the lymph system. In the cutaneous (skin) form, the disease enters through puncture wounds, cuts, or abrasions to the skin.

Clinical Signs

In the systemic form of protothecosis, the most common clinical sign is intermittent, bloody diarrhea or black, tarry feces. Weight loss, vomiting, and straining to defecate may also be seen. If the infection spreads to the eyes, one or more eye may be inflamed, painful, and blind. If the central nervous system (brain and spinal cord) is infected, neck pain, head tilt, lethargy, circling, ataxia (wobbly gait, lack of coordination), seizures, and weakness or partial paralysis may be seen.

The cutaneous form is less common than the systemic form in dogs. Cats develop only the skin form. Skin lesions consist of nodules and draining ulcers on the legs and trunk. Thickening of the outer layer of the skin may be seen. Occasionally, the infection may spread to nearby lymph nodes (glands), causing them to enlarge. In some dogs, the skin form of the disease transforms into a widespread infection.

Diagnostic Tests

Routine laboratory tests, abdominal x-rays, and fecal tests are often recommended when diarrhea and other GI signs are present. Microscopic evaluation of a rectal scraping may reveal algal organisms in rectal cells. An eye examination may reveal inflammation and retinal detachment.

The organism can sometimes be cultured from the urine, cerebrospinal fluid (obtained by spinal tap), or vitreous humor (the clear gel that fills the back of the eye, obtained by aspirating the eye). If the kidneys are involved, the organism may be seen on microscopic evaluation of the urine.

Biopsies of the colon are needed in some cases to demonstrate the organism. Immunologic testing may be recommended in some animals. Other tests may be needed to rule out more common causes of GI and ocular inflammation.

TREATMENT AND FOLLOW-UP

Treatment Options

Protothecosis is difficult to treat. Antifungal drugs, such as itraconazole and amphotericin, sometimes slow the progression of the systemic form of the disease, but they do not cure it. Amphotericin is given intravenously and is potentially toxic to the kidneys, so hospitalization is usually required when it is administered. Antibiotics and antifungal drugs have been used in combination in some cases. Prolonged therapy is needed.

Cutaneous protothecosis is sometimes treated by surgical removal of skin lesions combined with drug therapy.

Follow-up Care

Drug therapy is usually continued for at least 2-4 months, and for 3-4 weeks beyond the time that clinical signs seem to resolve. Some dogs require lifelong therapy. If infected eyes are painful, they may be removed to improve the quality of the dog's life. Removal of infected eyes does not alleviate the disease elsewhere in the body. Recheck visits and repeated laboratory testing are needed to monitor response to treatment, make modifications in therapy, and check for side effects of the medications.

Prognosis

Prognosis is very poor in most cases. Clinical signs may reappear after treatment is stopped, and most animals are not cured. Successful treatment of systemic protothecosis is rare. Animals suffering from the cutaneous form of the disease may have a slightly better prognosis than those with the systemic form. Animals with compromised immune systems have a grave prognosis, because they often succumb very quickly to the disease.

SPECIAL INSTRUCTIONS:

Pythiosis

Anisa D. Dunham, AS, RVT

BASIC INFORMATION

Description

Pythiosis is an uncommon infectious disease of dogs and cats. Most infections develop in dogs. Pythiosis occurs mainly in tropical and subtropical areas of the world. In the United States, it is present primarily along the Gulf of Mexico, mostly in southern Louisiana, Texas, Alabama, and Florida. Pythiosis has recently been reported in other eastern, western, and midwestern states.

Cause

Pythiosis is caused by *Pythium insidiosum,* which is related to fungi but not considered a true fungus. *Pythium* is found in warm water environments and enters the animal through damaged skin or mucous membranes, such as the lining of the nose, mouth, or stomach. The disease has three forms:

- The most common form of the disease occurs in the gastrointestinal (GI) tract of dogs. Any part of the GI tract may be affected, but the stomach and the upper small intestine are most commonly involved.
- Skin disease occurs less often in dogs and rarely in cats.
- Rarely, multiple organs can be affected in dogs.

Clinical Signs

Young, male, large-breed dogs are most likely to develop the GI form. Vomiting, weight loss, regurgitation, diarrhea, or bright red blood in the stools (hematochezia) may occur. Dogs usually remain bright and alert until late in the disease. Severe signs occur if intestinal obstruction or perforation develops.

Skin lesions may occur anywhere on the body and are slightly itchy nodules that may become ulcerated. Multiple holes or tracts in the skin may drain a clear or cloudy liquid. Animals with cutaneous pythiosis do not necessarily have involvement of other organs. Signs of nasal infection occur in cats with the skin form of the disease.

Diagnostic Tests

Pythiosis may be suspected in a young, large-breed dog living in an appropriate area with the clinical signs described. Sometimes, an abdominal mass may be felt by your veterinarian during the physical examination. Routine laboratory tests, abdominal x-rays, and an abdominal ultrasound are usually done when GI signs or a mass is present. Chest x-rays may also be recommended. These tests may reveal the following:

- The complete blood cell count and blood biochemistry profile may be normal.
- X-rays and ultrasound findings are variable. An abdominal mass may or may not be seen. An ultrasound may show thickening of the walls of the stomach or intestines.
- Chest x-rays may reveal megaesophagus (enlarged esophagus) resulting from esophagitis (inflammation of the lining of the esophagus).

The organism can be identified through microscopic examination of tissues removed from an affected animal by biopsy or sometimes by fine-needle aspiration. Special tests on the tissue may be necessary to find the organism. Culture of the organism may be tried. A test that measures antibodies to pythiosis in the blood of the animal (serology) can also be done to diagnose pythiosis.

TREATMENT AND FOLLOW-UP

Treatment Options

Surgical removal of localized infections is the preferred treatment. Most antifungal drugs are ineffective in treating the disease. When complete surgical removal cannot be accomplished, a combination of antifungal drugs (itraconazole and terbinafine) or intravenous amphotericin lipid complex (also an antifungal drug) can be tried. It may take several weeks to months of treatment before improvement is seen.

Follow-up Care

Resolution of clinical signs and weight gain are good signs. Repeated ultrasounds can be used to assess the size of any remaining abdominal masses. Serologic testing can be repeated after surgery to evaluate its effectiveness (antibody levels fall) and to monitor for recurrence of the disease (antibody levels rise again). Laboratory tests are frequently repeated throughout therapy to monitor for side effects of the medications. The frequency of recheck visits and repeated testing depends on the type and course of therapy used.

Prognosis

Prognosis is usually poor if complete surgical removal is not possible. Recurrence of disease is common.

SPECIAL INSTRUCTIONS:

Rabies

Lynn F. Guptill, DVM, PhD, DACVIM (Small Animal)

BASIC INFORMATION
Description
Rabies is a uniformly fatal infection that causes neurologic signs in infected animals. Rabies virus is maintained in various wildlife reservoirs around the world and can infect any mammal. Wildlife reservoirs vary by geographic location. In the United States, the most commonly infected wildlife species are bats, raccoons, skunks, and foxes. Rabies can be prevented in dogs and cats by vaccination.

Cause
Rabies is caused by a virus that is most commonly transmitted through saliva via a bite wound. It can also be transmitted by contact with the virus in saliva through an open wound or scratch, or through mucous membranes such as the gums of the mouth or the conjunctiva of the eyes. It is rarely transmitted by contact with other body fluids. The rabies virus spreads from the site of entry along nerves to the central nervous system (primarily the brain) and then to the salivary glands. Once in the central nervous system, the virus causes damage to nerve cells and to nerves that supply various tissues.

Clinical Signs
Neurologic signs are the main manifestation of rabies. Two different syndromes are described, a *furious* form and a *dumb* or *paralytic* form. Signs of both syndromes can occur in the same animal. The onset of signs is variable and may occur from 1-2 weeks to several months after exposure.

Initially, affected animals may appear anxious or restless or exhibit other behavioral changes. In the furious form of rabies, infected animals become irritable and aggressive and may bite or attack without provocation. Disorientation, weakness, and a wobbly gait are usually seen. These signs may last a few days, and then seizures may occur that are followed by death.

In the paralytic form, the initial anxious phase is usually followed by progressive weakness that eventually involves the muscles associated with swallowing and breathing. Excessive salivation may occur from inability to swallow normally. A change in bark or meow may be noticed. These signs are usually followed in a few days by coma and respiratory failure, which lead to death.

Diagnostic Tests
A history of a recent bite wound or other exposure to a potentially rabid animal, in combination with the clinical signs listed, are suggestive of rabies. A diagnosis of rabies should be considered in any animal with neurologic signs that has a history of possible exposure to a rabid (having rabies) animal.

No good diagnostic test is available to definitively diagnose rabies in a living animal. Testing of brain tissue after euthanasia remains the best diagnostic test. Testing of brain tissue is done at state diagnostic laboratories. Other tests may be recommended to rule out other diseases that can cause similar clinical signs.

TREATMENT AND FOLLOW-UP
Treatment Options
There is no effective treatment for rabies.

Follow-up Care
If rabies is suspected, extreme caution must be exercised when handling the animal, to avoid exposure to saliva or other bodily fluids. It is very important to avoid being bitten. Any bite wounds or potentially exposed open surfaces should be washed as soon as possible with warm, soapy water, and your health care provider should be contacted immediately.

Animals exposed to rabid animals must be carefully examined and then placed under close observation or quarantine, depending on the circumstances and whether they are currently vaccinated for rabies. Specific rules exist regarding the handling of animals exposed to rabies, and these rules are updated yearly in the *Compendium of Animal Rabies Control*, available at *http://www.nasphv.org*. Excellent information on rabies is also available from the Centers for Disease Control (*http://www.cdc.gov*).

States and local municipalities have laws regarding rabies control, including vaccination requirements and rules for handling domestic animals exposed to other animals known or suspected of being rabid.

Prognosis
Rabies is uniformly fatal. It is imperative that all cats and dogs be vaccinated for this disease, in accordance with local and state regulations.

SPECIAL INSTRUCTIONS:

Rocky Mountain Spotted Fever

Lynn F. Guptill, DVM, PhD, DACVIM (Small Animal)

BASIC INFORMATION
Description
Rocky Mountain spotted fever is a systemic disease of dogs in North, Central, and South America. It also affects humans.
Cause
Rocky Mountain spotted fever is caused by the bacteria *Rickettsia rickettsii,* which is transmitted by ticks. The disease may occur in dogs without prior known exposure to ticks.

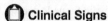 Clinical Signs
Some infected animals have no clinical signs. The most common clinical findings include the following:
- Fever, lethargy, decreased appetite, and possible weight loss
- Vomiting, diarrhea, coughing
- Inflammation and hemorrhages within the eyes
- Joint and muscle pain, joint swelling, lameness
- Neurologic signs, such as seizures, pain along the neck and back, uncoordinated movement (ataxia), head tilt, falling, and others

Diagnostic Tests
Routine laboratory tests are commonly recommended to investigate the clinical signs. Numerous abnormalities may be discovered, including the following:
- A complete blood count (CBC) may show low numbers of red blood cells (anemia), platelets, and white blood cells.
- A biochemistry profile may reveal low blood protein levels (especially albumin) and elevated cholesterol, liver, and kidney function tests.
- Urinalysis may show abnormally high protein in the urine.

X-rays of the abdomen, chest, and joints may be recommended, depending on the animal's clinical signs. Fluid may be aspirated from swollen joints and submitted for analysis. When neurologic signs are present, computed tomography (CT scan) or magnetic resonance imaging (MRI) may be considered. A spinal tap and collection of cerebrospinal fluid for analysis may also be recommended.

Blood tests for antibodies to *R. rickettsii* are commonly done. These tests may be performed twice, 2-4 weeks apart, to determine whether antibody levels are rising, which would indicate an active infection. Polymerase chain reaction (PCR) assays for *R. rickettsii* DNA may be done on blood or other tissues in some cases.

TREATMENT AND FOLLOW-UP
Treatment Options
The antibiotic, doxycycline, is the most commonly recommended treatment for Rocky Mountain spotted fever. Other antibiotics (tetracycline, enrofloxacin) may also be used. These drugs may cause gastrointestinal tract upset (decreased appetite, vomiting, diarrhea), so they are commonly given with food. Treatment with steroids is sometimes recommended for the inflammation associated with the immune response to this rickettsial agent, but this must be done with caution. Seriously ill animals often require hospitalization, with intravenous fluids, symptomatic medications that are appropriate for the clinical signs, and other supportive care.

Follow-up Care
Resolution or substantial improvement of the signs often occurs within the first 48-72 hours after starting treatment, especially when therapy is begun early in the course of the illness. Periodic examinations and repeated laboratory testing are often used to monitor response to treatment. Animals that have Rocky Mountain spotted fever are commonly exposed to other diseases transmitted by ticks, so institution of a strict, comprehensive tick control program is very important.
Prognosis
Prognosis is generally good for animals that are mildly affected. Prognosis is more guarded (uncertain) to poor for animals with severe neurologic signs, anemia, or other organ dysfunction.
Public Health Information
Rocky Mountain spotted fever is potentially zoonotic (transmissible from animals to humans), but transmission does not occur directly from animals to people. Instead, it takes place through a vector (intermediate host), such as a tick. If an animal is suspected of having Rocky Mountain spotted fever, people in the vicinity should take precautions to prevent tick bites.

SPECIAL INSTRUCTIONS:

Tetanus

Anisa D. Dunham, AS, RVT
Lynn F. Guptill, DVM, PhD, DACVIM (Small Animal)

BASIC INFORMATION

Description

Tetanus is a disease of warm-blooded animals. The clinical signs associated with this disease are caused by tetanospasmin, a potent bacterial neurotoxin (a toxin that acts on nerve cells). Muscle stiffness and spasms are typical of the disease. Tetanus is uncommon in dogs and cats.

Cause

Tetanus is caused by *Clostridium tetani*. These bacteria produce spores that persist in the environment, such as in dirt and debris. The spores are resistant to boiling and to many disinfectants. Spores of *C. tetani* enter wounds, where they multiply and produce tetanospasmin. Tetanospasmin affects the transmission of information from nerves to muscles, which leads to muscle stiffness.

Clinical Signs

Signs usually develop 5-21 days after a wound is infected with the bacteria. Signs may affect only one area of the body, such as increased stiffness in a group of muscles or an entire limb. Signs may gradually worsen and involve the entire nervous system (generalized tetanus). Generalized signs include facial muscle spasms ("lockjaw"), protrusion of the third eyelids, increased salivation, difficulty swallowing, extreme muscle stiffness of the legs, elevated body temperature, and altered heart and respiratory rates. Spasms of the muscles of the voice box (larynx), chest, and diaphragm may make breathing difficult. Animals may appear to have increased sensitivity to sound and touch.

Facial muscle spasms may cause wrinkling of the forehead and retraction of the lips, as if the animal is smiling or grimacing. This facial appearance is known as *risus sardonicus*. Extreme rigidity (stiffness) of the legs may give the animal a saw-horse stance, or cause it to fall over and be unable to walk. The legs are often held straight and are difficult to bend.

Diagnostic Tests

Diagnosis is usually based on the clinical signs and a history of a bite, wound, or surgical procedure performed within the previous 3 weeks. Culture of the organism from an affected animal is very difficult and is not usually done.

TREATMENT AND FOLLOW-UP

Treatment Options

Mildly affected animals may recover with treatment involving antibiotics that kill *Clostridium* species and wound management. Wounds are thoroughly cleaned, and dead material is removed, to minimize any further reproduction of the bacteria and to decrease the production of tetanospasmin. Severely affected animals require, in addition, intensive supportive care and prolonged hospitalization. Supportive treatment may include intravenous fluids, indwelling feeding tubes for supplying adequate nutrition, and assisted ventilation with a mechanical ventilator. Good nursing care is needed for animals that are unable to sit up or walk.

Sedatives and muscle relaxants may be needed. An injectable antitoxin may be used to neutralize toxin that is not bound to nerves. Once the toxin acts at the nerve-muscle junction, it cannot be removed, and supportive care must be provided until new nerve-muscle junctions can be generated.

Follow-up Care

Continuous supportive care is essential for successful recovery of animals with generalized tetanus. Intensive monitoring is needed in severely affected animals while they are hospitalized. Following discharge from the hospital, continued care is usually needed at home for some time. Recheck visits are used to monitor the animal's progress and recovery. Because the disease is so rare in dogs and cats, vaccination is not recommended.

Prognosis

Prognosis for recovery from tetanus is variable, depending on the severity of clinical signs at the time treatment is started. Animals with localized tetanus have a better prognosis than those with generalized tetanus. Recovery from generalized tetanus can take weeks to months.

SPECIAL INSTRUCTIONS:

Toxoplasmosis

Anisa D. Dunham, AS, RVT
Lynn F. Guptill, DVM, PhD, DACVIM (Small Animal)

BASIC INFORMATION

Description

Toxoplasmosis is a zoonotic disease (a disease that can be transmitted from animals to humans) that is caused by a protozoan parasite (a microscopic, one-celled organism). Toxoplasmosis can infect many different organs and cause serious signs of illness. Toxoplasmosis may also infect an animal without causing obvious clinical signs.

Cause

Toxoplasmosis is caused by *Toxoplasma gondii*, which infects almost all species of warm-blooded animals. Cats are the only animals that can excrete oocysts (infectious forms) in their feces. The most common mode of transmission is eating raw or undercooked meat that contains tissue cysts or oocysts. Transmission across the placenta or through the mother's milk is also possible.

When cats ingest tissue cysts, parasites are released and multiply in their gastrointestinal tract. Oocysts are shed in the cat's feces for 1-3 weeks after its first exposure to the parasite. The oocysts become infective after 24 or more hours outside the cat's body. Any animal may then become infected by eating them.

The parasites multiply within intestinal cells and can spread throughout the body. Parasites may enter any tissue and cause illness. In addition, cysts may form in muscles. Cysts may remain dormant for the life of the animal, or they may become activated and cause illness at a later time.

Cats that are shedding oocysts in feces usually appear healthy. Cats with other forms of the parasite in their tissues may become ill.

Clinical Signs

Clinical signs may develop more often in animals that are young, are immune suppressed, or have another infection. Signs are quite variable, depending on the organ or tissues involved. Weakness, incoordination, and other neurologic problems may be noted. Respiratory signs may occur, such as difficulty breathing, increased respiratory rate, and coughing. Inflammation of one or both eyes (uveitis) is a common manifestation in cats. If the liver and pancreas are affected, signs may include fever, decreased appetite, vomiting, weight loss, and jaundice (yellow color to the skin and gums). Multiple signs may be seen if the whole body is affected.

Diagnostic Tests

Diagnosis of clinical toxoplasmosis can be made based on a combination of several laboratory tests:

- Blood and urine tests are often needed to determine how the body is affected by the infection.
- Tests for antibodies to toxoplasmosis can be performed on serum (from blood), cerebrospinal fluid (from a spinal tap), or aqueous humor (fluid from the eye).
- X-rays of the chest and abdomen and an abdominal ultrasound may be recommended.
- Microscopic examinations of tissue samples or of cells from cerebrospinal fluid and the respiratory tract may be helpful in identifying the organism.
- Cats that are ill do not shed oocysts in their feces, because their illness is a result of parasites in other tissues, not in the intestinal tract.
- Other tests may be needed to rule out diseases that cause similar clinical signs.

TREATMENT AND FOLLOW-UP

Treatment Options

Drugs usually suppress multiplication of *T. gondii* organisms but do not clear all of the organisms from the body. Clindamycin (an antibiotic) is often the drug of choice. Additional supportive care in the hospital may be needed, depending on the severity of the clinical signs.

Follow-up Care

Nervous system and ocular signs are often slow to respond. Vision is often diminished or lost if uveitis is severe. Transmission of *T. gondii* can be reduced by limiting exposure to oocysts and tissue cysts. Feed cats only fully cooked commercial foods. Keep cats inside to prevent hunting.

Public Health Information

Toxoplasmosis is usually transmitted to humans by ingestion of undercooked meats or, less commonly, food or water contaminated with oocysts. The disease is rarely transmitted by direct contact with cats. People can be exposed by contact with sporulated (infective) oocysts from litter boxes, gardens, or sandboxes.

To prevent exposure to people, practice good hygiene in food preparation and cook meats thoroughly. Litter boxes should be cleaned and treated with boiling water daily, so that oocysts do not have time to sporulate. Pregnant women and immune-suppressed people are the most susceptible to toxoplasmosis, so they should wear gloves and possibly a mask when changing litter boxes, or the task should be performed by someone else in the household.

Prognosis

Prognosis for animals with widespread systemic disease is guarded (uncertain). Prognosis may only be determined in some cats by their response to initial treatment.

SPECIAL INSTRUCTIONS:

Tritrichomoniasis in Cats

Anisa D. Dunham, AS, RVT
Lynn F. Guptill, DVM, PhD, DACVIM (Small Animal)

BASIC INFORMATION

Description

Tritrichomoniasis is an infection with *Tritrichomonas foetus,* a microscopic, single-celled, protozoan parasite. *T. foetus* is well known for causing reproductive tract infections in naturally bred cattle and has recently been found to cause diarrhea in cats.

Cause

T. foetus is present all over the world. It is spread by close, direct contact. Infections are most common in young cats that are housed together with other cats.

Clinical Signs

Increased frequency of defecation and semiformed to liquid feces that sometimes contain fresh blood or mucus are the most common clinical signs. Diarrhea is most common in young cats. Adult cats may not develop diarrhea when infected.

Fecal incontinence and anal ulceration may occur if the diarrhea is present for long periods. The diarrhea associated with *T. foetus* may resolve over time. Whether *T. foetus* causes reproductive disease in cats is unclear.

Diagnostic Tests

Routine laboratory and fecal tests may be recommended to investigate the diarrhea. Diagnosis of tritrichomoniasis can be made by a number of different methods, including the following:

- Microscopic examination of a fresh fecal sample may reveal the organism.
- Special culture techniques exist for culturing the organism from feces of infected cats.
- An abdominal ultrasound may show an abnormal appearance of the large bowel and enlargement of local lymph nodes (glands), but these changes are not specific for tritrichomoniasis.

TREATMENT AND FOLLOW-UP

Treatment Options

T. foetus is resistant to many antiprotozoal drugs. Antibiotics are not recommended, because they may prolong the shedding of

T. foetus in the feces and do not resolve the problem. Ronidazole may be an effective treatment. This drug is not licensed for use in cats and should be used with caution. It may cause lethargy, ataxia (wobbliness, lack of coordination), tremors, and, occasionally, seizures.

Since most cats suffer no significant adverse effects from a *T. foetus* infection and the diarrhea often resolves over time, it may not be necessary or advisable to treat all affected cats with ronidazole. Feeding a highly digestible diet may be sufficient to control clinical signs in some cats. Any other accompanying intestinal parasites should be treated with appropriate medications.

Follow-up Care

Affected cats are monitored for dehydration if the diarrhea is profuse and persists. Prevention and control of the spread of *T. foetus* are important. Avoid overcrowding of cats, and practice good hygiene when multiple cats are housed together.

Public Health Information

It is not known whether *T. foetus* can infect humans. Because of close contact between infected cats and their owners, however, precautions should be taken. People in contact with infected cats should wear gloves and wash their hands thoroughly after cleaning litter boxes. Cat scratches and bites should be washed immediately. People with weakened immune systems may be more susceptible to infection, so they should always wash their hands after handling infected cats.

Prognosis

The long-term prognosis for infected cats is generally good. Most cats eventually overcome the infection, but this may take a long time (average, 9 months). Some cats have persistent diarrhea for 2 years, whereas in others signs resolve in only 4 months. Most infected cats continue to shed low numbers of organisms in their feces for many months after the diarrhea resolves.

SPECIAL INSTRUCTIONS:

SECTION 16

Behavioral Disorders

Section Editor: Rhea V. Morgan, DVM, DACVIM (Small Animal), DACVO

Aggression Among Household Cats
Dominance Aggression in Dogs
Elimination Problems in Cats
Elimination Problems in Dogs
Fear and Anxiety Disorders in Dogs

Petting Intolerance and Status Aggression
   in Cats
Play Aggression in Cats
Possessive and Territorial Aggression in Dogs

Aggression Among Household Cats

Rhea V. Morgan, DVM, DACVIM (Small Animal), DACVO

BASIC INFORMATION
Description
Cats are highly social and form discrete social groups and hierarchies. Intercat aggression can arise in a number of circumstances when cats are expected to live in the same environment. Aggression is common between intact males because of the competition for potential mates. Although this type of aggression is considered normal, it is usually unacceptable in confined cats and is a major reason why domesticated male cats are castrated.

Aggression can also arise when a new (strange) cat is introduced to the environment or when one cat attempts to dominate another.

Causes
Intercat aggression may develop in relation to social maturity issues or environmental changes within the household that are independent of the drive to mate. Cats that live in isolation from an early age or for much of their life may have poor social skills. Aggression is common toward new cats, because they are recognized as foreign to the established social group. The presence of a new cat also upsets the existing social hierarchy and may trigger dominance aggression among cats that got along well previously.

Other environmental disruptions can trigger dominance aggression, including temporary removal of a high-ranking cat from the environment (such as for a hospital stay) and failure of other cats to recognize or acknowledge the cat's prior status when it returns. Disruptive events in the household can precipitate fighting that may alter the normal social balance among cats. Genetic factors may also play a role in dominance aggression.

Clinical Signs
With the introduction of a new cat, the current cats in the household may hiss, spit, or attack the new one. With regard to dominance aggression, cats that got along well previously may begin to behave in a dominant or submissive fashion. The dominant cat approaches the subordinate one with the base of the tail elevated and the rest of the tail drooping. Its walk is stiff-legged. It may stare at the other cat or slowly rock its head from side to side. If the subordinate cat runs, the dominant cat may launch an attack. The victim may hide and actively avoid social encounters with the aggressor.

Diagnostic Tests
Diagnosis of dominance aggression is usually made from a thorough history. It is necessary to distinguish this form of aggression from play aggression and from redirected aggression by a highly aroused cat that cannot reach its preferred target (such as an outside animal). The circumstances that precipitate these other disorders may seem similar, but careful scrutiny of the events and clinical signs often reveals characteristic differences.

TREATMENT AND FOLLOW-UP
Treatment Options
The following measures are often helpful when introducing a new cat to the household:
- Initially, isolate the new cat in its own room, with its own food and water bowls and litter pan.
- Gradually introduce the cats through a glass or screened door or by cracking a solid door open 1-2 inches.
- Share bedding or cloths rubbed against the cats' faces to familiarize them with each other's scent.
- Once the cats appear to be acclimated to each other, allow them physical access for gradually increasing periods, under close supervision. A harness can be used on one of cats to provide some control.

For dominance and other intercat aggression, the following can be done:
- Separate the cats when they are unsupervised.
- Make sure that all cats have access to enough litter pans and food and water dishes so that they do not have to interact to fulfill their essential needs.
- Rotate cats that get along with both parties in the conflict, so that the aggressive situation does not progress to involve more cats.
- Desensitization and counter-conditioning techniques, as outlined by your veterinarian, can be tried in some neutral location within the house.

For both situations, medical therapy with fluoxetine, sertraline, clomipramine, amitriptyline, or other similar agents may be tried in refractory cases.

Follow-up Care
Repeated consultations may be needed with your veterinarian to monitor the cat's response to modifications made in the environment and to any medications used. Report any escalation in aggression to your veterinarian.

Prognosis
With regard to introducing a new cat, well-socialized, friendly cats may accept each other within hours or days. Poorly socialized cats may require weeks to months, and in rare instances, they may never accept each other.

Prognosis for dominance aggression is poor. Resolution is possible with weeks to months of consistent treatment but does not always occur.

SPECIAL INSTRUCTIONS:

Dominance Aggression in Dogs

Elizabeth A. Shull, DVM, DACVB, DACVIM (Neurology)

BASIC INFORMATION

Description

Dominance aggression (social, competitive, owner-directed) involves threatening postures and behaviors directed toward family members or other familiar people by a dog that perceives itself to be more dominant than the person. It is particularly disturbing because the aggression seems to be unprovoked and unpredictable.

Use of the term *dominance aggression* has been questioned, because the concept of dominance in dogs has been widely misused; dominance aggression has been overdiagnosed; and there is concern that the terminology suggests the dog should be domineered to manage the aggression.

Causes

Dominance aggression has its roots in the social organization of wolves, the domestic dog's closest wild relative. Within the wolf pack, there is a social hierarchy in which the dominant individuals have first access to critical resources. Among domestic dogs, dominance threats and overt aggression are exhibited in the contexts of competition over "resources" or in response to challenges and dominance signals.

People frequently do not understand how a dominant dog interprets their actions and gestures, so, from the dog's perspective, people can be confusing and inconsistent. Lavishing gratuitous affection on the dog, giving in to its demands for attention, or even unintentionally mimicking canine submissive signals (such as kissing the dog on its face) are contradictory behaviors to expecting the dog to do what the owner wishes. Inconsistency and unpredictability in social interactions with family members can result in anxiety and instability in the dog's social relationships, which in turn can escalate social competition and dominance aggression.

Clinical Signs

The highest incidence of dominance aggression occurs in intact males, followed by castrated males, spayed females, and unspayed females. Purebred dogs, especially the English springer spaniel, Lhasa apso, cocker spaniels, Doberman pinscher, toy poodle, and terriers, have a higher incidence than other breeds. Onset typically occurs at 1-3 years of age. Onset may seem sudden, but early, subtle signs may not be recognized.

Diagnostic Tests

A complete medical history, physical examination, and comprehensive laboratory tests are recommended to look for possible medical factors that can contribute to or complicate management of the aggression.

The behavioral diagnosis of canine aggression is determined by context and the specific stimulus or trigger, the target, behavioral components, and the age, sex, and breed of the dog.

- *Context and triggers*: Aggression may occur when the dog's dominance has been challenged by a dominance signal (petting, hugging, staring at, standing over, commanding, scolding, punishing, or forcing the dog to do something) or when a family member "competes" for a "critical resource" (such as food or a prized object).
- *Target*: Dominance aggression is most often directed toward the dog's owners and other familiar people and may be preferentially directed to certain individuals.
- *Behavioral components*: Snarling, growling, lunging, snapping, biting, and assumption of a dominant posture (erect or stiff body, ears, and tail; raised hackles; direct stare) may occur. Some dogs exhibit varying degrees of both dominance and fear, indicating that there is some anxiety or ambivalence in the dog's motivation.

Treatment Options

Because of the dangerous and complex nature of dominance aggression, specific treatment by a professional with knowledge and experience in the management of canine aggression is advised. The following are only general recommendations:

- Human safety is the first consideration. It is particularly dangerous to keep these dogs in homes with children. *Young* children are especially at risk.
- The aggression triggers should be identified and avoided. Head halters and basket muzzles may help reduce biting risk, but they are not guaranteed to prevent injury. Physical punishment is dangerous and counterproductive.
- Castration of intact males reduces dominance aggression, but the benefit may not occur for several months. Spaying of intact females may increase aggression.
- Obedience training is important to develop commands that can be used in behavior modification programs. "Nothing in Life is Free," a nonconfrontational method that requires the dog to defer by obeying commands before every interaction (attention, food, petting, play), can lessen the dog's dominant position. Specific desensitization techniques can reduce the dog's reaction to certain aggression triggers.
- Changes should be made in the way the family interacts with the dog to alter the dog's perception of its status. Temporarily withdrawing attention from the dog, as well as changes in feeding routine, exercise schedule, and sleeping or resting sites, may be recommended.
- Serotonergic drugs and drugs that improve impulse control may be beneficial for some dogs.

Prognosis

Dominance aggression is rarely, if ever, cured. In many instances, the severity can be reduced, but when the potential for serious injury is great, euthanasia should be considered.

SPECIAL INSTRUCTIONS:

Elimination Problems in Cats

Elizabeth A. Shull, DVM, DACVB, DACVIM (Neurology)

BASIC INFORMATION
Description
Elimination problems are the most common behavior problems of cats. They involve voluntary urination, defection, or both, outside the litter box and expression of urine while marking (spraying). Pet cats may mark with feces (middening), but this occurs rarely.

Any age, sex, or breed of cat may be affected, but long-haired cats may have an increased tendency for inappropriate defecation. Intact males spray urine the most, followed by neutered males and then intact and spayed females.

Causes
Behavioral causes of elimination problems include inappropriate elimination or toileting, urine marking, separation anxiety, and occasionally other types of fears. Medical abnormalities can also cause eliminations outside the litter box. Cats do not urinate, defecate, or urine mark out of spite.

- Inappropriate elimination is a common cause and often results from an aversion to something associated with the litter or litter box, or from an attraction or preference for something outside the litter box.
- Cats can have an aversion to the litter, the litter box, or the location of the litter box. Litter aversion may be related to texture or scent of the litter, presence of a deodorizer, depth of litter, inadequate cleaning, or a previous negative experience (such as pain or fear) associated with the litter.
- Litter box aversion may be related to the type (open, covered, self-cleaning) or size of the box, location of the box (high traffic area, isolated, poor accessibility, vulnerable to surprise attacks by other cats), presence or absence of a liner, type or scent of cleaner used in the box, and previous negative experiences.
- Conversely, cats may seek other surfaces and locations for elimination because of a preference for a particular surface or association of a specific type of surface or location with the act of eliminating. Fabric is a commonly chosen alternative surface.
- Urine marking is normal cat communication behavior. It may be motivated by sexual, territorial, or conflict situations involving other cats, and it may be triggered by social and environmental factors such as residual urine odors, unfamiliar odors, or the presence of unfamiliar animals or people. Cats outside the home may trigger spraying around doors, windows, air vents, and fireplaces. The more cats in a household, the greater the probability that spraying will occur.

Clinical Signs
Inappropriate elimination involves evacuation of a normal volume of urine or feces on a horizontal surface while the cat is in a squatting posture. Signs of litter or litter box aversion include complete avoidance of the litter, approaching the box hesitantly, perching on the edge of the box, not scratching in the litter, spraying while in the litter box, eliminating just outside the box, quickly running away from the box, and shaking of paws or meowing on exiting the box.

- A surface preference is suspected when a cat predominantly eliminates on a particular type of surface; a location preference is suggested when a cat frequently eliminates in one room or region of a room.
- Inappropriate elimination due to separation anxiety is suspected if the elimination occurs in the owner's absence. Urinating on the owner's bed is a common manifestation of separation anxiety.

Urine marking involves expression of a small volume of urine on a vertical surface by a cat in a standing position with a raised, quivering tail. Less commonly, cats may mark while squatting. Urine may be sprayed on established marking posts or on sites or objects that have social significance.

Diagnostic Tests
A thorough examination and routine laboratory tests are done, and additional laboratory tests, x-rays, and other imaging procedures may be recommended depending on the initial findings. After medical problems are excluded, behavioral diagnoses and treatment rely on descriptions of the behavioral problem and historical information.

Be sure to relay all pertinent information, such as the duration and frequency of the occurrences, location of the elimination, litter box information, relationships with other pets and people in the household, correction methods that have been tried, and medications being administered. Drawing a diagram of the floor plan of the house and indicating the locations and surfaces upon which elimination is occurring, as well as the locations of windows, doors, food and water bowls, and litter boxes, is often helpful.

In multiple-cat households, it must be determined which cat or cats are involved. Isolating the cats one at a time may reveal which one is responsible. Sometimes, a fluorescein chemical is given or scrapings of different-colored nontoxic crayons are placed into each cat's food to identify which cat is urinating or defecating inappropriately.

Continued

Elimination Problems in Cats—*cont'd*

Elizabeth A. Shull, DVM, DACVB, DACVIM (Neurology)

TREATMENT AND FOLLOW-UP

℞ Treatment Options

Treatment of inappropriate elimination or toileting involves increasing the appeal of the litter and litter box while decreasing the attractiveness and/or accessibility of the inappropriate location.

- Inadequate cleaning of the litter is a common reason for inappropriate elimination. Scooping and refreshing of litter should be done at least once daily, and fastidious cats may require more frequent scooping. Litter boxes are completely emptied and washed with plain soap (no fragrance) and hot water at least once weekly. In multiple-cat households, provide one box per cat, plus one extra box. Disperse the boxes throughout the home. Make the boxes easily accessible, but do not place them where the cat may be startled by household activities or other pets.
- For litter or litter box aversion, provide the cat with a different type of litter and box. In general, cats prefer scoopable, finely granular litter that has no scent, as well as open boxes. Individual cats vary in their preferences, so systematic trials may be required. Providing a smorgasbord of litter choices may be necessary to identify the type of litter most appealing to the cat.
- Large and overweight cats need boxes that are larger than the typical commercial litter box.
- Trimming hair between footpads, under the tail, and around the rear end of long-haired cats helps prevent litter and stool from attaching to the hair.
- For a surface preference, place the preferred type of surface temporarily in the litter box to re-establish the habit of using the box. For a location preference, either place the box at the preferred location; block the cat from that location; or make the location less appealing by covering it with a surface that is aversive or by applying an unappealing scent (such as citrus-scented air freshener).
- Clean inappropriate sites of elimination thoroughly with plain soap and water, and apply an effective odor eliminator. Avoid ammonia-based cleaners.
- If the cat is not using a litter box because of separation anxiety, fear, or anxiety or conflict with another cat, then those behavioral issues must also be addressed. Antianxiety medication may also be recommended to reduce arousal and anxiety associated with conflict and stress.
- Punishment is not helpful. Scolding or punishing the cat and then putting it in the litter box is especially detrimental and increases the likelihood that the cat will permanently avoid the litter box in the future.

Urine marking is treated by reducing the motivation for spraying and managing any environmental and social triggers:

- Neutering decreases spraying in 90% of intact males and in 95% of intact females.
- Reducing the number of cats in a multi-cat household also decreases the incidence of spraying; however, this is not always an acceptable treatment. Alternatively, try to treat the conflicts among household cats. (See handout on **Aggression Among Household Cats.**)
- Triggers from outside cats may be reduced by blocking the inside cat's view of the outside and by discouraging outside cats through the use of repellents such as *The Scarecrow*, a motion-activated water sprinkler.
- A urine odor eliminator is also used to remove residual urine odor from sites that have been sprayed. Placement of citrus-scented air fresheners may help break the habit of spraying on a particular spot. *Feliway* (a synthetic facial pheromone available as a plug-in diffuser and as a spray) may induce a cat to mark by facial rubbing rather than spraying. Providing scratching posts near a spraying site may stimulate marking by scratching instead of spraying.
- Adequate litter box cleaning helps reduce anxiety about the box that may trigger spraying in some cats.
- Antianxiety medication may be recommended to relieve anxiety associated with conflict. Punishment is counterproductive and only increases the cat's anxiety, which has the potential of increasing spraying.

🐾 Follow-up Care

Usually, when treating elimination problems in cats, a plan is developed for a few initial changes or treatments, and the cat's response is monitored for at least 1-2 weeks to determine the success of the plan. Based on the effectiveness of the initial plan, additional treatments may be recommended. If behavioral drugs are prescribed, monitoring is needed for adverse side effects, and follow-up laboratory tests may be recommended.

Prognosis

Response to appropriate, systematic treatment is often favorable, especially in uncomplicated cases, although gradual improvement over several days to weeks is more likely than an immediate response. Treatment outcomes are less favorable when the diagnosis or contributing factors have not been correctly identified or when treatments are randomly applied.

SPECIAL INSTRUCTIONS:

Elimination Problems in Dogs

Elizabeth A. Shull, DVM, DACVB, DACVIM (Neurology)

BASIC INFORMATION

Description

Urinating and/or defecating inside the home is a common behavioral problem of dogs. If the problem is not rectified, the dog may be removed from the household by being banished to the yard, relinquished to an animal shelter, or even euthanized.

Causes

The major causes of inappropriate elimination are incomplete house-training, urine marking, anxiety disorders (separation anxiety and noise phobia), submissive urination, excitement or greeting urination, and inappropriate elimination because of underlying medical disorders.

Clinical Signs

Dogs that are incompletely house-trained deposit urine and/or stool at inappropriate locations within the home. It is common in puppies and young dogs but can become a long-term problem.

Urine marking is the deposition of urine to indicate home ranges and territories and to locate and identify females that are in heat. It often occurs in territorial, sexual, and conflict situations. Dogs may urine mark inside the home despite being otherwise well house-trained. Intact males and females in heat mark most frequently. Urine marking usually does not develop until a dog has reached sexual maturity (at about 1 year of age).

Dogs with separation anxiety or noise phobias may exhibit inappropriate elimination when they are anxious. The inappropriate elimination done by dogs with separation anxiety is easily misinterpreted as spiteful behavior.

Submissive urination is manifested in response to perceived threats or dominance signals from other dogs or humans.

Excitement or greeting urination occurs when the dog is very excited, often when owners return home and when greeting new individuals.

Many medical disorders result in house-soiling because of alterations in function of the urinary or digestive systems or decreased mobility, control, or awareness.

Diagnosis

An accurate behavioral diagnosis of the type of elimination problem is necessary for successful treatment. Diagnosis is based on the age and sex of the dog, a description of the elimination behavior, and the circumstances in which it occurs. Possible underlying medical problems must be ruled out with laboratory and other tests before a behavioral diagnosis is made.

TREATMENT AND FOLLOW-UP

Treatment Options

The ideal treatment for incomplete house-training is prevention. If the dog is never given an opportunity to eliminate in the house, it quickly learns to eliminate only outside. A successful training program consists of taking the dog to an appropriate location for elimination on a regular schedule, using positive reinforcement, providing constant supervision when the dog is loose in the house, and confining the animal when it is unsupervised.

Inappropriate elimination that occurs because of anxiety is treated by managing the underlying anxiety. (See **Fear and Anxiety Disorders in Dogs**.) In some cases, remedial house-training is also required.

Castration improves urine marking in 70% of intact male dogs, and spaying usually resolves heat-related marking in female dogs. When possible, remove or minimize the dog's exposure to arousing stimuli. If the dog marks at one or two places, turn those sites into water and feeding stations. Clean and apply an enzymatic odor eliminator to the marked surfaces. *DAP*, a synthetic appeasing pheromone, may be helpful in some dogs to decrease anxiety and arousal level. In difficult cases, antianxiety medications may be tried.

Inappropriate management of submissive urination frequently makes it worse. In many cases, this type of urination spontaneously resolves with maturity. In general, the behavior should be ignored! Do not punish or reassure the dog. Avoid unintentional threatening and dominance gestures, and institute various management techniques. Desensitization therapy may be necessary if management changes are inadequate. Medications to relieve anxiety or increase urethral tone may be considered in cases that do not resolve with behavioral methods.

If the dog exhibits excitement or greeting urination, greeting should not be eliminated; however, the greeting routine can be changed to reduce the consequences. Make inside greetings low-key and calm. If possible, call the dog outside and greet it there. Redirect excitement and exuberance to running and playing. Greeting urination often resolves with maturity. If it does not, specific desensitization training may be necessary. Medications to relieve anxiety or increase urethral tone may be considered in cases that do not resolve with behavioral methods.

Prognosis

Prognosis for many elimination problems is good as long as the correct diagnosis is determined and appropriate treatment is implemented. Urine marking significantly improves in most dogs with neutering, over several weeks to months. Submissive and excitement or greeting urination cases that do not resolve with maturity are challenging and may require additional evaluation. Inappropriate elimination resulting from anxiety disorders is more problematic, because permanently resolving separation anxiety or noise phobia is unlikely.

SPECIAL INSTRUCTIONS:

Fear and Anxiety Disorders in Dogs

Elizabeth A. Shull, DVM, DACVB, DACVIM (Neurology)

BASIC INFORMATION

Description

Separation anxiety and noise phobias are prevalent fear-related disorders of dogs. Dogs with separation anxiety experience distress when left alone or when separated from a favorite person. Dogs with noise phobia experience fear in response to certain noises, especially loud, percussive sounds such as thunder, firecrackers, and gunshots.

Causes

Risk factors for separation anxiety include adoption from a shelter, rescue group, or prior home; prior life as a stray; having a noise phobia; moving to a different location; changes in the people or pets in the home; changes in household schedule; living with a single owner; and living in an urban environment. Problem behaviors associated with separation anxiety are not caused by spite.

Noise phobias are more common in herding breeds and hounds. Dogs with inadequate socialization; dogs that experienced a traumatic event when young; dogs living with another phobic dog; and concurrent separation anxiety are also contributing factors.

Clinical Signs

Separation anxiety has a slightly greater incidence in male and mixed-breed dogs. Many noise phobias develop before 1 year of age, and most are present by 5 years of age.

Signs of separation anxiety include anxiousness as the owner prepares to leave, excessive vocalization, digging, chewing, and rearranging household objects. Some dogs may aggressively growl and bite in an attempt to prevent the person from leaving. Self-injury, especially broken teeth, cuts in the mouth, and broken nails, may occur from attempts to escape. Some dogs also urinate, defecate, salivate, pant, tremble, or do not eat or drink (while the owner is away).

Dogs with noise phobias become more active and restless in response to the noise. They may pace, vocalize, jump against windows or doors, chew, dig, tremble, salivate, pant, eliminate inappropriately, have increased heart rates, and constantly seek to be close to the owner. In some dogs, the fear reaction is dramatic and can lead to activities that are destructive to the home or themselves.

Diagnostic Tests

Diagnosis is based on the presence of clinical signs and exclusion of other behavioral causes. A medical history, physical examination, and laboratory tests are done to exclude possible contributing conditions, such as urinary tract, gastrointestinal, hormonal, metabolic, or seizure disorders.

Separation anxiety can be challenging to diagnose, because many possible causes exist for the behaviors that occur with separation anxiety. Most noise phobias are easy to diagnose; however, if only the dog hears the sound or if the sound is not recognized by the owner, it may appear as if the dog is having a spontaneous panic attack. With thunderstorm phobia, it is common for the dog to act fearful before people are aware a storm is approaching.

It may be difficult to differentiate these two conditions if the dog is afraid of noises only when it is alone.

TREATMENT AND FOLLOW-UP

Treatment Options

Treatment for separation anxiety includes the following:

- Increase exercise and play, such as agility training.
- Encourage independence; discourage constant close contact.
- Ignore pestering and demanding behaviors; reinforce calm behaviors.
- Make arrivals and departures low-key; ignore the dog for 30 minutes before departure.
- Stop punishment, because it increases the dog's anxiety level.
- Consider alternative measures, such as pet-sitters, doggy day care, or taking the dog along.
- Consider behavioral modification training, as outlined by your veterinarian.
- Antianxiety medications are often beneficial. Two drugs, clomipramine (*Clomicalm*) and fluoxetine (*Reconcile*) are approved for treating separation anxiety.
- Nonpharmaceutical antianxiety products, such as *Anxiety Wrap* (a stretchy body suit) and *DAP* (a synthetic calming pheromone), may be tried.

Treatment for noise phobia includes the following:

- Ignore the fear behavior.
- Avoid both punishment and reassurance.
- Establish a safe, dark place where sounds are muffled; provide pleasant, calm experiences there.
- Play music with similar tones to mask the phobic sound.
- Consider behavioral modification techniques, such as desensitization and counter-conditioning.
- Antianxiety medications may be beneficial, but no drugs are approved specifically for this condition.
- Nonpharmaceutical antianxiety products (*DAP, Anxiety Wrap, Storm Defender, Thunderband,* and *Mutt Muffs*) may be tried.

Follow-up Care

Maintain a record of the occurrence and its severity to assess response to treatment. Laboratory tests are periodically done in dogs on long-term behavioral medications to monitor for possible side effects.

Prognosis

Many cases significantly improve with treatment; however, several weeks to months are often needed to achieve a satisfactory response. Systematic trials of treatments are commonly needed to determine which strategies and medications are most beneficial for an individual dog.

SPECIAL INSTRUCTIONS:

Petting Intolerance and Status Aggression in Cats

Rhea V. Morgan, DVM, DACVIM (Small Animal), DACVO

BASIC INFORMATION

Description

Petting intolerance is manifested by growling, biting, and scratching at the time of petting. These behaviors may occur when a person initiates petting, when a certain type of petting is performed, or when petting ceases.

Because cats often include humans in their social hierarchy, some assertive cats may also attempt to control people by being "pushy" or "bossy" when held or petted. These latter behaviors may indicate status aggression, especially if they are directed only toward people who do not hold a position of control or leadership over the cat.

Causes

The cause of petting intolerance is not well understood. Genetics may play a role, because some cats are more likely to exhibit intolerance to petting than others. In some instances, the cat may object to petting performed on one or more parts of the body, such as the back or stomach. When cats groom each other, they usually concentrate on the head and neck, so stroking other parts of the body may be foreign to them and may trigger a defensive reaction.

Owner interactions can vary widely with cats that exhibit petting intolerance. In some instances, the owner may have minimal physical contact with the cat, whereas in other situations the owner may attempt to hold and pet the cat for long periods. In some cases, the cat accepts petting for a period of time, but when some threshold is met the cat no longer wants to be petted.

Clinical Signs

With petting intolerance, the cat becomes aggressive only when it is handled and petted. The petting is commonly initiated by the person. The cat may provide subtle clues of its intention to bite or scratch before it acts aggressively. Such clues may include twitching of the tail or ears, rippling of the skin, licking, dilation of the pupils, and low-volume growling.

With status aggression, the cat may actually seek out the owner, block the owner's path, and manifest behaviors that indicate a desire for attention, such as head butting and rubbing. Assertive behaviors may occur, including unwillingness to be moved from a resting place, blocking access to doorways, and mock predatory actions as people pass by.

Diagnostic Tests

The behavioral history commonly indicates that some form of petting intolerance is present, but careful examination of the situation and behaviors may be needed to determine whether status aggression is a component of the condition.

TREATMENT AND FOLLOW-UP

Treatment Options

If certain actions trigger petting intolerance, they should be avoided. For example, if the cat has a certain threshold for duration of petting, then limit the time of petting. If petting a certain area of the body induces aggression, then avoid that area. If the cat becomes aggressive only when the human initiates petting, do not lift, hold, or pet the cat unless it seeks the attention.

Try to separate all petting from physical restraint, so that the two situations are not connected in the cat's mind. Desensitization and counter-conditioning techniques may be tried to improve the cat's acceptance of petting. These techniques can be outlined by your veterinarian.

With status aggression, it is important for the people involved to take a stronger leadership role with the cat. Punishment is inappropriate, but positive reinforcement techniques may be used. With positive reinforcement, rewards are given when the cat behaves in a compliant, appropriate fashion. Your veterinarian can also provide you with techniques for either ignoring or interrupting assertive behaviors. For cats that become highly aroused, medical therapy with fluoxetine, sertraline, clomipramine, amitriptyline, or other similar agents may be tried.

Follow-up Care

It is important to have clear goals about improving petting intolerance. Discuss these goals with your veterinarian, and make sure you understand which corrective actions are appropriate for you to take. Follow-up visits are helpful in providing feedback and making modifications in how you approach the situation. Inadvertent or inappropriate responses on the part of people can make the cat's aggression escalate.

Prognosis

If the cat's needs and tolerance levels can be clearly defined, petting intolerance can often be resolved by modifying how humans interact with the cat. Resolving status aggression requires time, patience, and persistence, but if the cat can be taught to be subordinate to people in the household, then the prognosis is good. In some instances, the owner(s) and the cat may be a poor match, so adoption of another cat with a preference for petting or a less assertive personality may be considered.

SPECIAL INSTRUCTIONS:

Play Aggression in Cats

Rhea V. Morgan, DVM, DACVIM (Small Animal), DACVO

BASIC INFORMATION

Description

During an incidence of causal play, the cat may suddenly begin biting and scratching. The playfulness escalates to an unacceptable level of aggressiveness. The aggressiveness is most often directed toward other cats or humans but may occasionally be directed toward dogs.

Causes

Inadequate or inappropriate socialization of kittens to people and other cats may be a cause. Cats that are bottle-raised have not been taught what is appropriate during play by their mother or littermates. They may not realize that their behavior is unacceptable.

When people use their hands or feet as toys, they may inadvertently teach the cat that it is acceptable to bite or claw those appendages. Genetics may also play a role, because some cats seem to become more aroused than normal when they play.

Clinical Signs

The cat may stalk, chase, and leap onto people, then bite or claw them. The bites can be deep. Prior to the attack, the cat may assume a predatory posture. It may stare at the person or other animal, the pupils may dilate, and the tail may twitch. Moving targets are attacked more often than stationary ones. An episode of apparently normal play between two cats may escalate into fighting.

Diagnostic Tests

The diagnosis is usually made from a careful and thorough history. It is necessary to distinguish this form of aggression from dominance aggression between cats, redirected aggression by a highly aroused cat that cannot reach its preferred target, and intolerance of petting. The circumstances that precipitate these other disorders and the clinical signs associated with them may seem similar, but careful scrutiny of the circumstances and signs often reveals characteristic differences.

TREATMENT AND FOLLOW-UP

Treatment Options

Providing adequate amounts of exercise and time for play helps to prevent this form of aggression. Make sure the cat has a variety of toys. Gently correct young kittens when their behavior becomes unacceptable, and redirect them to playing with their toys.

Discourage cats from batting at your hands or feet during play. If a predatory body posture is seen, stop playing with the cat and avoid any jumping, running, or shouting. Interrupt play between cats that appears to be escalating into more aggressive wrestling or fighting.

For cats that become highly aroused, medical therapy with fluoxetine, sertraline, clomipramine, amitriptyline, or other similar agents may be tried. During the initial phase of therapy, people who may be targets of the attacks should wear protective clothing until the cat's behavior can be trusted.

Follow-up Care

Recheck visits are often scheduled to monitor the cat's response to modifications made to its environment and to any medications used. Some cats can be weaned from medications within 1-3 weeks, whereas others require long-term therapy. Laboratory tests may be recommended to monitor for drug side effects if they are used for a prolonged period. It is important to report any escalation in the cat's aggression to your veterinarian. Some aggressive cats can do serious harm to people.

Prognosis

Prognosis is generally good if appropriate, consistent intervention is applied to the situation. In some cats, the signs resolve completely. In other cats, play aggression can be triggered by anyone who does not follow the steps needed to interrupt and de-escalate the situation. All people who come into contact with these cats should be warned of their behavior and taught the most effective methods of interacting with them.

Be honest with your veterinarian about your feelings toward the cat. If you are afraid of the cat, then discuss other options, such as placing the cat in a different home.

SPECIAL INSTRUCTIONS:

Possessive and Territorial Aggression in Dogs

Rhea V. Morgan, DVM, DACVIM (Small Animal), DACVO

BASIC INFORMATION

Description

Possessive aggression occurs when the dog is defending a cherished object (toy, bone, food). Control of important resources is somewhat normal in dogs, but possessive aggression exceeds the tolerated limits of this behavior.

Territorial aggression is defensive behavior of a geographic area. Although it is normal for dogs to bark at strangers and other animals approaching their home turf, territorial aggression usually involves an unacceptable escalation of protective behaviors. Territorial aggression can involve small spaces (a favored resting place, a room, an automobile) or large ones (yards, farms).

Causes

Dogs that have lived as strays or were allowed to roam free may develop possessive aggression as a means of survival. Lack of appropriate training and behavioral modification of puppies that manifest defense of desired objects can reinforce their possessive behavior, and the behavior can worsen over time.

A combination of genetics and learning probably contributes to territorial aggression. Fear aggression can accompany territorial aggression, and both conditions may worsen at maturity.

Clinical Signs

Possessive aggression occurs only when the dog is defending an object. Signs of possessive and territorial aggression can be a component of dominance aggression, but other signs should also be noted (such as dominance toward the owner and other dogs) with the latter condition.

Signs of territorial aggression include persistent, loud barking; growling; snapping; and biting. These signs occur despite lack of threat by the approaching person or animal. Usually, the aggression is directed toward non–family members, but occasionally the behaviors are directed toward members of the household (human and animal) when certain areas of the house are entered.

Territorial aggressiveness usually increases in intensity as the distance of the approaching individual decreases and does not abate despite attempts at intervention or correction, or signs of submission on the part of the approaching animal. Confinement of the dog to a small space (crate, dog house, chains, or runs) may intensify the signs. Intact male dogs commonly patrol their territories, but the behavior can also occur in neutered males and female dogs.

Diagnostic Tests

Diagnosis is often made based on the history and clinical signs. A detailed behavioral history and observation of the behavior may be needed to confirm the diagnosis. Routine laboratory tests may be recommended to rule out any contributing medical conditions (such as conditions that cause pain or increased appetite).

TREATMENT AND FOLLOW-UP

Treatment Options

Treatment of possessive aggression involves the following:
- If the coveted item can be identified and is nonessential, it can be removed from the environment.
- If the item cannot be removed, then behavioral modification techniques, such as desensitization and counter-conditioning, may be used. These techniques are designed to alter the dog's response to people and other animals that approach the coveted item.

Treatment of territorial aggression may involve the following:
- If possible, do not leave the dog outside unsupervised.
- Start obedience training, using positive reinforcement, and issue appropriate commands when the aggression begins.
- Keep the dog muzzled, on a leash, or confined to an area where it cannot see approaching visitors. Head collars (such as the *Gentle Leader*) may also be helpful when the animal is leashed.
- Neutering of sexually intact animals sometimes helps to decrease the signs, but surgery rarely solves the problem.
- Desensitization and counter-conditioning behavioral techniques may be tried to modify the dog's response to strangers approaching and entering its territory.

When instituting behavioral modification techniques for these two conditions, your veterinarian may establish a program for you or refer your dog to a veterinary behavioral specialist.

Follow-up Care

Behavioral modification techniques can be confusing at first, so check in frequently with your veterinarian if you are unsure how to proceed. After several days, the techniques usually become easier.

Prognosis

Prognosis for these behaviors is variable. Many cases of possessive aggression significantly improve with treatment; however, several weeks to months are often needed to achieve a satisfactory response. Territorial aggression can be more difficult to control and requires sustained, long-term diligence. Systematic trials of treatments are commonly needed to determine which strategies are most beneficial for an individual dog.

SPECIAL INSTRUCTIONS:

SECTION 17

Nutritional Disorders

Section Editor: Joseph W. Bartges, DVM, PhD, DACVIM (Small Animal), DACVN

Feeding Trials for Possible Food Allergy
Homemade Diets
Obesity in Cats

Obesity in Dogs
Overnutrition of Large-Breed Dogs
Taurine Deficiency

Feeding Trials for Possible Food Allergy

Joseph W. Bartges, DVM, PhD, DACVIM (Small Animal), DACVN
Donna M. Raditic, DVM, CVA

BASIC INFORMATION

Description

A food allergy is a reaction to food by the body's immune system. Food allergy is different from food intolerance (such as lactose intolerance) or other adverse reactions to food (such as dietary imbalances, toxicity, or irritation from ingested foreign bodies) that do not involve the immune system.

Causes

In most situations, protein in the food causes the immune reaction. Often the protein source is from animals (such as meat, eggs, or dairy products), but occasionally a carbohydrate source can also be involved. Common foods that induce allergies in dogs include beef, chicken, dairy products, wheat gluten, corn, and soy protein. In cats, common foods that induce allergies include beef, fish, wheat gluten, corn, and dairy products. Dogs and cats can be allergic to more than one food ingredient in a diet.

Clinical Signs

Itchiness, licking, and chewing of the paws, flank, groin, neck, and ears are common signs. Cats often scratch their faces and ears. The itching occurs during all seasons of the year. Some dogs may have recurrent ear inflammation or infections. Gastrointestinal signs such as chronic vomiting, diarrhea, belching, and frequent bowel movements may also occur. It is common for both skin signs and gastrointestinal problems to be present in the same animal, and these problems tend to persist or recur.

Diagnostic Tests

No single, specific test exists that can diagnose a food allergy. Although allergen blood testing is available, these tests are not very accurate and are not a predictably reliable way to diagnose a food allergy or to determine the ingredients to which your dog or cat may be allergic. It is important to provide your veterinarian with a thorough and complete history of all foods and treats your dog or cat eats, including table scraps, chew toys, and medications that are chewable or contain flavorings.

TREATMENT AND FOLLOW-UP

Treatment Options

A dietary food trial may be used to diagnose a food allergy. A food trial involves feeding an elimination diet for 2 to 4 months. The ideal elimination diet includes a new, highly digestible protein source, moderate protein content, and no food additives. Elimination diets include a homemade diet, a commercial diet containing a novel (never fed before) protein and/or carbohydrate source, or a commercial diet composed of hydrolyzed (broken into fragments) protein.

Homemade diets can be formulated by a veterinary nutritionist and are usually composed of a single protein, carbohydrate, and fat source. During the initial food trial phase, the diet does not have to be complete and balanced; however, if your dog or cat responds to this diet, it will need to be balanced if it is given for longer than 2 to 4 months.

Diets with unusual sources of protein and carbohydrate (duck and potato, white fish and rice, venison and potato, rabbit and green peas) can be obtained commercially that are complete, balanced, and designed to be fed long term.

Hydrolyzed protein diets contain proteins that are broken down into pieces that are too small to stimulate the immune system. These diets typically contain a single carbohydrate and fat source and are formulated to be complete and balanced for adult dogs and cats.

During the food trial, no other foods or treats can be fed, including table scraps. Medications that contain flavoring should be changed or discontinued. Your pet must be watched closely to make sure it does not get into the garbage, eat things outside, or obtain food from children in the house, neighbors, or friends. Although an elimination diet must be fed for at least 2 to 4 months, many clinical signs improve in about 6 weeks. Depending on the severity of the clinical signs, medications may initially be needed to decrease itching and inflammation or to treat any secondary bacterial skin infections.

Follow-up Care

For dogs and cats that respond to the initial elimination diet, the diet can be continued if it is complete and balanced and formulated to meet the requirements of an adult dog or cat. If a homemade diet has been given, then further consultation with a veterinary nutritionist may be needed to ensure that the diet is balanced and can be used long term. Eventually, many medications given to relieve signs of the allergy can be discontinued.

Prognosis

Prognosis for treating a food allergy is good as long as the dog or cat is not re-exposed to the food ingredient or ingredients that trigger the immune response.

SPECIAL INSTRUCTIONS:

Homemade Diets

Joseph W. Bartges, DVM, PhD, DACVIM (Small Animal), DACVN
Donna M. Raditic, DVM, CVA

BASIC INFORMATION
Description

Homemade diets are diets made for individual pets by pet owners. Recipes for these diets can be found in textbooks, in magazine articles, and on the Internet, or they can be acquired from a veterinary nutritionist (a specialist certified by the American College of Veterinary Nutrition). Most published recipes are unbalanced and/or incomplete, and consultation with a veterinary nutritionist is encouraged to evaluate the recipe or to formulate a homemade diet based on your and the pet's preferences.

Types of Diets

Homemade diets fall into two basic categories:
- Homemade diet combined with commercially available pet food
- Complete homemade diet, which can be further divided into diets made with raw ingredients, cooked ingredients, or a combination of the two

Rationale for Homemade Diets

There are several reasons to consider feeding a homemade diet:
- Food trial or long-term management of potential adverse food reactions
- Requirement for a special food to manage a disease or combination of diseases that cannot be achieved with commercially available therapeutic diets
- Personal preference by an owner because of negative information about commercial pet foods (erroneous information in most cases); the belief that home cooked foods are better (more natural) than commercial foods; the feeling of a stronger bond between the owner and pet by cooking for the pet; or the belief that home cooking is cheaper (not true in most cases).

Creating Homemade Diets

Several services are available to help owners with formulating and balancing a homemade diet. These resources include the following:

- Angell Memorial Animal Hospital, Boston MA: telephone consultations through (617) 588-7282
- BalanceIt.com
- Petdiets.com
- University of California Davis School of Veterinary Medicine, Nutrition Support Service: telephone consultations through (530) 752-1393
- University of Missouri College of Veterinary Medicine, Small Animal Nutrition: email consultations through datzc@missouri.edu
- University of Tennessee Veterinary Nutrition Service: email consultations through utvns@utk.edu
- Virginia-Maryland Regional College of Veterinary Medicine, Small Animal Nutrition Service: referrals made through (540) 231-7666

When making a homemade diet, do not deviate from the recipe provided to you, because this could make the diet unbalanced or incomplete. Veterinary nutritionists can formulate several versions of a homemade diet to provide variety for the pet. Personal hygiene is important when mixing or feeding these diets, especially when feeding raw ingredients. A separate set of food preparation equipment (bowls, mixing spoons, measuring cups, knives) should be used for preparing homemade diets for pets. Prepare the diet in a special area, away from where human food is prepared.

TREATMENT AND FOLLOW-UP

Follow-up Care

Dogs and cats that are fed a homemade diet are evaluated periodically by a physical examination and laboratory tests. Bowel movements should be reasonably formed, and animals should maintain body weight and body condition while on the diet. If any problems or abnormalities develop, consultation with a veterinary nutritionist is worthwhile to evaluate or re-evaluate a homemade diet. If necessary, a sample of the homemade diet can be sent to a food analysis laboratory to determine amounts of nutrients in the diet.

SPECIAL INSTRUCTIONS:

Obesity in Cats

Joseph W. Bartges, DVM, PhD, DACVIM (Small Animal), DACVN

BASIC INFORMATION

Description

Obesity is defined as body weight in excess of 15% above normal resulting from the accumulation of fat. It occurs in 25-50% of cats in the United States. Associated health risks include fatty liver syndrome, diabetes mellitus, musculoskeletal and cardiovascular diseases, high blood pressure, high fat levels in the blood, possible anesthetic and surgical complications, decreased heat tolerance and stamina, and reproductive problems.

Causes

Obesity occurs when energy intake exceeds energy expenditure and other risk factors are present, such as neutering and dietary factors. Feeding calorically dense, highly palatable, high-fat diets and free-choice feeding increase the risk of obesity.

Clinical Signs

Affected cats have excessive fat accumulation around their neck, over the tail-head, along the underside, and in the abdominal cavity. Difficulty moving or breathing, exercise intolerance, urinary or fecal incontinence, unkempt appearance, and pressure sores may occur.

Diagnostic Tests

Cats are usually tested for liver disease and diabetes mellitus (sugar diabetes). Other tests may be recommended to assess for obesity-related diseases in other organs.

TREATMENT AND FOLLOW-UP

Treatment Options

Weight reduction programs involve a multistep approach that includes good owner commitment, a feeding plan, and an exercise plan. In order for the animal to lose weight, it is necessary for energy expenditure to be greater than energy intake. This is accomplished by increasing exercise and by feeding a diet that is lower in fat and higher in fiber.

Nutrients in diets formulated for weight loss in cats are designed to decrease energy intake, so that weight loss occurs without inducing other nutrient deficiencies. In order to achieve weight loss, a diet is fed that meets resting energy requirements of the cat at its ideal weight. Weight loss is better achieved with meal feeding rather than free-choice feeding. It is also important to limit treats and not to allow access to other pets' food or to human food.

Alternatively, diets that are higher in fat and protein and lower in carbohydrates compared with adult maintenance foods can be fed. When feeding this type of diet, food intake must also be decreased. A low-fat, high-fiber diet can be started, and if weight loss is not achieved, the alternative diet can be tried.

Getting a cat to exercise can be difficult. It helps to place meals in locations that force the cat to climb up or down or to jump. Some cats will chase toys or lights, and feeders are available that force the cat to play with them in order to reach the food.

Getting a cat to lose weight in a multicat household where other cats are not obese is even more difficult. Feed the obese cat separately from the nonobese cats. The nonobese cats' food can be placed in a large box with a narrow opening that is too small to allow the obese cat to enter. Radiocontrolled devices can be used that allow the nonobese cats (who wear special collars) entry into areas through a gate that has a radio receiver. Pick up leftover food so that the obese cat does not eat the other cats' food.

Follow-up Care

Body weight is monitored every 2 weeks during weight loss, and the diet and exercise are adjusted to achieve a loss of 1-2% of body weight per week. Many cats lose weight in a stairstep fashion: They lose quite a bit over the first 2 weeks, do not lose much over the next 2 weeks, and then lose quite a bit again. Alterations in diet are not usually made unless weight has remained unchanged at two sequential examinations. Laboratory tests are done periodically. If the cat also has diabetes, fructosamine and glucose tests may be recommended. Insulin dosage may need to be decreased or discontinued over time as weight loss occurs.

When the desired target weight is reached, body weight is monitored monthly to ensure the ideal weight is maintained. The maintenance diet is usually an adult diet designed to maintain the lower weight. These diets are typically higher in fiber and lower in fat than most over-the-counter, adult maintenance diets. Certain diets labeled as *light* may be used, but they are not as effective. The alternative weight-loss diet (high fat and protein, low carbohydrate) can also be continued. Treats, snacks, and table scraps should comprise less than 5% of total caloric intake.

Prognosis

Weight loss is more difficult to achieve in obese cats than in obese dogs. Working with a veterinarian is important because of the many obesity-related diseases that occur in cats. Prevention of obesity in growing cats is also very important.

SPECIAL INSTRUCTIONS:

Obesity in Dogs

Joseph W. Bartges, DVM, PhD, DACVIM (Small Animal), DACVN

BASIC INFORMATION

Description

Obesity is defined as body weight in excess of 15% above normal resulting from an accumulation of fat. It occurs in 25-50% of dogs in the United States. Associated health risks include musculoskeletal and cardiovascular diseases, hypertension (high blood pressure), hyperlipidemia (excessive levels of fat in the bloodstream), higher incidences of bladder and mammary (breast) cancer, possible anesthetic and surgical complications, decreased heat tolerance and stamina, and reproductive problems.

Causes

Obesity occurs when energy intake exceeds energy expenditure and other risk factors are present. Certain breeds, such as the Labrador retriever, cairn terrier, American cocker spaniel, dachshund, basset hound, and beagle, as well as females and middle-aged animals, have an increased incidence of obesity. Neutering increases the risk of obesity. Dietary factors also play a role. Feeding calorically dense, highly palatable, high-fat diets and free-choice feeding increase the risk. Hypothyroidism (low thyroid levels) and hyperadrenocorticism (high blood cortisone levels) are also associated with obesity.

Clinical Signs

Dogs that are obese have excessive fat accumulation around the neck, over the tail-head, along the underside, and in the abdominal cavity. Obesity may be associated with difficulty moving or breathing, exercise intolerance, urinary or fecal incontinence, unkempt appearance, and pressure sores.

Diagnostic Tests

Dogs are usually tested for hypothyroidism and hyperadrenocorticism. Other tests may be recommended to assess for obesity-related diseases in other organs and to search for any underlying risk factors.

TREATMENT AND FOLLOW-UP

Treatment Options

If obesity is associated with hypothyroidism or hyperadrenocorticism, treatment is started for these conditions. Weight reduction programs involve a multistep approach that includes good owner commitment, a feeding plan, and an exercise plan. In order for the animal to lose weight, it is necessary for energy expenditure to be greater than energy intake. This is accomplished by increasing exercise (increased energy expenditure) and by feeding a diet that is lower in fat and higher in fiber (lower energy intake) than typical adult dog foods.

Nutrients in diets formulated for weight loss in dogs are designed to decrease energy intake so that weight loss occurs without inducing other nutrient deficiencies. In order to achieve weight loss, a diet is fed that meets resting energy requirements of the dog at its ideal weight. Weight loss is better achieved with the feeding of meals rather than free-choice feeding. It is also important to limit treats and not to allow access to other pets' food or human food.

An approved medication, dirlotapide (*Slentrol*), is available to facilitate weight loss in dogs. It induces weight loss by decreasing appetite. In clinical studies, it was found to be effective and safe, although some dogs may vomit when the drug is initially started. Dosages of dirlotapide are adjusted so that an average of 1% weight loss occurs per week until the desired target weight is reached. Once the target weight is reached, diet and exercise are adjusted and dirlotapide is continued until the target body weight remains stable. When the weight maintenance phase has been reached, dirlotapide is discontinued, and the dog is placed on a maintenance dietary and exercise regimen.

Follow-up Care

Body weight is monitored every 2 weeks, and the diet, exercise, and dirlotapide (if used) are adjusted to cause a 1-2% loss of weight per week. Many dogs lose weight in a stairstep fashion. They lose quite a bit over a 2-week period and then do not lose much over the next 2 weeks. Alterations in diet and dirlotapide are not usually done unless weight has not changed at two sequential examinations.

After the desired target weight is reached, body weight is monitored monthly to ensure that weight is maintained. The maintenance diet is usually an adult diet designed to help maintain the lower weight. This diet is typically higher in fiber and lower in fat than average over-the-counter adult diets, but it is not intended for weight loss. Certain diets labeled as *light* may be used, but they are not as effective. Treats, snacks, and table scraps should comprise less than 5% of the total caloric intake.

Prognosis

Weight loss is difficult to achieve in some dogs and requires prolonged dedication and dietary restrictions. Prevention of obesity in growing and adult animals is very important and is often easier to achieve than weight reduction.

SPECIAL INSTRUCTIONS:

Overnutrition of Large-Breed Dogs

Joseph W. Bartges, DVM, PhD, DACVIM (Small Animal), DACVN

BASIC INFORMATION

Description

Overnutrition of large- and giant-breed puppies during their rapid growth phase can result in developmental orthopedic disease (DOD).

Causes

The rate of growth, certain nutrients, food consumption, and feeding methods all affect the development of orthopedic disease. Excess energy intake results in rapid growth and obesity, which are associated with DOD, so it is important to maintain optimal body condition during growth. Excessive intake of calcium (greater than 3% of the dry matter of the diet) also increases the risk of DOD. Excessive intake can occur when supplemental calcium is given to large- and giant-breed dogs to promote skeletal growth. Free-choice feeding (compared with limited-meal feeding) has also been shown to increase the risk of DOD.

Clinical Signs

DOD can manifest as hip dysplasia, osteochondrosis dissecans, joint laxity, ligament laxity, or hyperextended joints. A common clinical sign of these diseases is often lameness of the affected leg or legs. For other signs, see the handouts on these individual diseases.

Diagnostic Tests

A history of high energy intake and/or calcium supplementation in a large- or giant-breed puppy with lameness often allows a suspicion of DOD. Various diagnostic tests are available for the diseases involved in DOD, but x-rays of the affected leg are often recommended.

TREATMENT AND FOLLOW-UP

Treatment Options

Treatment of DOD depends on the specific orthopedic problem present. Treatment options may involve medications or surgery. Physical therapy and changing the dog to an appropriate diet are also required. Diets formulated for large- and giant-breed dogs during growth are available that may help prevent DOD. These diets are typically lower in calories, fat, and calcium but contain similar protein content when compared with standard growth diets. Although calcium intake alone is important, the dietary calcium-to-phosphorus ratio is even more important. This ratio in the food should be between 1.1:1.0 and 1.5:1.0. Large- and giant-breed growth diets are usually fed until the dog is $1\frac{1}{2}$ to 2 years of age.

Follow-up Care

Periodic physical examinations are often performed to monitor body weight and condition. Additional follow-up testing and monitoring depend on the specific disease present and the treatments chosen for that condition.

Prognosis

Prognosis depends on the severity and location of the DOD problem. Even with treatment, degenerative arthritis may develop at a later date in affected joints.

SPECIAL INSTRUCTIONS:

Taurine Deficiency

Joseph W. Bartges, DVM, PhD, DACVIM (Small Animal), DACVN

BASIC INFORMATION
Description
Taurine is a beta-sulfonic amino acid that is an essential nutrient for cats and, in certain situations, for dogs. Taurine deficiency has been associated with heart disease in cats and in certain breeds of dogs. Cats cannot make taurine from other amino acids, and they lose taurine in their bile. Taurine is found primarily in animal-based products, and commercial cat foods have extra taurine added to them.

Causes
Taurine deficiency occurs in cats and dogs when loss of taurine exceeds the intake of taurine. In dogs, deficiency most commonly occurs when homemade vegetarian diets are fed, although some dogs have a breed-associated risk. Cats may become deficient if they eat foods formulated for dogs or if they do not absorb taurine for some reason.

Clinical Signs
In cats, taurine deficiency is associated with retinal degeneration, dilated cardiomyopathy (a disease of heart muscle), and reproductive problems. The retinal degeneration may result in blindness. In pregnant queens, taurine deficiency is associated with abortion, stillbirth, and birthing of kittens that do not survive. If live kittens are born to queens (mothers) that are taurine deficient, they often have skeletal abnormalities, such as a curved spine and small stature.

In certain breeds of dogs, taurine deficiency is associated with dilated cardiomyopathy. The American cocker spaniel, dogs that are prone to develop cystine or urate bladder stones (such as English bulldogs), and possibly the golden retriever and the Portuguese water dog may develop this type of heart disease. (These breeds are not the same as those that develop the large-breed–related form of dilated cardiomyopathy.)

Diagnostic Tests
Taurine deficiency may be suspected based on a dietary history and the presence of clinical signs. The retinal degeneration seen in cats begins with lesions in the retina that are unique to this disease and may be discovered on an eye examination. X-rays and a heart ultrasound (echocardiogram) are often needed to diagnose the presence of dilated cardiomyopathy in both dogs and cats. X-rays also help identify skeletal abnormalities. If reproductive problems are present, evaluation for other causes of decreased conception rates or stillbirths is needed.

Demonstration of low taurine levels in plasma (preferred in dogs) or in whole blood (dogs, preferred in cats) helps confirm the diagnosis. In cats, the plasma taurine concentration can decrease below the normal range after less than 24 hours of fasting; therefore, sampling of whole blood is preferred.

TREATMENT AND FOLLOW-UP

Treatment Options
Although taurine deficiency is now a rare cause of dilated cardiomyopathy in cats, taurine is inexpensive and safe, so it is often given orally for an 8-week trial when dilated cardiomyopathy is diagnosed. Taurine is also administered to any dog that develops cardiomyopathy and is not a common breed for the large-breed form of the disorder. Taurine is usually given two to three times daily, and the dose is based on the dog's body weight.

Commercial dry cat foods are required to contain 0.1% taurine on a dry matter basis, and canned foods are required to contain 0.2% on a dry matter basis. Canned diets are required to contain more taurine than dry diets because canned diets promote the growth of intestinal bacteria that degrade taurine.

Follow-up Care
For cats and dogs with dilated cardiomyopathy, clinical signs and echocardiography are typically monitored every 1 to 2 months. Notify your veterinarian if any signs related to the heart recur or worsen. Rechecks are also periodically needed to monitor retinal changes in affected cats. Measurement of taurine levels may be repeated to ensure that they are in the normal range and to make decisions regarding adjustment of medications.

Prognosis
Taurine-deficient dilated cardiomyopathy in cats can be cured with appropriate treatment. In dogs, the disease may improve, but it is not reversible.

Retinal changes that are present at the time of diagnosis are not reversible, but taurine supplementation does prevent further degeneration of the retina. Blindness associated with this deficiency is permanent.

SPECIAL INSTRUCTIONS:

SECTION 18

Toxicology

Section Editor: Petra A. Volmer, DVM, MS, DABVT, DABT

Acetaminophen Toxicosis
Amitraz Toxicosis
Antifreeze Poisoning
Avermectin Toxicosis
Bread Dough Poisoning
Chocolate and Methylxanthine Toxicosis
Cholecalciferol Rodenticide Poisoning
Grape and Raisin Toxicosis in Dogs
Herbal Poisonings
Lead Poisoning
Macadamia Nut Toxicosis in Dogs

Metaldehyde Poisoning
Nonsteroidal Anti-Inflammatory Drug Toxicosis
Organophosphorus and Carbamate Insecticide Poisoning
Paintball Toxicosis
Poisoning from Illicit Human Drugs: Depressants
Poisoning from Illicit Human Drugs: Opioids
   and Stimulants
Pyrethrin and Pyrethroid Toxicosis
Strychnine Poisoning
Xylitol Toxicosis in Dogs
Zinc Toxicosis

Acetaminophen Toxicosis

Petra A. Volmer, DVM, MS, DABVT, DABT

BASIC INFORMATION

Description

Acetaminophen is a non-aspirin pain reliever found in more than 200 formulations. The most recognized trade name is *Tylenol*. Acetaminophen is often found in combination with other drugs, such as antihistamines and decongestants.

Causes and Toxicity

Cats are most sensitive to the effects of acetaminophen, although dogs can also be poisoned. Cats lack an enzyme necessary to detoxify acetaminophen, so it can accumulate quickly. The ability of the blood to carry oxygen is most commonly affected in cats. The blood turns a brown or gray color and is unable to transport oxygen to body tissues. This condition is called *methemoglobinemia*. Dogs generally require higher doses to be poisoned, and the liver tends to be the most affected organ.

Clinical Signs

Within 2-4 hours after exposure, cats may develop a purplish-brown or gray discoloration to the gums, accompanied by weakness, rapid heart rate, and rapid breathing. In some cases, cats drool, vomit, or develop swelling of the face or paws. The blood may appear brown, gray, or black, and the urine may be discolored. Clinical signs of anemia and decreased urine production from kidney failure are also possible.

In dogs, vomiting and jaundice (yellow discoloration to the whites of the eyes and gums) may occur with liver toxicity. Dogs may also develop a reduction in the ability of the blood to carry oxygen, but at higher doses than those that cause liver failure. Occasionally, dogs develop dry eye (keratoconjunctivitis sicca) from decreased production of tears.

Diagnostic Tests

A tentative diagnosis is based on a history of exposure to acetaminophen, consistent clinical signs, and characteristic discoloration of the blood or urine. Laboratory tests often indicate an anemia in cats and liver damage in dogs. Specialized blood tests to detect methemoglobinemia or to measure acetaminophen levels can be performed by an outside laboratory. Other laboratory tests, x-rays, an abdominal ultrasound, and liver biopsy (in dogs) may be needed to rule out other diseases that cause similar clinical signs.

TREATMENT AND FOLLOW-UP

Treatment Options

Induction of vomiting may be recommended if the exposure was recent (within 1 hour). Vomiting should be induced only under the direction of a veterinarian. Activated charcoal may also be administered by mouth to help bind acetaminophen in the gut and prevent its absorption into the body. In many cases, hospitalization is required for intensive treatment and monitoring. Several medications (such as acetylcysteine, ascorbic acid, or cimetidine) may be administered to counter the effects of the acetaminophen by assisting the body in metabolizing and removing the acetaminophen. Supportive measures are usually needed and may include intravenous fluids, oxygen therapy, whole blood transfusions, and agents to assist the liver.

Follow-up Care

Laboratory tests are used to monitor for methemoglobinemia, anemia, jaundice, and liver and kidney function. Intensive monitoring may be required initially if liver or kidney failure occurs and may be continued for some time as the animal recovers. In dogs, tear production may also be monitored for several days. Keep all products containing acetaminophen out of the reach of pets.

Prognosis

For minor toxicoses, prognosis is good with prompt, aggressive treatment. For cases with prolonged or severe methemoglobinemia, anemia, liver damage, or kidney failure, prognosis is guarded (uncertain). The first 3-4 days following intoxication are critical, and animals that start to improve within that period have a higher chance of recovery.

SPECIAL INSTRUCTIONS:

Amitraz Toxicosis

Petra A. Volmer, DVM, MS, DABVT, DABT

BASIC INFORMATION

Description

Amitraz is used to control ticks, mites, and lice on dogs. It is available as a dip (*Mitaban*) and a collar (*Preventic*) and is an ingredient in a topical preparation (*Promeris*).

Causes and Toxicity

Clinical signs may develop following labeled use of the topical products on pets or from ingestion of the collars. Amitraz should not be used on cats. In general, toy and small-breed dogs are more susceptible to the adverse effects of amitraz even with appropriate use.

Clinical Signs

Signs usually begin within 2-4 hours but can be delayed as long as 12 hours following exposure. Signs can include vomiting, sedation, disorientation, unsteady gait, decreased gut movement (motility), slow heart rate, coma, and seizures. In severe cases, death may occur. Amitraz may also increase blood glucose levels, so care must be taken when using it on dogs that are diabetic.

Diagnostic Tests

Diagnosis is based on a history of exposure and the presence of consistent clinical signs. Analysis of amitraz may be performed on urine, plasma, skin, blood, or stomach contents. Such analyses cannot be performed at the veterinary hospital or clinic but require the use of an outside laboratory. Laboratory and other tests may be recommended to rule out other conditions that cause similar clinical signs.

TREATMENT AND FOLLOW-UP

Treatment Options

For topical exposures following use of a dip or topical formulation, the animal is bathed in a liquid dish detergent. Dogs that have ingested a collar may benefit from induction of vomiting under the guidance of a veterinarian. In some cases, retrieval of collar fragments from the stomach or intestines through endoscopy (use of a flexible viewing scope passed into the stomach through the mouth) or surgery (abdominal incision) may be warranted.

Treatment is symptomatic for the patient exhibiting clinical signs. The veterinarian may use a reversal agent, such as yohimbine or atipamezole, to hasten recovery. Animals exhibiting clinical signs usually require hospitalization for treatment and supportive care, such as intravenous fluids and anticonvulsants. Close monitoring is also required until the animal recovers.

Follow-up Care

Sedation following amitraz dips usually lasts about 24 hours but can persist up to 72 hours. If amitraz poisoning is diagnosed quickly and reversal agents are administered, recovery can occur within 24 hours in many animals. Recovery may be prolonged (several days) if treatment is delayed or ingested material is not removed from the gut. No residual effects are expected following recovery.

Prognosis

Prognosis is good for animals receiving prompt treatment. Those with prolonged or severe signs have a guarded (uncertain) prognosis.

SPECIAL INSTRUCTIONS:

Antifreeze Poisoning

Petra A. Volmer, DVM, MS, DABVT, DABT

BASIC INFORMATION
Description

Antifreeze products can contain ethylene glycol, propylene glycol, methanol, or a combination of these agents. Most automotive antifreeze liquids contain ethylene glycol and pose the greatest hazard to pets; they are often dyed a fluorescent green. Some relatively safe antifreeze products are available that contain propylene glycol, and they are dyed a blue or green color. Propylene glycol is considered a GRAS (generally recognized as safe) substance and is found in many food and pharmaceutical products, such as toothpaste and cosmetics. When ingested in large amounts, however, it can still cause illness. Methanol is present in windshield washer fluids as well as gasoline antifreezes.

Causes and Toxicity

All three compounds (ethylene glycol, propylene glycol, and methanol) are metabolized in the body to acids. Therefore, animals can develop a serious metabolic condition known as *acidosis* after drinking these fluids. In addition, all of these compounds can depress the brain and cause "drunken" behavior, mental depression, and coma.

Of the three compounds, ethylene glycol is of the most serious concern for pets. It is said to have a "sweet" taste that is attractive to dogs and cats. When it is metabolized by the body, crystals form that are deposited in the kidneys. It is not uncommon for this crystal formation to be so severe that kidney failure and subsequent death occurs.

Clinical Signs

Signs can occur within 1 hour after ingestion. Animals may appear "drunk" and wobbly. Vomiting and increased urination may occur initially. In many instances, mild, early signs are overlooked by animal caretakers, delaying life-saving treatment.

With ethylene glycol ingestion, dogs may appear to recover for a brief period, but cats often remain mentally depressed. Within 4-6 hours, more serious changes can develop, such as acidosis, rapid breathing, serious vomiting, decreased body temperature, heart arrhythmias (irregular heart rhythms), and severe depression or coma. Anywhere from 12-36 hours after ingestion, kidney failure may develop with decreased urine production. The kidney damage is often irreversible and fatal.

Diagnostic Tests

Diagnosis is based on a history of exposure and appropriate clinical signs. Because many ethylene glycol formulations contain a fluorescent dye, muzzles, paws, urine, and vomitus may fluoresce (glow) under ultraviolet (UV) light. Initial laboratory tests may show nonspecific changes or evidence of early metabolic and kidney abnormalities. Test kits are available that measure the concentration of ethylene glycol in the blood. In the absence of a commercial ethylene glycol test kit, a human hospital laboratory may be able to perform this analysis.

Later in the clinical course, laboratory tests may show severe abnormalities in kidney function. An ultrasound and/or biopsy of the kidney may be recommended to search for changes compatible with ethylene glycol poisoning. More tests may be indicated to rule out other diseases and toxins that can cause similar clinical signs.

TREATMENT AND FOLLOW-UP
Treatment Options

Because antifreeze products are rapidly absorbed, vomiting is induced only if no clinical signs are present and should be performed only under the direction of your veterinarian. Activated charcoal does not bind antifreeze well, so it is not usually indicated. Animals that exhibit signs of inebriation or have a positive ethylene glycol test are often hospitalized for monitoring of body temperature, breathing, heart rate and rhythm, and urine production. For propylene glycol and methanol ingestions, supportive care generally results in full recovery with no residual effects.

Because every moment that passes means further metabolism of ethylene glycol, all ethylene glycol exposures are considered to be medical emergencies. Animals are hospitalized for administration of intravenous fluids to protect the kidneys. Medications to prevent further metabolism of ethylene glycol (into products that harm the kidney) may be given, such as ethanol (grain alcohol) or fomepizole (*Antizol-Vet*). Fomepizole is approved for use only in dogs but has shown some success in cats as well. Intensive supportive treatment is usually needed for several days, especially if acute kidney failure develops. In severe cases, your veterinarian may recommend referral to a specialty facility for dialysis treatment, if it is available.

Follow-up Care

Intensive monitoring of urine output and laboratory tests are usually needed for several days. Animals that survive may have residual, chronic kidney damage that requires periodic monitoring.

Prognosis

Prognosis is good for animals ingesting methanol or propylene glycol. If the animal ingested a large amount of ethylene glycol or if treatment was delayed, the prognosis is grave and death is likely.

SPECIAL INSTRUCTIONS:

Avermectin Toxicosis

Petra A. Volmer, DVM, MS, DABVT, DABT

BASIC INFORMATION

Description

Avermectins are a group of antiparasite agents (parasiticides) used in the prevention of heartworm (*Dirofilaria immitis*) disease and in the treatment of infestations by mites such as scabies (sarcoptic mange), demodicosis (*Demodex* mites), and ear mites (*Otodectes* mites). Certain members of the avermectins can also be found in ant and roach baits. Some common avermectins are ivermectin (*Heartgard, Ivomec, Tri-Heart*), selamectin (*Revolution*), moxidectin (*Proheart*), milbemycin (*Interceptor*), and abamectin (*Avomec, Raid, Hot Shot MaxAttrax*).

Causes and Toxicity

The avermectins exert their effect by mimicking inhibitory neurotransmitters in the central nervous system (brain and spinal cord), which results in depression of brain activity and death of the parasite. Avermectins can have the same effect in animals. Most animals are quite resistant to the effects of these compounds, because they do not accumulate in the brains of animals. However, dogs with a deficiency in P-glycoprotein, an enzyme that helps remove avermectins from the brain, are exquisitely sensitive to these compounds. The avermectins accumulate and exert their inhibitory effect on the brain, and this action is reflected by the clinical signs.

In general, certain herding breeds of dogs are more likely to have the *MRD1* genetic mutation that causes a deficiency in P-glycoprotein. Such breeds include the collie, Australian shepherd, Shetland sheepdog, and border collie. Individuals of other breeds, such as the Old English sheepdog, German shepherd dog, long-haired whippet, and a variety of mixed-breed dogs, may also have the *MRD1* mutation and exhibit sensitivity to avermectins.

Most cases of avermectin toxicosis have resulted from administration of high doses of the drug (often of the oral livestock product) or from ingestion of horse dewormer paste by farm dogs. In some cases, the avermectin compound was injected subcutaneously as a treatment for mange.

Clinical Signs

Signs can occur within several hours after exposure. Initial signs include lethargy, pupil dilation, and staggered gait. These signs may be followed by apparent blindness (which is often reversible with time), tremors, decreased body temperature, slow heart rate, coma, and death. Seizures may also occur. Signs may persist for days or even weeks in severe cases.

Diagnostic Tests

Diagnosis is based on a history of exposure to an avermectin-containing product and consistent clinical signs. Breed predisposition also increases the likelihood of the diagnosis. There are no rapid tests for the avermectins that can be done in the veterinary clinic. Analyses may be performed on various body tissues by outside laboratories. Laboratory and other tests may be recommended to rule out other causes of similar clinical signs. A genetic test for the *MDR1* gene mutation is available on a cheek swab sample from a dog with suspected P-glycoprotein deficiency.

TREATMENT AND FOLLOW-UP

Treatment Options

Your veterinarian may induce vomiting in the animal if an avermectin-containing product has been ingested and the pet is not exhibiting clinical signs. This is followed by administration of activated charcoal to decrease absorption of the compound into the body. Administration of activated charcoal also hastens elimination of the avermectin.

If the dog is exhibiting clinical signs, treatment is directed at controlling those signs and may include assisting breathing (placing the animal on a ventilator), administering intravenous fluids, maintaining body temperature, and providing nutrition. In severe cases, the animal may be in a coma-like state for weeks and will require good nursing care to prevent the formation of bedsores.

Follow-up Care

The status of nervous and heart systems must be monitored continuously while the animal is showing clinical signs. Frequent follow-up visits may be needed after your pet is discharged to monitor its progress and to ensure that it continues to recover without complications.

Prognosis

A complete recovery is expected in animals receiving prompt and aggressive treatment, especially if the clinical signs are mild. Although signs may persist for prolonged periods (days to weeks), recovery can occur in many cases with appropriate treatment.

SPECIAL INSTRUCTIONS:

Bread Dough Poisoning

Petra A. Volmer, DVM, MS, DABVT, DABT

BASIC INFORMATION

Description

The ingestion of raw dough used for baking bread or pizza crusts can pose a hazard to dogs.

Causes and Toxicity

Dough containing yeast rises in the warm, humid environment of the stomach. Expanding dough can compromise blood flow to the stomach wall and decrease blood return to the heart. Yeast fermentation releases ethanol, an alcohol, which can make a dog act "drunk" or intoxicated.

Clinical Signs

Dogs may go through the motions of vomiting or retching without bringing up any stomach contents. The abdomen may become enlarged and distended. The dog may become mentally subdued and wobbly when walking, due to the production of ethanol. In severe cases, the dog may collapse and become comatose.

Diagnostic Tests

Diagnosis is based on evidence of ingestion of uncooked yeast dough and compatible clinical signs. X-rays of the abdomen may reveal foreign material in the stomach and help to rule out bloating and twisting of the stomach from other causes. Laboratory tests may be recommended to assess the effects on other organs and to rule out other causes of mental depression and collapse.

TREATMENT AND FOLLOW-UP

Treatment Options

Your veterinarian may recommend that vomiting be induced if the ingestion was recent (within 1-2 hours). This should be done only under the direction of a veterinarian. In severe cases, the animal may require hospitalization for fluid therapy and supportive care. The stomach may be pumped or surgery may be performed to remove the dough, if a large quantity was ingested.

Follow-up Care

Monitoring of the animal may be required for 1-3 days until it returns to normal. Keep all yeast dough out of the reach of dogs that are prone to ingesting foreign objects.

Prognosis

If the animal is treated early, the prognosis is excellent for a full recovery. If a large amount of yeast dough was consumed or if treatment was delayed, then the prognosis is less favorable.

SPECIAL INSTRUCTIONS:

Chocolate and Methylxanthine Toxicosis

Petra A. Volmer, DVM, MS, DABVT, DABT

BASIC INFORMATION

Description

Chocolate contains caffeine and theobromine, both of which are members of the methylxanthine group of compounds. Another member of this class is theophylline. The methylxanthines occur naturally in several plants, such as the leaves of *Thea sinensis* (used to make tea), the seeds of *Theobroma cacao* (used to make chocolate), and the fruit of *Coffea arabica* (used to make coffee). Theophylline is present in tea and some medications. Caffeine is found in coffee, tea, chocolate, colas, the herb guarana, and some human stimulant drugs. Theobromine is present in chocolate, cocoa beans, cocoa bean hulls (cocoa bean mulch), colas, and tea.

Causes and Toxicity

Methylxanthines as a group act as central nervous system stimulants. They are rapidly absorbed from the gastrointestinal tract. The most common cause of poisoning in small animals is eating (ingestion of) chocolate, although toxicity has occurred following ingestion of coffee grounds, tea bags, or human medications. In addition to their stimulant effects, many chocolate products contain high levels of fat that may cause gastrointestinal upset and pancreatitis. Cocoa powder contains the highest amounts of caffeine and theobromine, followed by unsweetened baker's chocolate, semisweet chocolate, and milk chocolate. White chocolate contains negligible amounts of methylxanthines but can still pose a risk of gastrointestinal upset and pancreatitis.

Clinical Signs

The most common signs are restlessness and hyperactivity, vomiting, diarrhea, increased drinking and urinating, and a rapid heart rate. Animals may begin pacing and are unable to sit still. They may pant and appear anxious. Hyperactivity may progress to tremors and seizures if large amounts are ingested.

Diagnostic Tests

Diagnosis is based on a history of recent ingestion along with consistent clinical signs. The vomitus may contain evidence of the substance ingested. Various body tissues can be analyzed for methylxanthines; however, this test cannot be performed at the veterinary hospital or clinic, and samples must be sent to an outside laboratory. Laboratory and other tests may be recommended to rule out other causes of similar clinical signs.

TREATMENT AND FOLLOW-UP

Treatment Options

In some cases, your veterinarian may recommend that you induce vomiting at home. This should be done only under the direction of your veterinarian. Depending on the amount ingested and signs the animal is exhibiting, activated charcoal may be administered. Activated charcoal helps prevent absorption of the methylxanthine agent from the gut. Clinical signs are treated symptomatically and may require intravenous fluids, as well as medications to control hyperactivity, seizures, vomiting, and a rapid heart rate.

Follow-up Care

Care must be taken to ensure that methylxanthine-containing products are not accessible to pets. Chocolate poisoning is especially a risk during holidays such as Halloween, Christmas, Valentine's Day, and Easter.

Prognosis

In most cases, recovery occurs within 24-48 hours with appropriate treatment. The prognosis is guarded (uncertain) if large amounts are ingested, if treatment is delayed, or if the animal is exhibiting severe signs.

SPECIAL INSTRUCTIONS:

Cholecalciferol Rodenticide Poisoning

Petra A. Volmer, DVM, MS, DABVT, DABT

BASIC INFORMATION

Description

Cholecalciferol is also known as *vitamin D3*. It is formulated into rat and mouse baits and marketed under brand names such as *Rampage, Quintox, Rat-B-Gon,* and *Mouse-B-Gon.* Ingestion of (eating) these baits can result in life-threatening illness and even death in pets.

In most cases, the cholecalciferol found in vitamin supplements is not considered a serious risk for companion animals, even when massive ingestion has occurred.

Causes and Toxicity

Cholecalciferol is converted in the liver and kidneys to its active form. The active form causes calcium and phosphorus levels in the blood to rise through a series of interactions in the intestines, kidneys, and bone. Severe elevations in calcium and phosphorus can result in mineralization (deposition of calcium or calcification) within soft tissues such as the kidneys, gut, tendons, heart, and blood vessels. As little as ½ tablespoon of cholecalciferol bait can be enough to cause signs in a 20-pound (9.5-kg) dog.

Clinical Signs

Lethargy, vomiting, diarrhea (sometimes bloody), lack of appetite, and possibly an increase in drinking and urination are usually seen within 36-48 hours but can appear as soon as 12 hours after ingestion of the bait. Acute kidney failure with inability to produce urine may occur by 24-48 hours following large ingestions. Sudden death may occur, in an animal that previously appeared to recover, due to soft tissue mineralization and rupture of a calcified blood vessel such as the aorta.

Diagnostic Tests

Diagnosis is based on a history of exposure, consistent clinical signs, and laboratory findings. After the ingestion, there is a rapid (within 12-72 hours) and moderate increase in the blood phosphorus level, followed in a few hours by a more severe increase in calcium. Soft tissue mineralization may occur at this time and may sometimes be detected with x-rays or an ultrasound. Measurement of the active component of cholecalciferol may be done at certain laboratories. Other tests may be recommended to rule out other causes of elevated calcium, elevated phosphorus, and acute kidney failure.

TREATMENT AND FOLLOW-UP

Treatment Options

Treatment is aimed at removal of the poison (known as *decontamination*), reduction of calcium and phosphorus levels, and treatment of any kidney failure. If the ingestion occurred recently, vomiting may be induced to remove all the poison in the stomach, and activated charcoal may be given to prevent the poison from entering the bloodstream.

Intravenous administration of saline is used to lower blood calcium and may be given for several days or until calcium returns to normal. Other drugs, such as diuretics (furosemide) and steroids (prednisone), may also be tried to lower the calcium level. Drugs that bind phosphorus may be given if phosphorus remains high. Sometimes blood calcium does not respond to these therapies, and more aggressive measures may be considered. (See also the handout on **Acute Kidney Failure**.)

Follow-up Care

Depending on the levels of blood calcium and phosphorus, treatment may be required for weeks. Blood calcium, phosphorus, and kidney values are monitored for a minimum of several days, and then as needed until they return to normal.

Prognosis

The prognosis is good in animals that are promptly decontaminated and treated. Prognosis is more uncertain if soft tissue mineralization occurs, because it is often irreversible and can lead to structural and functional damage in various organs.

SPECIAL INSTRUCTIONS:

Grape and Raisin Toxicosis in Dogs

Petra A. Volmer, DVM, MS, DABVT, DABT

BASIC INFORMATION

Description

A syndrome of kidney failure in dogs is associated with eating (ingestion of) commercially available grapes and raisins. Any type of grape or raisin, as well as pulp from wine pressings, can pose a hazard. Only dogs are affected.

Causes and Toxicity

All breeds of dogs are susceptible. Ingestion of as few as 4-5 raisins can cause the disease.

Clinical Signs

Dogs may develop vomiting, with or without diarrhea, within the first 6-8 hours following ingestion. Vomiting is closely followed by a decrease in activity and lack of appetite. Affected dogs may drink and urinate more. As the disease progresses, the kidneys may stop producing urine, and death can result.

Diagnostic Tests

Diagnosis of grape or raisin poisoning is based on a history or evidence of ingestion and consistent clinical signs. There are no specific tests available to confirm grape or raisin poisoning. Laboratory tests reveal abnormal kidney function. Evidence of grapes or raisins may be found in the vomitus or stool. Other tests (laboratory tests, x-rays, ultrasound) may be needed to rule out other causes of kidney failure.

TREATMENT AND FOLLOW-UP

Treatment Options

Ingestion of grapes or raisins should be considered a medical emergency and treated immediately. Your veterinarian may recommend that vomiting be induced if the ingestion was recent (within 4 hours). Activated charcoal may be given by mouth to bind with the material and prevent absorption into the body. Daily monitoring, with repeated laboratory testing, is done for 3-4 days to watch for any changes in kidney function that warrant further treatment. If needed, the dog may be hospitalized for intravenous fluid therapy and other supportive measures and to monitor urine output. In severe cases, your veterinarian may recommend referral to a specialty facility for dialysis treatment, if it is available.

Follow-up Care

Laboratory tests are repeated periodically to monitor the recovery of kidney function. Monitoring may be required for days to weeks as kidney function returns to normal. If chronic kidney failure develops, then long-term monitoring is usually needed. All sources of grapes or raisins should be removed from the pet's environment.

Prognosis

If treated early, dogs with no clinical signs have a good prognosis. If treatment is delayed or if evidence of kidney failure develops, then the prognosis is guarded (uncertain). Recovery of kidney function may take days to weeks, and in some dogs it never returns to normal.

SPECIAL INSTRUCTIONS:

Herbal Poisonings

Petra A. Volmer, DVM, MS, DABVT, DABT

EPHEDRINE AND PSEUDOEPHEDRINE
Description and Causes
Ephedrine and pseudoephedrine are naturally found in the plants *Ephedra sinica* (ma huang, yellow horse, sea grape plant) and *Sida cordifolia* (Indian common mallow). These compounds are used medicinally for weight loss and as decongestants, and they are used illicitly as herbal ecstasy and as precursors for methamphetamine.
Toxicity
They are rapidly acting central nervous system stimulants.

Clinical Signs
Initial signs can include restlessness, agitation, pacing, panting, and vocalizing. Changes in heart rate can occur. Muscle tremors and seizures are common and are associated with increased body temperature. Death can occur.

Diagnostic Tests
Diagnosis is based on a history of exposure and compatible clinical signs. Pseudoephedrine can be identified in blood and urine.

Treatment Options
Signs can develop quickly, so vomiting is induced only under the direction of a veterinarian, and only if no clinical signs are apparent. Activated charcoal may be administered. In severe cases, hospitalization is required for monitoring of heart rate and rhythm and to provide treatments such as anticonvulsants or sedatives.
Prognosis
Prognosis is good for animals that receive prompt treatment.

GUARANA
Description and Causes
Guarana is an herbal stimulant derived from *Paullinia cupana* seeds, which contain 3-5% caffeine. Guarana is used as a caffeine source by the soft drink industry. Some herbal stimulants contain combinations of ma huang and guarana, which enhances their toxicity.
Toxicity
Caffeine is a rapidly acting central nervous system stimulant.

Clinical Signs
Initial signs include vomiting, hyperactivity, and increased drinking, urination, and heart rate. Muscle tremors and seizures are common. Death can occur.

Diagnostic Tests
Diagnosis is based on a history of ingestion and consistent clinical signs. Caffeine can be detected in stomach contents, blood, or urine.

Treatment Options
Signs can occur quickly, so vomiting is induced only under the direction of a veterinarian, and only if no signs are apparent.

Administration of activated charcoal binds the caffeine and prevents further absorption. Hospitalization for monitoring and treatment is necessary for animals with severe exposures. Anticonvulsants, sedatives, medications to correct heart arrhythmias, and intravenous fluids may be administered.
Prognosis
Prognosis is good for animals receiving prompt treatment. If treatment is delayed or prolonged or severe signs occur, prognosis is poor.

ST. JOHN'S WORT
Description and Causes
St. John's wort (*Hypericum perforatum*) contains hypericin and pseudohypericin, compounds that act on the central nervous system. Other common names are rosin rose and Klamath weed.
Toxicity
St. John's wort stimulates a number of neurotransmitters in the brain.

Clinical Signs
Initial signs can include vomiting, diarrhea, and lethargy. Vocalizing, increased body temperature, muscle tremors, and seizures can occur with large ingestions. In rare cases, the liver may be affected.

Diagnostic Tests
Diagnosis is based on a history of exposure and consistent clinical signs.

Treatment Options
Vomiting is induced only under the direction of a veterinarian, and only if the animal is not exhibiting signs. Activated charcoal is beneficial if large amounts were consumed. Hospitalization may be needed for administration of medications to control tremors or seizures, excessive vomiting, or diarrhea and to support the liver.
Prognosis
Mild signs usually resolve in 24 hours. Animals with liver disease require periodic monitoring.

ECHINACEA
Description and Cause
Echinacea purpurea (purple cone flower, scurvy root) is used as an immune stimulant.

Clinical Signs
Echinacea has a wide margin of safety. The most common signs are vomiting or diarrhea. Although it is uncommon, a severe allergic response (anaphylaxis) is possible.

Continued

Herbal Poisonings—*cont'd*

Petra A. Volmer, DVM, MS, DABVT, DABT

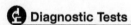 **Diagnostic Tests**

Diagnosis is based on a history of exposure and consistent clinical signs.

Treatment Options

Most exposures do not require any treatment. For large ingestions, vomiting can be induced as directed by your veterinarian. Most gastrointestinal signs are self-limited.

Prognosis

Prognosis is excellent.

VALERIAN

Description and Causes

The root of *Valerian officinalis* is used as a sedative and sleeping aid. Other common names are all-heal, vandal root, and heliotrope.

Toxicity

The compounds in Valerian root produce sedation.

Clinical Signs

Valerian root has a wide margin of safety. Clinical signs can include drowsiness and weakness.

Diagnostic Tests

Diagnosis is based on a history of exposure and consistent clinical signs.

Treatment Options

The sedative effects from most ingestions are short-lived and do not require treatment. Affected animals should be confined to prevent self-injury (such as falling from furniture or down stairs). For large ingestions, vomiting can be induced under the direction of your veterinarian, provided the animal is not exhibiting signs. Activated charcoal may be administered.

Prognosis

Since valerian root has a wide margin of safety and clinical signs in most cases are of short duration and self-limited, the prognosis is excellent.

SPECIAL INSTRUCTIONS:

Lead Poisoning

Petra A. Volmer, DVM, MS, DABVT, DABT

BASIC INFORMATION
Description

Lead is a heavy metal that was banned from residential paints in 1977 and restricted in gasolines and oils in order to reduce environmental contamination. Despite these measures, lead is still readily present in the environment. Sources of lead include fishing sinkers, curtain weights, artist paints, outdoor paints, lead solder, wire shielding, automotive batteries, plumbing caulk, old leaded pipes, linoleum, computer equipment, old or contaminated toys, roofing felt, improperly glazed pottery, lead arsenate pesticides, lead shot for guns, and wine cork covers. Older houses may still contain leaded paint that is exposed on renovation of the home.

Causes and Toxicity

Lead fumes and fine particles, such as those resulting from sanding of old leaded paint surfaces, can be absorbed into the lungs. Larger particles can be coughed up, swallowed, and absorbed from the gut. Ingestion (eating the material) is the most common route of exposure. Once in the body, lead can be deposited in a number of tissues, resulting in various clinical effects. Lead is bound to red blood cells as it is carried to tissues. The highest concentrations of lead occur within bone, teeth, liver, lungs, kidneys, brain, and spleen. Lead can also cross the placenta, putting the unborn fetus at risk, and pass into the milk of the mother, posing a hazard for nursing animals.

Once in the body, lead can interfere with a number of cellular functions. It can inhibit red blood cell production and may alter nerve transmission. Lead poisoning can occur in all companion animals, but dogs and birds are affected more often than cats. Lead poisoning occurs most commonly in young animals, because they have a greater tendency to play with and swallow foreign objects that may contain lead. Young animals also absorb lead more readily than adults do.

Clinical Signs

Gastrointestinal and neurologic signs occur most often, but signs can be vague and nondistinct. Decreased appetite, vomiting, abdominal pain and colic, diarrhea, decreased activity level, unsteady gait, tremors, and/or seizures may occur. Chronic signs can include weight loss, anemia, behavioral changes, and seizures.

Diagnostic Tests

A diagnosis of lead poisoning is based on evidence of exposure to lead-containing objects, compatible clinical signs, and supportive laboratory test results. Ingested or aspirated objects containing lead may be visible on abdominal or chest x-rays. Lead lines may be seen in bone x-rays, and lead pellets may be discovered in soft tissues. Lead pellets in most soft tissues (in muscle, under the skin) are usually stable and do not contribute to lead poisoning. However, lead that is located in acidic environments such as the stomach, intestines, joints, or abscesses is absorbed into the body and may be associated with lead poisoning. Routine laboratory tests may be recommended to look for changes that are compatible with lead poisoning. Measurement of lead levels in the blood allows confirmation of the diagnosis.

TREATMENT AND FOLLOW-UP

Treatment Options

Treatment involves controlling any severe clinical signs, removing lead from the gastrointestinal tract, performing chelation therapy to bring blood lead levels down, and eliminating lead from the environment. Lead remaining in the gut must be removed to prevent further absorption, especially since some chelation agents may enhance the absorption of lead. Several drugs are available for the chelation of lead in the body, including calcium EDTA, D-penicillamine (*Cuprimine*), and succimer (*Chemet*). Which agent is chosen depends on factors such as availability, severity of clinical signs, expense, and preferred route of administration.

The pet's environment must also be cleared of the source of lead to prevent re-exposure. This may involve removal of leaded objects, paints, dust from remodeling projects, and so on. If no obvious lead-containing object is identified, analysis of the pet's water supply may be considered.

Follow-up Care

Blood lead levels are usually rechecked 2 weeks after chelation therapy. Re-treatment may be necessary if levels remain high. It is important to take any diagnosis of lead poisoning in a companion animal seriously, because pets act as sentinels for exposure to humans. Owners should consider having themselves, their children, and other pets in the home tested for lead following a positive diagnosis in a family pet. After treatment, notify your veterinarian if any signs recur, because they may indicate that lead still exists in the environment.

Prognosis

Prognosis for animals with mild to moderate signs that receive appropriate therapy is favorable, providing the source of lead is found and eliminated. Those animals exhibiting severe signs have a more uncertain prognosis.

SPECIAL INSTRUCTIONS:

Macadamia Nut Toxicosis in Dogs

Petra A. Volmer, DVM, MS, DABVT, DABT

BASIC INFORMATION

Description

Macadamia nuts are harvested from Hawaiian *Macadamia integrifolia* and *Macadamia tetraphylla* trees. They are commonly eaten roasted and used in baked goods. The nut is 75% oil.

Causes and Toxicity

The mechanism of action of the toxin is not understood, but ingestion of nuts can result in temporary weakness and tremors of the rear legs in dogs. As little as 1.8 tablespoons of nuts ingested by a 25-pound (12-kg) dog may result in toxicity.

Clinical Signs

Signs are usually seen within 12 hours. Dogs may vomit, act lethargic, be shaky or weak, seem lame, or be unable to rise. Usually, the rear legs are more affected than the forelegs. Often these signs are accompanied by a mild fever (104° F, 40° C). Pancreatitis may arise because of the high fat content in the nuts. Signs usually resolve within 48-72 hours with only supportive treatment.

Diagnostic Tests

There are no specific tests available to confirm macadamia nut poisoning. Diagnosis is based on evidence of exposure and clinical signs. Nut fragments may be found in the vomitus and stool. Laboratory tests, x-rays, and an ultrasound may be recommended to rule out diseases that can cause similar signs (especially if there is no history of ingestion of the nuts) or to determine whether pancreatitis is developing.

TREATMENT AND FOLLOW-UP

Treatment Options

Induction of vomiting may be recommended if the ingestion was recent and the dog is not showing any clinical signs. Vomiting should be induced only under the direction of a veterinarian. Activated charcoal may be administered to bind the material and prevent its absorption into the body. Most animals recover with minimal or supportive treatment. In some cases, an enema may hasten recovery. In severe cases in which tremors occur, the animal may be hospitalized for intravenous medications and fluid therapy.

Follow-up Care

No long-term effects are expected, as long as severe tremors and pancreatitis do not occur. Laboratory tests may be repeated if pancreatitis is present.

Prognosis

The prognosis is excellent in most cases.

SPECIAL INSTRUCTIONS:

Metaldehyde Poisoning

Petra A. Volmer, DVM, MS, DABVT, DABT

BASIC INFORMATION

Description

Metaldehyde is the active ingredient in many snail and slug baits. Formulations include pelleted bait, granules, liquids, and wettable powders, and some are dyed blue or green. Certain ingredients added to the baits, such as molasses, apples, rice, soybeans, and oats, may make them palatable (tasty) to species other than snails and slugs. Brand names include *Deadline, Prozap, Snarol, Turf King, Eliminator, Terminide,* and *Ortho Bug-geta.*

Causes and Toxicity

Metaldehyde acts on the animal's nervous system, causing intense stimulation. As little as 1 teaspoon of bait can be lethal to a 5-pound (2.5-kg) dog.

Clinical Signs

Signs can occur 1-4 hours after ingestion (after eating the bait). Initially, the animal may appear anxious and may drool (salivate) excessively. Then tremors, panting, a rapid heart rate, increased body temperature, and seizures may occur. Death is also possible. In some animals that survive, signs of liver failure may be seen 2-3 days later.

Diagnostic Tests

Diagnosis is based on a history of exposure and consistent clinical signs. In some cases, it may be possible to detect metaldehyde in stomach contents, bait, urine, and plasma, although this analysis takes several days and therefore does not help with an immediate diagnosis. Routine laboratory tests and x-rays may be recommended to assess organ damage and to rule out other causes of similar clinical signs.

TREATMENT AND FOLLOW-UP

Treatment Options

Induction of vomiting can be performed under the direction of a veterinarian if the ingestion was very recent. Administration of activated charcoal by mouth helps bind metaldehyde in the gut so that it is not absorbed into the body.

A number of drugs, such as muscle relaxers, sedatives, and antiseizure medications, can be used by your veterinarian to treat animals with clinical signs. In many cases, these treatments are accompanied by supportive measures such as intravenous fluids and oxygen therapy.

Follow-up Care

Signs can last up to 5 days, but most resolve over 12-72 hours with appropriate treatment. Laboratory tests may be repeated in patients with evidence of liver damage.

Prognosis

The prognosis is good for animals that receive prompt, aggressive treatment. Although permanent liver changes have been reported in some cases, most animals make a full recovery with no residual effects.

SPECIAL INSTRUCTIONS:

Nonsteroidal Anti-Inflammatory Drug Toxicosis

Petra A. Volmer, DVM, MS, DABVT, DABT

BASIC INFORMATION
Description
Nonsteroidal anti-inflammatory drugs (NSAIDs) act against pain, fever, and inflammation. A number of prescription and over-the-counter NSAIDs are available for human use. The following NSAIDs are approved for use in dogs under the direction of a veterinarian: carprofen (*Rimadyl*), meloxicam (*Metacam*), deracoxib (*Deramaxx*), tepoxalin (*Zubrin*), etodolac (*EtoGesic*), ketoprofen (*Anafen*). Only Metacam is approved for use in cats in the United States.

Causes and Toxicity
NSAIDs reduce prostaglandin synthesis by inhibiting the cyclo-oxygenase enzymes known as *COX-1* and *COX-2*. The COX-1 enzyme regulates a number of important functions of the gut, platelets, and kidneys. The COX-2 enzyme regulates inflammation, pain, and fever. Many of the NSAIDs currently available are selective for COX-2 and therefore produce less adverse effects on the stomach and kidneys. With ingestion of large doses, however, the COX-1 enzyme is also affected. The end result is that the gut and the kidneys can be damaged. Dogs and cats are very sensitive to the effects of NSAIDs, and seemingly small ingestions can pose problems.

Clinical Signs
Initially, animals may exhibit vomiting that sometimes contains blood. Diarrhea, abdominal pain, and lethargy may be noted. Sudden collapse and death may result from perforated stomach ulcers. Adverse effects on the kidneys can cause increased drinking and urinating and, eventually, a reduction in urine production if kidney failure occurs. If urine production stops entirely, death will result.

Diagnostic Tests
Diagnosis is based on evidence of ingestion and consistent clinical signs. Laboratory tests may reveal abnormalities in kidney function tests. Examination of the urine may show blood as well as increased white blood cells and protein. Endoscopic examination (passage of a flexible fiberoptic viewing scope) of the stomach may reveal ulcers. Identification of the actual NSAID ingested may be possible through an outside laboratory; however, the analysis is not usually available in time to be of much benefit. Other tests may be recommended to rule out other diseases and toxins that can cause similar signs.

TREATMENT AND FOLLOW-UP
Treatment Options
Your veterinarian may recommend induction of vomiting if the ingestion was recent and the animal is not showing any clinical signs. Vomiting should be induced only under the direction of a veterinarian. Activated charcoal may be administered to bind with the material in the gut and prevent its absorption into the body.

Hospitalization may be recommended in some cases for administration of intravenous fluids to rehydrate and improve kidney function and medications to protect the gut. Other therapy and supportive care may be indicated for stomach ulcers and bleeding into the gut. In severe cases with unresponsive kidney damage, your veterinarian may recommend referral to a specialty facility for dialysis treatment, if it is available.

Follow-up Care
Laboratory tests are repeated periodically to monitor recovery of kidney function. Urine output may also be monitored, especially while your pet is hospitalized. Monitoring may be required for several days until kidney function returns to normal. If chronic kidney failure develops, then long-term monitoring is usually needed. Keep all NSAIDs out of the reach of pets. Do not administer NSAIDs to pets unless they are prescribed by a veterinarian.

Prognosis
Prognosis is favorable for animals that receive prompt and aggressive treatment. For large ingestions and for animals that develop kidney damage, the prognosis is guarded (uncertain), and severe cases may result in death.

SPECIAL INSTRUCTIONS:

Organophosphorus and Carbamate Insecticide Poisoning

Petra A. Volmer, DVM, MS, DABVT, DABT

BASIC INFORMATION

Description

An insecticide is a compound that is designed to kill insects. Organophosphorus and carbamate insecticides act on the nervous systems of both insects and animals, so they can produce adverse affects in exposed animals. These insecticides are formulated as sprays, powders, dips, and granules and are used to control a number of agricultural, garden, and residential insect pests.

Causes and Toxicity

These insecticides bind to an enzyme called *acetylcholinesterase* that normally breaks down a transmitter substance in the nervous system. Binding of the enzyme results in overstimulation of the nervous system. Most insecticides in this class of agents are well absorbed by any route (skin, mouth, gastrointestinal tract). The degree of toxicity can vary widely, depending on the compound involved and its formulation. Some organophosphorus and carbamate insecticides are highly toxic, and small amounts can be deadly. Others have a much wider margin of safety. Brand names include *Bonide/Ortho Systemic Rose* and *Flower Care* (disulfoton), *Dursban* and *Lorsban* (chlorpyrifos), *Paramite* (phosmet), *Orthene* (acephate), and *Golden Malrin* (methomyl).

Clinical Signs

These insecticides may cause a number of signs in animals, including drooling, tearing, increased urination, diarrhea, difficulty breathing, vomiting, increased or decreased heart rate, and pupil constriction. In some cases, muscle weakness, tremors, and seizures may be noted. Death can occur. Depending on the insecticide involved, its potency, and whether exposure was by ingestion (via eating) or by absorption through the skin, signs may be seen within minutes to days. Rarely, a delayed neurologic syndrome may develop 1-4 weeks after exposure that results in permanent muscle weakness and decreased sensation (feeling), progressing to varying degrees of paralysis.

Diagnostic Tests

Diagnosis is based on a history of exposure, appropriate clinical signs, a measured decrease in whole blood cholinesterase activity on laboratory testing, and finding the chemical in body tissues as well as the suspect feed or bait. No specific changes are expected on routine laboratory tests or x-rays, but these tests may be needed to rule out other causes of similar clinical signs. Unfortunately, the measurement of cholinesterase activity and analysis for the chemical in suspected poisons may take several days to weeks, so they do not help with an immediate diagnosis.

TREATMENT AND FOLLOW-UP

Treatment Options

Animals that have eaten one of these insecticides may be treated by inducing vomiting to remove any residual poison from the stomach. Vomiting should be induced under the direction of a veterinarian. Vomiting may be followed by administration of activated charcoal to bind the agent, depending on the compound, when it was ingested, and whether the animal is showing clinical signs. Exposure of the skin is usually treated with bathing to remove the product.

Animals that are showing signs may be treated with a number of drugs that help counteract the effects of the insecticides and decrease the clinical signs or provide support for the animal. Oxygen therapy may be required for animals with breathing problems.

Follow-up Care

Recovery times can vary from 12-24 hours to weeks, depending on the insecticide involved and the extent of signs.

Prognosis

The prognosis is favorable for animals that are treated rapidly and aggressively. No permanent changes are expected. Animals that have eaten large amounts of a rapidly acting insecticide and those with long-standing signs before treatment have a poorer prognosis.

SPECIAL INSTRUCTIONS:

Paintball Toxicosis

Petra A. Volmer, DVM, MS, DABVT, DABT

BASIC INFORMATION

Description

Paintballs are marble-sized balls filled with paint that are used in warlike games. They are generally labeled as nontoxic. Dogs commonly chew on the balls and have been known to eat several hundred. As many as 1000 paintballs may come in one container.

Causes and Toxicity

The paint solution in the balls contains osmotically active substances that can draw water from the bloodstream into the gut. As a result, blood components, particularly sodium, can become elevated. In some cases, smaller, osmotically active substances can be absorbed from the paint into the body and cause depression of the central nervous system (especially the brain).

Clinical Signs

Clinical signs can occur as early as 1 hour after ingestion and include vomiting, diarrhea, and weakness. Tremors and seizures may also develop. Paint may be noted in the vomitus or on the fur.

Diagnostic Tests

Diagnosis is based on evidence of exposure and consistent clinical signs. An elevated serum sodium concentration is the most common laboratory abnormality. Other laboratory tests and x-rays may be recommended to rule out other diseases that cause similar clinical signs and laboratory abnormalities.

TREATMENT AND FOLLOW-UP

Treatment Options

Your veterinarian may recommend induction of vomiting for recent ingestions in dogs that are not exhibiting clinical signs. Vomiting should be induced under the direction of a veterinarian. For ingestion of very large numbers of paintballs, the dog's stomach may need to be pumped. Animals may require hospitalization for treatment of serious signs and for monitoring of blood sodium levels. Intravenous fluids and enemas may be given to lower the blood sodium concentration.

Follow-up Care

Blood sodium measurements and other laboratory tests are monitored until they return to normal. Keep paintballs out of reach of dogs.

Prognosis

Prognosis is good for dogs receiving prompt and aggressive treatment.

SPECIAL INSTRUCTIONS:

Poisoning from Illicit Human Drugs: Depressants

Petra A. Volmer, DVM, MS, DABVT, DABT

BASIC INFORMATION

Animal exposures to illicit drugs are uncommon but are usually emergency situations when they do occur. In most cases, ingestion of the owner's prescription products occurs; however, drugs manufactured in clandestine laboratories may also be consumed. Most street drugs contain impurities that can confuse the diagnosis. In many instances, animal caretakers are reluctant to provide information surrounding the exposure. In general, the most common drugs of abuse are the depressants (barbiturates, benzodiazepines, marijuana), opioids, and stimulants (amphetamines and cocaine).

BARBITURATES
Description
Sources of barbiturates include amobarbital (*Amytal*), aprobarbital (*Alurate*), butabarbital (*Busodium, Butalan, Butisol*), mephobarbital (*Mebaral*), pentobarbital (*Nembutal*), phenobarbital (*Solfoton, Luminal, Barbita*), and secobarbital (*Seconal*). Barbiturates are controlled substances whose distribution is regulated by the U.S. Drug Enforcement Administration (DEA). Street names include barbs, downers, red devils, goof balls, yellow jackets, block busters, pinks, reds and blues, and Christmas trees. Secondary poisoning can occur from ingestion of carcasses of animals euthanized with pentobarbital.
Causes and Toxicity
The principal effect of barbiturates is depression of the central nervous system, especially the brain.

 ### Clinical Signs

Barbiturates cause weakness, drowsiness, incoordination, and, in severe cases, coma, depression of respiration (diminished breathing), and death.

 ### Diagnostic Tests

Diagnosis is based on a history of exposure and compatible clinical signs. Barbiturates can be detected in stomach contents, blood, urine, and feces; however, testing must be performed at outside laboratories.

Treatment Options

If exposure was recent and the animal is not showing any clinical signs, vomiting can be induced under the direction of a veterinarian. Your veterinarian may administer activated charcoal to help bind the barbiturate in the gut and prevent its absorption into the body. For severe ingestions, the animal may be hospitalized for monitoring of the heart and lungs, as well as administration of intravenous fluids and supportive care.
Prognosis
For animals with recent ingestions that are treated rapidly, the prognosis is good.

BENZODIAZEPINES
Description
Benzodiazepines are prescription antianxiety, anticonvulsant, and sedative drugs. They are controlled substances, whose distribution is regulated by the DEA. Common names include lorazepam (*Ativan*), clorazepate (*Tranxene*), prazepam (*Centrax*), clonazepam (*Klonopin*), flurazepam (*Dalmane*), triazolam (*Halcion*), chlordiazepoxide (*Librium*), halazepam (*Paxipam*), temazepam (*Restoril*), oxazepam (*Serax*), diazepam (*Valium*), and alprazolam (*Xanax*). Flunitrazepam (*Rohypnol*) is referred to as the *date rape drug*; it is illegal in the United States. Some street names include downers, V (for valium), rophies, roofies, roach, and rope (flunitrazepam).
Causes and Toxicity
Benzodiazepines bind to receptors in the brain and cause central nervous system (mental) depression. Benzodiazepines have a wide margin of safety between doses that cause drowsiness and doses that are lethal.

 ### Clinical Signs

Low doses can cause weakness, disorientation, and depression. At higher doses, vocalization, restlessness, tremors, and seizures are possible.

 ### Diagnostic Tests

Diagnosis is based on a history of exposure and consistent clinical signs. Analysis of urine or blood for benzodiazepines can be performed by an outside laboratory.

 ### Treatment Options

Animals exhibiting signs must be monitored and protected from injury (such as falling downstairs or off furniture). Your veterinarian may recommend induction of vomiting if the exposure was recent and a large amount of drug was ingested. Activated charcoal may be administered to bind with the drug and prevent its absorption into the body. For severe exposures, hospitalization may be required for administration of intravenous fluids and supportive care. Flumazenil (*Romazicon*), an antidote for the benzodiazepines, may be administered in severe cases if it is available.
Prognosis
Prognosis for most benzodiazepine ingestions is good.

MARIJUANA
Description
All parts of the marijuana plant (*Cannabis sativa*) are toxic. Marijuana is available as the dried herb, a resin (hash or hashish), or a sticky liquid (hash oil). Street names include hemp, pot, grass, Mary Jane, sinsemilla, hash, hashish, Bhang, Ganja, charas, Thai stick, reefer, and wacky-backy.

Continued

Poisoning from Illicit Human Drugs: Depressants—*cont'd*

Petra A. Volmer, DVM, MS, DABVT, DABT

Causes and Toxicity

The toxic constituents in marijuana act on the brain and influence the interpretation of stimuli from sensory organs. A wide margin of safety exists between doses that cause early behavioral effects and doses that are lethal.

Clinical Signs

Affected animals may be restless, nervous, and disoriented. Vomiting, diarrhea, tremors, incoordination, weakness, and dilated pupils may occur. Signs may last 18-72 hours.

Diagnostic Tests

Diagnosis is based on a history of exposure and compatible clinical signs. Marijuana compounds may be detected in urine.

Treatment Options

Induction of vomiting may be recommended, and activated charcoal may be administered following large ingestions. Animals showing signs should be protected from injury (such a falling off furniture) and given supportive care.

Prognosis

Prognosis in most cases is excellent, with most effects being temporary.

SPECIAL INSTRUCTIONS:

Poisoning from Illicit Human Drugs: Opioids and Stimulants

Petra A. Volmer, DVM, MS, DABVT, DABT

BASIC INFORMATION

Animal exposures to illicit drugs are uncommon but are usually emergency situations when they do occur. In most cases, ingestion of the owner's prescription products occurs; however, drugs manufactured in clandestine laboratories may also be consumed. Most street drugs contain impurities that can confuse the diagnosis. In many instances, animal caretakers are reluctant to provide information surrounding the exposure. In general, the most common drugs of abuse are the depressants (barbiturate, benzodiazepines, marijuana), opioids, and stimulants (amphetamines and cocaine).

OPIOIDS
Description

Opioids are derived from the poppy plant (*Papaver somniferum*). There are a number of legal and illegal compounds in this category, including apomorphine, hydromorphone, codeine, meperidine, fentanyl, methadone, morphine, oxycodone, hydrocodone, oxymorphone, buprenorphine, and butorphanol. Some street names include M, morph, and Miss Emma for morphine; smack, skag, hammer, H, horse, rock, white, slow, Harry cone, and China white for heroin; T-threes and schoolboy for codeine; dollies for methadone; and dillies for hydromorphone.

Causes and Toxicity

These drugs affect the brain, gastrointestinal tract, heart, and kidneys.

Clinical Signs

The most common signs include vomiting, drooling, weakness, and sedation. The heart rate may increase or decrease. With large exposures, breathing can be compromised, body temperature may drop, and tremors, seizures, and coma can occur.

Diagnostic Tests

Diagnosis is based on a history of exposure and compatible clinical signs. Some opioids can be detected in urine and blood.

Treatment Options

Vomiting is induced only under the direction of a veterinarian, and only if the animal is not showing any signs. Activated charcoal may be administered. For severe cases, hospitalization may be necessary to monitor breathing and heart functions and to provide supportive care, such as intravenous fluids. An antidote, such as naloxone, may be given to reverse or shorten the clinical signs.

Prognosis

Prognosis is good if the animal is treated early and aggressively. It is guarded (uncertain) if seizures occur.

AMPHETAMINES
Description

Amphetamines are used to treat narcolepsy, obesity, and attention deficit disorders. Examples include methamphetamine (*Methadrine, Desoxyn*), dexamphetamine (*Dexedrine*), amphet-amine (*Benzedrine, Adderall*), and methylphenidate (*Ritalin*). Street names include speed, bennies, meth, crank, crystal, chalk, snow seals (cocaine plus amphetamine), b-bombs, and ice.

Causes and Toxicity

Amphetamines are central nervous system stimulants. They are rapidly absorbed and have a rapid onset of action.

Clinical Signs

Hyperexcitability and agitation can occur within 1-2 hours after ingestion. Animals may have dilated pupils, a rapid heart rate, heart arrhythmias, and panting. With large ingestions, tremors, shaking, and seizures can occur.

Diagnostic Tests

Diagnosis is based on a history of exposure and consistent clinical signs. Amphetamines can be detected in urine and blood.

Treatment Options

Because signs can develop very quickly, induction of vomiting should be done only under the direction of a veterinarian. Activated charcoal may be administered. Animals showing signs may be hospitalized for monitoring and treatment. Tremors and seizures can be treated with a variety of anticonvulsants. Intravenous fluids promote the elimination of the amphetamines via the urine and protect the kidneys.

Prognosis

Animals receiving early and aggressive treatment have a good prognosis. Those animals with prolonged or severe signs (such as seizures) have a poor prognosis.

COCAINE
Description

Cocaine is a central nervous system stimulant derived from the coca plant (*Erythroxylum* spp.). It is found in two forms, the hydrochloride salt, which is a powder, and the free base (crack cocaine), which is often smoked. Street names include beam, big C, blow, Carrie Nation, coke, girl, her, lady, leaf, nose candy, snow, snowbirds, stardust, white, crack, flake, rock (crack cocaine), banano, and bazooka.

Causes and Toxicity

Cocaine is a rapidly absorbed and acts as a stimulant.

Clinical Signs

Hyperexcitability and agitation can occur within 1-2 hours after ingestion. Animals may have dilated pupils, a rapid heart rate, heart arrhythmias, and panting. With large ingestions, tremors, shaking, and seizures can occur.

Diagnostic Tests

Diagnosis is based on a history of exposure and compatible clinical signs. Cocaine can be detected in blood, stomach contents, and urine.

Continued

Poisoning from Illicit Human Drugs: Opioids and Stimulants—*cont'd*

Petra A. Volmer, DVM, MS, DABVT, DABT

℞ Treatment Options

Because signs can develop very quickly, induction of vomiting should be done only under the direction of a veterinarian. Activated charcoal may be administered. Animals showing signs may be hospitalized for monitoring and treatment. Tremors and seizures can be treated with a variety of anticonvulsants and sedatives. Intravenous fluids promote the elimination of the cocaine via the urine and protect the kidneys.

Prognosis

Prognosis is good for animals receiving prompt and aggressive therapy. It is guarded (uncertain) for those with prolonged signs or if treatment is delayed.

SPECIAL INSTRUCTIONS:

Pyrethrin and Pyrethroid Toxicosis

Petra A. Volmer, DVM, MS, DABVT, DABT

BASIC INFORMATION

Description

The natural pyrethrins are a group of six insecticides derived from the flowers of the *Chrysanthemum* plant. Pyrethroids are synthetic compounds similar to pyrethrins, with a longer duration of action, higher toxicity to insects, and greater stability than their natural counterparts. Pyrethrins and pyrethroids are readily available as flea treatments for dogs and cats and for killing insects in homes. Concentrations and formulations vary and can include sprays, liquids, topical solutions (applied to the fur on the back or neck areas), foggers, and gels.

Causes and Toxicity

Pyrethroids act on the nervous system of insects, causing hyperexcitability. Toxicity to pets can occur from appropriate or inappropriate use of pyrethrin- or pyrethroid-containing products. Cats tend to be more sensitive to the pyrethrins and pyrethroids than dogs. In cats, flea treatments containing less than 2% pyrethrins are not expected to cause severe clinical signs. Topical treatments labeled for dogs may contain 36-65% pyrethroids, so these formulations can result in severe signs (including death) in cats.

Dogs are generally more tolerant of exposure to these compounds, and clinical signs, if they appear at all, are infrequent and less pronounced.

Clinical Signs

Dermal exposure of cats to a flea spray containing less than 2% pyrethrins or pyrethroids may cause the animal to twitch the ears and skin, flick the tail, shake the paws, walk abnormally, hide, or exhibit other behavioral abnormalities. These types of signs usually resolve in 24-48 hours. If cats lick these products through grooming, they may develop excessive drooling and an upset stomach. In rare cases, dogs may exhibit similar signs.

Topical flea treatments labeled for dogs often contain concentrated pyrethroids; when applied to a cat, they can result in severe signs requiring immediate treatment. Cats may seem uneasy or restless, cry out, and then develop tremors and seizures within 12-18 hours. Immediate treatment by a veterinarian is required, because death may occur unless aggressive therapy is instituted. In some cases, exposure and clinical signs may occur in cats if they are in close association with recently treated dogs, especially if the cat grooms or licks the dog before the product has dried.

Diagnostic Tests

A history of exposure and consistent clinical signs are often sufficient to make a diagnosis. Animals exposed to a flea product may have a greasy appearance to the fur at the application site, as well as a chemical odor. Analyses for pyrethrins or pyrethroids can be performed on fur by outside laboratories. Laboratory and other tests may be recommended to rule out other causes of similar clinical signs. Be sure to take any containers associated with these products with you to the veterinary hospital so that the veterinarian can read the ingredient list.

TREATMENT AND FOLLOW-UP

Treatment Options

Animals exhibiting signs following application of a flea spray are bathed with a liquid dish detergent to remove the residue from the spray. Animals are then dried thoroughly and kept warm so that they do not become chilled. Signs usually resolve within several hours after bathing. Liquid vitamin E applied to affected areas may help reduce skin irritation. Those animals showing only drooling can be given a tasty treat, such as canned pet food, to remove the bad taste from the mouth.

Contact your veterinarian immediately if your cat is exposed to concentrated pyrethroid products, such as many of the topical solutions. Treatment for these products is done only under the direction of a veterinarian and may consist of bathing to remove the product and administration of intravenous medications to help control tremors and seizures. Supportive care (intravenous fluids, correcting body temperature) may also be warranted. Many cats require hospitalization. Signs usually resolve in 24-72 hours following treatment, if they are not severe.

Follow-up Care

Cats with severe signs require continuous monitoring while hospitalized. Animals receiving timely and appropriate treatment usually make a full recovery, if they are not severely ill.

Prognosis

Prognosis is good for many cats receiving prompt, aggressive treatment. If treatment is delayed or signs are severe, prognosis is guarded (uncertain). The concentrated products can be lethal to cats.

SPECIAL INSTRUCTIONS:

Strychnine Poisoning

Petra A. Volmer, DVM, MS, DABVT, DABT

BASIC INFORMATION

Description

Strychnine is a bitter alkaloid substance that is extracted from the seeds of *Strychnos nux vomica* trees. Strychnine is used to control populations of ground squirrels, meadow and deer mice, prairie dogs, rats, porcupines, chipmunks, rabbits, and pigeons. Baits containing strychnine are often dyed red, green, or blue and are combined with grain. Availability of over-the-counter versions of the poison varies across the country. Some formulations are available only through licensed pest control operators.

Causes and Toxicity

Strychnine is quickly absorbed from the gastrointestinal tract, causing rapid onset of clinical signs. Strychnine acts on the animal's nervous system to cause profound stimulation with severe muscle spasms and seizures. Strychnine is highly toxic to all animals.

Clinical Signs

Clinical signs are similar among all animals and can develop as quickly as 10 minutes after ingestion (eating the bait). Initially, animals may appear anxious or nervous, have a rapid rate of breathing, and have excessive salivation (drooling). Vomiting is uncommon. These signs can rapidly progress to generalized muscle stiffness, tremors, and seizures. The jaw may be clamped shut and the neck arched back. The signs may be continuous, or there may be brief intervals of relaxation between episodes. Death occurs from impaired breathing secondary to muscle stiffness. Depending on the dose ingested, death can occur within minutes to hours.

Diagnostic Tests

Diagnosis is based on a history of exposure, consistent clinical signs, and finding strychnine in bait and/or stomach contents on analysis. There are no specific blood (laboratory) abnormalities that arise following strychnine ingestion. In some cases, strychnine may be found in urine.

TREATMENT AND FOLLOW-UP

Treatment Options

Because strychnine can cause a very rapid onset of clinical signs, the opportunity to induce vomiting (in order to remove the poison from the stomach) is often lost. Once clinical signs are present, vomiting is not induced, because it could cause more harm than good. In some cases, your veterinarian may administer activated charcoal to try and prevent absorption of the poison.

Most affected animals must be hospitalized for emergency treatment. Muscle stiffness, tremors, and seizures can sometimes be managed with injectable drugs such as anticonvulsants and muscle relaxants. Supportive care may include administration of intravenous fluids; correction of high body temperatures induced by the muscle tremors and seizures; and respiratory support with oxygen or more aggressive measures.

Follow-up Care

Most poisoned animals must be hospitalized for at least 24-72 hours as they receive treatment. Care should be taken to remove all bait sources from the animal's environment.

Prognosis

Prognosis depends on the amount of strychnine ingested and how soon the animal receives treatment. If the animal eats a large amount or if treatment is delayed until the animal exhibits severe signs, the prognosis is poor. Many animals die before they receive appropriate treatment because of the rapid onset of signs. If a smaller amount is eaten and/or aggressive treatment is started right away, the prognosis is better.

SPECIAL INSTRUCTIONS:

Xylitol Toxicosis in Dogs

Petra A. Volmer, DVM, MS, DABVT, DABT

BASIC INFORMATION

Description

Xylitol is an artificial sweetener found in sugar-free chewing gums, candies, mints, and baked goods, as well as some toothpastes and mouthwashes. Xylitol is also available as a granular powder for use as a sweetener in baked goods, drinks, and cereals.

Causes and Toxicity

In dogs, xylitol causes the release of large amounts of insulin. Subsequently, exposed animals can develop a rapid and profound drop in blood sugar. This effect only occurs in dogs; xylitol is safe for human use. In some cases, the liver may also be affected in dogs that have ingested (eaten) xylitol-containing products. In many cases, the development of liver failure is not preceded by hypoglycemia (low blood sugar).

Clinical Signs

Dogs may initially develop vomiting or diarrhea. Following ingestion of some xylitol-containing products, blood glucose may drop in as little as 30-60 minutes. If the drop in blood sugar is profound, weakness, difficulty walking, collapse, and seizures may occur. Ingestion of chewing gum can result in delayed hypoglycemia about 12 hours after ingestion. The low blood sugar may persist for 24-36 hours. Acute liver failure can develop in 24-72 hours, with signs of jaundice, lethargy, and abnormal bleeding tendencies.

Diagnostic Tests

Diagnosis is based on evidence of recent ingestion of xylitol-containing products, together with compatible clinical signs and laboratory results (decreased blood sugar, elevated liver tests). Other laboratory tests, abdominal x-rays, and/or an ultrasound may be recommended to rule out other causes of low blood sugar and liver disease.

TREATMENT AND FOLLOW-UP

Treatment Options

Your veterinarian may recommend that vomiting be induced if the ingestion was recent and the animal is not exhibiting any clinical signs. Induction of vomiting should be done only under the direction of a veterinarian, especially since clinical signs may develop rapidly following ingestion of xylitol. Hospitalization may be required if blood sugar is low, so that intravenous dextrose (a form of sugar) can be administered as needed, or if liver failure occurs. Intensive supportive care and other therapy for liver failure may be indicated.

Follow-up Care

Blood sugar and liver tests may be repeated periodically for 2-3 days or until they return to normal. Other monitoring tests may be recommended, based on the presence of other abnormalities that may develop with xylitol toxicosis (such as low potassium or liver failure–induced blood clotting problems). Remove any xylitol-containing products from the dog's environment.

Prognosis

For recent ingestions that produce only hypoglycemia and are treated promptly, the prognosis is good. The prognosis is guarded (uncertain) for dogs that develop liver failure.

SPECIAL INSTRUCTIONS:

Zinc Toxicosis

Petra A. Volmer, DVM, MS, DABVT, DABT

BASIC INFORMATION

Description

The most common source of zinc for small animals is eating (ingestion of) pennies minted after 1982. During that year, the composition of United States pennies changed from all copper to a zinc core with copper cladding (exterior coating). Other sources include zinc, brass, and galvanized steel hardware (nuts, bolts) and topical zinc oxide ointments.

Causes and Toxicity

Elemental zinc is released from metallic objects by the action of stomach acid. Once absorbed into the bloodstream, zinc can cause the red blood cells of dogs and cats to rupture. Zinc oxide ointment is directly irritating to the lining of the stomach, causing vomiting. If zinc oxide ointment is frequently licked by the pet (following daily application to the skin of the pet) for weeks or months, a zinc toxicosis can also develop.

Because younger animals are more likely to ingest foreign bodies, they are at increased risk for zinc toxicosis. The severity of clinical signs depends on the amount of zinc ingested and the duration of the object's presence in the stomach. As little as one penny can poison a dog or cat.

Clinical Signs

Affected animals may have vomiting, lethargy, weakness, diarrhea, and abdominal pain. Destruction of red blood cells results in anemia, reddish-colored urine, and yellowish skin (jaundice). The pigments released on rupture of the red blood cells can be toxic to the kidneys, leading to kidney (renal) failure in severe cases.

Diagnostic Tests

Diagnosis is based on evidence of ingestion of metallic objects along with consistent clinical signs. Metallic objects may be visible on abdominal x-rays. Zinc levels can be measured in the blood (serum), but this analysis usually cannot be performed at the veterinary hospital or clinic, and blood samples must be sent to an outside laboratory. Laboratory and other tests may be recommended to rule out other causes of acute anemia and similar clinical signs.

TREATMENT AND FOLLOW-UP

Treatment Options

Metallic objects in the gastrointestinal tract may be removed with the use of endoscopy (in which a flexible tube is passed into the stomach through the mouth) or surgery (via an abdominal incision). Serum zinc levels usually decrease rapidly after the source of zinc is removed. Blood transfusions may be administered for animals with severe anemia. In most cases, animals require hospitalization to receive symptomatic and supportive treatment, such as intravenous fluids and medications to control vomiting and protect the kidneys.

Follow-up Care

Laboratory tests may be repeated to monitor improvement in the anemia. X-rays may be repeated to ensure that all metallic material has been removed. Frequent follow-up visits are often needed if kidney failure or severe anemia has occurred. It is also important to remove all zinc-containing objects from the pet's environment.

Prognosis

Animals that receive prompt, thorough treatment, with removal of the zinc material, have a good prognosis. Those animals exhibiting severe or prolonged signs have a guarded (uncertain) prognosis, because renal failure or death may occur.

SPECIAL INSTRUCTIONS:

SECTION 19

Environmental Disorders

Section Editor: Rhea V. Morgan, DVM, DACVIM (Small Animal), DACVO

Burns
Electrical Cord Injury
Heat Prostration

Shock
Venomous Snake Bites

Burns

Rhea V. Morgan, DVM, DACVIM (Small Animal), DACVO

BASIC INFORMATION
Description
Burns may occur from exposure to heat or flames (thermal burns), caustic chemicals, or electrical currents. (See handout on **Electrical Cord Injury**.) The severity of the burn is determined by the depth and extent of the injury. The extent of the burn is estimated as a percentage of total body surface area (TBSA) affected.

Burns are classified as superficial (first-degree) burns if only the skin and fur are affected. Partial-thickness (second-degree) burns involve the skin, its glands, and superficial tissue. Full-thickness (third-degree) burns destroy all the layers of the skin and nearby tissues and may destroy fat, muscles, and bone.

Causes
Several types of thermal burns may occur and have a variety of causes:
- Dry, direct heat injuries may be caused by heating pads and lamps, radiators, stoves, light bulbs, and other hot surfaces.
- Wet, direct heat injuries may be caused by hot water, steam, hot tar, oils, or other liquids.
- Common sources of flame-induced injuries include house or barn fires, campfires, forest fires, and malicious burnings.

Chemical injuries may involve several classes of materials, as in the following examples:
- Acids: some toilet bowl cleaners, battery acid, metal and concrete cleaners, rust removers
- Alkaline bases: bleach, drain and oven cleaners, ammonia, Lysol, certain pool chemicals, lime
- Oxidizing agents: bleach, peroxide, manganates
- Solvents: turpentine, paint thinners, gasoline, kerosene

Clinical Signs
Superficial burns cause redness, swelling, and ulceration of the skin, with singeing or loss of fur. Partial-thickness burns cause these signs as well as blistering, edema, and thickening of the skin. Deeper partial-thickness burns may be yellow or whitish in color, dry, and less sensitive to touch. Full-thickness burns may be charred and have a leathery texture, with no recognizable normal skin. Most burns are painful, but full-thickness burns may initially be nonpainful, because nerve endings are destroyed. Depending on the source of the burn, other serious signs may be present as a result of smoke inhalation, electrical current exposure, shock, and damage to other organs.

Diagnostic Tests
Diagnosis is often determined by the history and physical examination. If the animal was exposed to chemicals, bring the container to the veterinary hospital. Numerous diagnostic tests may be recommended for animals with severe burns, because they can cause problems with the lungs, heart, gut, urinary system, and overall circulation.

TREATMENT AND FOLLOW-UP
Treatment Options
Treatment involves care of burn wounds and all the other systemic changes caused by the burns. In general, the treatment of shock, respiratory distress, and cardiac problems takes priority over treatment of the wounds. Seriously injured animals may require oxygen, fluid therapy with crystalloid or colloid solutions, and blood or plasma transfusions. (See the handouts for each of these therapies.) Fluids may be supplemented with electrolytes and glucose (sugar), because many metabolic problems arise with burns. Intensive nursing care, prevention of hypothermia, pain control, and therapy for liver and kidney damage may all be needed.

Proper wound care is important to prevent infections and decrease the amount of body fluids lost by evaporation. Wound care often involves applications of ointments, such as silver sulfadiazine, silver nitrate, and mafenide acetate, and frequent bandaging. Bandage changes must be done carefully, using a sterile technique.

Burned tissue changes a lot over the first several days, and areas that are not going to survive become more obvious over time. Dead skin and tissue must be softened and removed. In some cases, medicated ointments or hydrotherapy (such as a gentle whirlpool bath) can be used, but in other cases repeated surgical procedures are necessary. Once all tissue death has occurred and the dead material has been removed, large burn sites may be prepared for grafting. If skin grafts are anticipated, your pet may be referred to a veterinary surgery specialist for this procedure.

Nutritional support is very important during the recovery period, because the body must expend a great deal of energy to heal itself from burns. A high-calorie, high-protein diet is often recommended.

Follow-up Care
With severe burns, intensive monitoring and repeated laboratory testing are often needed for days. Close monitoring of body weight and nutritional status may be continued for weeks to months.

Prognosis
Prognosis is inversely proportional to the severity of the burn. Other organs are likely to be affected with burns that involve more than 20% of the TBSA, and animals rarely survive if more than 50% of the TBSA is burned. Healing of severe burn wounds may take up to 6 months, and multiple surgeries may be needed.

SPECIAL INSTRUCTIONS:

Electrical Cord Injury

Rhea V. Morgan, DVM, DACVIM (Small Animal), DACVO

BASIC INFORMATION

Description

These injuries usually occur when animals chew on live electrical cords. Puppies and kittens are affected most often, because the cords make attractive play items. Electrical energy is transformed into heat at the point where the exposed wires touch tissues, so a local burn results. Electrical current can also travel into the body, disrupting many normal functions. The severity of injury is proportional to the duration of exposure and the intensity of the electrical current.

Causes

Exposed electrical cords are the most common source of injury. Cords that are temporarily located in open areas, such as those used to power Christmas tree lights, floor fans, space heaters, or outdoor tools, may draw an animal's interest and attention. Although uncommon in small companion animals, lightning strikes and exposure to live power lines can also cause electrical injuries.

Clinical Signs

When electrical cords are bitten, pale yellow, tan, or gray burns may be present on the lips and tongue. With high arcing currents, copper deposits are also left at the site. Systemic effects of the electrical current include muscle spasms and seizures; irregular heart rhythms (arrhythmias) and cardiac arrest; respiratory distress and arrest; vomiting and abdominal pain; and unconsciousness. The gums of the mouth may be pale or blue (cyanotic) in color.

Filling of the lungs with fluid (pulmonary edema) is a delayed effect of electrical cord injuries that may produce coughing of bloody or pink fluid and difficulty breathing 12-36 hours after exposure. Arrhythmias may also occur hours after the injury.

Diagnostic Tests

The diagnosis may be obvious if the injury was witnessed or the animal was found unconscious, convulsing, or in respiratory distress near a damaged electrical cord. The presence of oral burns and other compatible clinical signs may allow a presumptive diagnosis, especially in a young animal. Laboratory tests may be recommended to rule out other diseases that cause similar clinical signs; the results of these tests are usually normal in animals with electrical cord injuries. Chest x-rays are often performed if pulmonary edema is suspected.

TREATMENT AND FOLLOW-UP

Treatment Options

Disconnect the electricity before touching the animal! Remove the animal from the source of current, and clear its mouth and nostrils of any mucus or fluid. If the animal is not breathing, start mouth-to-nose breathing. Seek veterinary care immediately if the animal is having muscle spasms, seizures, difficulty breathing, or weakness or is collapsed or unconscious.

At the veterinary clinic, therapy for shock is started with oxygen, intravenous fluids, and cardiopulmonary resuscitation (CPR), as needed. (See the handouts on **Shock** and **Cardiopulmonary Resuscitation**.) If the animal is not breathing on its own, it may be attached to a mechanical ventilator, if one is available.

Hospitalization may be recommended, even for animals with minimal clinical signs, so that they may be closely monitored for 24-48 hours to observe for the onset of pulmonary edema and cardiac arrhythmias. Therapy for the edema may include oxygen therapy, diuretics (such as furosemide), and drugs to dilate the airways (such as terbutaline or aminophylline). Anti-arrhythmic medications are administered as needed.

Minor oral burns are often cleaned with an antiseptic solution. Most burns heal without surgery, but severe, full-thickness (third-degree) burns may require surgery if the tissue dies and becomes necrotic. Hard foods, chew toys, and treats are avoided until the burns have healed. Antibiotics may be given for secondary infections, and pain medications are administered as needed.

Follow-up Care

Animals with only mild signs that require no treatment should be kept quiet and carefully observed for signs of pulmonary edema for 24-48 hours. Most animals in shock or cardiac arrest require intensive monitoring throughout the initial therapy and for a few days, if they survive. Monitoring may include measurements of blood pressure, pulse quality, gum color, heart rate and rhythm, breathing rate, blood oxygen levels, body temperature, neurologic reflexes, and urine output. Continuous electrocardiography may be needed if arrhythmias develop. (See handout on **Electrocardiography: Intermittent and Continuous**.) Laboratory tests may be recommended for seriously injured animals to detect problems that may arise in other organs from the effects of shock and cardiac arrest. Chest x-rays are usually performed if signs of pulmonary edema develop, and they are periodically repeated until all edema has resolved.

Prognosis

Most animals found in cardiac arrest or unconscious do not survive. Survival rates for animals that develop pulmonary edema range from 39% to 85%. Prognosis is good for animals with only oral burns or other mild clinical signs.

SPECIAL INSTRUCTIONS:

Heat Prostration

Rhea V. Morgan, DVM, DACVIM (Small Animal), DACVO

BASIC INFORMATION
Description
Heat prostration (heat stroke) can occur when body temperatures rise to 104-106° F (greater than 40° C). Heat stroke usually involves exposure to high environmental temperatures and can be precipitated by various medical conditions. Exertional heat stroke occurs when internal heat generated by strenuous exercise is not adequately dissipated and body temperature rises to dangerous levels. Exertional heat stroke occurs most often in racing and sporting dogs.

Causes
Causes generally fall into two categories: those that decrease the ability to dissipate heat and those that increase heat production. External factors that decrease heat dissipation include confinement in a poorly ventilated space, sudden exposure to high environmental temperatures, increased humidity, and limited access to water. Internal factors include obesity, heart and brain diseases, upper airway diseases, and thick hair coats or jackets.

External factors that increase generation of heat include certain medications and the ingestion of macadamia nuts or hops. Internal factors include prolonged muscle spasms or seizures, certain hormonal problems, exercise, and fever.

Clinical Signs
Signs vary depending on the degree and duration of temperature elevation. Panting and elevated temperatures (hyperthermia) are the most common signs. The animal may be dull, weak and wobbly, collapsed, convulsing, or in a coma. Respiratory and heart rates are usually high, and breathing may be very noisy. Gums of the mouth may be bright red or blue (cyanotic). Pulses may be weak. Vomiting and diarrhea may occur.

Bleeding tendencies may be noted, with small hemorrhages in the gums or skin and blood in the feces, urine, or vomitus. Exertional heat stroke may turn the urine a dark brown. Other signs may be present, depending on underlying diseases or contributing factors. Delayed signs may develop 3-5 days after apparent recovery, such as decreased urine production (kidney failure), jaundice (liver failure), infection (sepsis), severe respiratory distress, widespread bleeding, or sudden death from heart arrhythmias.

Diagnostic Tests
Diagnosis is based on finding an extremely high body temperature, a history of exposure to heat, and compatible clinical signs. Laboratory tests and chest x-rays are often recommended to assess the effect of the hyperthermia on various body organs and to search for contributing causes. Common laboratory changes caused by hyperthermia include dehydration, prolonged blood clotting, abnormal kidney and liver tests, low blood sugar, and electrolyte abnormalities.

TREATMENT AND FOLLOW-UP
Treatment Options
Heat prostration is an emergency! The goals of therapy are to lower body temperature, treat shock (if present) and other organ damage, and correct precipitating or contributing factors. As soon as you realize your pet has heat prostration, remove it from the source of heat and wet it with cool tap water. Wrap the animal in a cool, wet towel and transport it to the veterinary hospital immediately.

Cooling methods that may be used at the hospital include submersing the animal in a lukewarm water bath; applying alcohol to the footpads or ice to the groin; and placing the animal in front of fans. Cooling methods should not be extreme, because the body temperature could fall too low (hypothermia).

Treatment for shock may involve insertion of a breathing tube, oxygen therapy, and administration of intravenous (IV) fluids, supplemental electrolytes, and glucose (sugar). IV medications may be given to control muscle spasms and seizures, arrhythmias, and brain edema. If the animal is not breathing on its own, it may be attached to a mechanical ventilator, if one is available. If blood clotting tests are abnormal, plasma may be transfused.

Aggressive therapy is continued until the body temperature begins to decrease and the animal becomes stable. Treatment is then modified to address damage to various organs and any contributing factors or diseases.

Follow-up Care
Most animals with heat prostration require intensive monitoring throughout the initial therapy and for a few days after the emergency has resolved. During therapy, blood pressure, pulse quality, gum color, heart rate and rhythm, breathing rate, blood oxygen levels (pulse oximetry), body temperature, and urine output are commonly monitored. In the hours and days after the crisis, laboratory tests and chest x-rays may be performed to detect problems that may arise in other organs from the effects of hyperthermia.

Prognosis
Prognosis depends on the severity and duration of hyperthermia and the presence of secondary organ failure. Survival is poor for comatose animals and for those with kidney or liver failure or unresponsive bleeding. Animals that survive heat stroke are prone to a recurrence if exposed to a similar situation in the future, so preventive measures are important.

SPECIAL INSTRUCTIONS:

Shock

Rhea V. Morgan, DVM, DACVIM (Small Animal), DACVO

BASIC INFORMATION

Description

Shock is a state of circulatory collapse with inadequate delivery of oxygen to the tissues of the body. In most cases of shock, blood pressure falls to dangerously low levels. If shock lasts for very long, the body cannot compensate for the low blood pressure, and irreversible damage can occur to multiple organs.

Causes

Shock can be classified into three types:

* *Hypovolemic shock* occurs from low circulating blood volume. Common causes include external or internal bleeding, severe vomiting and/or diarrhea, excessive urine production (diuresis), loss of fluid from the bloodstream secondary to low circulating protein levels (especially hypoalbuminemia), and loss of fluids into the gastrointestinal tract (such as with bloating and twisting of the stomach).
* *Cardiogenic shock* occurs with certain heart diseases. Examples include congestive heart failure, arrhythmias, cardiomyopathies, pericardial effusion, pulmonary thrombosis, and certain congenital heart defects.
* *Vasculogenic shock* occurs when blood vessels lose muscle tone and acutely dilate. It may arise with heat stroke, anaphylaxis (a life-threatening allergic reaction), and sepsis (a severe, generalized bacterial infection).

Clinical Signs

Weakness, restlessness, high heart rates (tachycardia), weak pulses, rapid breathing, and reduced urine production are all signs of shock. The gums are usually pale but may be bright red with vasculogenic shock. With prolonged shock, body temperature usually falls (except during heat stroke); the animal becomes mentally dull and often collapses. Coma, cardiac arrest, and dilated pupils are signs that death is near.

Diagnostic Tests

Shock is usually diagnosed based on the physical findings along with a history that provides evidence of one of the precipitating causes. Several quick screening tests, such as packed cell volume and total proteins, blood pressure, pulse oximetry (measurement of oxygen levels in the blood), and an electrocardiogram, may be performed to evaluate the immediate status of the animal. Blood may also be drawn for further testing, but treatment is not delayed while laboratory tests are pending. Other tests may be recommended to identify and better characterize the underlying cause of shock, after therapy is underway.

TREATMENT AND FOLLOW-UP

Treatment Options

The presence of shock is an emergency, and immediate treatment is needed. Treatment has three main goals: to support breathing, to control any bleeding, and to expand the circulating blood volume. Treatment involves the following measures:

* Any active bleeding is stopped with direct pressure, bandages, tourniquets, or surgical ligation of blood vessels.
* Oxygen therapy is started to increase oxygen delivery to the tissues. (See handout on **Oxygen Therapy**.)
* An intravenous (IV) catheter is inserted, and fluid therapy with crystalloid fluids is begun immediately. Supplemental electrolytes and glucose (sugar) may be added to the fluids. Large amounts of fluids are usually needed and are given at very fast rates. In some cases, more than one IV catheter may be inserted, so that more fluids can be given quickly. Blood or plasma transfusions or colloid solutions may also be administered. (See handouts on **Transfusion Therapy in Dogs, Transfusion Therapy in Cats,** and **Fluid Therapy**.)
* A number of IV medications may be given, such as steroids, vasoactive drugs to improve blood pressure, sodium bicarbonate (especially if the animal is in cardiac arrest), and antibiotics (especially for sepsis).
* Other therapies depend on the underlying cause of shock and may include lowering body temperature during heat stroke, removing air from a bloated stomach, administering medications for arrhythmias, removing any air from a traumatized chest cavity, and other measures.

Follow-up Care

Most animals in shock require intensive monitoring throughout the initial therapy and for a few days after shock has resolved. Monitoring during therapy may include measurements of blood pressure, pulse quality, gum color, heart rate and rhythm, breathing rate, blood oxygen levels, body temperature, neurologic reflexes, and urine output. In the hours and days after therapy, laboratory tests and chest x-rays may be performed to detect problems that may arise in other organs from the effects of shock.

Prognosis

Prognosis varies depending on the duration of shock, the underlying cause, and secondary changes caused by the circulatory collapse. If the underlying cause is treatable, if shock is quickly reversed with therapy, and if there are no major effects on other organs, then the prognosis is good. If shock is difficult to reverse or leads to damage in the kidneys, brain, and gut, then the animal may not survive. Likewise, if the underlying cause of shock is severe and life-threatening, such as with serious trauma, major burns, or irreversible heart and lung disease, the prognosis is also grave.

SPECIAL INSTRUCTIONS:

Venomous Snake Bites

Rhea V. Morgan, DVM, DACVIM (Small Animal), DACVO

BASIC INFORMATION

Description

Snake envenomation occurs when poisonous material is injected into the victim during a bite. Of the 120 species of snakes that live in the United States, only 25 are venomous. Alaska, Maine, and Hawaii are the only states without venomous snakes. With the exception of the coral snake, all venomous snakes in the United States are pit vipers. Pit vipers include rattlesnakes, cottonmouths, and copperheads.

Causes

The composition of snake venom varies by species and age of the snake, season of the year, geographic location, and time since the snake's last bite. Venom is not injected with every bite. In up to 25% of pit viper bites and 50% of coral snake bites, venom is not released.

Pit viper venom kills cells at the site of the bite, and may cause hypovolemic shock, destruction of red blood cells, and abnormal bleeding. Neurotoxins in the venom may produce muscle weakness and respiratory paralysis.

Coral snake venom causes less local tissue damage, but it contains a neurotoxin that causes progressive weakness and respiratory failure. Destruction of red blood cells can also occur.

Clinical Signs

Signs usually develop within 30 minutes after a pit viper bite. Puncture wounds that ooze bloody liquid and pain and swelling at the bite site are common. Evidence of shock may be present, with high heart and respiratory rates, weak pulses, pale gums, weakness, and mental dullness. Widespread microscopic blood clot formation within the body may consume all available circulating clotting proteins, with subsequent serious bleeding from many body sites. Abnormal effects on red blood cells may occur within 24 hours, and platelet numbers may decrease within 2 weeks. Progressive muscle weakness and respiratory paralysis may develop. Severe tissue death around the bite wound may occur within 6-24 hours. Muscle destruction, with secondary kidney failure, may also occur.

Fang wounds are not as obvious with coral snake bites, and less local tissue damage occurs. Generalized muscle weakness or tremors, drowsiness, disorientation, drooling, and trouble swallowing may occur within 3 hours. Difficulty breathing and aspiration pneumonia may develop. Death from respiratory failure can occur within 4 hours. Sometimes the onset of weakness and paralysis is delayed for up to 48 hours.

Diagnostic Tests

Diagnosis is often made by observation of the bite, discovery of bite wounds, and the presence of compatible clinical signs. No diagnostic tests are available to confirm the presence of venom in the body; rather, laboratory tests are used to assess damage to blood cells and other body organs.

TREATMENT AND FOLLOW-UP

Treatment Options

No effective measures exist to prevent spread of the venom from the bite site, so cutting and sucking on the wounds, applying a tourniquet, and applying ice are not recommended. If a snake bite is suspected, transport your pet to a veterinary hospital immediately!

Treatment of pit viper bites involves intravenous (IV) fluid therapy and other medications for shock, administration of pain medications, and local cleansing of the wound. If the animal is in respiratory failure, a mechanical ventilator may be used and oxygen therapy started. Antivenin (antivenom) is available from two different manufacturers. Cottonmouth and copperhead bites are less likely to require antivenom than bites from the Eastern diamondback, Western diamondback, or Mojave rattlesnake. Antivenin is added to the IV fluids and may be repeated as needed, depending on the response induced. Severe tissue death at the wound site may require surgery at a later date.

Following a coral snake bite, most animals are hospitalized for at least 48 hours, because clinical signs can be delayed for 10-18 hours. Treatment is primarily supportive, with IV fluids, oxygen therapy, and mechanical ventilation as needed. No commercial coral snake antivenin is currently available in the United States. Antivenin produced for Australian tiger snake and Mexican coral snake bites may be helpful and can be considered for suspected coral snake bites.

Follow-up Care

Frequent monitoring is needed for 24-48 hours. During initial therapy, blood pressure, pulse quality, gum color, heart rate and rhythm, breathing rate, blood oxygen levels (pulse oximetry), neurologic reflexes, body temperature, and urine output may be monitored. In the following days, laboratory tests and chest x-rays may be performed to detect problems that may arise in other organs from the effects of the venom.

Prognosis

Prognosis depends on the location of the bite on the animal (legs are best; head and face are the worst sites), amount of venom injected, and availability of antivenin. Many dogs survive with appropriate, intensive therapy; however, signs of neurotoxicity may not be reversible.

SPECIAL INSTRUCTIONS:

INDEX

A

AA subluxation. *See* Atlantoaxial (AA) subluxation.
Abscess(es)
  orbital, 372
    prostatic, in dogs, 207
      subcutaneous, 341
Acetaminophen toxicosis, 444
  causes and toxicity of, 444
  clinical signs of, 444
  description of, 444
  diagnostic tests for, 444
  follow-up care for, 444
  prognosis of, 444
  treatment options for, 444
Acne, in cats, 307
  causes of, 307
  clinical signs of, 307
  description of, 307
  diagnostic tests for, 307
  follow-up care for, 307
  prognosis of, 307
  treatment options for, 307
Acute lymphocytic leukemia (ALL), 242
  causes of, 242
  clinical signs of, 242
  description of, 242
  diagnostic tests for, 242
  follow-up care for, 242
  prognosis of, 242
  treatment options for, 242
Acute renal failure (ARF), 187
  causes of, 187
  chronic *vs.*, 10
  clinical signs of, 187
  description of, 187
  diagnostic tests for, 187
  follow-up care for, 187
  prognosis of, 187
  treatment options for, 187
Acute respiratory distress syndrome (ARDS), 69
  causes of, 69
  clinical signs of, 69
  description of, 69
  diagnostic tests for, 69
  follow-up care for, 69
  prognosis of, 69
  treatment options for, 69
Addison's disease, 183
Adenitis, sebaceous, in dogs, 338
Adenocarcinoma, 148, 159
Adenomas
  renal, 210
  sebaceous, in dogs, 312
Adverse reactions; *See* Allergies/allergic reactions Anaphylaxis.
AF. *See* Atrial fibrillation (AF).
Agalactia, 217
  causes of, 217
  clinical signs of, 217
  description of, 217
  diagnostic tests for, 217

Agalactia (*Continued*)
  follow-up care for, 217
  prognosis of, 217
  treatment options for, 217
Aggression
  dominance
    in cats, 427
    in dogs, 428
  in household cats, 427
    causes of, 427
    clinical signs of, 427
    description of, 427
    diagnostic tests for, 427
    follow-up care for, 427
    petting intolerance and, 433
    play and, 434
    prognosis of, 427
    status and, 433
    treatment options for, 427
  play, in cats, 434
  possessive, in dogs, 435
  status, in cats, 433
  territorial, in dogs, 435
Airway obstruction, 6, 72, 78, 97
ALDs. *See* Angular limb deformities (ALDs).
ALL. *See* Acute lymphocytic leukemia (ALL).
Allergic dermatitis, flea, 324
Allergies/allergic reactions, 269
  causes of, 269
  clinical signs of, 269
  description of, 269
  diagnostic tests for, 269
  drug, 269
  follow-up care for, 269
  food, 325, 437
  prognosis of, 269
  treatment options for, 269
Alopecia, cyclical (seasonal) flank, 318
Alopecia X, 309
  causes of, 309
  clinical signs of, 309
  description of, 309
  diagnostic tests for, 309
  follow-up care for, 309
  prognosis of, 309
  treatment options for, 309
Amitraz toxicosis, 445
  causes and toxicity of, 445
  clinical signs of, 445
  description of, 445
  diagnostic tests for, 445
  follow-up care for, 445
  prognosis of, 445
  treatment options for, 445
Amphetamine toxicity, 462
Amputation, limb, 2
  complications of, 2
  follow-up care for, 2
  indications for, 2
  poor candidates for, 2
  postoperative care for, 2
  preparation for, 2

Amputation, limb (*Continued*)
  purpose of, 2
  technique for, 2
Amyloidosis, 208
Anal sac diseases, 134
  causes of, 134
  clinical signs of, 134
  description of, 134
  diagnostic tests for, 134
  follow-up care for, 134
  prognosis of, 134
  treatment options for, 134
Anaphylaxis, 269
Anaplasmosis, in dogs, 404
  causes of, 404
  clinical signs of, 404
  description of, 404
  diagnostic tests for, 404
  follow-up care for, 404
  prognosis of, 404
  public health information on, 404
  treatment options for, 404
Anconeal process, ununited disease of, 305
Anemia, 243
  aplastic, 245
  causes of, 243, 273
  of chronic kidney disease, 188
  clinical signs of, 243
  description of, 243
  diagnostic tests for, 243
  follow-up care for, 243
  hemolytic, immune-mediated, 255
  infectious, feline, 251
  prognosis of, 243
  treatment options for, 243
Anesthesia, general
  preoperative evaluation for, 23
  prognosis of, 23
  risk classification for, 23
  treatment options for, 23
Angular limb deformities (ALDs), in dogs, 275
  causes of, 275
  clinical signs of, 275
  description of, 275
  diagnostic tests for, 275
  follow-up care for, 275
  prognosis of, 275
  treatment options for, 275
Anterior uveitis, 348
  causes of, 348
  clinical signs of, 348
  description of, 348
  diagnostic tests for, 348
  follow-up care for, 348
  prognosis of, 348
  treatment options for, 348
Anticoagulant rodenticide toxicity, 244
  causes of, 244
  clinical signs of, 244
  description of, 244
  diagnostic tests for, 244

Anticoagulant rodenticide toxicity (*Continued*)
  follow-up care for, 244
  prognosis of, 244
  treatment options for, 244
Antifreeze poisoning, 446
  causes and toxicity of, 446
  clinical signs of, 446
  description of, 446
  diagnostic tests for, 446
  follow-up care for, 446
  prognosis of, 446
  treatment options for, 446
Anxiety disorders, in dogs, 432
  causes of, 432
  clinical signs of, 432
  description of, 432
  diagnostic tests for, 432
  follow-up care for, 432
  prognosis of, 432
  treatment options for, 432
Aortic arch, persistent right, 54
APCs. *See* Atrial premature contractions (APCs).
Aplastic anemia, 245
  causes of, 245
  clinical signs of, 245
  description of, 245
  diagnostic tests for, 245
  follow-up care for, 245
  prognosis of, 245
  treatment options for, 245
ARDS. *See* Acute respiratory distress
    syndrome (ARDS).
ARF. *See* Acute renal failure (ARF).
Arrhythmias. *See also specific rhythm.*
  diagnostic tests for, 12, 58
  ventricular, with cardiomyopathy, 34, 43,
    44, 50
Arrhythmogenic cardiomyopathy, in Doberman
    pinschers, 50
Arrhythmogenic right ventricular cardiomyo-
    pathy (ARVC), in boxers, 34
  causes of, 34
  clinical signs of, 34
  description of, 34
  diagnostic tests for, 34
  follow-up care for, 34
  prognosis of, 34
  treatment options for, 34
Arterial thromboembolism, peripheral, 35
  causes of, 35
  clinical signs of, 35
  description of, 35
  diagnostic tests for, 35
  follow-up care for, 35
  prognosis of, 35
  treatment options for, 35
Arthritis
  degenerative, 295
  erosive, 289
  immune-mediated, 289
  rheumatoid, 289
  septic, 302
Arthrodesis, 3
  complications of, 3
  postoperative/follow-up care for, 3
  preparation for, 3
  purpose of, 3
  technique for, 3

ARVC. *See* Arrhythmogenic right ventricular
    cardiomyopathy (ARVC).
ASD. *See* Atrial septal defect (ASD).
AT. *See* Atrial tachycardia (AT).
Atlantoaxial (AA) subluxation, in dogs, 100
  causes of, 100
  clinical signs of, 100
  description of, 100
  diagnostic tests for, 100
  follow-up care for, 100
  prognosis of, 100
  treatment options for, 100
Atopic dermatitis, in dogs, 310
  causes of, 310
  clinical signs of, 310
  description of, 310
  diagnostic tests for, 310
  follow-up care for, 310
  prognosis of, 310
  treatment options for, 310
Atrial fibrillation (AF), 36
  causes of, 36, 51, 64
  clinical signs of, 36
  description of, 36
  diagnostic tests for, 36
  with dilated cardiomyopathy, 43, 44
  follow-up care for, 36
  prognosis of, 36
  treatment options for, 36
Atrial premature contractions (APCs), 37
  causes of, 37
  clinical signs of, 37
  description of, 37
  diagnostic tests for, 37
  follow-up care for, 37
  prognosis of, 37
  treatment options for, 37
Atrial septal defect (ASD), 65
  causes of, 65
  clinical signs of, 64, 65
  description of, 65
  diagnostic tests for, 65
  follow-up care for, 65
  prognosis of, 65
  treatment options for, 65
Atrial standstill, 58
  causes of, 58
  clinical signs of, 58
  description of, 58
  diagnostic tests for, 58
  follow-up care for, 58
  prognosis of, 58
  treatment options for, 58
Atrial tachycardia (AT), 37
  causes of, 37
  clinical signs of, 37
  description of, 37
  diagnostic tests for, 37
  follow-up care for, 37
  prognosis of, 37
  treatment options for, 37
Atrioventricular valve (AV), in dogs,
    degeneration of, 38
  causes of, 38
  clinical signs of, 38
  description of, 38
  diagnostic tests for, 38
  follow-up care for, 38

Atrioventricular valve (AV), in dogs,
    degeneration of (*Continued*)
  prognosis of, 38
  treatment options for, 38
Aural hematoma, 385
  causes of, 385
  clinical signs of, 385
  description of, 385
  diagnostic tests for, 385
  follow-up care for, 385
  prognosis of, 385
  treatment options for, 385
Avascular necrosis, of femoral head, 291
Avermectin toxicosis, 447
  causes and toxicity of, 447
  clinical signs of, 447
  description of, 447
  diagnostic tests for, 447
  follow-up care for, 447
  prognosis of, 447
  treatment options for, 447
Avulsions, brachial plexus, 102

B
Babesia infection, in dogs, 246
  causes of, 246
  clinical signs of, 246
  description of, 246
  diagnostic tests for, 246
  follow-up care for, 246
  prognosis of, 246
  treatment options for, 246
Barbiturates toxicity, 460
Bartonellosis, 391
  causes of, 391
  clinical signs of, 391
  description of, 391
  diagnostic tests for, 391
  follow-up care for, 391
  prognosis of, 391
  treatment options for, 391
Benign prostatic hypertrophy (BPH), in
    dogs, 189
  causes of, 189
  clinical signs of, 189
  description of, 189
  diagnostic tests for, 189
  follow-up care for, 189
  prognosis of, 189
  treatment options for, 189
Benign skin tumors, in dogs, 312
  causes of, 312
  clinical signs of, 312
  description of, 312
  diagnostic tests for, 312
  follow-up care for, 312
  prognosis of, 312
  treatment options for, 312
Benzodiazepines toxicity, 460
Bicipital tendinopathy (BT), 276
  causes of, 276
  clinical signs of, 276
  description of, 276
  diagnostic tests for, 276
  follow-up care for, 276
  prognosis of, 276
  treatment options for, 276
Biliary mucocele, 145

Bladder cancer, 190
  causes of, 190
  clinical signs of, 190
  description of, 190
  diagnostic tests for, 190
  follow-up care for, 190
  prognosis of, 190
  treatment options for, 190
Bladder inflammation. *See* Cystitis.
Bladder stones
  in cats, 191
    causes of, 191
    clinical signs of, 191
    description of, 191
    diagnostic tests for, 191
    follow-up care for, 191
    prognosis of, 191
    treatment options for, 191
  in dogs, 192
    causes of, 192
    clinical signs of, 192
    description of, 192
    diagnostic tests for, 192
    follow-up care for, 192
    prognosis of, 192
    treatment options for, 192
Bladder trauma, 193
  causes of, 193
  clinical signs of, 193
  description of, 193
  diagnostic tests for, 193
  follow-up care for, 193
  prognosis of, 193
  treatment options for, 193
Blastomycosis, 392
  cause of, 392
  clinical signs of, 392
  description of, 392
  diagnostic tests for, 392
  follow-up care for, 392
  prognosis of, 392
  treatment options for, 392
Blood pressure (BP) measurement,
       indirect, 4
  complications of, 4
  equipment for, 4
  interpretation of, 4
  preparation for, 4
  purpose of, 4
  technique for, 4
Blood urea nitrogen (BUN), as kidney
       function test, 19
Bone disease. *See also specific disease, e.g.,*
       Osteochondrosis (OC).
  degenerative, 119, 295
  nutritional, 294
Bone marrow aspiration, 5
  complications of, 5
  follow-up care for, 5
  preparation for, 5
  purpose of, 5
  technique for, 5
Bone tumors, 277
  causes of, 277
  clinical signs of, 277
  description of, 270, 277
  diagnostic tests for, 277
  follow-up care for, 277

Bone tumors (*Continued*)
  prognosis of, 277
  treatment options for, 277
Borreliosis, 393
  causes of, 393
  clinical signs of, 393
  description of, 393
  diagnostic tests for, 393
  follow-up care for, 393
  prognosis of, 393
  treatment options for, 393
Botulism, 101
  causes of, 101
  clinical signs of, 101
  description of, 101
  diagnostic tests for, 101
  follow-up care for, 101
  prognosis of, 101
  treatment options for, 101
Boxers, right ventricular cardiomyopathy
       in, 34
BP. *See* Blood pressure (BP) measurement.
BPH. *See* Benign prostatic hypertrophy (BPH).
Brachial plexus avulsion, 102
  causes of, 102
  clinical signs of, 102
  description of, 102
  diagnostic tests for, 102
  follow-up care for, 102
  prognosis of, 102
  treatment options for, 102
Brachycephalic syndrome, 72
  causes of, 72
  clinical signs of, 72, 78
  description of, 72
  diagnostic tests for, 72
  follow-up care for, 72
  prognosis of, 72
  treatment options for, 72
Bradycardia, sinus, 60
Brain injury
  ischemic, 118
  traumatic, 111
Brain tumors, 103
  causes of, 103
  clinical signs of, 103
  description of, 103
  diagnostic tests for, 103
  follow-up care for, 103
  prognosis of, 103
  treatment options for, 103
Bread dough poisoning, 448
  causes and toxicity of, 448
  clinical signs of, 448
  description of, 448
  diagnostic tests for, 448
  follow-up care for, 448
  prognosis of, 448
  treatment options for, 448
Bronchitis
  acute, 73
    causes of, 73
    clinical signs of, 73
    description of, 73
    diagnostic tests for, 73
    follow-up care for, 73
    prognosis of, 73
    treatment options for, 73

Bronchitis (*Continued*)
  allergic
    in cats, 70
      acute *vs.* chronic, 70
      causes of, 70
      clinical signs of, 70
      description of, 70
      diagnostic tests for, 70
      follow-up care for, 70
      prognosis of, 70
      treatment options for, 70
    in dogs, 71
      causes of, 71
      clinical signs of, 71
      description of, 71
      diagnostic tests for, 71
      follow-up care for, 71
      prognosis of, 71
      treatment options for, 71
  chronic, 74
    causes of, 74
    clinical signs of, 74
    description of, 74
    diagnostic tests for, 74
    follow-up care for, 74
    prognosis of, 74
    treatment options for, 74
  infectious, in dogs, 397
Bronchoscopy, 6
  complications of, 6
  follow-up care for, 6
  preparation for, 6
  purpose of, 6
  technique for, 6
Brucellosis, in dogs, 394
  cause of, 394
  clinical signs of, 394
  description of, 394
  diagnostic tests for, 394
  follow-up care for, 394
  prevention of, 394
  prognosis of, 394
  treatment options for, 394
BT. *See* Bicipital tendinopathy (BT).
Bullous lung disease, 75
  causes of, 75
  clinical signs of, 75
  description of, 75
  diagnostic tests for, 75
  follow-up care for, 75
  treatment options for, 75
BUN (blood urea nitrogen), as kidney function
       test, 19
Burns, 469
  causes of, 469, 470
  classification of, 469
  clinical signs of, 469
  description of, 469
  diagnostic tests for, 469
  follow-up care for, 469
  prognosis of, 469
  treatment options for, 469

C

Calcaneal (Achilles) tendon injury, 278
  causes of, 278
  clinical signs of, 278
  description of, 278

Calcaneal (Achilles) tendon injury (*Continued*)
  diagnostic tests for, 278
  follow-up care for, 278
  prognosis of, 278
  treatment options for, 278
Campylobacteriosis, 395
  causes of, 395
  clinical signs of, 395
  description of, 395
  diagnostic tests for, 395
  follow-up care for, 395
  prognosis of, 395
  treatment options for, 395
Carbamate insecticide poisoning, 458
  causes of, 458
  clinical signs of, 458
  description of, 458
  diagnostic tests for, 458
  follow-up care for, 458
  prognosis of, 458
  treatment options for, 458
Carcinoma. *See also specific type, e.g.,*
      Squamous cell carcinoma.
  bladder, 190
  bone marrow aspiration for, 5
  chemotherapy for, 9
  gastric, 148
  hypercalcemia related to, 254
  intestinal, 159
  laryngeal and tracheal, 80
  limb, amputation and, 2
  lung, 83
  nasal, 86
  orbital, secondary, 373
  prostate, in dogs, 205
  renal, 210
Cardiac arrest, 66
  causes of, 66, 470
  clinical signs of, 66
  description of, 66
  diagnostic tests for, 66
  follow-up care for, 66
  prognosis of, 66
  treatment options for, 40, 66
Cardiac tumors, 39
  causes of, 39
  clinical signs of, 39, 52
  description of, 39
  diagnostic tests for, 39
  follow-up care for, 39
  heart base, 39, 52, 84
  prognosis of, 39
  treatment options for, 39
Cardiomyopathy
  arrhythmogenic (occult), in Doberman
      pinschers, 50
  arrhythmogenic right ventricular, in
      boxers, 34
  dilated. *See* Dilated cardiomyopathy (DCM).
  hypertrophic, in cats, 49
  taurine-deficiency. *See* Taurine-deficiency
      cardiomyopathy.
Cardiopulmonary resuscitation (CPR), 40
  causes of, 40
  clinical signs of, 40
  description of, 40, 66
  diagnostic tests for, 40
  follow-up care for, 40

Cardiopulmonary resuscitation (CPR) (*Continued*)
  prognosis of, 40
  treatment options for, 40, 356
Carpal hyperextension/hyperflexion disorder,
      juvenile, 290
Carpal shearing injuries, 279
  causes of, 279
  clinical signs of, 279
  description of, 279
  diagnostic tests for, 279
  follow-up care for, 279
  prognosis of, 279
  treatment options for, 279
Castration
  of male cats, 7
    complications of, 7
    follow-up care for, 7
    postoperative care for, 7
    preparation for, 7
    purpose of, 7
    technique for, 7
  of male dogs, 8
    complications of, 8
    follow-up care for, 8
    postoperative care for, 8
    preparation for, 8
    purpose of, 8
    technique for, 8
Casts, for fracture repair, 15
  complications of, 15
  follow-up care for, 15
  postoperative care for, 15
  preparation for, 15
  purpose of, 15
  technique for, 15
Cataracts, 349
  causes of, 349
  classification of, 349
  clinical signs of, 349
  description of, 349
  diagnostic tests for, 349
  follow-up care for, 349
  prognosis of, 349
  treatment options for, 349
Caudal cervical spondylopathy, 105
  causes of, 105
  clinical signs of, 105
  description of, 105
  diagnostic tests for, 105
  follow-up care for, 105
  prognosis of, 105
  treatment options for, 105
Caudal occipital malformation, 106
  causes of, 106
  clinical signs of, 106
  description of, 106
  diagnostic tests for, 106
  follow-up care for, 106
  prognosis of, 106
  treatment options for, 106
Caval syndrome, in dogs, 47–48
CCL. *See* Cranial cruciate ligament (CCL) disease.
CEA. *See* Collie eye anomaly (CEA).
Cellulitis, 341
  causes of, 341
  clinical signs of, 341
  description of, 341
  diagnostic tests for, 341

Cellulitis (*Continued*)
  follow-up care for, 341
  juvenile, 326
  orbital, 372
  prognosis of, 341
  treatment options for, 341
Cervical spondylopathy, caudal, 105
Chemotherapy, 9
  common agents for, 9
  complications of, 9
  follow-up care for, 9
  preparation for, 9
  purpose of, 9
  technique for, 9
Cheyletiellosis, 313
  causes of, 313
  clinical signs of, 313
  description of, 313
  diagnostic tests for, 313
  follow-up care for, 313
  prognosis of, 313
  treatment options for, 313
Chiari-like malformation, 106
Chocolate toxicosis, 449
  causes and toxicity of, 449
  clinical signs of, 449
  description of, 449
  diagnostic tests for, 449
  follow-up care for, 449
  prognosis of, 449
  treatment options for, 449
Cholangiohepatitis, in cats, 135
  causes and toxicity of, 135
  clinical signs of, 135
  description of, 135
  diagnostic tests for, 135
  follow-up care for, 135
  forms of, 135
  prognosis of, 135
  treatment options for, 135
Cholecalciferol rodenticide poisoning, 450
  causes and toxicity of, 450
  clinical signs of, 450
  description of, 450
  diagnostic tests for, 450
  follow-up care for, 450
  prognosis of, 450
  treatment options for, 450
Chorioretinitis, 350
  causes of, 350
  clinical signs of, 350
  description of, 350
  diagnostic tests for, 350
  follow-up care for, 350
  prognosis of, 350
  treatment options for, 350
Chronic kidney disease (CKD)
  anemia of, 188
    causes of, 188
    clinical signs of, 188
    description of, 188
    diagnostic tests for, 188
    follow-up care for, 188
    prognosis of, 188
    treatment options for, 188
  in cats, 194
    causes of, 194
    clinical signs of, 62, 194

Chronic kidney disease (CKD) (*Continued*)
    description of, 194
    diagnostic tests for, 194
    follow-up care for, 194
    prognosis of, 194
    treatment options for, 194
    in dogs, 195
        causes of, 195
        clinical signs of, 62, 195
        description of, 195
        diagnostic tests for, 195
        follow-up care for, 195
        prognosis of, 195
        treatment options for, 195
    nutritional management of, 20
        changing diets in, 20
        dietary components in, 20
        follow-up care for, 20
        indications for, 20
        purpose of, 20
Chronic lymphocytic leukemia
    (CLL), 247
    causes of, 247
    clinical signs of, 247
    description of, 247
    diagnostic tests for, 247
    follow-up care for, 247
    prognosis of, 247
    treatment options for, 247
Cilia, ectopic, 354
Claw disease
    asymmetrical, 314
        causes of, 314
        clinical signs of, 314
        description of, 314
        diagnostic tests for, 314
        follow-up care for, 314
        prognosis of, 314
        treatment options for, 314
    symmetrical, 315
        causes of, 315
        clinical signs of, 315
        description of, 315
        diagnostic tests for, 315
        follow-up care for, 315
        prognosis of, 315
        treatment options for, 315
Cleft palate, 136
    causes of, 136
    clinical signs of, 136
    description of, 136
    diagnostic tests for, 136
    follow-up care for, 136
    prognosis of, 136
    treatment options for, 136
CLL. *See* Chronic lymphocytic leukemia
    (CLL).
Coagulopathy
    disseminated, 249
    liver disease association with, 248
        causes of, 248
        clinical signs of, 248
        description of, 248
        diagnostic tests for, 248
        follow-up care for, 248
        prognosis of, 248
        treatment options for, 248
    von Willebrand disease as, 267

Cocaine toxicity, 462–463
Coccidioidomycosis, 399
    cause of, 399
    clinical signs of, 399
    description of, 399
    diagnostic tests for, 399
    follow-up care for, 399
    prognosis of, 399
    treatment options for, 399
Coccidiosis, enteric, 400
Colitis
    acute, 137
        causes of, 137
        clinical signs of, 137
        description of, 137
        diagnostic tests for, 137
        follow-up care for, 137
        prognosis of, 137
        treatment options for, 137
    chronic, 138
        causes of, 138
        clinical signs of, 138
        description of, 138
        diagnostic tests for, 138
        follow-up care for, 138
        prognosis of, 138
        treatment options for, 138
Collie eye anomaly (CEA), 351
    causes of, 351
    clinical signs of, 351
    description of, 351
    diagnostic tests for, 351
    follow-up care for, 351
    prognosis of, 351
    treatment options for, 351
Congestive heart failure, in dogs
    left-sided, 41
        causes of, 41
        clinical signs of, 41
        description of, 41
        diagnostic tests for, 41
        follow-up care for, 41
        prognosis of, 41
        treatment options for, 38, 41
    right-sided, 42
        causes of, 42
        clinical signs of, 42
        description of, 42
        diagnostic tests for, 42
        follow-up care for, 42
        prognosis of, 42
        treatment options for, 42
Conjunctivitis, 352
    causes of, 352
    clinical signs of, 352
    description of, 352
    diagnostic tests for, 352
    follow-up care for, 352
    prognosis of, 352
    treatment options for, 352
Copper storage hepatopathy, in dogs, 139
    causes of, 139
    clinical signs of, 139
    description of, 139
    diagnostic tests for, 139
    follow-up care for, 139
    prognosis of, 139
    treatment options for, 139

Corneal erosions, persistent, 375
    causes of, 375
    clinical signs of, 375
    description of, 375
    diagnostic tests for, 375
    follow-up care for, 375
    prognosis of, 375
    treatment options for, 375
Corneal sequestration, feline, 358
    causes of, 358
    clinical signs of, 358
    description of, 358
    diagnostic tests for, 358
    follow-up care for, 358
    prognosis of, 358
    treatment options for, 358
Corneal ulceration, 353
    causes of, 353
    clinical signs of, 353
    description of, 353
    diagnostic tests for, 353
    follow-up care for, 353
    persistent, 375
    prognosis of, 353
    treatment options for, 353
Coronavirus, feline, 405
    causes of, 405
    clinical signs of, 405
    description of, 405
    diagnostic tests for, 405
    follow-up care for, 405
    prognosis of, 405
    treatment options for, 405
Coronoid process, medial, fragmented disease
    of, 284
CPR. *See* Cardiopulmonary resuscitation
    (CPR).
Cranial cruciate ligament (CCL)
    disease, 280
    causes of, 280
    clinical signs of, 280
    description of, 280
    diagnostic tests for, 280
    follow-up care for, 280
    prognosis of, 280
    treatment options for, 280
Creatinine/creatinine clearance test, as kidney
    function test, 19
Cryptococcosis, 401
    causes of, 401
    clinical signs of, 401
    description of, 401
    diagnostic tests for, 401
    follow-up care for, 401
    prognosis of, 401
    treatment options for, 401
Cryptorchidism, 218
    causes of, 218
    clinical signs of, 218
    description of, 218
    diagnostic tests for, 218
    follow-up care for, 218
    prognosis of, 218
    treatment options for, 218
Cryptosporidiosis, 402
    causes of, 402
    clinical signs of, 402
    description of, 402

Cryptosporidiosis (*Continued*)
  diagnostic tests for, 402
  follow-up care for, 402
  prognosis of, 402
  treatment options for, 402
Cushing's disease, 179, 309
Cutaneous lupus erythematosus, 316
  clinical signs of, 316
  description of, 316
  diagnostic tests for, 316
  exfoliative, 323
  follow-up care for, 316
  prognosis of, 316
  treatment options for, 316
Cutaneous T-cell lymphoma, 317
  causes of, 317
  clinical signs of, 317
  description of, 317
  diagnostic tests for, 317
  follow-up care for, 317
  prognosis of, 317
  treatment options for, 317
Cyclical flank alopecia, 318
  causes of, 318
  clinical signs of, 318
  description of, 318
  diagnostic tests for, 318
  follow-up care for, 318
  prognosis of, 318
  treatment options for, 318
Cyst(s)
  iridociliary, 367
  mediastinal, 84
  prostatic and paraprostatic, in
      dogs, 206
  renal, 203, 210
Cystitis
  cats, 196
    causes of, 196
    clinical signs of, 196
    description of, 196
    diagnostic tests for, 196
    follow-up care for, 196
    prognosis of, 196
    treatment options for, 196
  in dogs, 197
    causes of, 197
    clinical signs of, 197
    description of, 197
    diagnostic tests for, 197
    follow-up care for, 197
    prognosis of, 197
    treatment options for, 197
Cytauxzoonosis, 403
  causes of, 403
  clinical signs of, 403
  description of, 403
  diagnostic tests for, 403
  follow-up care for, 403
  prognosis of, 403
  treatment options for, 403

D
Deafness, 386
  causes of, 386
  classifications of, 386
  clinical signs of, 386
  description of, 386

Deafness (*Continued*)
  diagnostic tests for, 386
  follow-up care for, 386
  prognosis of, 386
  treatment options for, 386
Defecation problems, 144, 163,
      429–430, 431
Degenerative joint disease (DJD), 295
Degenerative lumbosacral disease, 119
Degenerative myelopathy, 107
  causes of, 107
  clinical signs of, 107
  description of, 107
  diagnostic tests for, 107
  follow-up care for, 107
  prognosis of, 107
  treatment options for, 107
Degenerative valve disease, atrioventricular,
      in dogs, 38
Demodicosis, in dogs, 320
  causes of, 320
  clinical signs of, 320
  description of, 320
  diagnostic tests for, 320
  follow-up care for, 320
  prognosis of, 320
  treatment options for, 320
Depigmentation, nasal, 331
Depressants poisoning, 460–461
Dermatitis
  acute moist, in dogs, 308
  atopic, in dogs, 310
  flea allergic, 324
  foot pad, in cats, 335
  Malassezia, 328
Dermatophytosis, 321
  causes of, 321
  clinical signs of, 321
  description of, 321
  diagnostic tests for, 321
  follow-up care for, 321
  prognosis of, 321
  treatment options for, 321
Dermatosis
  lupoid, 323
  vitamin A–responsive, 345
  zinc-responsive, 346
Developmental orthopedic disease (DOD), of
      large-breed dogs
  causes of, 441
  clinical signs of, 441
  description of, 441
  diagnostic tests for, 441
  follow-up care for, 441
  prognosis of, 441
  treatment options for, 441
Diabetes insipidus (DI), 176
  causes of, 176
  clinical signs of, 176
  description of, 176
  diagnostic tests for, 176
  follow-up care for, 176
  prognosis of, 176
  treatment options for, 176
Diabetes mellitus (DM)
  in cats, 177
    causes of, 177
    clinical signs of, 177

Diabetes mellitus (DM) (*Continued*)
    description of, 177
    diagnostic tests for, 177
    follow-up care for, 177
    prognosis of, 177
    treatment options for, 177
  in dogs, 178
    causes of, 178
    clinical signs of, 178
    description of, 178
    diagnostic tests for, 178
    follow-up care for, 178
    prognosis of, 178
    treatment options for, 178
Dialysis, 10
  complications of, 10
  follow-up care for, 10
  preparation for, 10
  purpose of, 10
  technique for, 10
    hemodialysis, 10
    peritoneal, 10
Diaphragmatic hernia, 76
  causes of, 76
  clinical signs of, 76
  description of, 53, 76
  diagnostic tests for, 76
  follow-up care for, 76
  prognosis of, 76
  treatment options for, 76
DIC. *See* Disseminated intravascular
      coagulation (DIC).
Diet(s). *See also* Food *entries;* Nutritional
      management.
  homemade, 438
Dilated cardiomyopathy (DCM)
  in cats, 43
    causes of, 43
    clinical signs of, 43
    description of, 43
    diagnostic tests for, 43
    follow-up care for, 43
    prognosis of, 43
    treatment options for, 43
  in dogs, 44
    causes of, 34, 44
    clinical signs of, 44
    description of, 44
    diagnostic tests for, 44
    follow-up care for, 44
    prognosis of, 44
    treatment options for, 44
Discoid lupus erythematosus, 316
  causes of, 316
  clinical signs of, 316
  diagnostic tests for, 316
  follow-up care for, 316
  prognosis of, 316
  treatment options for, 316
Discospondylitis, 108
  causes of, 108
  clinical signs of, 108
  description of, 108
  diagnostic tests for, 108
  follow-up care for, 108
  prognosis of, 108
  treatment options for, 108
Dislocations. *See* Luxation(s).

Disseminated intravascular coagulation
(DIC), 249
causes of, 249
clinical signs of, 249
description of, 249
diagnostic tests for, 249
follow-up care for, 249
prognosis of, 249
treatment options for, 249
Distemper virus
canine, 396
cause of, 396
clinical signs of, 396
description of, 396
diagnostic tests for, 396
follow-up care for, 396
neurologic disease related to, 104
causes of, 104
clinical signs of, 104
description of, 104
diagnostic tests for, 104
follow-up care for, 104
prognosis of, 104
treatment options for, 104
prognosis of, 396
treatment options for, 396
feline, 417. *See also* Parvovirus.
Distichiasis, 354
causes of, 354
clinical signs of, 354
description of, 354
diagnostic tests for, 354
follow-up care for, 354
prognosis of, 354
treatment options for, 354
DJD (degenerative joint disease), 295
DM. *See* Diabetes mellitus (DM).
Doberman pinschers, occult cardiomyopathy
in, 50
DOD. *See* Developmental orthopedic disease
(DOD).
Dominance aggression
in dogs, 428
causes of, 428
clinical signs of, 428
description of, 428
diagnostic tests for, 428
prognosis of, 428
treatment options for, 428
in household cats, 427
Drug allergies, 269
Drug indications. *See specific pathology.*
Drug toxicities, 202. *See also specific drug,*
e.g., Amitraz toxicosis.
human. *See also specific drug, e.g.,*
Acetaminophen toxicosis.
illicit, 460–461, 462–463. *See also specific*
drug, e.g., Depressants poisoning.
Dry eye, 369
Ductus arteriosus, disorders of, 51, 54
Dystocia, 219
causes of, 219
clinical signs of, 219
description of, 219
diagnostic tests for, 219
follow-up care for, 219
prognosis of, 219
treatment options for, 219

E
Ear mites, 387
ECG. *See* Electrocardiogram (ECG).
Echinacea toxicity, 452–453
Echocardiography, 11
complications of, 11
follow-up care for, 11
indications for. *See specific pathology, e.g.,*
Cardiomyopathy.
preparation for, 11
purpose of, 11
technique for, 11
types of, 11, 35, 61, 65
Eclampsia, in dogs, 220
causes of, 220
clinical signs of, 220
description of, 220
diagnostic tests for, 220
follow-up care for, 220
prognosis of, 220
treatment options for, 220
Ectopic cilia, 354
causes of, 354
clinical signs of, 354
description of, 354
diagnostic tests for, 354
follow-up care for, 354
prognosis of, 354
treatment options for, 354
Ectopic ureter, in dogs, 198
causes of, 198
clinical signs of, 198
description of, 198
diagnostic tests for, 198
follow-up care for, 198
prognosis of, 198
treatment options for, 198
Ectropion, 355
causes of, 355
clinical signs of, 355
description of, 355
diagnostic tests for, 355
follow-up care for, 355
prognosis of, 355
treatment options for, 355
Edema, pulmonary, 93
Effusions
pericardial, 52
pleural, 87
Ehrlichiosis, in dogs, 404
causes of, 404
clinical signs of, 404
description of, 404
diagnostic tests for, 404
follow-up care for, 404
prognosis of, 404
public health information on, 404
treatment options for, 404
Elbow
dysplasia of, 284
in fragmented medial coronoid process
disease, 284
in ununited anconeal process disease,
305
Elbow incongruency, 281
causes of, 281
clinical signs of, 281
description of, 281

Elbow incongruency (*Continued*)
diagnostic tests for, 281
follow-up care for, 281
prognosis of, 281
treatment options for, 281
Elbow luxation, traumatic, 282
causes of, 282
clinical signs of, 282
description of, 282
diagnostic tests for, 282
follow-up care for, 282
prognosis of, 282
treatment options for, 282
Electrical cord injury, 470
causes of, 470
clinical signs of, 470
description of, 470
diagnostic tests for, 470
follow-up care for, 470
prognosis of, 470
treatment options for, 470
Electrocardiogram (ECG), 12
complications of, 12
follow-up care for, 12
indications for. *See specific pathology, e.g.,*
Congestive heart failure.
interpretation of. *See specific rhythm, e.g.,*
Atrial tachycardia.
preparation for, 12
purpose of, 12
technique for, 11, 12
Elimination problems
in cats, 429–430
causes of, 429
clinical signs of, 429
description of, 429
diagnostic tests for, 429
follow-up care for, 430
prognosis of, 430
treatment options for, 430
in dogs, 215, 431
causes of, 431
clinical signs of, 431
description of, 431
diagnostic tests for, 431
prognosis of, 431
treatment options for, 431
fecal, 144, 163
Embolic myelopathy, fibrocartilaginous,
109
Embolus, 266
Emergency care. *See specific pathology, e.g.,*
Heat prostration.
Encephalitis, necrotizing, 110
Encephalopathy, hepatic, 154
Endocarditis, 45
causes of, 45
clinical signs of, 45
description of, 45
diagnostic tests for, 45
follow-up care for, 45
prognosis of, 45
treatment options for, 45
Enteric coccidiosis, 400
causes of, 400
clinical signs of, 400
description of, 400
diagnostic tests for, 400

Enteric coccidiosis (*Continued*)
  follow-up care for, 400
  prognosis of, 400
  treatment options for, 400
Enteropathy, protein-losing, 173
Entropion, 356
  causes of, 356
  clinical signs of, 356
  description of, 356
  diagnostic tests for, 356
  follow-up care for, 356
  prognosis of, 356
  treatment options for, 356
Eosinophilic granuloma complex,
      in cats, 322
  causes of, 322
  clinical signs of, 322
  description of, 322
  diagnostic tests for, 322
  follow-up care for, 322
  prognosis of, 322
  treatment options for, 322
Eosinophilic keratitis, feline, 359
  causes of, 359
  clinical signs of, 359
  description of, 359
  diagnostic tests for, 359
  follow-up care for, 359
  prognosis of, 359
  treatment options for, 359
Ephedrine toxicity, 452
EPI. *See* Exocrine pancreatic insufficiency
      (EPI).
Epitheliomas, sebaceous, in dogs, 312
Epulis, in dogs, 140
  causes of, 140
  clinical signs of, 140
  description of, 140
  diagnostic tests for, 140
  follow-up care for, 140
  prognosis of, 140
  treatment options for, 140
ESF. *See* External skeletal fixation
      (ESF).
Esophageal foreign body, 141
  causes of, 141
  clinical signs of, 141
  description of, 141
  diagnostic tests for, 141
  follow-up care for, 141
  prognosis of, 141
  treatment options for, 141
Esophageal stricture, 142
  causes of, 142
  clinical signs of, 142
  description of, 142
  diagnostic tests for, 142
  follow-up care for, 142
  prognosis of, 142
  treatment options for, 142
Esophagitis, 142
  causes of, 142
  clinical signs of, 142
  description of, 142
  diagnostic tests for, 142
  follow-up care for, 142
  prognosis of, 142
  treatment options for, 142

Exfoliative cutaneous lupus erythematosus, 323
  causes of, 323
  clinical signs of, 323
  description of, 323
  diagnostic tests for, 323
  prognosis of, 323
  treatment options for, 323
Exocrine pancreatic insufficiency
      (EPI), 143
  causes of, 143
  clinical signs of, 143
  description of, 143
  diagnostic tests for, 143
  follow-up care for, 143
  prognosis of, 143
  treatment options for, 143
External skeletal fixation (ESF), for fracture
      repair, 16
  complications of, 16
  follow-up care for, 16
  postoperative care for, 16
  preparation for, 16
  purpose of, 16
  technique for, 16
Extramedullary plasmacytoma, 270
  causes of, 270
  clinical signs of, 270
  description of, 270
  diagnostic tests for, 270
  follow-up care for, 270
  prognosis of, 270
  treatment options for, 270
Eye
  collie anomaly of, 351
  dry, 369
  proptosis of, 379
  tumors of, 366, 373
Eyelid
  rolling of, inward *vs.* outward, 355, 356
  third, prolapse of gland of, 378
  tumors of, 357
    causes of, 357
    clinical signs of, 357
    description of, 357
    diagnostic tests for, 357
    follow-up care for, 357
    prognosis of, 357
    treatment options for, 357

F
Facial nerve paralysis, idiopathic, 113
  causes of, 113
  clinical signs of, 113
  description of, 113
  follow-up care for, 113
  prognosis of, 113
  treatment options for, 113
Fanconi syndrome, in dogs, 199
  causes of, 199
  clinical signs of, 199
  description of, 199
  diagnostic tests for, 199
  follow-up care for, 199
  prognosis of, 199
  treatment options for, 199
FCEM. *See* Fibrocartilaginous embolic
      myelopathy (FCEM).
Fear disorders, in dogs, 432

Fecal incontinence, 144
  causes of, 144
  clinical signs of, 144
  description of, 144
  diagnostic tests for, 144
  follow-up care for, 144
  prognosis of, 144
  treatment options for, 144
Fecal retention, in cats, 163
Femoral head and neck ostectomy (FHO), 13
  complications of, 13
  follow-up care for, 13
  postoperative care for, 13
  preparation for, 13
  purpose of, 13, 291
  technique for, 13
Femoral head, avascular necrosis of, 291
Fever of unknown origin (FUO), 250
  causes of, 250
  clinical signs of, 250
  description of, 250
  diagnostic tests for, 250
  follow-up care for, 250
  prognosis of, 250
  treatment options for, 250
Fibrocartilaginous embolic myelopathy
      (FCEM), 109
  causes of, 109
  clinical signs of, 109
  description of, 109
  diagnostic tests for, 109
  follow-up care for, 109
  prognosis of, 109
  treatment options for, 109
Fibrotic myopathies, 283
  causes of, 283
  clinical signs of, 283
  description of, 283
  diagnostic tests for, 283
  follow-up care for, 283
  prognosis of, 283
  treatment options for, 283
Fistula, perianal, in dogs, 169
Flail chest, 77
  causes of, 77
  clinical signs of, 77
  description of, 77
  diagnostic tests for, 77
  follow-up care for, 77
  treatment options for, 77
Flank alopecia, cyclical (seasonal), 318
Flea allergic dermatitis, 324
  causes of, 324
  clinical signs of, 324
  description of, 324
  diagnostic tests for, 324
  follow-up care for, 324
  prognosis of, 324
  treatment options for, 324
Fluid therapy, 14
  complications of, 14
  equipment for, 14
  follow-up care for, 14
  preparation for, 14
  purpose of, 14. *See also specific pathology
      or procedure.*
  techniques for, 14. *See also* Subcutaneous
      (SC, SQ) fluid administration

FMCP. *See* Fragmented medial coronoid
  process (FMCP) disease.
Folliculitis, superficial bacterial, 342
  causes of, 342
  clinical signs of, 342
  description of, 342
  diagnostic tests for, 342
  follow-up care for, 342
  prognosis of, 342
  treatment options for, 342
Food allergies, 325
  causes of, 325
  clinical signs of, 325
  description of, 325
  diagnostic tests for, 325
  feeding trials for, 437
    causes of, 437
    clinical signs of, 437
    description of, 437
    diagnostic tests for, 437
    follow-up care for, 437
    prognosis of, 437
    treatment options for, 437
  follow-up care for, 325
  prognosis of, 325
  treatment options for, 325
Food toxicities, 202. *See also specific food,*
  e.g., Bread dough poisoning.
Foot pad disease, plasma cell, in cats, 335
Foreign body(ies)
  airway, 6, 97
  esophageal, 141
  gastric, 147
Fracture repair
  casts and splints for, 15
  external skeletal fixation for, 16
  internal skeletal fixation for, 17
Fractures
  mandibular, 292
  rib, flail chest with, 77
Fragmented medial coronoid process (FMCP)
  disease, 284
  causes of, 284
  clinical signs of, 284
  description of, 284
  diagnostic tests for, 284
  follow-up care for, 284
  prognosis of, 284
  treatment options for, 284
FUO. *See* Fever of unknown origin (FUO).
Furunculosis, deep bacterial, 319
  causes of, 319
  clinical signs of, 319
  description of, 319
  diagnostic tests for, 319
  follow-up care for, 319
  prognosis of, 319
  treatment options for, 319

G
Gabapentin *(Neurotin),* for seizures, 126
Gall bladder disease
  in cats, cholangiohepatitis as, 135
  in dogs, 145
    causes of, 145
    clinical signs of, 145
    description of, 145
    diagnostic tests for, 145

Gall bladder disease (*Continued*)
    follow-up care for, 145
    prognosis of, 145
    treatment options for, 145
Gastric foreign body, 147
  causes of, 147
  clinical signs of, 147
  description of, 147
  diagnostic tests for, 147
  follow-up care for, 147
  prognosis of, 147
  treatment options for, 147
Gastric neoplasia, 148
  causes of, 148
  clinical signs of, 148
  description of, 148
  diagnostic tests for, 148
  follow-up care for, 148
  prognosis of, 148
  treatment options for, 148
Gastritis
  acute, 149
    causes of, 149
    clinical signs of, 149
    description of, 149
    diagnostic tests for, 149
    follow-up care for, 149
    prognosis of, 149
    treatment options for, 149
  chronic, 150
    causes of, 150, 410
    clinical signs of, 150
    description of, 150
    diagnostic tests for, 150
    follow-up care for, 150
    prognosis of, 150
    treatment options for, 150
Gastroenteritis, hemorrhagic, in dogs, 153
Gastrointestinal ulceration, 151
  causes of, 151
  clinical signs of, 151
  description of, 151
  diagnostic tests for, 151
  follow-up care for, 151
  prognosis of, 151
  treatment options for, 151
GFR (glomerular filtration rate), as kidney
  function test, 19
Giardiasis, 409
  causes of, 409
  clinical signs of, 409
  description of, 409
  diagnostic tests for, 409
  follow-up care for, 409
  prognosis of, 409
  public health information on, 409
  treatment options for, 409
Gingivitis, 152
  causes of, 152
  clinical signs of, 152
  description of, 152
  diagnostic tests for, 152
  follow-up care for, 152
  prognosis of, 152
  treatment options for, 152
Glaucoma
  in cats, 361
    causes of, 361

Glaucoma (*Continued*)
    clinical signs of, 361
    description of, 361
    diagnostic tests for, 361
    follow-up care for, 361
    prognosis of, 361
    treatment options for, 361
  in dogs, 362
    causes of, 362
    clinical signs of, 362
    description of, 362
    diagnostic tests for, 362
    follow-up care for, 362
    prognosis of, 362
    treatment options for, 362
Glomerular filtration rate (GFR), as kidney
  function test, 19
Granuloma complex, eosinophilic, in cats, 322
Granulomatous meningoencephalitis (GME),
  110
  causes of, 110
  clinical signs of, 110
  description of, 110
  diagnostic tests for, 110
  follow-up care for, 110
  prognosis of, 110
  treatment options for, 110
Grape toxicosis, in dogs, 451
  causes and toxicity of, 451
  clinical signs of, 451
  description of, 451
  diagnostic tests for, 451
  follow-up care for, 451
  prognosis of, 451
  treatment options for, 451
Guarana toxicity, 452

H
Hair follicles
  eyelid, abnormal development of, 354
  growing disorder of, 309
  mite infestation of, 320
  plugged, in cats, 307
  superficial bacterial infection of, 342
  tumors of, in dogs, 312
HCM. *See* Hypertrophic cardiomyopathy
  (HCM).
Head trauma, 111
  causes of, 111
  clinical signs of, 111
  description of, 111
  diagnostic tests for, 111
  follow-up care for, 111
  prognosis of, 111
  treatment options for, 111
Hearing loss. *See* Deafness.
Heart block, second- and third-degree, 57
Heart failure. *See* Congestive heart failure.
Heartworm (HW) disease
  in cats, 46
    causes of, 46
    clinical signs of, 46
    description of, 46
    diagnostic tests for, 46
    follow-up care for, 46
    preventive drugs for, 46
    prognosis of, 46
    treatment options for, 46

Heartworm (HW) disease (*Continued*)
  in dogs, 47–48
    causes of, 47
    clinical signs of, 47
    description of, 47
    diagnostic tests for, 47
    follow-up care for, 48
    physiologic effects of, 47
    preventive drugs for, 48
    prognosis of, 48
    treatment options for, 48
Heat prostration, 471
  causes of, 471
  clinical signs of, 471
  description of, 471
  diagnostic tests for, 471
  follow-up care for, 471
  prognosis of, 471
  treatment options for, 471
Helicobacteriosis, 410
  causes of, 410
  clinical signs of, 410
  description of, 410
  diagnostic tests for, 410
  follow-up care for, 410
  prognosis of, 410
  treatment options for, 410
Hemangiosarcoma
  cardiac, 39
    pericardial effusion with, 39, 52
    right atrial, in dogs, 39
  spinal cord, 128
  splenic, 262
Hematoma, ear flap, 385
Hemobartonellosis, in cats, 251
  causes of, 251
  clinical signs of, 251
  description of, 251
  diagnostic tests for, 251
  follow-up care for, 251
  treatment options for, 251
Hemolytic anemia, immune-mediated, 255
Hemophilia A, 252
  causes of, 252
  clinical signs of, 252
  description of, 252
  diagnostic tests for, 252
  follow-up care for, 252
  prognosis of, 252
  treatment options for, 252
Hemophilia B, 253
  causes of, 253
  clinical signs of, 253
  description of, 253
  diagnostic tests for, 253
  follow-up care for, 253
  prognosis of, 253
  treatment options for, 253
Hemorrhagic gastroenteritis, in dogs, 153
  causes of, 153
  clinical signs of, 153
  description of, 153
  diagnostic tests for, 153
  follow-up care for, 153
  prognosis of, 153
  treatment options for, 153
Hepatic encephalopathy, 154
  causes of, 154

Hepatic encephalopathy (*Continued*)
  clinical signs of, 154
  description of, 154
  diagnostic tests for, 154
  follow-up care for, 154
  treatment options for, 154
Hepatic lipidosis, in cats, 155
  causes of, 155
  clinical signs of, 155
  description of, 155
  diagnostic tests for, 155
  follow-up care for, 155
  prognosis of, 155
  treatment options for, 155
Hepatitis, chronic, in dogs, 156
  causes of, 156
  clinical signs of, 156
  description of, 156
  diagnostic tests for, 156
  follow-up care for, 156
  prognosis of, 156
  treatment options for, 156
Hepatozoonosis, in dogs, 411
  causes of, 411
  clinical signs of, 411
  description of, 411
  diagnostic tests for, 411
  follow-up care for, 411
  prognosis of, 411
  treatment options for, 411
Herbal poisonings, 452–453
Hernia
  diaphragmatic, 76
  hiatal, 72, 78
  perineal, in dogs, 171
  peritoneopericardial diaphragmatic, 53
Herpesvirus, feline, eye disorders related to,
    359, 360
Hip arthroplasty, total, 28
Hip dysplasia, in dogs, 285
  causes of, 285
  clinical signs of, 285
  description of, 285
  diagnostic tests for, 285
  follow-up care for, 285
  prognosis of, 285
  treatment options for, 285
  triple pelvic osteotomy for, 31
Hip luxation, 286
  causes of, 286
  clinical signs of, 286
  description of, 286
  diagnostic tests for, 286
  follow-up care for, 286
  prognosis of, 286
  treatment options for, 286
Histiocytic sarcoma (HS), 271
  causes of, 271
  clinical signs of, 271
  description of, 159, 271
  diagnostic tests for, 271
  follow-up care for, 271
  prognosis of, 271
  treatment options for, 271
Histiocytosis, malignant, 271
Histoplasmosis, 412
  cause of, 412
  clinical signs of, 412

Histoplasmosis (*Continued*)
  description of, 412
  diagnostic tests for, 412
  follow-up care for, 412
  prognosis of, 412
  treatment options for, 412
HO. *See* Hypertrophic osteopathy (HO).
HOD. *See* Hypertrophic osteodystrophy (HOD).
Homemade diets, 438
  creating, 438
  description of, 438
  follow-up care for, 438
  rationale for, 438
  types of, 438
Horner's syndrome, 363
  causes of, 363
  clinical signs of, 85, 363
  description of, 363
  diagnostic tests for, 363
  follow-up care for, 363
  prognosis of, 363
  treatment options for, 363
Household product/substance toxicities, 202.
          See also specific product, e.g.,
          Antifreeze poisoning.
HS. *See* Histiocytic sarcoma (HS).
HW. *See* Heartworm (HW) disease.
Hydrocephalus, 112
  causes of, 112
  clinical signs of, 112
  description of, 112
  diagnostic tests for, 112
  follow-up care for, 112
  prognosis of, 112
  treatment options for, 112
Hyperadrenocorticism, in dogs, 179
  causes of, 179
  clinical signs of, 179
  description of, 179
  diagnostic tests for, 179
  follow-up care for, 179
  pituitary-dependent, 179
  prognosis of, 179
  treatment options for, 179
Hypercalcemia, 180
  cancer association with, 254
    causes of, 254
    clinical signs of, 254
    description of, 254
    diagnostic tests for, 254
    follow-up care for, 254
    prognosis of, 254
    treatment options for, 254
  causes of, 180
  clinical signs of, 180
  description of, 180
  diagnostic tests for, 180
  follow-up care for, 180
  prognosis of, 180
  treatment options for, 180
Hyperlipidemia, 181
  causes of, 181
  clinical signs of, 181
  description of, 181
  diagnostic tests for, 181
  follow-up care for, 181
  prognosis of, 181
  treatment options for, 181

Hyperparathyroidism, 180
   cancer and, 254
   nutritional secondary, 294
Hypertension, 4
   pulmonary, 55
   systemic, 62
Hypertensive retinopathy, 364
   causes of, 364
   clinical signs of, 364
   description of, 364
   diagnostic tests for, 364
   follow-up care for, 364
   prognosis of, 364
   treatment options for, 364
Hyperthyroidism, in cats, 182
   causes of, 182
   clinical signs of, 182
   description of, 182
   diagnostic tests for, 182
   follow-up care for, 182
   prognosis of, 182
   treatment options for, 182
Hypertrophic cardiomyopathy (HCM), in cats, 49
   causes of, 49
   clinical signs of, 49
   description of, 49
   diagnostic tests for, 49
   follow-up care for, 49
   prognosis of, 49
   treatment options for, 49
Hypertrophic osteodystrophy (HOD), in dogs, 287
   causes of, 287
   clinical signs of, 287
   description of, 287
   diagnostic tests for, 287
   follow-up care for, 287
   prognosis of, 287
   treatment options for, 287
Hypertrophic osteopathy (HO), in dogs, 288
   causes of, 288
   clinical signs of, 288
   description of, 288
   diagnostic tests for, 288
   follow-up care for, 288
   prognosis of, 288
   treatment options for, 288
Hypervitaminosis A, 294
Hyphema, 365
   causes of, 365
   clinical signs of, 365
   description of, 365
   diagnostic tests for, 365
   follow-up care for, 365
   prognosis of, 365
   treatment options for, 365
Hypoadrenocorticism, 183
   causes of, 183
   clinical signs of, 183
   description of, 183
   diagnostic tests for, 183
   follow-up care for, 183
   prognosis of, 183
   treatment options for, 183
Hypoglycemia, 184
   causes of, 184
   clinical signs of, 184
   description of, 184
   diagnostic tests for, 184

Hypoglycemia (*Continued*)
   follow-up care for, 184
   prognosis of, 184
   treatment options for, 184
Hypotension, 4
Hypothyroidism, in dogs, 185
   causes of, 185
   clinical signs of, 185
   description of, 185
   diagnostic tests for, 185
   follow-up care for, 185
   prognosis of, 185
   treatment options for, 185
Hypovitaminosis D, 294

I
IBD. *See* Inflammatory bowel disease (IBD).
Idiopathic peripheral vestibular disease, 114
   causes of, 114
   clinical signs of, 114
   description of, 114
   diagnostic tests for, 114
   follow-up care for, 114
   prognosis of, 114
   treatment options for, 114
Illicit human drug poisonings
   basic information on, 460–461, 462–463
   specific drugs of, 460–461, 462–463
Immune-mediated arthritis, 289
   causes of, 289
   clinical signs of, 289
   description of, 289
   diagnostic tests for, 289
   follow-up care for, 289
   prognosis of, 289
   treatment options for, 289
Immune-mediated hemolytic anemia (IMHA), 255
   cause of, 255
   clinical signs of, 255
   description of, 255
   diagnostic tests for, 255
   follow-up care for, 255
   prognosis of, 255
   treatment options for, 255
Immune-mediated thrombocytopenia (ITP), 256
   causes of, 256
   clinical signs of, 256
   description of, 256
   diagnostic tests for, 256
   follow-up care for, 256
   prognosis of, 256
   treatment options for, 256
Immunodeficiency virus, feline, 406
   causes of, 406
   clinical signs of, 406
   description of, 406
   diagnostic tests for, 406
   follow-up care for, 406
   prognosis of, 406
   treatment options for, 406
Incontinence
   fecal, 144
   urinary, in dogs, 215
Infection(s)
   antibiotic resistant, 415
   bacteria. *See also specific infection, e.g.,*
      Campylobacteriosis.
      deep, in pyoderma and furunculosis, 319

Infection(s) (*Continued*)
   of joints, 302
   superficial, of hair follicles, 342
   fungus. *See also specific infection, e.g.,*
      Blastomycosis.
   skin, 321, 340
   parasite. *See also specific infestation, e.g.,*
      Heartworm (HW) disease.
   intestinal, 161
   pathology associated with. *See specific
      anatomy or pathology, e.g.,*
      Laryngotracheitis.
   public health information on, 404,
      409, 415, 421, 422, 424, 425
   virus. *See specific virus, e.g.,* Distemper
      virus.
   yeast
      ear, external *vs.* middle, 387, 389
      skin, 328
Infectious anemia, feline, 251
Infectious tracheobronchitis (ITB),
      canine, 397
   causes of, 397
   clinical signs of, 397
   description of, 397
   diagnostic tests for, 397
   follow-up care for, 397
   prognosis of, 397
   treatment options for, 397
Infertility
   in bitches, 221
      causes of, 221
      clinical signs of, 221
      description of, 221
      diagnostic tests for, 221
      prognosis of, 221
      treatment options for, 221
   in male dogs, 222
      causes of, 222
      clinical signs of, 222
      description of, 222
      diagnostic tests for, 222
      prognosis of, 222
      treatment options for, 222
   in queens, 223
      causes of, 223
      clinical signs of, 223
      description of, 223
      diagnostic tests for, 223
      prognosis of, 223
      treatment options for, 223
   in toms, 224
      causes of, 224
      clinical signs of, 224
      description of, 224
      diagnostic tests for, 224
      prognosis of, 224
      treatment options for, 224
Inflammatory bowel disease (IBD)
   in cats, 157
      causes of, 157
      clinical signs of, 157
      description of, 157
      diagnostic tests for, 157
      follow-up care for, 157
      prognosis of, 157
      treatment options for, 157
   cholangiohepatitis with, 135

Inflammatory bowel disease (IBD) (*Continued*)
  in dogs, 158
    causes of, 158
    clinical signs of, 158
    description of, 158
    diagnostic tests for, 158
    follow-up care for, 158
    prognosis of, 158
    treatment options for, 158
Influenza, canine, 398
  cause of, 398
  clinical signs of, 398
  description of, 398
  diagnostic tests for, 398
  follow-up care for, 398
  prognosis of, 398
  treatment options for, 398
Infraspinatus tendinopathy (IT), 283
Insecticides poisoning, 458
Insulin, 177, 178
Internal skeletal fixation, for fracture repair, 17
  complications of, 17
  follow-up care for, 17
  postoperative care for, 17
  preparation for, 17
  purpose of, 17
  technique for, 17
Intertrigo, 339
Intervertebral disc disease (IVDD), 116–117
  causes of, 116
  clinical signs of, 108, 116
  description of, 109, 116, 119
  diagnostic tests for, 116
  follow-up care for, 117
  prognosis of, 117
  treatment options for, 117
Intestinal neoplasia, 159
  causes of, 159
  clinical signs of, 159
  description of, 159
  diagnostic tests for, 159
  follow-up care for, 159
  prognosis of, 159
  treatment options for, 159
Intestinal obstruction, 160
  causes of, 160
  clinical signs of, 160
  description of, 160
  diagnostic tests for, 160
  follow-up care for, 160
  prognosis of, 160
  treatment options for, 160
Intestinal parasites, 161
  causes of, 161
  clinical signs of, 161
  description of, 161
  diagnostic tests for, 161
  follow-up care for, 161
  prognosis of, 161
  treatment options for, 161
Intraocular tumors, 366
  causes of, 366
  clinical signs of, 366
  description of, 366
  diagnostic tests for, 366
  follow-up care for, 366
  prognosis of, 366
  treatment options for, 366

Intravenous fluids. *See* Fluid therapy.
Iohexol clearance test, for kidney function, 19
Iridociliary cysts, 367
  causes of, 367
  clinical signs of, 367
  description of, 367
  diagnostic tests for, 367
  follow-up care for, 367
  prognosis of, 367
  treatment options for, 367
Iris melanosis, of cats, 368
  causes of, 368
  clinical signs of, 368
  description of, 368
  diagnostic tests for, 368
  follow-up care for, 368
  prognosis of, 368
  treatment options for, 368
Ischemic brain injury, 118
  causes of, 118
  clinical signs of, 118
  description of, 118
  diagnostic tests for, 118
  follow-up care for, 118
  prognosis of, 118
  treatment options for, 118
IT (infraspinatus tendinopathy), 283
ITB. *See* Infectious tracheobronchitis (ITB).
ITP. *See* Immune-mediated thrombocytopenia (ITP).
IVDD. *See* Intervertebral disc disease (IVDD).

J

Juvenile carpal hyperextension/hyperflexion disorder, 290
  causes of, 290
  clinical signs of, 290
  description of, 290
  diagnostic tests for, 290
  follow-up care for, 290
  prognosis of, 290
  treatment options for, 290
Juvenile cellulitis, 326
  causes of, 326
  clinical signs of, 326
  description of, 326
  diagnostic tests for, 326
  follow-up care for, 326
  prognosis of, 326
  treatment options for, 326

K

Kennel cough, in dogs, 397
Keppra. *See* Levetiracetam *(Keppra)*.
Keratitis
  in cats
    eosinophilic, 359
    necrotizing, 358
  chronic superficial, 374
  pigmentary, 376
Keratoconjunctivitis, feline herpesvirus, 360
  causes of, 360
  clinical signs of, 360
  description of, 360
  diagnostic tests for, 360
  follow-up care for, 360
  prognosis of, 360
  treatment options for, 360

Keratoconjunctivitis sicca (KCS), 369
  causes of, 369
  clinical signs of, 369
  description of, 369
  diagnostic tests for, 369
  follow-up care for, 369
  prognosis of, 369
  treatment options for, 369
Keratopathy, lipid, 371
Kidney disease
  in cats, polycystic, 204
  chronic. *See* Chronic kidney disease (CKD).
  in dogs
    protein-losing, 208
    systemic lupus erythematosus and, 273
    urine protein assays for, 32
  neoplasia as, 210
Kidney dysplasia, in dogs, 200
  causes of, 200
  clinical signs of, 200
  description of, 200, 210
  diagnostic tests for, 200
  follow-up care for, 200
  prognosis of, 200
  treatment options for, 200
Kidney failure
  acute. *See* Acute renal failure (ARF).
  chronic
    acute *vs.*, 10
    transplantation for, 18
  dialysis for, 10
Kidney function
  Fanconi syndrome and, 199
  laboratory tests of, 19
Kidney infection, 209
Kidney stones, 10
  in cats, 201
    causes of, 201
    clinical signs of, 201
    description of, 201
    diagnostic tests for, 201
    follow-up care for, 201
    prognosis of, 201
    treatment options for, 201
Kidney toxins, 202
  causes of, 202
  clinical signs of, 202
  description of, 202
  diagnostic tests for, 202
  follow-up care for, 202
  treatment options for, 202
Kidney transplantation, in cats, 18
  complications of, 18
  follow-up care for, 18
  postoperative care for, 18
  preparation for, 18
  purpose of, 18
  technique for, 18
Knee (stifle) luxation, 304
  patella luxation *vs.*, 299

L

Laboratory tests
  indications for. *See specific pathology, e.g.,* Cardiomyopathy.
  preoperative, 23

Laryngeal collapse, in dogs, 78
  causes of, 78
  clinical signs of, 78
  description of, 78
  diagnostic tests for, 78
  follow-up care for, 78
  prognosis of, 78
  treatment options for, 78
Laryngeal neoplasia, 80
  causes of, 80
  clinical signs of, 80
  description of, 80
  diagnostic tests for, 80
  follow-up care for, 80
  prognosis of, 80
  treatment options for, 80
Laryngeal paralysis, 79
  causes of, 79
  clinical signs of, 79
  description of, 79
  diagnostic tests for, 79
  follow-up care for, 79
  prognosis of, 79
  treatment options for, 79
Laryngitis, 81
Laryngotracheitis, 81
  causes of, 81
  clinical signs of, 81
  description of, 81
  diagnostic tests for, 81
  follow-up care for, 81
  prognosis of, 81
  treatment options for, 81
Lead poisoning, 454
  causes of, 454
  clinical signs of, 454
  description of, 454
  diagnostic tests for, 454
  follow-up care for, 454
  prognosis of, 454
  treatment options for, 454
Legg-Calvé-Perthes disease, 291
  causes of, 291
  clinical signs of, 291
  description of, 291
  diagnostic tests for, 291
  follow-up care for, 291
  prognosis of, 291
  treatment options for, 291
Leishmaniasis, 413
  causes of, 413
  clinical signs of, 413
  description of, 413
  diagnostic tests for, 413
  follow-up care for, 413
  prognosis of, 413
  treatment options for, 413
Lens luxation/subluxation, 370
  causes of, 370
  clinical signs of, 370
  description of, 370
  diagnostic tests for, 370
  follow-up care for, 370
  prognosis of, 370
  treatment options for, 370
Leptospirosis, 414
  causes of, 414
  clinical signs of, 414

Leptospirosis (Continued)
  description of, 414
  diagnostic tests for, 414
  follow-up care for, 414
  prognosis of, 414
  treatment options for, 414
Leukemia
  acute lymphocytic, 242
  chronic lymphocytic, 247
  mast cell, 260
Leukemia virus, feline, 407
  cause of, 407
  clinical signs of, 407
  description of, 407
  diagnostic tests for, 407
  follow-up care for, 407
  treatment options for, 407
Levetiracetam (Keppra), for seizures, 126
Limb (leg)
  amputation of, 2
  angular deformities of, in dogs, 275
Lipid keratopathy, 371
  causes of, 371
  clinical signs of, 371
  description of, 371
  diagnostic tests for, 371
  follow-up care for, 371
  prognosis of, 371
  treatment options for, 371
Lipidosis, hepatic, in cats, 155
Lipomas, in dogs, 327
  causes of, 327
  clinical signs of, 327
  description of, 327
  diagnostic tests for, 327
  follow-up care for, 327
  prognosis of, 327
  treatment options for, 327
Liver disease. See also Hepatic entries.
  cholangiohepatitis as, 135
  coagulopathy associated with, 248
  copper storage, in dogs, 139
LSA. See Lymphosarcoma (LSA).
Lumbosacral disease, degenerative, 119
  causes of, 119
  clinical signs of, 119
  description of, 119
  diagnostic tests for, 119
  follow-up care for, 119
  prognosis of, 119
  treatment options for, 119
Lung disease. See also Pulmonary entries;
    Respiratory entries.
  bullous, 75
Lung lobe torsion, 82
  causes of, 82
  clinical signs of, 82
  description of, 82
  diagnostic tests for, 82
  follow-up care for, 82
  prognosis of, 82
  treatment options for, 82
Lung tumors, 83
  causes of, 83
  clinical signs of, 83
  description of, 83
  diagnostic tests for, 83
  follow-up care for, 83

Lung tumors (Continued)
  prognosis of, 83
  treatment options for, 83
Lupus erythematosus
  cutaneous, 316
    exfoliative, 323
  discoid, 316
  systemic
    dermatologic aspects of, 343
    sysemic aspects of, 273
Luxation(s)
  atlantoaxial, in dogs, 100
  elbow, 282
  hip, 286
  knee (stifle), 304
  lens, 370
  patellar, 299
  sacroiliac joint, 300
  shoulder, 303
  shoulder blade (scapula), 301
Lyme disease, 393
Lymphedema, 257
  causes of, 257
  clinical signs of, 257
  description of, 257
  diagnostic tests for, 257
  follow-up care for, 257
  prognosis of, 257
  treatment options for, 257
Lymphocytic leukemia
  acute, 242
  chronic, 247
Lymphoma
  in cats, 258
    causes of, 258
    clinical signs of, 258
    description of, 258
    diagnostic tests for, 258
    follow-up care for, 258
    prognosis of, 258
    treatment options for, 258
  cutaneous T-cell (epitheliotropic), 317
  in dogs, 259
    causes of, 259
    clinical signs of, 259
    description of, 259
    diagnostic tests for, 259
    follow-up care for, 259
    prognosis of, 259
    treatment options for, 259
  gastric, 148
  intestinal, 159
  intraocular, 366
  orbital, 373
Lymphoplasmacytic stomatitis, in cats, 162
  causes of, 162
  clinical signs of, 162
  description of, 162
  diagnostic tests for, 162
  follow-up care for, 162
  prognosis of, 162
  treatment options for, 162
Lymphosarcoma (LSA), 258, 259
  cardiac, 39
  laryngeal and tracheal, 80
  mediastinal, 84
  nasal, 86
  renal, 210

M

Macadamia nut toxicosis, in dogs, 455
  causes of, 455
  clinical signs of, 455
  description of, 455
  diagnostic tests for, 455
  follow-up care for, 455
  prognosis of, 455
  treatment options for, 455
Malassezia dermatitis, 328
  causes of, 328
  clinical signs of, 328
  description of, 328
  diagnostic tests for, 328
  follow-up care for, 328
  prognosis of, 328
  treatment options for, 328
Malignant histiocytosis (MH), 271
  causes of, 271
  clinical signs of, 271
  description of, 271
  diagnostic tests for, 271
  follow-up care for, 271
  prognosis of, 271
  treatment options for, 271
Mammary fibroadenomatous hyperplasia,
      225
  causes of, 225
  clinical signs of, 225
  description of, 225
  diagnostic tests for, 225
  follow-up care for, 225
  prognosis of, 225
  treatment options for, 225
Mammary tumors
  in cats, 226
    causes of, 226
    clinical signs of, 226
    description of, 226
    diagnostic tests for, 226
    follow-up care for, 226
    prognosis of, 226
    treatment options for, 226
  in dogs, 227
    causes of, 227
    clinical signs of, 227
    description of, 227
    diagnostic tests for, 227
    follow-up care for, 227
    prognosis of, 227
    treatment options for, 227
Mandibular fractures, 292
  causes of, 292
  clinical signs of, 292
  description of, 292
  diagnostic tests for, 292
  follow-up care for, 292
  prognosis of, 292
  treatment options for, 292
Mandibular nerve paralysis, idiopathic
      bilateral, 115
Mange
  notoedric, 332
  sarcoptic, 337
Marijuana toxicity, 460–461
Mass(es). *See also* Tumor(s).
  mediastinal, 84
  polyps as, nasal and nasopharyngeal, 85

Mast cell tumors (MCT)
  in cats, 329
    causes of, 329
    clinical signs of, 329
    description of, 329
    diagnostic tests for, 329
    follow-up care for, 329
    prognosis of, 329
    treatment options for, 329
  in dogs, 330
    causes of, 330
    clinical signs of, 330
    description of, 330
    diagnostic tests for, 330
    follow-up care for, 330
    prognosis of, 330
    treatment options for, 330
  orbital, 373
  systemic, 260
Masticatory myositis
  causes of, 293
  clinical signs of, 293
  description of, 293
  diagnostic tests for, 293
  follow-up care for, 293
  prognosis of, 293
  treatment options for, 293
Mastitis, 228
  causes of, 228
  clinical signs of, 228
  description of, 228
  diagnostic tests for, 228
  follow-up care for, 228
  prognosis of, 228
  treatment options for, 228
Mastocytosis, 260
  in cats, 329
  causes of, 260
  clinical signs of, 260
  description of, 260
  diagnostic tests for, 260
  in dogs, 330
  follow-up care for, 260
  prognosis of, 260
  treatment options for, 260
MCT. *See* Mast cell tumors (MCT).
Medial coronoid process, fragmented disease
      of, 284
Mediastinal masses, 84
  causes of, 84
  clinical signs of, 84
  description of, 84
  diagnostic tests for, 84
  follow-up care for, 84
  prognosis of, 84
  treatment options for, 84
Megacolon, in cats, 163
  causes of, 163
  clinical signs of, 163
  description of, 163
  diagnostic tests for, 163
  follow-up care for, 163
  prognosis of, 163
  treatment options for, 163
Megaesophagus, 164
  causes of, 164
  clinical signs of, 164
  description of, 164

Megaesophagus (*Continued*)
  diagnostic tests for, 164
  follow-up care for, 164
  prognosis of, 164
  treatment options for, 164
Melanoma, 165, 366
Melanosis, iris, in cats, 368
Meningeal arteritis, steroid-responsive, 130
Meningoencephalitis, granulomatous, 110
Metaldehyde poisoning, 456
  causes of, 456
  clinical signs of, 456
  description of, 456
  diagnostic tests for, 456
  follow-up care for, 456
  prognosis of, 456
  treatment options for, 456
Metaphyseal disorders, 287
Methicillin-resistant *Staphylococcus* infections
      (MRS), 415
  causes of, 415
  clinical signs of, 415
  description of, 415
  diagnostic tests for, 415
  follow-up care for, 415
  prognosis of, 415
  public health information on, 415
  treatment options for, 415
Methylxanthine toxicosis, 449
  causes and toxicity of, 449
  clinical signs of, 449
  description of, 449
  diagnostic tests for, 449
  follow-up care for, 449
  prognosis of, 449
  treatment options for, 449
MG. *See* Myasthenia gravis (MG).
MH. *See* Malignant histiocytosis (MH).
Mite infestation, 313, 320, 332, 337
Mitral valve
  degeneration of, in dogs, 38
  dysplasia of, 64
    causes of, 64
    clinical signs of, 64
    description of, 64
    diagnostic tests for, 64
    follow-up care for, 64
    prognosis of, 64
    treatment options for, 64
  infection of, 45
Moist dermatitis, acute, in dogs, 308
  causes of, 308
  clinical signs of, 308
  description of, 308
  diagnostic tests for, 308
  follow-up care for, 308
  prognosis of, 308
  treatment options for, 308
Mouth
  inflammation of. *See* Stomatitis.
  neoplasms of, 140, 165, 166
MRS. *See* Methicillin-resistant
      Staphylococcus infections (MRS).
Mucocele
  biliary, 145
  salivary, in dogs, 174
Multiple myeloma, 272
  causes of, 272

Multiple myeloma (*Continued*)
  clinical signs of, 272
  description of, 272
  diagnostic tests for, 272
  follow-up care for, 272
  prognosis of, 272
  treatment options for, 272
Myasthenia gravis (MG), 120
  causes of, 120
  clinical signs of, 120
  description of, 120
  diagnostic tests for, 120
  follow-up care for, 120
  forms of, 120
  prognosis of, 120
  treatment options for, 120
Mycobacteriosis, atypical, 311
  causes of, 311
  clinical signs of, 311
  description of, 311
  diagnostic tests for, 311
  follow-up care for, 311
  prognosis of, 311
  treatment options for, 311
Myeloma, multiple, 272
Myelopathy
  degenerative, 107
  fibrocartilaginous embolic, 109
Myopathies, fibrotic, 283
Myositis
  atrophic, 293
  eosinophilic, 293
  masticatory, 293

N

Nasal depigmentation, 331
  causes of, 331
  clinical signs of, 331
  description of, 331
  diagnostic tests for, 331
  follow-up care for, 331
  prognosis of, 331
  treatment options for, 331
Nasal polyps, in cats, 85
  causes of, 85
  clinical signs of, 85
  description of, 85
  diagnostic tests for, 85
  follow-up care for, 85
  prognosis of, 85
  treatment options for, 85
Nasal tumors, malignant, 86
  causes of, 86
  clinical signs of, 86
  description of, 86
  diagnostic tests for, 86
  follow-up care for, 86
  prognosis of, 86
  treatment options for, 86
Nasopharyngeal polyps, in cats, 85
Necrotizing encephalitis (NE), 110
  causes of, 110
  clinical signs of, 110
  description of, 110
  diagnostic tests for, 110
  follow-up care for, 110
  prognosis of, 110
  treatment options for, 110

Neoplasia
  benign. *See specific tumor, e.g.,* Adenomas.
  gastric, 148
  intestinal, 159
  laryngeal and tracheal, 80
  malignant. *See specific malignancy, e.g.,*
      Carcinoma.
  renal, 210
Neosporosis, in dogs, 416
  cause of, 416
  clinical signs of, 416
  description of, 416
  diagnostic tests for, 416
  follow-up care for, 416
  prognosis of, 416
  treatment options for, 416
Nephrotoxicosis, 202
Nerve sheath tumors, peripheral, 121
Neuritis
  acute polyradiculoneuritis, in dogs, 122
  optic, 350
Neuropathy
  canine distemper, 104
  cranial nerve, 113, 114, 115
  disc disease causing. *See* Intervertebral disc
      disease (IVDD).
  Horner's syndrome and, 363
  trigeminal, idiopathic, 115
Neurotin. *See* Gabapentin *(Neurotin).*
Noise phobias, in dogs, 432
Nonsteroidal anti-inflammatory drug
      (NSAID) toxicosis, 457
  causes of, 457
  clinical signs of, 457
  description of, 457
  diagnostic tests for, 457
  follow-up care for, 457
  prognosis of, 457
  treatment options for, 457
Notoedric mange, 332
  causes of, 332
  clinical signs of, 332
  description of, 332
  diagnostic tests for, 332
  follow-up care for, 332
  prognosis of, 332
  treatment options for, 332
Nutritional bone diseases, 294
  causes of, 294
  clinical signs of, 294
  description of, 294
  diagnostic tests for, 294
  follow-up care for, 294
  prognosis of, 294
  treatment options for, 294
Nutritional management
  of burns, 469
  of chronic kidney disease, 20
  of diabetes mellitus, 177, 178
  of food allergy. *See* Food allergies.
  of heart disease, 43, 44
    in dogs, 38, 41, 42
    taurine and. *See* Taurine-deficiency
        cardiomyopathy.
  homemade diets for, 438
  overnutrition *vs.,* of large-breed dogs,
      441
  for weight loss

Nutritional management (*Continued*)
  in cats, 439
  in dogs, 440
Nutritional secondary hyperparathyroidism, 294

O

OA. *See* Osteoarthritis (OA).
Obesity
  in cats, 439
    causes of, 439
    clinical signs of, 439
    description of, 439
    diagnostic tests for, 439
    follow-up care for, 439
    prognosis of, 439
    treatment options for, 439
  in dogs, 440
    causes of, 440
    clinical signs of, 440
    description of, 440
    diagnostic tests for, 440
    follow-up care for, 440
    prognosis of, 440
    treatment options for, 440
Obstructions *See specific anatomy, e.g.,*
      Urethral obstruction (UO).
OC. *See* Osteochondrosis (OC).
Occipital malformation, caudal, 106
Occult cardiomyopathy (OC), in Doberman
      pinschers, 50
  causes of, 50
  clinical signs of, 50
  description of, 50
  diagnostic tests for, 50
  follow-up care for, 50
  prognosis of, 50
  treatment options for, 50
OCD (osteochondritis dissecans), 296
Opioids poisoning, 462
Optic neuritis, 350
  causes of, 350
  clinical signs of, 350
  description of, 350
  diagnostic tests for, 350
  follow-up care for, 350
  prognosis of, 350
  treatment options for, 350
Oral melanoma, in dogs, 165
  causes of, 165
  clinical signs of, 165
  description of, 165
  diagnostic tests for, 165
  follow-up care for, 165
  prognosis of, 165
  treatment options for, 165
Orbital abscessation, 372
  causes of, 372
  description of, 372
  diagnostic tests for, 372
  follow-up care for, 372
  prognosis of, 372
  treatment options for, 372
Orbital cellulitis, 372
  causes of, 372
  clinical signs of, 372
  description of, 372
  diagnostic tests for, 372
  follow-up care for, 372

Orbital cellulitis (*Continued*)
 prognosis of, 372
 treatment options for, 372
Orbital tumors, 373
 causes of, 373
 clinical signs of, 373
 description of, 373
 diagnostic tests for, 373
 follow-up care for, 373
 prognosis of, 373
 treatment options for, 373
Organophosphorus insecticide poisoning, 458
 causes of, 458
 clinical signs of, 458
 description of, 458
 diagnostic tests for, 458
 follow-up care for, 458
 prognosis of, 458
 treatment options for, 458
Ostectomy, of femoral head and neck, 13
Osteoarthritis (OA), 295
 causes of, 295
 clinical signs of, 295
 description of, 295
 diagnostic tests for, 295
 follow-up care for, 295
 prognosis of, 295
 treatment options for, 295
Osteochondritis dissecans (OCD), 296
Osteochondroma, laryngeal and tracheal, 80
Osteochondrosis (OC), 296
 causes of, 296
 clinical signs of, 296
 description of, 296
 diagnostic tests for, 296
 follow-up care for, 296
 prognosis of, 296
 treatment options for, 296
Osteodystrophy
 hypertrophic, in dogs, 287
 types 1 and 2, 287
Osteomyelitis, 297
 causes of, 297
 clinical signs of, 297
 description of, 297, 298
 diagnostic tests for, 297
 follow-up care for, 297
 prognosis of, 297
 treatment options for, 297
Osteopathy
 hypertrophic, in dogs, 288
 metaphyseal, 287
Osteosarcoma
 bone, 277
 laryngeal and tracheal, 80
 orbital, 373
 spinal cord, 128
Otitis externa, 387
 causes of, 387
 clinical signs of, 387
 description of, 387
 diagnostic tests for, 387
 follow-up care for, 387
 prognosis of, 387
 treatment options for, 387
Otitis interna, 388
 causes of, 388
 clinical signs of, 388

Otitis interna (*Continued*)
 description of, 388
 diagnostic tests for, 388
 follow-up care for, 388
 prognosis of, 388
 treatment options for, 388
Otitis media, 389
 causes of, 389
 clinical signs of, 85, 389
 description of, 389
 diagnostic tests for, 389
 follow-up care for, 389
 prognosis of, 389
 treatment options for, 389
Ovarian remnant syndrome, 229
 causes of, 229
 clinical signs of, 229
 description of, 229
 diagnostic tests for, 229
 follow-up care for, 229
 prognosis of, 229
 treatment options for, 229
Overnutrition, of large-breed dogs, 441
 causes of, 441
 clinical signs of, 441
 description of, 441
 diagnostic tests for, 441
 follow-up care for, 441
 prognosis of, 441
 treatment options for, 441
Oxygen therapy, 21
 complications of, 21
 equipment for, 21
 follow-up care for, 21
 indications for. *See specific pathology, e.g.,*
  Pneumonia.
 preparation for, 21
 purpose of, 21
 technique for, 21

P
Paintball toxicosis, 459
 causes of, 459
 clinical signs of, 459
 description of, 459
 diagnostic tests for, 459
 follow-up care for, 459
 prognosis of, 459
 treatment options for, 459
Pancreatic insufficiency, exocrine, 143
Pancreatitis
 in cats, 167
  causes of, 167
  clinical signs of, 167
  description of, 167
  diagnostic tests for, 167
  follow-up care for, 167
  prognosis of, 167
  treatment options for, 167
 cholangiohepatitis with, 135
 in dogs, 168
  causes of, 168
  clinical signs of, 168
  description of, 168
  diagnostic tests for, 168
  follow-up care for, 168
  prognosis of, 168
  treatment options for, 168

Panleukopenia, feline, 417
Pannus, 374
 causes of, 374
 clinical signs of, 374
 description of, 374
 diagnostic tests for, 374
 follow-up care for, 374
 prognosis of, 374
 treatment options for, 374
Panosteitis, 298
 causes of, 298
 clinical signs of, 298
 description of, 298
 diagnostic tests for, 298
 follow-up care for, 298
 prognosis of, 298
 treatment options for, 298
Paralysis
 acute polyradiculoneuritis causing,
  122
 facial, idiopathic, 113, 115
 laryngeal, 79
 spinal nerve. *See* Intervertebral disc disease
  (IVDD).
 ticks causing, 131
Paraphimosis, in dogs, 230
 causes of, 230
 clinical signs of, 230
 description of, 230
 diagnostic tests for, 230
 follow-up care for, 230
 prognosis of, 230
 treatment options for, 230
Paraprostatic cysts, in dogs, 206
 causes of, 206
 clinical signs of, 206
 description of, 206
 diagnostic tests for, 206
 follow-up care for, 206
 prognosis of, 206
 treatment options for, 206
Parvovirus
 canine, 418
  cause of, 418
  clinical signs of, 418
  description of, 418
  diagnostic tests for, 418
  follow-up care for, 418
  prognosis of, 418
  treatment options for, 418
 feline, 417
  cause of, 417
  clinical signs of, 417
  description of, 417
  diagnostic tests for, 417
  follow-up care for, 417
  prevention of, 417
  prognosis of, 417
  treatment options for, 417
Patella luxation, 299
 causes of, 299
 clinical signs of, 299
 description of, 299
 diagnostic tests for, 299
 follow-up care for, 299
 knee (stifle) luxation *vs.*, 304
 prognosis of, 299
 treatment options for, 299

Patent ductus arteriosus (PDA), 51
  causes of, 51
  clinical signs of, 51
  description of, 51
  diagnostic tests for, 51
  follow-up care for, 51
  prognosis of, 51
  treatment options for, 51
Pemphigus complex, 333
  causes of, 333
  clinical signs of, 333
  description of, 333
  diagnostic tests for, 333
  follow-up care for, 333
  prognosis of, 333
  treatment options for, 333
Penile tumors, in dogs, 231
  causes of, 231
  clinical signs of, 231
  description of, 231
  diagnostic tests for, 231
  follow-up care for, 231
  prognosis of, 231
  transmissible venereal, 231
  treatment options for, 231
Perianal fistula, in dogs, 169
  causes of, 169
  clinical signs of, 169
  description of, 169
  diagnostic tests for, 169
  follow-up care for, 169
  prognosis of, 169
  treatment options for, 169
Perianal tumors, 170
  causes of, 170
  clinical signs of, 170
  description of, 170
  diagnostic tests for, 170
  follow-up care for, 170
  prognosis of, 170
  treatment options for, 170
Pericardial effusion, 52
  causes of, 39, 52
  clinical signs of, 52
  description of, 52
  diagnostic tests for, 52
  follow-up care for, 52
  prognosis of, 52
  treatment options for, 39, 52
Perineal hernia, in dogs, 171
  causes of, 171
  clinical signs of, 171
  description of, 171
  diagnostic tests for, 171
  follow-up care for, 171
  prognosis of, 171
  treatment options for, 171
Perinephric pseudocysts, in cats, 203
  causes of, 203
  clinical signs of, 203
  description of, 203
  diagnostic tests for, 203
  follow-up care for, 203
  prognosis of, 203
  treatment options for, 203
Periodontal disease, 152
Peripheral nerve sheath tumors (PNSTs),
      121
  causes of, 121

Peripheral nerve sheath tumors (PNSTs)
      (Continued)
  clinical signs of, 121
  description of, 121
  diagnostic tests for, 121
  follow-up care for, 121
  prognosis of, 121
  treatment options for, 121
Peripheral vestibular disease, idiopathic, 114
Peritoneopericardial diaphragmatic hernia
      (PPDH), 53
  causes of, 53, 76
  clinical signs of, 53
  description of, 53
  diagnostic tests for, 53
  follow-up care for, 53
  prognosis of, 53
  treatment options for, 53
Persistent right aortic arch (PRAA), 54
  causes of, 54
  clinical signs of, 54
  description of, 54
  diagnostic tests for, 54
  follow-up care for, 54
  prognosis of, 54
  treatment options for, 54
Petting intolerance, in cats, 433
  causes of, 433
  clinical signs of, 433
  description of, 433
  diagnostic tests for, 433
  follow-up care for, 433
  prognosis of, 433
  treatment options for, 433
PH. See Pulmonary hypertension (PH).
Phenobarbital, for seizures, 125
Phimosis, 232
  causes of, 232
  clinical signs of, 232
  description of, 232
  diagnostic tests for, 232
  follow-up care for, 232
  prognosis of, 232
  treatment options for, 232
Physical examination, preoperative, 23
Physical rehabilitation, 22
  complications of, 22
  follow-up care for, 22
  preparation for, 22
  purpose of, 16–17, 22
  technique of, 22
Physical therapy, exercise and modalities
      for, 22
Pigmentary keratitis, 376
  causes of, 376
  clinical signs of, 376
  description of, 376
  diagnostic tests for, 376
  follow-up care for, 376
  prognosis of, 376
  treatment options for, 376
Pinnal seborrhea, 334
  causes of, 334
  clinical signs of, 334
  description of, 334
  diagnostic tests for, 334
  follow-up care for, 334
  prognosis of, 334
  treatment options for, 334

PKD. See Polycystic kidney disease (PKD).
Placental sites, subinvolution of, in dogs, 236
Plant toxicities, 202. See also specific plant,
      e.g., Grape toxicosis.
Plasma cell pododermatitis, in cats, 335
  causes of, 335
  clinical signs of, 335
  description of, 335
  diagnostic tests for, 335
  follow-up care for, 335
  prognosis of, 335
  treatment options for, 335
Plasmacytoma
  extramedullary, 270
  gastric, 148
  intestinal, 159
Play aggression, in cats, 434
  causes of, 434
  clinical signs of, 434
  description of, 434
  diagnostic tests for, 434
  follow-up care for, 434
  prognosis of, 434
  treatment options for, 434
PLE. See Protein-losing enteropathy (PLE).
Pleural effusion, 87
  causes of, 87
  clinical signs of, 87
  description of, 87
  diagnostic tests for, 87
  follow-up care for, 87
  prognosis of, 87
  treatment options for, 87
PLN. See Protein-losing nephropathy (PLN).
Pneumonia
  aspiration, 88
    causes of, 88
    clinical signs of, 88
    description of, 88
    diagnostic tests for, 88
    follow-up care for, 88
    prognosis of, 88
    treatment options for, 88
  bacterial, 89
    causes of, 89
    clinical signs of, 89
    description of, 89
    diagnostic tests for, 89
    follow-up care for, 89
    prognosis of, 89
    treatment options for, 89
  fungal, 90
    causes of, 90
    clinical signs of, 90
    description of, 90
    diagnostic tests for, 90
    follow-up care for, 90
    prognosis of, 90
    treatment options for, 90
  lobar, 89
Pneumothorax, 91
  with bullous lung disease, 75
  causes of, 91
  clinical signs of, 91
  description of, 91
  diagnostic tests for, 91
  follow-up care for, 91
  tension, 91
  treatment options for, 91

PNSTs. *See* Peripheral nerve sheath tumors (PNSTs).
Pododermatitis, plasma cell, in cats, 335
Poisoning(s). *See also* Toxins/toxicities.
  herbal, 452–453
  insecticides, 458
  lead, 454
  metaldehyde, 456
  rodenticides, 36, 244, 450
  strychnine, 465
Polycystic kidney disease (PKD), in cats, 204
  causes of, 204
  clinical signs of, 204
  description of, 204
  diagnostic tests for, 204
  follow-up care for, 204
  prognosis of, 204
  treatment options for, 204
Polycythemia, 261
  causes of, 261
  classifications of, 261
  clinical signs of, 261
  description of, 261
  diagnostic tests for, 261
  follow-up care for, 261
  prognosis of, 261
  treatment options for, 261
Polyps, nasal and nasopharyngeal, in cats, 85
Polyradiculoneuritis, acute, in dogs, 122
  causes of, 122
  clinical signs of, 122
  description of, 122
  diagnostic tests for, 122
  follow-up care for, 122
  prognosis of, 122
  treatment options for, 122
Portosystemic vascular anomalies, 172
  causes of, 172
  clinical signs of, 172
  description of, 172
  diagnostic tests for, 172
  follow-up care for, 172
  prognosis of, 172
  treatment options for, 172
Possessive aggression, in dogs, 435
  causes of, 435
  clinical signs of, 435
  description of, 435
  diagnostic tests for, 435
  follow-up care for, 435
  prognosis of, 435
  treatment options for, 435
Potassium bromide, for seizures, 125
PPDH. *See* Peritoneopericardial diaphragmatic hernia (PPDH).
PRA. *See* Progressive retinal atrophy (PRA).
PRAA. *See* Persistent right aortic arch (PRAA).
Pregnancy
  eclampsia during, in dogs, 220
  labor difficulties with, 219
  loss of, in bitches, 233
    causes of, 233
    clinical signs of, 233
    description of, 233
    diagnostic tests for, 233
    false, 234
    follow-up care for, 233
    prognosis of, 233
    treatment options for, 233

Premature contractions
  atrial, 37
  ventricular, 67
Preoperative evaluation, 23
  anesthetic risk classification in, 23
  description of, 23
  prognosis in, 23
  testing in, 23
  treatment options in, 23
Primary seborrhea, 336
  causes of, 336
  clinical signs of, 336
  description of, 336
  diagnostic tests for, 336
  follow-up care for, 336
  prognosis of, 336
  treatment options for, 336
Progressive retinal atrophy (PRA), 377
  causes of, 377
  clinical signs of, 377
  description of, 377
  diagnostic tests for, 377
  follow-up care for, 377
  prognosis of, 377
  treatment options for, 377
Prolapse
  of third eyelid gland, 378
  urethral, in dogs, 213
  uterine, 238
Proptosis, of eye, 379
  causes of, 379
  clinical signs of, 379
  description of, 379
  diagnostic tests for, 379
  follow-up care for, 379
  prognosis of, 379
  treatment options for, 379
Prostate cancer, in dogs, 205
  causes of, 205
  clinical signs of, 205
  description of, 205
  diagnostic tests for, 205
  follow-up care for, 205
  prognosis of, 205
  treatment options for, 205
Prostatic abscessation, in dogs, 207
  causes of, 207
  clinical signs of, 207
  description of, 207
  diagnostic tests for, 207
  follow-up care for, 207
  prognosis of, 207
  treatment options for, 207
Prostatic cysts, in dogs, 206
  causes of, 206
  clinical signs of, 206
  description of, 206
  diagnostic tests for, 206
  follow-up care for, 206
  prognosis of, 206
  treatment options for, 206
Prostatic hypertrophy, benign, in dogs, 189
Prostatitis, in dogs, 207
  causes of, 207
  clinical signs of, 207
  description of, 207
  diagnostic tests for, 207
  follow-up care for, 207

Prostatitis, in dogs (*Continued*)
  prognosis of, 207
  treatment options for, 207
Protein-losing enteropathy (PLE), 173
  causes of, 173
  clinical signs of, 173
  description of, 173
  diagnostic tests for, 173
  follow-up care for, 173
  prognosis of, 173
  treatment options for, 173
Protein-losing nephropathy (PLN), in dogs, 208
  causes of, 208
  clinical signs of, 208
  description of, 208
  diagnostic tests for, 208
  follow-up care for, 208
  prognosis of, 208
  treatment options for, 208
Protothecosis, in dogs, 419
  causes of, 419
  clinical signs of, 419
  description of, 419
  diagnostic tests for, 419
  follow-up care for, 419
  prognosis of, 419
  treatment options for, 419
PS. *See* Pulmonic stenosis (PS).
Pseudocyesis, 234
  causes of, 234
  clinical signs of, 234
  description of, 234
  diagnostic tests for, 234
  follow-up care for, 234
  prognosis of, 234
  treatment options for, 234
Pseudocysts, perinephric, in cats, 203
Pseudoephedrine toxicity, 452
Public health information. *See* Zoonoses; *specific disease, e.g.,* Ehrlichiosis.
Pulmonary contusions, 92
  causes of, 92
  clinical signs of, 92
  description of, 92
  diagnostic tests for, 92
  follow-up care for, 92
  prognosis of, 92
  treatment options for, 92
Pulmonary edema, 93
  causes of, 93, 470
  clinical signs of, 93
  description of, 93
  diagnostic tests for, 93
  follow-up care for, 93
  prognosis of, 93
  treatment options for, 93
Pulmonary hypertension (PH), 55
  causes of, 47, 55
  clinical signs of, 55
  description of, 55
  diagnostic tests for, 55
  follow-up care for, 55
  prognosis of, 55
  treatment options for, 55
Pulmonic stenosis (PS), 56
  causes of, 56, 63
  clinical signs of, 56
  description of, 56

Pulmonic stenosis (PS) (*Continued*)
  diagnostic tests for, 56
  follow-up care for, 56
  prognosis of, 56
  treatment options for, 56
Pyelonephritis, 209
  causes of, 209
  clinical signs of, 209
  description of, 209
  diagnostic tests for, 209
  follow-up care for, 209
  prognosis of, 209
  treatment options for, 209
Pyoderma
  deep bacterial, 319
    causes of, 319
    clinical signs of, 319
    description of, 319
    diagnostic tests for, 319
    follow-up care for, 319
    prognosis of, 319
    treatment options for, 319
  skin fold, 339
Pyometra complex, 235
  causes of, 235
  clinical signs of, 235
  description of, 235
  diagnostic tests for, 235
  follow-up care for, 235
  prognosis of, 235
  treatment options for, 235
Pyrethrin/pyrethroid toxicosis, 464
  causes of, 464
  clinical signs of, 464
  description of, 464
  diagnostic tests for, 464
  follow-up care for, 464
  prognosis of, 464
  treatment options for, 464
Pythiosis, 420
  cause of, 420
  clinical signs of, 420
  description of, 420
  diagnostic tests for, 420
  follow-up care for, 420
  prognosis of, 420
  treatment options for, 420

Q
Quadriceps contracture (QC), 283

R
RA (rheumatoid arthritis), 289
Rabies, 421
  cause of, 421
  clinical signs of, 421
  description of, 421
  diagnostic tests for, 421
  follow-up care for, 421
  prognosis of, 421
  treatment options for, 421
Radiography, indications for. *See specific pathology or procedure.*
Raisin toxicosis, in dogs, 451
  causes and toxicity of, 451
  clinical signs of, 451
  description of, 451
  diagnostic tests for, 451

Raisin toxicosis, in dogs (*Continued*)
  follow-up care for, 451
  prognosis of, 451
  treatment options for, 451
Renal neoplasia, 210
  causes of, 210
  clinical signs of, 210
  description of, 210
  diagnostic tests for, 210
  follow-up care for, 210
  prognosis of, 210
  treatment options for, 210
Renal scintigraphy, as kidney function test, 19
Respiratory arrest, cardiopulmonary resuscitation for, 40
Respiratory distress, acute syndrome of, 69
Respiratory infection, upper, in cats, 408
Retinal degeneration (retinopathy)
  hypertensive, 364
  progressive, 377
  sudden acquired, 382
  taurine-deficiency, 383, 442
Retinal detachment, 380
  causes of, 380
  clinical signs of, 380
  description of, 380
  diagnostic tests for, 380
  follow-up care for, 380
  prognosis of, 380
  treatment options for, 380
Retinal dysplasia, 381
  causes of, 381
  clinical signs of, 381
  description of, 381
  diagnostic tests for, 381
  follow-up care for, 381
  prognosis of, 381
  treatment options for, 381
Rhabdomyoma, laryngeal, 80
Rheumatoid arthritis (RA), 289
Rhinitis, 94, 95
Rhinoscopy, 24
  complications of, 24
  follow-up care for, 24
  preparation for, 24
  purpose of, 24, 94, 95
  technique for, 24
Rhinosinusitis
  allergic, 94, 95
  in cats, 94
    causes of, 94
    clinical signs of, 94
    description of, 94
    diagnostic tests for, 94
    follow-up care for, 94
    prognosis of, 94
    treatment options for, 94
  in dogs, 95
    causes of, 95
    clinical signs of, 95
    description of, 95
    diagnostic tests for, 95
    follow-up care for, 95
    prognosis of, 95
    treatment options for, 95
Rocky Mountain spotted fever, 422
  cause of, 422

Rocky Mountain spotted fever (*Continued*)
  clinical signs of, 422
  description of, 422
  diagnostic tests for, 422
  follow-up care for, 422
  prognosis of, 422
  public health information on, 422
  treatment options for, 422
Rodenticides poisoning, 202, 244, 450

S
Sacroiliac luxation, 300
  causes of, 300
  clinical signs of, 300
  description of, 300
  diagnostic tests for, 300
  follow-up care for, 300
  prognosis of, 300
  treatment options for, 300
St. John's wort toxicity, 452
Salivary mucocele, in dogs, 174
  causes of, 174
  clinical signs of, 174
  description of, 174
  diagnostic tests for, 174
  follow-up care for, 174
  prognosis of, 174
  treatment options for, 174
Sarcoma. *See also specific type, e.g., Histiocytic sarcoma (HA).*
  bone, 277
  gastric, 148
  intestinal, 159
  intraocular, 366
  orbital, 373
  spinal cord, 128
Sarcoptic mange, 337
  causes of, 337
  clinical signs of, 337
  description of, 337
  diagnostic tests for, 337
  follow-up care for, 337
  prognosis of, 337
  treatment options for, 337
SARD. *See* Sudden acquired retinal degeneration (SARD).
SAS. *See* Subaortic stenosis (SAS).
SC. *See* Subcutaneous (SC, SQ) fluid administration.
Scapular luxation, 301
  causes of, 301
  clinical signs of, 301
  description of, 301
  diagnostic tests for, 301
  follow-up care for, 301
  prognosis of, 301
  treatment options for, 301
SCC. *See* Squamous cell carcinoma (SCC).
Sebaceous adenitis, in dogs, 338
  causes of, 338
  clinical signs of, 338
  description of, 338
  diagnostic tests for, 338
  follow-up care for, 338
  prognosis of, 338
  treatment options for, 338
Sebaceous gland tumors, in dogs, 312

Seborrhea
  pinnal, 334
  primary, 336
Second-degree heart block, 57
  causes of, 57
  clinical signs of, 57
  description of, 57
  diagnostic tests for, 57
  follow-up care for, 52
  prognosis of, 57
  treatment options for, 57
Seizures, 123
  causes of, 123, 220
  clinical signs of, 123
  description of, 123
  diagnostic tests for, 123
  follow-up care for, 123, 126
  idiopathic, 124
    causes of, 124
    clinical signs of, 124
    description of, 124
    diagnostic tests for, 124
    follow-up care for, 124
    prognosis of, 124
    treatment options for, 124
  prognosis of, 123
  resistant cases of, 126
    antiepileptic drugs for, 126
    emergency drugs for, 126
  treatment of
    drugs for, 125
    follow-up care for, 126
    options for, 123, 125
    resistant cases in, 126
Separation anxiety, in dogs, 432
Septal defects, atrial *vs.* ventricular, 63, 65
Septic arthritis, 302
  causes of, 302
  clinical signs of, 302
  description of, 302
  diagnostic tests for, 302
  follow-up care for, 302
  treatment options for, 302
Sequestration, corneal, in cats, 358
SH. *See* Systemic hypertension (SH).
Shearing injuries
  carpal, 279
  tarsal, 279
SHM. *See* Syringohydromyelia (SHM).
Shock, 472
  causes of, 47, 470, 471, 472
  classification of, 472
  clinical signs of, 472
  description of, 472
  diagnostic tests for, 472
  follow-up care for, 472
  prognosis of, 472
  treatment options for, 472
Shoulder luxation, 303
  causes of, 303
  clinical signs of, 303
  description of, 303
  diagnostic tests for, 303
  follow-up care for, 303
  prognosis of, 303
  treatment options for, 303
Sick sinus syndrome, 58
  causes of, 58

Sick sinus syndrome (*Continued*)
  clinical signs of, 58
  description of, 58
  diagnostic tests for, 58
  follow-up care for, 58
  prognosis of, 58
  treatment options for, 58
Sinus arrhythmia, 59
  causes of, 59
  clinical signs of, 59
  description of, 59
  diagnostic tests for, 59
  follow-up care for, 59
  prognosis of, 59
  treatment options for, 59
Sinus bradycardia, 60
  causes of, 60
  clinical signs of, 60
  description of, 60
  diagnostic tests for, 60
  follow-up care for, 60
  prognosis of, 60
  treatment options for, 60
Sinusitis
  in cats, 94
  in dogs, 95
  recurrent, 94
SIPS. *See* Subinvolution of placental sites (SIPS).
Skin fold pyoderma, 339
  causes of, 339
  clinical signs of, 339
  description of, 339
  diagnostic tests for, 339
  follow-up care for, 339
  prognosis of, 339
  treatment options for, 339
SLE. *See* Systemic lupus erythematosus (SLE).
Snake bites, venomous, 473
Solitary osseous plasmacytomas (SOP), 270
Spinal cord
  compression of, 105, 116, 117
  degenerative myelopathy of, 107
  inflammation of covering of, 130, 132
  ischemia/infarction of, 109
Spinal cord trauma, 127
  causes of, 127
  clinical signs of, 127
  description of, 127
  diagnostic tests for, 127
  follow-up care for, 127
  prognosis of, 127
  treatment options for, 127
Spinal cord tumors, 128
  causes of, 128
  clinical signs of, 128
  description of, 128
  diagnostic tests for, 128
  follow-up care for, 128
  prognosis of, 128
  treatment options for, 128
Splenic hemangiosarcoma, 262
  causes of, 262
  clinical signs of, 262
  description of, 262
  diagnostic tests for, 262
  follow-up care for, 262
  prognosis of, 262
  treatment options for, 262

Splenic torsion, 263
  causes of, 263
  clinical signs of, 263
  description of, 263
  diagnostic tests for, 263
  follow-up care for, 263
  prognosis of, 263
  treatment options for, 263
Splenomegaly, 264
  causes of, 264
  clinical signs of, 264
  description of, 264
  diagnostic tests for, 264
  follow-up care for, 264
  treatment options for, 264
Splints
  for flail chest, 77
  for fracture repair, 15
Spondylopathy, caudal cervical, 105
Spondylosis deformans, 129
  causes of, 129
  clinical signs of, 129
  description of, 129
  diagnostic tests for, 129
  follow-up care for, 129
  prognosis of, 129
  treatment options for, 129
Sporotrichosis, 340
  causes of, 340
  clinical signs of, 340
  description of, 340
  diagnostic tests for, 340
  follow-up care for, 340
  prognosis of, 340
  treatment options for, 340
SQ. *See* Subcutaneous (SC, SQ) fluid
  administration.
Squamous cell carcinoma (SCC), oral, in cats,
  166
  causes of, 166
  clinical signs of, 166
  description of, 166
  diagnostic tests for, 166
  follow-up care for, 166
  prognosis of, 166
  treatment options for, 166
SRMA. *See* Steroid-responsive meningeal
  arteritis (SRMA).
Staphylococcus infection,
  methicillin-resistant, 415
Status aggression, in cats, 433
  clinical signs of, 433
  description of, 433
  diagnostic tests for, 433
  prognosis of, 433
  treatment options for, 433
Sterilization, elective
  of female cats, 25
    complications of, 25
    follow-up care for, 25
    postoperative care for, 25
    preparation for, 25
    purpose of, 25
    technique for, 25
  of female dogs, 26
    complications of, 26
    follow-up care for, 26
    postoperative care for, 26

Sterilization, elective (*Continued*)
    preparation for, 26
    purpose of, 26
    technique for, 26
Steroid-responsive meningeal arteritis
    (SRMA), 130
    causes of, 130
    clinical signs of, 130
    description of, 130
    diagnostic tests for, 130
    follow-up care for, 130
    prognosis of, 130
    treatment options for, 130
Stifle (knee) luxation, 304
    causes of, 304
    clinical signs of, 304
    description of, 304
    diagnostic tests for, 304
    follow-up care for, 304
    prognosis of, 304
    treatment options for, 304
Stimulants poisoning, 462
Stomatitis, 162
    lymphoplasmacytic, in cats, 162
Stones. *See* Bladder stones; Kidney stones.
Stricture, esophageal, 142
Stroke
    heat, 471
    ischemic, 118
Strychnine poisoning, 465
    causes of, 465
    clinical signs of, 465
    description of, 465
    diagnostic tests for, 465
    follow-up care for, 465
    prognosis of, 465
    treatment options for, 465
Subaortic stenosis (SAS), 61
    causes of, 61
    clinical signs of, 61
    description of, 61
    diagnostic tests for, 61
    follow-up care for, 61
    prognosis of, 61
    treatment options for, 61
Subcutaneous abscess, 341
    causes of, 341
    clinical signs of, 341
    description of, 341
    diagnostic tests for, 341
    follow-up care for, 341
    prognosis of, 341
    treatment options for, 341
Subcutaneous (SC, SQ) fluid administration, 27
    dosage for, 27
    equipment for, 27
    purpose of, 27
    technique for, 14, 27
Subinvolution of placental sites (SIPS), in
    dogs, 236
    causes of, 236
    clinical signs of, 236
    description of, 236
    diagnostic tests for, 236
    follow-up care for, 236
    prognosis of, 236
    treatment options for, 236

Sudden acquired retinal degeneration
    (SARD), 382
    causes of, 382
    clinical signs of, 382
    description of, 382
    diagnostic tests for, 382
    follow-up care for, 382
    prognosis of, 382
    treatment options for, 382
Swallowing disorders, 88
Syringohydromyelia (SHM), 106
    clinical signs of, 106
    description of, 106
    diagnostic tests for, 106
    follow-up care for, 106
    prognosis of, 106
    treatment options for, 106
Systemic hypertension (SH), 62
    causes of, 62
    clinical signs of, 62
    description of, 62
    diagnostic tests for, 62
    follow-up care for, 62
    prognosis of, 62
    treatment options for, 62
Systemic lupus erythematosus (SLE), in
    dogs
    dermatologic aspects of, 343
        causes of, 343
        clinical signs of, 343
        description of, 343
        diagnostic tests for, 343
        follow-up care for, 343
        prognosis of, 343
        treatment options for, 343
    systemic aspects of, 273
        causes of, 273
        clinical signs of, 273
        description of, 273
        diagnostic tests for, 273
        follow-up care for, 273
        prognosis of, 273
        treatment options for, 273

T

Tachycardia
    atrial, 37
    ventricular, 67
Tarsal shearing injuries, 279
    causes of, 279
    clinical signs of, 279
    description of, 279
    diagnostic tests for, 279
    follow-up care for, 279
    prognosis of, 279
    treatment options for, 279
Taurine deficiency, 442
    causes of, 442
    clinical signs of, 442
    description of, 442
    diagnostic tests for, 442
    follow-up care for, 442
    prognosis of, 442
    treatment options for, 442
    in cats, 43
    in dogs, 44
Taurine-deficiency retinopathy, 383

Taurine-deficiency retinopathy (*Continued*)
    causes of, 383, 442
    clinical signs of, 383
    description of, 383
    diagnostic tests for, 383
    follow-up care for, 383
    prognosis of, 383
    treatment options for, 383
T-cell lymphoma, cutaneous, 317
Tendinopathy
    bicipital, 276
    calcaneal (Achilles), traumatic,
        278
    infraspinatus, 283
Territorial aggression, in dogs, 435
    causes of, 435
    clinical signs of, 435
    description of, 435
    diagnostic tests for, 435
    follow-up care for, 435
    prognosis of, 435
    treatment options for, 435
Testes
    failure to descend, 218
    removal of. *See* Castration.
    retained, 237
Testicular tumors, in dogs, 237
    causes of, 237
    clinical signs of, 237
    description of, 237
    diagnostic tests for, 237
    follow-up care for, 237
    prognosis of, 237
    treatment options for, 237
Tetanus, 423
    cause of, 423
    clinical signs of, 423
    description of, 423
    diagnostic tests for, 423
    follow-up care for, 423
    prognosis of, 423
    treatment options for, 423
Tetralogy of Fallot, 63
    causes of, 63
    clinical signs of, 63
    description of, 63
    diagnostic tests for, 63
    follow-up care for, 63
    prognosis of, 63
    treatment options for, 63
THA. *See* Total hip arthroplasty (THA).
Third eyelid, prolapse of gland
    of, 378
    causes of, 378
    clinical signs of, 378
    description of, 378
    diagnostic tests for, 378
    follow-up care for, 378
    prognosis of, 378
    treatment options for, 378
Third-degree heart block, 57
    causes of, 57
    description of, 57
    diagnostic tests for, 57
    follow-up care for, 57
    prognosis of, 57
    treatment options for, 57

Thrombocytopenia, 265
  causes of, 265, 273
  clinical signs of, 265
  description of, 265
  diagnostic tests for, 265
  follow-up care for, 265
  immune-mediated, 256
  prognosis of, 265
  treatment options for, 265
Thromboembolism, peripheral
    arterial, 35
Thrombosis, 266
  causes of, 49, 266
  clinical signs of, 266
  description of, 266
  diagnostic tests for, 266
  follow-up care for, 266
  prognosis of, 266
  treatment options for, 266
Thymomas, mediastinal, 84
Tick paralysis, 131
  causes of, 131
  clinical signs of, 131
  description of, 131
  diagnostic tests for, 131
  follow-up care for, 131
  prognosis of, 131
  treatment options for, 131
Toenail disease. See Claw disease.
Torsion
  lung lobe, 82
  splenic, 263
Total hip arthroplasty (THA), 28
  complications of, 28
  follow-up care for, 28
  postoperative care for, 28
  preparation for, 28
  purpose of, 28
  technique for, 28
Toxins/toxicities. See also Poisoning(s).
  drug. See Drug toxicities.
  food, 202. See also specific food, e.g.,
      Grape toxicosis.
  household product, 202. See also
      specific product, e.g., Paintball
      toxicosis.
  kidney, 202
Toxoplasmosis, 424
  cause of, 424
  clinical signs of, 424
  description of, 424
  diagnostic tests for, 424
  follow-up care for, 424
  prognosis of, 424
  public health information on, 424
  treatment options for, 424
TPO. See Triple pelvic osteotomy (TPO)
Tracheal collapse, in dogs, 96
  cause of, 96
  clinical signs of, 96
  description of, 96
  diagnostic tests for, 96
  follow-up care for, 96
  prognosis of, 96
  treatment options for, 96
Tracheal neoplasia, 80
  causes of, 80

Tracheal neoplasia (Continued)
  clinical signs of, 80
  description of, 80
  diagnostic tests for, 80
  follow-up care for, 80
  prognosis of, 80
  treatment options for, 80
Tracheal obstruction, 97
Tracheal trauma, 98
  causes of, 98
  clinical signs of, 98
  description of, 98
  diagnostic tests for, 98
  follow-up care for, 98
  prognosis of, 98
  treatment options for, 98
Tracheitis, 81
Tracheobronchitis, infectious, in
    dogs, 397
Tracheostomy, care of, 78
Transfusion therapy
  in cats, 29
    complications of, 29
    follow-up care for, 29
    preparation for, 29
    purpose of, 29
    technique for, 29
  in dogs, 30
    complications of, 30
    follow-up care for, 30
    preparation for, 30
    purpose of, 30
    technique for, 30
Transmissible venereal tumor
    (TVT), 231
Trauma. See specific anatomy or injury, e.g.,
    Burns.
Tremor syndrome, 132
  causes of, 132
  clinical signs of, 132
  description of, 132
  diagnostic tests for, 132
  follow-up care for, 132
  prognosis of, 132
  treatment options for, 132
Tricuspid dysplasia, 64
  causes of, 64
  clinical signs of, 64
  description of, 64
  diagnostic tests for, 64
  follow-up care for, 64
  prognosis of, 64
  treatment options for, 64
Trigeminal neuropathy, idiopathic, 115
  causes of, 115
  clinical signs of, 115
  description of, 115
  diagnostic tests for, 115
  follow-up care for, 115
  prognosis of, 115
  treatment options for, 115
Triple pelvic osteotomy (TPO), for hip
    dysplasia, 31
  complications of, 31
  follow-up care for, 31
  postoperative care for, 31
  preparation for, 31

Triple pelvic osteotomy (TPO), for hip
    dysplasia (Continued)
  purpose of, 31
  technique for, 31
Tritrichomoniasis, in cats, 425
  cause of, 425
  clinical signs of, 425
  description of, 425
  diagnostic tests for, 425
  follow-up care for, 425
  prognosis of, 425
  public health information on, 425
  treatment options for, 425
Tumor(s). See also Neoplasia.
  bone, 277
  brain, 103
  extramedullary plasmacytoma as, 270
  eye, 366, 373
  eyelid, 357
  fat cell, in dogs, 327
  heart, 39
  intraocular, 366
  kidney, 210
  lung, 83
  mammary, in cats, 226
  mast cell, 260
  mediastinal, 84
  mouth, in dogs, 140
  nasal
    benign, 85
    malignant, 86
  orbital, 373
  parathyroid, 36
  penile, in dogs, 231
  perianal, 170
  peripheral nerve sheath, 121
  skin, in dogs, 312
  spinal cord, 128
  testes, in dogs, 237
TVT (transmissible venereal tumor), 231

U
Ulceration(s)
  corneal, 353
    persistent, 375
  gastrointestinal, 138, 151
  skin, lupus erythematosus as, 316, 343
Ultrasound
  for blood pressure measurement, 4, 62
  cardiac. See Echocardiography.
  indications for. See specific pathology.
Ununited anconeal process (UAP)
    disease, 305
  causes of, 305
  clinical signs of, 305
  description of, 305
  diagnostic tests for, 305
  follow-up care for, 305
  prognosis of, 305
  treatment options for, 305
UO. See Urethral obstruction (UO).
Upper respiratory infection (URI), feline, 408
  causes of, 408
  clinical signs of, 408
  description of, 408
  diagnostic tests for, 408
  follow-up care for, 408

Upper respiratory infection (URI), feline
(*Continued*)
prognosis of, 408
treatment options for, 408
Ureter, ectopic, in dogs, 198
Ureteral obstruction, in cats, 211
causes of, 211
clinical signs of, 211
description of, 211
diagnostic tests for, 211
follow-up care for, 211
prognosis of, 211
treatment options for, 211
Urethral obstruction (UO), in cats, 212
causes of, 212
clinical signs of, 212
description of, 212
diagnostic tests for, 212
follow-up care for, 212
prognosis of, 212
treatment options for, 212
Urethral prolapse, in dogs, 213
causes of, 213
clinical signs of, 213
description of, 213
diagnostic tests for, 213
follow-up care for, 213
prognosis of, 213
treatment options for, 213
Urethritis, 214
causes of, 214
clinical signs of, 214
description of, 214
diagnostic tests for, 214
follow-up care for, 214
prognosis of, 214
treatment options for, 214
URI. *See* Upper respiratory infection (URI).
Urinary incontinence, in dogs, 215
causes of, 215
clinical signs of, 215
description of, 215
diagnostic tests for, 215
follow-up care for, 215
prognosis of, 215
treatment options for, 215
Urination problems
in cats, 429–430
in dogs, 215, 431
Urine protein assays, 208
in dogs, 32
complications of, 32
description of, 32
preparation for, 32
purpose of, 32
Urine specific gravity, as kidney function test, 19
Uterine prolapse, 238
causes of, 238
clinical signs of, 238
description of, 238
diagnostic tests for, 238
follow-up care for, 238
prognosis of, 238
treatment options for, 238
Uterus
pus-filled, 235
removal of. *See* Sterilization.
Uveitis, anterior, 348

V
Vaccine-associated vasculitis, in
dogs, 344
causes of, 344
clinical signs of, 344
description of, 344
diagnostic tests for, 344
follow-up care for, 344
prognosis of, 344
treatment options for, 344
Vaccines. *See specific disease, e.g.,* Kennel
cough.
Vaginal edema, in dogs, 239
causes of, 239
clinical signs of, 239
description of, 239
diagnostic tests for, 239
prognosis of, 239
treatment options for, 239
Vaginitis, in dogs, 240
causes of, 240
clinical signs of, 240
description of, 240
diagnostic tests for, 240
follow-up care for, 240
prognosis of, 240
treatment options for, 240
Valerian root toxicity, 453
Vascular anomalies, portosystemic, 172
Vasculitis, vaccine-associated, in
dogs, 344
Venomous snake bites, 473
causes of, 473
clinical signs of, 473
description of, 473
diagnostic tests for, 473
follow-up care for, 473
prognosis of, 473
treatment options for, 473
Ventricular fibrillation (VF), 66
causes of, 66
clinical signs of, 66
description of, 66
diagnostic tests for, 66
follow-up care for, 66
prognosis of, 66
treatment options for, 40, 66, 73
Ventricular premature contractions
(VPCs), 67
causes of, 34, 50, 67
clinical signs of, 67
description of, 67
diagnostic tests for, 67
follow-up care for, 67
prognosis of, 67
treatment options for, 67
Ventricular septal defect (VSD), 63, 65
Ventricular tachycardia (VT), 67
causes of, 34, 50, 67
clinical signs of, 67
description of, 67
diagnostic tests for, 67
follow-up care for, 67
treatment options for, 67
Vertebrae
cervical, 100
malformation-malarticulation of, 105
subluxation of, in dogs, 100

Vertebrae (*Continued*)
lumbosacral, degenerative disease of, 119
spondylosis deformans of, 129
Vestibular disease
idiopathic peripheral, 114
inner ear inflammation and, 388
VF. *See* Ventricular fibrillation (VF).
Vitamin A–responsive dermatosis, 345
causes of, 345
clinical signs of, 345
description of, 345
diagnostic tests for, 345
follow-up care for, 345
prognosis of, 345
treatment options for, 345
Vitamin imbalances, in dogs
bone diseases related to, 294
scurvy as, 287
Vocal cords, 78, 79, 81
Von Willebrand disease (VWD), 267
causes of, 267
clinical signs of, 267
description of, 267
diagnostic tests for, 267
follow-up care for, 267
prognosis of, 267
treatment options for, 267
VPCs. *See* Ventricular premature contractions
(VPCs).
VSD (ventricular septal defect), 63, 65
VT. *See* Ventricular tachycardia (VT).

W
Weight reduction programs, 439, 440
Wobbler syndrome, 105

X
Xylitol toxicosis, in dogs, 466
causes of, 466
clinical signs of, 466
description of, 466
diagnostic tests for, 466
follow-up care for, 466
prognosis of, 466
treatment options for, 466

Z
Zinc toxicosis, 467
causes of, 467
clinical signs of, 467
description of, 467
diagnostic tests for, 467
follow-up care for, 467
prognosis of, 467
treatment options for, 467
Zinc-responsive dermatosis, 346
causes of, 346
clinical signs of, 346
description of, 346
diagnostic tests for, 346
follow-up care for, 346
prognosis of, 346
treatment options for, 346
Zonisamide (*Zonegran*), for seizures, 126
Zoonoses
bacterial, 404, 414, 422
mites as, 332, 337
parasitic, 402, 409, 413, 424, 425